Clinical Medicine for the MRCP PACES Volume 1

Core clinical skills

Edited by

Gautam Mehta

Specialist Registrar in Gastroenterology
Wellcome Trust Research Fellow
Institute of Hepatology
University College London

Bilal Iqbal

Specialist Registrar in Cardiology
Hammersmith Hospital
Imperial College London

Forewords by

Professor Sir Graeme Catto

President, General Medical Council (2002–9)

Professor Sir Kenneth Calman

Chief Medical Officer (1991–8)

OXFORD
UNIVERSITY PRESS

Great Clarendon Street, Oxford OX2 6DP

Oxford University Press is a department of the University of Oxford.
It furthers the University's objective of excellence in research, scholarship,
and education by publishing worldwide in

Oxford New York

Auckland Cape Town Dar es Salaam Hong Kong Karachi
Kuala Lumpur Madrid Melbourne Mexico City Nairobi
New Delhi Shanghai Taipei Toronto

With offices in

Argentina Austria Brazil Chile Czech Republic France Greece
Guatemala Hungary Italy Japan Poland Portugal Singapore
South Korea Switzerland Thailand Turkey Ukraine Vietnam

Oxford is a registered trade mark of Oxford University Press
in the UK and in certain other countries

Published in the United States
by Oxford University Press Inc., New York

© Oxford University Press, 2010

The moral rights of the authors have been asserted
Database right Oxford University Press (maker)

First published 2010

British Library Cataloguing in Publication Data
Data available

Library of Congress Cataloguing in Publication Data
Data available

Typeset by Glyph International, Bangalore, India
Printed in Great Britain
by Ashford Colour Press Ltd., Gosport, Hampshire

ISBN 978–0–19–954255–0

10 9 8 7 6 5 4 3 2 1

Foreword

The message is loud and clear. Patients, the public and the medical profession itself expect doctors to practise safe and high quality medicine. Of course, how we perform in practice is inevitably influenced by the knowledge, skills, and behaviours we acquire—and that in turn depends on appropriate assessment procedures. Over the last few years, the Royal Colleges of Physicians have revised the way they assess candidates for the MRCP (UK), an almost essential prerequisite to becoming a consultant physician in the UK. The new PACES examinations remain clinically relevant while ensuring greater objectivity in marking.

These two volumes adopt an innovative approach to help the postgraduate student prepare for these new assessments. Based on a selection of clinical cases from the various systems of the body, the authors emphasize the importance of communication skills and ethical considerations. What make these books different, however, are the *clinical notes* sections which not only guide the candidate through the technique of clinical examination but also integrate investigative results and consider relevant differential diagnoses. Each section also includes a number of questions commonly asked by examiners.

The authors are senior registrars and medical educators with experience of preparing candidates for the MRCP PACES examination. They have produced two volumes packed with the information needed to pass PACES and to practise high quality medicine. While written specifically for those aspiring to be physicians, these volumes deserve to be widely read by all with an interest in clinical medicine. Candidates in particular and patients have good reason to welcome these volumes.

Professor Sir Graeme Catto

Foreword

Ask any patient what matters about their care, and communication is likely to be near the top of their agenda. The communication they need is not just about the language used, and the depth of the explanation, but about the way in which the process is conducted. Communication allows the transmission of empathy, compassion, and care as well as facts about the illness and possible treatment. It is also about listening, not just hearing, what the patient says.

One of the privileges of being a doctor is to be allowed to share the stories of patients. These allow the doctor to become involved and by listening enabled to interpret the story, understand it and make some sense of it. That is a very particular skill and is at the heart of the consultation. Add to this the need to consider a wide variety of ethical issues and the task becomes even more complex. Discussions on consent, or on whether to proceed with treatment, are not easy. But it is what doctors do, and the newer methods of learning to communicate, and not just to be dropped in at the deep end, can make a difference. This is what this book is about.

Patients have huge experience of their illness and their symptoms and what they mean to them. The privilege is being allowed to share that and to have an opportunity of changing things for the better. Two lessons have been important for me. First, the mantra of not getting involved with patients, was one that was taught to me as an undergraduate. I don't think it works. Empathy, kindness, and compassion require involvement and professionalism does not mean that one cannot feel concern for a patient or a family and want to make a difference. I read somewhere of the patient who asked, 'my story is broken, can you help me fix it?' To do that effectively does require active listening and participation.

The second is that patients are highly sophisticated and can teach doctors a lot about how to behave. As an oncologist many years ago, I set up a series of cancer support groups. I like to think that they made contribution to helping patients and their families. However what I am sure of is that they helped the clinical staff understand better what the problems really were. We benefited as least as much as the patients did, if not more, and I have always been grateful for all that they taught me.

Finally, a word on equanimity. This was the subject of one of Sir William Osler's great essays. It means the ability to be able to keep a clear head, provide a way forward and give confidence and calmness when things get difficult. It too is part of the communication which is so important between patient and doctor.

Kenneth C Calman

Preface

'Progress is impossible without change, and those who cannot change their minds cannot change anything.'

George Bernard Shaw

This is a time of unprecedented change in medical training in the UK. Over recent years, the Modernising Medical Careers (MMC) initiative has completely altered the landscape of postgraduate medical education and assessment. New medical graduates are required to complete a two-year Foundation programme (F1 and F2) acquiring generic skills and then progress through a two-year Core Medical Training programme (CT1 and CT2). This is followed by a Higher Specialist Training programme (ST3 onwards), which is of variable duration depending on the chosen specialty. The completion of higher specialist training, and the award of a certificate of completion of postgraduate training (CCT), is essential for eligibility for consultant posts in the UK.

Patient safety and quality in healthcare are at the heart of developments in postgraduate medical education, and these two volumes are designed to help the candidate meet the demands of modern healthcare. The emphasis of MMC is towards competency-based training, requiring doctors to demonstrate competence prior to career progression. The principles of competency-based assessment are based upon the recognition that assessment of basic knowledge and clinical skills do not necessarily relate to the complex behaviours and interactions that physicians demonstrate during everyday practice.

This revolution in postgraduate medical education has been reflected in changes to the MRCP examination. Until recently, the MRCP (PACES) was not mandatory for progression to specialty training. However, from August 2011, the full MRCP (UK) Diploma will be mandatory requirements for ST3 entry into the medical specialties. Therefore, the MRCP (PACES) is increasingly viewed as a valid, high-stakes assessment to regulate entrance to specialty training.

The MRCP clinical examination has evolved to meet the demands of a broad and detailed examination of clinical performance and professionalism. The MRCP (PACES) examination was introduced in 2001, comprising 5 stations: Station 1 (Respiratory and Abdominal Systems); Station 2 (History Taking Skills); Station 3 (Cardiovascular and Central Nervous System); Station 4 (Communication Skills); and Station 5 (Skin, Eye, Locomotor, and Endocrine Systems). Since October 2009, Station 5 has been replaced by the new Station 5 (Integrative Clinical Assessment), which involves two 10-minute encounters, each known as a 'Brief Clinical Consultation'. The candidate has a brief introductory explanatory referral and then has 8 minutes to undertake a focused history and examination to solve the clinical problem, answer any questions the patient may have, and to explain their investigation and/or management plan to the patient. The remaining 2 minutes are spent with the examiners, to relate the findings and differential diagnosis, and to provide an outline of investigation and management plans, in greater detail than that given to the patient. The focused history and examination does not necessarily have to be taken in a specific order, but should rather be seen as an opportunity for integrative assessment, as seen on a post-take ward round. The purpose of this change is to push the boundaries of assessment away from basic knowledge and technique, and towards the higher-order skills that define professionalism and performance. Therefore, the new Station 5 does not simply assess the candidate's aptitude with a stethoscope or tendon hammer, or knowledge of differential diagnoses, but rather considers their global performance as a professional.

Additionally, from October 2009 a new marking system has been introduced that is centred around seven core clinical skills: (A) Physical examination; (B) Identifying physical signs; (C) Clinical communication; (D) Differential diagnosis; (E) Clinical judgement; (F) Managing patients' concerns; and (G): Managing patient welfare. Stations 1–4 will assess four to five core clinical skills, but since the new Station 5 is a global assessment, it will take account of all seven core clinical skills. Each of the skills assessed at every encounter is marked on a scale of Unsatisfactory (0 marks), Borderline (1 mark), or Satisfactory (2 marks). Given that there are two examiners who mark each clinical skill from 0–2, the total number of marks available is 172. Therefore, since Station 5 tests all the core clinical skills, this station comprises 56 out of the possible 172, almost a third of the total marks! Appropriate preparation for this unique station is consequently of utmost importance.

This two-volume textbook is focused upon the needs of candidates preparing for the MRCP (PACES) examination. This volume provides clinical cases with a unique style of presentation, where each classical case presentation is accompanied by a systematic set of easy-to-follow clinical notes. This is followed by common questions asked by examiners, with evidence-based answers. This synthesis of clinical examination and presentation techniques, followed by a focused case-based discussion is ideal for understanding and learning. Moreover, this is the only textbook to extensively review the new MRCP (PACES) Station 5. We have included a compilation of 20 cases that reflect the new Station 5 format, providing a conceptual framework for structuring the history and clinical examination in the limited time provided in the examination, and developing differential diagnoses, preliminary investigations, and management plans.

Although the new Station 5 replaces the skin, eyes, endocrine, and locomotor stations, it is likely that the majority of Station 5 encounters will still relate to one of these four systems. For this reason, cases from these four systems are found in the supplementary section of this volume. However, it is important for candidates to prepare for cases relating to the other stations and areas not previously covered in the examination, for example acute medicine, haematology, infectious disease, and elderly medicine. They should also be prepared to encounter medical problems that are met in everyday practice without pertaining to a specific diagnosis, such as chest pain, hypotension, or deterioration in renal function. Thus, it is conceivable that some patients may not display a wealth of clinical signs, and the candidate will need to focus on addressing the clinical problem through integrated clinical assessment within the boundaries of safe and professional practice.

The final aspect of performance in the MRCP (PACES) examination, and often that most feared by candidates, is the final case presentation to the examiner. This relays to the examiner the clinical competence and the level of confidence of the candidate. This presentation may set the tone for the entire examination, and may sometimes make a difference between a pass and a fail. Although body language, eye contact, and confidence in your clinical skills are the essentials for elegant presentation, the case presentations included in this book reflect a uniform and systematic style of presentation that spans the examination routine. Clearly, presentation styles vary from individual to individual, and of course the styles preferred by examiners may also vary. However, the advantage of a systematic approach is that one will not forget to mention important positive and negative signs. Most examiners are content with this presentation strategy, but others may ask you just to give the diagnosis followed by positive clinical signs. We believe that by adopting a presentation strategy as given in this book such a prompted change in presentation style should not pose a problem. However, this may not be true in reverse. What is most important is to adopt your own consistent and systematic style for presentation.

This book comprehensively covers the knowledge, techniques, and performance required for success in clinical examinations. Although it primarily serves as a revision tool for the MRCP (PACES) examination, this book will also be useful for candidates preparing for undergraduate examinations, MBBS and USMLE (US), and other postgraduate examinations, FRACP (Australia) and FCCP (Canada). However, a textbook can never replace clinical practice, and this book is not designed to do so. This book should be used alongside thorough clinical exposure and practice. As Vince Lombardi, the legendary Miami Dolphins coach said, 'Practice does not make perfect. Only perfect practice makes perfect.'

Acknowledgements

First, I would like to thank my co-authors Bilal and Deborah for their never-ending patience and effort. Without their spirit and enthusiasm, this project would have been filed along with most of my other great ideas! Many thanks also to the other contributors—Fatima, Paul, and Rimona for their sterling work.

No work of this magnitude is possible without mentorship, and I am particularly indebted to Andrew Thillainayagam for his unwavering support and guidance. It was those memorable first words from my first post-take ward round, 'Gautam, are you sure you want to be a physician?' that inspired me to pursue excellence in my chosen field. I also owe a debt of gratitude to Ian Curran, and my medical education colleagues at the London Deanery and Barts & Royal London, for introducing me to the concepts of learning and teaching that underpin this book.

I am grateful to all those at Oxford University Press for making this idea a reality—Fiona Goodgame, Christopher Reid, Stephanie Ireland, and Joanna Hardern to name but a few.

Whatever the weaknesses of these books, they would have been far greater without the help of my friends Mathena and Samer, who reviewed the manuscript more times than they care to remember. Special thanks also to Alex for never-ending support and inspiration.

Finally, these books are dedicated to my parents, to whom I owe so much. My mother for her love and affection, and my father for being my role-model in medicine and in life.

Gautam Mehta

First, I would like to thank my co-authors Gautam and Deborah for all their hard work, time and patience, without which this venture would never have been completed. I would like to thank Fatima, Paul, and Rimona for their contributions and feedback.

I am forever indebted to Chris Wathen for his invaluable advice, support, and guidance in orientating this project, especially at such a time of unprecedented change to the curriculum and structure of the MRCP (PACES) examination.

If it were not for Oxford University Press, our concepts for novel MRCP (PACES) textbooks would have remained as such, and would never have become a reality. I would particularly like to thank our colleagues, Fiona, Stephanie, Chris, and Joanna at Oxford University Press for their friendly advice, support, and patience throughout every stage of this project.

I cannot be grateful enough to Nabila and Adam for their everlasting support, resilience and patience at home, without which, I would never have been able to complete this, for what once felt like a never-ending project.

Finally, I would like to dedicate these books to my parents, as it if were not for their affection and inspiration at every stage of my life and career, I would not be where I am today.

Bilal Iqbal

List of Contributors

Paul Bentley
Clinical Senior Lecturer and Honorary Consultant Neurologist
Imperial College London, UK

Rimona Weil
Specialist Registrar in Neurology
Royal Free Hospital
University College London, UK

Structure of the MRCP (PACES) examination

Structure of the examination

The 5 stations comprising the MRCP (PACES) examinations are set up such that, at any one time, 5 candidates can be examined. The duration of each station is 20 minutes. Stations 2 and 4 are designated 20 minutes each, whereas stations 1, 3, and 5 are further split into two 10-minute clinical encounters. Each station is preceded by a 5-minute interval. This is particularly useful for stations 2, 4, and 5, where the initial candidate information that outlines the scenario(s) can be used to gather your thoughts, organize your history taking approach, and develop preliminary differential diagnoses.

Skills tested in the examination

From October 2009, the marking scheme for the MRCP (PACES) examination has changed. There are now seven clinical skills tested in the examination. The Clinical Skills tested are:

A. Physical Examination

B. Identifying Physical Signs

C. Clinical Communication

D. Differential Diagnosis

E. Clinical Judgement

F. Managing Patients' Concerns

G. Maintaining Patient Welfare

The marking scheme

Each skill is designated a mark: 0 (unsatisfactory), 1 (borderline), and 2 (satisfactory).

Station	Encounter	Time (min)	A	B	C	D	E	F	G	Maximum marks (per examiner)
1	Abdomen	10	•	•		•	•		•	10
1	Respiratory	10	•	•		•	•		•	10
2	History	20			•	•	•	•	•	10
3	Cardiovascular	10	•	•		•	•		•	10
3	Nervous system	10	•	•		•	•		•	10
4	Communication	20			•		•	•	•	8
5	Brief Clinical Consultation (1)	10	•	•	•	•	•		•	•	14
5	Brief Clinical Consultation (2)	10	•	•	•	•	•		•	•	14

Examiners are no longer required to award an overall judgement mark for each encounter. Given that 2 examiners will each score the candidate, the total marks are 172. Station 5 now constitutes 56 marks—that's almost a third of the total marks.

For specific mark sheets and further information about the MRCP (PACES) structure, please visit

(a) www.mrcpuk.org/PACES/Pages/PacesMarkSheets.aspx

(b) www.mrcpuk.org/PACES/Pages/PacesFormat.aspx

Contents

List of Abbreviations

↑	raised
↓	lowered
A&E	Accident and Emergency Department
AAFB	acid-alcohol fast bacilli
ABCD score	Age, Blood pressure, Clinical features, and Duration of symptoms
ABPA	allergic bronchopulmonary aspergillosis
ABVD	adriamycin, bleomycin, vinblastine, dacrabazine
AC	air conduction
ACC	American College of Cardiology
ACE	angiotensin converting enzyme
ACR	American College of Rheumatology
ACTH	adrenocorticotrophic hormone
ADA	Adenosine deaminase activity
ADH	antidiuretic hormone
ADPKD	autosomal dominant polycystic kidney disease
AF	atrial fibrillation
AFLP	acute fatty liver of pregnancy
AFP	alpha-fetoprotein
AHA	American Heart Association
AICA	anterior inferior cerebellar artery infarction
AIDP	acute inflammatory demyelinating polyradiculoneuropathy
AIDS	aquired immunodeficiency syndrome
AIP	acute interstitial pneumonia
ALP	alkaline phosphatase
ALT	alanine aminotransferase
AML	acute myeloid leukaemia
AMPA	α-amino-hydroxy-5-methylisoxasole-4 propionic acid
AMTS	abbreviated mental test score
ANA	antinuclear autoantibody
ANCA	anti-neutrophil cytoplasmic antibody
anti-CCP	Anti-cyclic citrullinated peptide
anti-GBM	anti-glomerular basement membrane antibody
anti-RNP	anti-ribonucleoprotein antibody
AP	anterio-posterior
APC	adenomatous polyposis coli
APTT	activated partial thromboplastin time
APUD	amine precursor uptake and decarboxylation
ARDS	acute respiratory distress syndrome
A-R-P	Accommodation Reflex Preserved
ARPKD	Autosomal recessive polycystic kidney disease
ASA	atrial septal aneurysm
ASD	atrial septal defect
ATS	American Thoracic Society
AVM	arteriovenous malformations
AVNRT	atrioventricular nodal re-entry tachycardia
AVRT	atrioventricular re-entry tachycardia
BC	bone conduction

BCC	basal cell carcinoma
BEACOPP	bleomycin, etoposide, doxorubicin, cyclophosphamide, Oncovin, prednisolone, procarabazine
BMD	Becker's muscular dystrophy
BMI	body mass index
BNF	British National Formulary
BNP	brain natriuretic peptide
BP	blood pressure
bpm	beats per minute
BPPV	benign paroxysmal positional vertigo
CAB	Citizens Advice Bureau
CABG	coronary artery bypass graft
CADASIL	cerebral autosomal dominant arteriopathy with subcortical infarcts and leucoencephalopathy
CAM	Confusion Assessment Method
cAMP	cyclic adenosine monophosphate
c-ANCA	cytoplasmic anti-neutrophil cytoplasmic antibody
CAT	computerized axial tomography
CHD	coronary heart disease
CIDP	chronic inflammatory demyelinating polyneuropathy
CINCA	Chronic Infantile, Neurologic, Cutaneous, and Articular
CJD	Creutzfeldt-Jakob disease
CK	creatinine kinase
CML	chronic myeloid leukaemia
CMV	cytomegalovirus
CNS	central nervous system
COMT	catechol-O-methyl transferase
COP	cryptogenic organizing pneumonia
COPD	chronic obstructive pulmonary disease
COPP	cyclophosphamide, Oncovin (vincristine), prednisolone, procarbazine
CPA	cerebellopontine angle
CPEO	chronic progressive external ophthalmoplegia
CPR	cardiopulmonary resuscitation
CRC	colorectal cancer
CRH	corticotrophin releasing hormone
CRP	C-reactive protein
CSF	cerebrospinal fluid
CT	computed tomography
CT KUB	CT— kidneys, ureters, bladder
CXR	chest X-ray
D-AB	Dorsal-ABduct
DAFNE	Dose Adjustment for Normal Eating programme
DCCT	Diabetes Control and Complications Trial
DDAVP	desmopressin acetate (synthetic analogue of vasopressin)
DHS	Drug Hypersensitivity Syndrome
DI	diabetes insipidus
DIC	disseminated intravascular coagulation
DIP	desquamative interstitial pneumonia
DIP	distal interphalangeal
DKA	diabetic ketoacidosis

DMARDs	disease modifying anti-rheumatic drugs
DMD	Duchenne's muscular dystrophy
DNAR	do not attempt resuscitation
DNCB	dinitrochlorobenzene
DPA	Data Protection Act (1998)
DPCP	diphenylcypropenone
DPP-IV	dipeptidyl peptidase IV
DRESS	Drug Reaction with Eosinophilia and Systemic Symptoms
DVLA	Driver and Vehicle Licensing Agency
DVT	deep vein thrombosis
EAA	extrinsic allergic alveolitis
EBV	Epstein-Barr virus
ECCE	extracapsular cataract extraction
ECG	electrocardiogram
EDIC	Epidemiology of Diabetes Interventions and Complications trial
EDTA	ethylenediaminetetraacetic acid
EEG	electroencephalogram
EIA	enzyme immunoassay
EMG	electromyography
ENA	extractable nuclear antigen
ENT	ear, nose, and throat
EPS	electrophysiological studies
ERCP	endoscopic retrograde cholangiopancreatography
ERG	electroretinogram
ERS	European Respiratory Society
ESR	erythrocyte sedimentation rate
FAP	famililal adenomatous polyposis
FBC	full blood count
FDA	Food and Drug Administration
FDR	first-degree relative
FET	forced expiratory time
FEV	forced expiratory volume
FH	family history
FNA	fine-needle aspiration
FOB	faecal occult blood
FRC	functional residual capacity
FSH	follicle stimulating hormone
FTA	fluorescent treponemal antibody
FVC	forced vital capacity
GALS	gait, arms. legs. spine
GBS	Guillain-Barré syndrome
GFR	glomerular filtration rate
GGT	gamma glutamyl transpeptidase
GH	growth hormone
GHRH	growth hormone-releasing hormone
GI	gastrointestinal
GIST	gastrointestinal stromal tumour
GLP-1	Glucagon-like peptide 1
GMC	General Medical Council
GN	glomerulonephritis

GORD	gastrooesophageal reflux disease
GTN	glyceryl trinitrate
HAART	highly active anti-retroviral therapy
Hb	haemoglobin
HCC	hepatocellular cancer
hCG	human chorionic gonadotrophin
HCV	hepatitis C virus
HDL	high density lipoprotein
HELLP	Haemolysis, Elevated Liver enzymes, Low Platelets
HHT	hereditary haemorrhagic telangiectasia
HHV-6	human herpesvirus 6
HIV	human immunodeficiency virus
HL	Hodgkin's lymphoma
HMSN	hereditary motor and sensory neuropathies
HNPCC	hereditary nonpolyposis colorectal cancer
HNPP	hereditary neuropathy with pressure palsy
HONK	hyperosmolar hyperglycaemic non-ketotic
HR	heart rate
HRA	Human Rights Act (1998)
HRCT	high resolution CT (scan)
HSMN	hereditary motor and sensory neuropathy
HSV	herpes simplex virus
HTLV-1	human T-lymphotropic virus-1
IBD	inflammatory bowel disease
IBS	irritable bowel syndrome
ICAS	Independent Complaints Advocacy Service
ICD	implantable cardioverter defibrillator
ICCE	intracapsular cataract extraction
ICU	Intensive Care Unit
IDA	iron-deficiency anaemia
IGF-1	insulin-like growth factor-I
IH	immunohistochemistry
IM	intramuscular
IMCA	independent mental capacity advocates
INO	internuclear ophthalmoplegia
INR	international normalized ratio
IPV	inactivated polio virus
IV	intravenous
IVC	inferior vena cava
IVIG	intravenous immunoglobulin
IVTA	Intravitreal triamcinolone acetonide
JVP	jugular venous pressure
LA	left atrium
LABA	long acting β_2 agonist
LACI	lacunar circulation stroke
LADA	latent autoimmune disease of the adult
LDH	lactate dehydrogenase
LDL	low density lipoprotein
LEMS	Lambert-Eaton myasthenic syndrome
LFT	liver function tests

LIST OF ABBREVIATIONS

LH	luteinising hormone
LIP	lymphoid interstitial pneumonia
LLZ	left lower zone
LMN	lower motor neurone
LP	lumbar puncture
LPHs	lipotropins
LUZ	left upper zone
LV	left ventricle
MALT	mucosal-associated lymphoid tissue
MCA	middle cerebral artery
MCP	metacarpophalangeal
MDR TB	multi-drug resistant tuberculosis
MEN	mulitple endocrine neoplasia
MGUS	Monoclonal gammopathy of undetermined significance
MI	myocardial infarction
MMSE	Mini Mental State Examination
MND	motor neurone disease
MPTP	1-methyl-4-phenyl-1,2,3,6-tetrahydropridine
MPZ	myelin protein zero gene
MRA	magnetic resonance angiogram
MRCP	magnetic resonance cholangiopancreatography
MRI	magnetic resonance imaging
MRSA	methicillin-resistant Stephylococcus aureus
MRV	magnetic resonance venography
MSA	multiple systems atrophy
MSH	melanocyte-stimulating hormone
MSI	microsatellite instability
MSM	men who have sex with men
MuSK	muscle-specific kinase
NAAT	nucleic acid amplification test
nAChR	nicotinic acetylcholine receptors
NAFLD	non-alcoholic fatty liver disease
NCS	nerve conduction studies
NHL	non-Hodgkin's lymphoma
NICE	National Institute for Health and Clinical Excellence
NMDA	N-methyl-D-aspartic acid
NO	nitric oxide
NSAID	nonsteroidal anti-inflammatory drug
NSCLC	non-small cell carcinoma
NSIP	non-specific interstitial pneumonia
NSTEMI	non-ST segment elevation myocardial infarction
NYHA	New York Heart Association
OA	osteoarthritis
OIs	opportunistic infections
OGD	oesophago-gastro-duodenoscopy
OPV	oral live attenuated polio virus
PA	pulmonary artery
PACI	partial anterior circulation infarct
P-AD	Palmar-ADduct
p-ANCA	perinuclear anti-neutrophil cytoplasmic antibody

PALS	Patient Advocacy and Liaison
PAN	polyarteritis nodosa
PBC	primary biliary cirrhosis
PCI	percutaneous coronary intervention
PCP	pneumocystis jiroreci pneumonia
PCR	polymerase chain reaction
PCWP	pulmonary capillary wedge pressure
PDA	patent ductus arteriosus
PE	pulmonary embolism
PEG	percutaneous gastronomy
PFO	patent foramen ovale
PFT	pulmonary function test
PI	protease inhibitor
PICA	posterior inferior cerebellar artery
PIP	proximal interphalangeal
PJS	Peutz-Jehgers syndrome
PMF	pulmonary massive fibrosis
PMP22	peripheral myelin protein-22 gene
POCI	posterior circulation infarct
POEMS	Polyneuropathy, Organomegaly, Endocrinopathy, Monoclonal gammopathy, and Skin changes
POMC	proopiomelanocortin
PSP	progressive supranuclear palsy
PPD	purified protein derivative
PR	per rectum
PSA	Prostate Specific Antigen
PSC	primary sclerosing cholangitis
PSP	progressive supranuclear palsy
PTH	parathyroid hormone
PTU	propylthiouracil
PVS	persistent vegetative state
QALYS	Quality Adjusted Life Years
RA	rheumatoid arthritis
RA	right atrium
RAPD	relative afferent pupillary defects
RBC	red blood cell
RB-ILD	respiratory bronchiolitis-interstitial lung disease
REM	rapid eye movement
RhF	Rheumatoid factor
RLZ	right lower zone
RNA	ribonucleic acid
RNP	ribonuclear protein
RPGN	Rapidly Progressive Glomerulonephritis
RPR	Rapid Plasmin Reagin
RUZ	right upper zone
RV	right ventricle
SADBE	squaric acid dinitryl ester
SAH	subarachnoid haemorrhage
SCC	squamous cell carcinoma
SCLC	small cell carcinoma

SHBG	sex hormone-binding globulin
SHO	Senior House Officer
SIADH	syndrome of inappropriate anti-diuretic hormone
SLE	systemic lupus erythematosus
SPECT	Single Photon Emission Computed Tomography
SSRI	selective serotonin reuptake inhibitor
STEMI	ST segment elevation myocardial infarction
STI	sexually transmitted infection
SUDEP	Sudden Unexpected Death in Epilepsy
SVC	superior vena cava
SVTs	supraventricular tachycardias
TACI	total anterior circulation infarct
TB	tuberculosis
TED	thrombo-embolus deterrent
TGF	transforming growth factor
TIA	transient ischaemic attack
TIPS	transjugular intrahepatic portosystemic shunt
TLC	total lung capacity
TNF	tumour necrosis factor
TNM	classification system: spread of primary tumour (T); extent of lymph node involvment (N); and presence or absence of metastases (M)
TPHA	*T pallidum* haemagglutination
TTP	thrombotic thrombocytopenic purpura
TSH	thyroid stimulating hormone
TSI	thyroid stimulating immunoglobulin
TVO	transient visual obscurations
U&E	urea and electrolytes
UC	ulcerative colitis
UIP	usual interstitial pneumonia
UKPDS	UK Prospective Diabetes Study
UMN	upper motor neurone
USA	unstable angina
VDRL	Venereal Disease Reference Laboratory
VEGF	vascular endothelial growth factor
VF	ventricular fibrillation
VHFs	viral haemorrhagic fevers
V-Q	ventilation-perfusion
VSD	ventricular septal defect
VT	ventricular tachychardia
VZV	varicella zoster virus
WBC	white blood cell
WCC	white cell count
WHO	World Health Organization
WPW	Wolff-Parkinson-White syndrome

Station 1 ◆ (Abdomen System)

(Respiratory System)

Abdomen System

Case 1 ♦ **Chronic Liver Disease**

CASE PRESENTATION

This patient is **icteric**,[1] with **cachexia**[2] and **abdominal distension**. There is no evidence of **anaemia**.[3] There is **clubbing**,[4] **leuconychia**,[5] and **palmar erythema**.[6] Multiple **spider naevi**[7] are present on the trunk and face. There are multiple **petechiae** and **ecchymoses**.[8] There is **gynaecomastia** and **loss of body hair**.[9] On examination of the abdomen,[10] **caput medusae**[11] are present. There is **hepatosplenomegaly**[12] and **ascites**.[13] There is a **hepatic venous hum**.[14] There are no hepatic bruits.[15] There is **peripheral oedema**.[16] There are no signs of hepatic encephalopathy.[17]

The diagnosis is **cirrhosis of the liver** with **portal hypertension**.[18]

Clinical notes

1. Jaundice is a marker of severity of liver disease, as well as a consequence of decompensation. Yellow discolouration is not usually seen until the serum bilirubin is >40µmol/L (twice the upper limit of normal), although the earliest signs of jaundice can be detected in the periphery of the conjunctivae, or in the buccal mucosa. Remember, there are other causes of jaundice in liver disease, such as Zieve's syndrome (haemolysis and hyperlipidaemia in alcohol misuse), or biliary obstruction.

2. Cachexia can be established by demonstrating muscle and fat loss. Wasting of the temporalis muscle is an early sign of generalized muscle atrophy. A reduced triceps skin-fold thickness is a marker of loss of fat stores. This can be demonstrated by palpating for redundant skin over the triceps area between your thumb and forefingers.

3. Anaemia is most reliably demonstrated by looking for conjunctival pallor. This is thought to be more sensitive than looking for pallor of skin creases, nails, or other mucosal membranes. If there is no evidence of anaemia, it is an important negative to mention to the examiner. The principal causes of anaemia in chronic liver disease are blood loss from portal hypertensive gastropathy, alcohol excess causing bone marrow suppression and poor nutrition.

4. Other gastrointestinal (GI) causes of clubbing include inflammatory bowel disease (IBD), coeliac disease, GI lymphoma and rare causes of malabsorption such as tropical sprue and Whipple's disease.

5. Leuconychia is a non-specific finding which is associated with hypoalbuminaemia as well as other conditions such as heart failure, renal disease, Hodgkin's lymphoma (HL) and diabetes mellitus (see Case 8—Nephrotic Syndrome).

6. Palmar erythema reflects the vasodilated state of cirrhosis. Other causes of palmar erythema include hypercapnoea, rheumatoid arthritis, thyrotoxicosis, pregnancy, fever, and exercise.

7. Spider naevi are vascular lesions, with a central arteriole that supplies smaller surrounding vessels. Generally, the number and size correlate with the severity of liver disease, although they may occur in normal individuals and pregnancy. Spider naevi, palmar erythema, gynaecomastia, and loss of body hair are thought to be the consequence of altered sex hormone metabolism, and an increase in the oestradiol:free testosterone ratio. Carefully inspect the superior vena cava (SVC) distribution, and remember not to miss inspecting the patient's back!

8. Petechiae and echymoses are a consequence of coagulopathy and thrombocytopenia. Thrombocytopenia may occur due to both hypersplenism and alcohol-related marrow suppression.

9. Gynaecomastia and loss of body hair are also thought to be the consequence of altered sex hormone metabolism (oestradiol:free testosterone ratio). In male patients, the gynaecomastia may be evident, but it is best to examine and palpate the areolar regions in all male patients to clearly demonstrate your understanding to the examiner. Gynaecomastia can be identified by palpating glandular tissue beneath the nipple and areolar region—it is often a firm and mobile disc of tissue.

10. Before proceeding to palpation and percussion, carefully inspect the abdomen. Many useful clinical signs can be identified in patients with chronic liver disease. In particular, note the following:
    - Scars suggesting paracentesis or liver biopsies
    - Surgical scars, i.e. Chevron (roof top) modification incision or Mercedes-Benz modification suggesting previous pancreatic, gastric, or hepatobiliary surgery
    - Fullness of the flanks suggesting ascites
    - Distended abdominal wall veins (see below)

11. Caput medusae are a result of umbilical vein recannalization due to portal hypertension. This leads to prominence of abdominal wall veins. The appearance is thought to resemble the head (caput) of the Medusa. The direction of flow in abdominal wall vessels distinguishes portal hypertension from inferior vena cava obstruction. In portal hypertension, the flow is AWAY from the umbilicus.

12. The cirrhotic liver may be small or enlarged. In most cases, a cirrhotic liver is small and shrunken, but in cases where it is due to alcohol or non-alcoholic fatty liver disease (NAFLD) hepatomegaly may be present. Always comment on the liver edge. Tender hepatomegaly suggests stretch of the liver capsule, by a process that has caused *recent* hepatic enlargement, such as infective hepatitis, alcoholic hepatitis, or malignancy. A hard irregular liver edge suggests malignancy. Cirrhosis due to alcohol or NAFLD may cause hepatomegaly due to fat deposition.

13. Volume status must be assessed in all patients with ascites (see Case 2—Ascites). This can be done at the end of the examination, after sitting the patient forward to inspect the back and palpate cervical lymph nodes. Cirrhosis is typically associated with systemic vasodilatation, hence the cardiac filling pressure is low or normal. However, congestive cardiac failure is a rare cause of hepatic congestion and cirrhosis. These patients may have an elevated venous pressure and associated tricuspid regurgitation.

14. The hepatic venous hum is a murmur that is audible in portal hypertension or hepatocellular carcinoma. It results from collateral formation between the portal system and remnant of the umbilical vein. It is best appreciated over the epigastrium.

15. A hepatic bruit over the liver can be heard with alcoholic hepatitis or hepatic carcinoma (primary or secondary). Other rare causes include hepatic arteriovenous malformations, intestinal arteriovenous malformations, hepatic haemangioma, and TIPS (transjugular intrahepatic portosystemic shunt).

16. The mechanism for oedema is hypoalbuminaemia and stimulation of the rennin-angiotensin system.

17. Asterixis is a frequent finding in hepatic encephalopathy. The flapping tremor is best elicited in outstretched, dorsiflexed hands. Flexion and extension movements of the fingers and wrists are seen, with the flexion phase being more rapid than the extension phase, which returns the fingers and wrists to the initial position. The spectrum of clinical features of hepatic encephalopathy begins with disturbance in the diurnal sleep pattern (insomnia and hypersomnia), which precedes overt neurological signs. Bradykinesia and asterixis subsequently occur, preceding hyperreflexia, transient decerebrate posturing and coma. Asterixis is not specific for hepatic encephalopathy, but may also occur in other toxic encephalopathies such as uraemia or respiratory failure. Asterixis is almost always bilateral; unilateral asterixis suggests a structural neurological lesion.

18. Specific signs to suggest an underlying cause of liver disease are rare, but the candidate should be prepared to mention them if the examiner asks about further examination findings.
    - **Alcohol**: Dupuytren's contractures, parotid enlargement (see signs of alcohol misuse below)
    - **Chronic hepatitis B and C infection**: tattoos, signs of intravenous drug use. Hepatitis C is also associated with porphyria cutanea tarda and type III cryoglobulinaemia (palpable purpura and livedo reticularis).
    - **Primary biliary cirrhosis**: hyperpigmentation, xanthelesma, tendon xanthomata, excoriation marks

- **Haemochromatosis**: bronze pigmentation, arthropathy, finger tip skin pricks (glucose testing in diabetes)
- **Congestive cardiac failure**: raised venous pressure, third heart sound
- **Wilson's disease**: Kayser-Fleischer rings (only seen on slit-lamp examination), akinetic-rigid syndrome
- **α$_1$-antitrypsin deficiency**: lower zone emphysema
- **Budd-Chiari syndrome**: loss of hepatic jugular reflux (due to inferior cava involvement)

Questions commonly asked by examiners

What are the causes of cirrhosis?
- **Alcohol**
- **Viral**
  - Hepatitis B
  - Hepatitis C
- **Autoimmune**
  - Primary Biliary Cirrhosis (PBC)
  - Primary Sclerosing Cholangitis (PSC)
  - Autoimmune hepatitis
- **Metabolic**
  - Non-alcoholic steatohepatitis
  - Haemachromatosis
  - α$_1$ Antitrypsin deficiency
  - Wilson's disease
  - Cystic Fibrosis
- Drugs
  - Methotrexate
  - Isoniazid
  - Amiodarone
  - Phenytoin

What are the signs of alcohol misuse?
- Cachexia
- Tremor
- Parotid enlargement
- Dupuytren's contracture
- Cerebellar syndrome
- Peripheral neuropathy
- Myopathy

What are the consequences of cirrhosis?
- **Consequences of portal hypertension**
  - Oesophageal varices
  - Ascites
  - Hypersplenism/thrombocytopenia
- **Consequences of liver dysfunction**
  - Coagulopathy
  - Encephalopathy

- ◆ Jaundice
- ◆ Hypoalbuminaemia
- Hepatocellular carcinoma

What are the causes of decompensation in cirrhosis?

- Infection
- Spontaneous bacterial peritonitis
- Hypokalaemia——decreases renal ammonia clearance
- Gastrointestinal bleeding
- Sedatives
- Hepatocellular carcinoma

How do you classify the severity of hepatic encephalopathy?

Hepatic encephalopathy is defined as reversible neurological dysfunction or coma due to liver disease.

Grade 1—Insomnia/reversal of day-night sleep pattern
Grade 2—Lethargy/disorientation
Grade 3—Confusion/somnolescence
Grade 4—Coma

Asterixis may be present at any stage

How do you assess the severity of cirrhosis?

The Childs–Pugh score assesses disease severity and prognosis.

Score	1	2	3
Bilirubin (mmol/L)	<35	35–52	>50
Ascites	Nil	Mild	Moderate
Encephalopathy	Nil	1–2	3–4
PT (sec prolonged)	1–4	4–6	>7
Albumin (g/L)	>35	28–35	<28

Child–Pugh >10 (grade C)—33% 1 year mortality
Child–Pugh 7–9 (grade B)—80% survive 5 years
Child–Pugh 5–6 (grade A)—90% survive 5 years

Are you aware of any strategies for the management of cirrhosis?

Slowing or reversing liver disease

Treatment depends on the underlying disease. Abstinence in alcoholic liver disease, antiviral therapy in viral hepatitis, and immunosuppression in autoimmune hepatitis, all improve liver fibrosis.

Preventing superimposed liver damage

Abstinence from alcohol improves prognosis in viral hepatitis and chronic liver disease.
All patients should be immunized against hepatitis A, and hepatitis B if risk factors are present.
Pneumococcal and yearly influenza vaccines should also be considered.

Preventing complications

Surveillance for hepatoma involves 6-monthly abdominal ultrasound and alpha-fetoprotein (AFP) measurement, although a survival benefit from this approach has not been conclusively demonstrated. All patients should undergo endoscopy as surveillance for oesophageal varices. Patients with medium or large varices, or any varices in the context of advanced (Child–Pugh C)

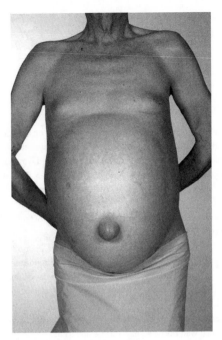

Figure 1.1 A patient with decompensated chronic liver disease. There is gross ascites with an umbilical hernia. Note the mild degree of gynaecomastia.

liver disease are treated with <u>non-selective beta blockers</u> as primary prophylaxis. Following an episode of spontaneous bacterial peritonitis, prophylactic antibiotics are indicated.

Liver transplantation

The decision to proceed to liver transplantation is taken by a transplant centre. Selection is a balance of the severity of liver disease, against the presence of co-morbidity, which would affect outcome. Most centres advocate 6 months of abstinence from alcohol, and age under 65 years. Alcohol abstinence is insisted upon not to 'ration' organs, but because liver function may improve considerably following alcohol cessation. Some conditions are considered for transplantation independent of disease severity, due to the presence of symptoms that affect quality of life. Examples include intractable pruritus in PBC, or recurrent cholangitis in PSC.

Case 2 ◆ Ascites

CASE PRESENTATION

*This patient is not cachectic. There is no evidence of lymphadenopathy[1] or stigmata of chronic liver disease.[2] The **abdomen is** distended,[3] but is soft and non-tender. The **umbilicus is** everted.[4] There are no collateral vessels visible on the abdominal wall.[5] There is no evidence of hepatosplenomegaly. The abdomen is **dull to percussion** in the flanks, with **shifting** dullness.[6] A **fluid thrill** can be demonstrated.[7]*

The venous pressure is not elevated,[8] and there is no peripheral oedema. There are no signs of hepatic encephalopathy.[9]

*The diagnosis is **ascites**.[10]*

Clinical notes

1. Lymphadenopathy in the presence of ascites suggests malignancy or infection such as tuberculosis. Haematological malignancy is associated with extra-hepatic portal vein thrombosis causing portal hypertension and ascites. Furthermore, other causes of generalized lymphadenopathy (infectious mononucleosis, cytomegalovirus (CMV), toxoplasmosis, HIV, HHV-6, Bartonella, systemic lupus erythematosus (SLE) and sarcoidosis) may cause ascites if retroperitoneal lymph nodes affect lymphatic duct drainage.

2. Cirrhosis is the most common cause of ascites; therefore it is important to look carefully for the signs of chronic liver disease (see Case 1 Chronic Liver Disease).

3. There are several causes of abdominal distension: obesity, ascites, abdominal mass, gravid uterus, intestinal obstruction, or constipation. The *absence* of abdominal tenderness makes intestinal obstruction unlikely. The candidate should palpate for an abdominal or pelvic mass carefully. Obesity and ascites may be difficult to distinguish, however, patients with significant ascites should demonstrate a fluid thrill or shifting dullness.

4. An everted umbilicus occurs when ascites is tense, due to fluid within a hernial sac. Para-umbilical herniae, or other abdominal wall herniae, may also be apparent.

5. Prominent abdominal wall collateral vessels may be a consequence of portal hypertension, termed caput medusae, or of inferior vena caval obstruction. These can be distinguished by occluding the vessels below the umbilicus. The direction of flow in caput medusae is away from the umbilicus, towards the legs. In inferior vena caval obstruction, flow is towards the head.

6. Ascites can be detected clinically by assessing for *shifting dullness* to percussion or a *fluid thrill*. The absence of flank dullness on percussion has been shown to be the most accurate predictor of ascites (probability of ascites without flank dullness is less than 10%). Approximately 1500mL of fluid must be present before dullness is present. Once dullness has been demonstrated in the flanks, the patient is asked to roll *towards* the examiner (to prevent the patient falling off the bed), and after 15 seconds percussion is repeated to demonstrate a change in note to resonant.

7. A fluid thrill is elicited by tapping the abdomen on one side, and feeling the transmitted wave by placing the other hand flat on the other side of the abdomen. Large volume ascites is required for a fluid thrill to be present. Only one of these tests need be performed, i.e. shifting dullness need not be performed if a fluid thrill is present.

8. Assessment of the jugular venous pressure (JVP) need not be performed routinely during the abdominal examination. However, if ascites of unknown cause is found, volume status must be assessed. Cirrhosis is typically associated with systemic vasodilatation, hence the cardiac filling pressure is low or normal. An elevated venous pressure, in the absence of tense ascites or renal insufficiency, suggests heart failure, atrial myxoma, or constrictive pericarditis as the cause of ascites.

9. Signs of hepatic encephalopathy suggest the presence of liver failure. This is an important negative to mention, since ascites may occur due to reversible *acute-on-chronic liver failure* in which encephalopathy is invariably present. This should be distinguished from progressive liver disease and portal hypertension, which is irreversible although encephalopathy may not be present.

10. When presenting a diagnosis of ascites, it is important to consider the underlying cause and consider potential aetiologies. Mentioning relevant negative findings demonstrates to the examiner your lateral thinking and active thought processes. Remember hypoalbuminaemia can be caused by malnutrition, chronic liver disease and nephrotic syndrome. Throughout your general observations, note the presence of rheumatological disease, i.e. rheumatoid arthritis and SLE, as this can result in nephrotic syndrome (membranous glomerulonephritis).

Questions commonly asked by examiners

What are the most common causes of ascites in developed countries?

- Cirrhosis (75%)
- Malignancy (10%)
- Heart failure (3%)
- Tuberculosis (2%)
- Pancreatitis (1%)

What initial investigations would you request to determine the aetiology of the ascites?

- **Diagnostic paracentesis**
  - ascitic fluid albumin and total protein
  - ascitic fluid differential white cell count
  - ascitic fluid gram stain and culture (for conventional microbes and acid-fast bacilli)
  - ascitic fluid cytology
- **Abdominal ultrasound**
  - to exclude liver or intra-abdominal mass lesions suggestive of malignancy
  - splenomegaly suggests portal hypertension
  - hepatic vein and portal vein doppler should be performed to exclude thrombosis
- **Blood tests**
  - liver function tests (LFTs)
  - prothrombin time
  - full blood count (FBC) (thrombocytopenia suggests hypersplenism and portal hypertension)

How do you classify transudative and exudative ascites?

Since many patients with ascites also have decreased serum albumin levels, comparing the ascitic fluid albumin with the serum albumin is superior to comparing the ascitic fluid albumin with a fixed value (i.e. 25g/L). The serum ascites———albumin gradient (SA–AG) is calculated as:

$$SA–AG = \text{serum albumin (g/L)}—\text{ascitic fluid albumin (g/L)}$$

SA–AG > 11g/L suggests transudative ascites, and SA–AG < 11g/L suggests exudative ascites.

What is the pathophysiology of ascites and oedema in cirrhosis?

Ascites only occurs in cirrhosis following the development of portal hypertension. One cause of ascites is disruption of portal blood flow in the liver due to fibrosis, causing fluid to accumulate in the peritoneum. Another cause is vasodilatation of the splanchnic circulation.

The diseased liver produces vasodilatory compounds, which cause splanchnic vasodilatation, an increase in blood flow through the portal vein, and consequently an increase in portal vein pressure. This also causes a decrease in systemic vascular resistance, and consequently a decrease in effective circulating volume and blood pressure. This leads to activation of the renin-angiotensin-aldosterone systems, and the sympathetic nervous system. This is also the reason why the cardiac filling pressure is low, and the venous pressure is not elevated.

The net result is avid sodium and water retention, propagating the development of ascites and oedema.

What is the initial therapy for ascites in cirrhosis?

Therapy is directed towards reversing these physiological abnormalities.

- Dietary sodium restriction
- fluid restriction
- Diuretic therapy——initially with aldosterone antagonists, such as spironolactone. Once a naturesis has been achieved (confirm by measuring urinary sodium), a loop diuretic can be added to increase diuresis.

How does this relate to the development of the hepatorenal syndrome?

The hepatorenal syndrome is the end stage of the spectrum of ascites and portal hypertension. Since systemic vasodilatation causes a progressive decrease in effective circulating volume, this results in the activation of vasoconstrictor systems which reduce renal blood flow. This reduces glomerular filtration rate, and causes progressive renal dysfuction in end-stage liver disease, despite structurally normal kidneys.

Case 3 ◆ **Hepatomegaly**

CASE PRESENTATION 2

*This patient is **cachectic**.[1] There is no evidence of anaemia,[2] icterus, or stigmata of chronic liver disease.[3] There is no lymphadenopathy.[4] The abdomen is not distended,[5] and there is no clinical evidence of ascites.[6] There is **hepatomegaly** with a non-tender liver edge palpable 4cm below the costal margin.[7] There is also a palpable **umbilical nodule**.[8] There is no evidence of splenomegaly. There are no audible bruits or a hepatic venous hum.[9] There are no signs of encephalopathy to suggest hepatic failure.[10]*

*This patient has **hepatomegaly**. The presence of **cachexia** and an **umbilical nodule** suggests **malignancy** as the most likely cause.*

CASE PRESENTATION 2

*This patient is **well-nourished**.[1] There is no evidence of anaemia,[2] icterus, or stigmata of chronic liver disease.[3] There is no lymphadenopathy.[4] The abdomen is not distended,[5] and there is no clinical evidence of ascites.[6] There is **hepatomegaly** with a **tender liver edge** palpable 4cm below the costal margin.[7] There is no evidence of splenomegaly. There are no audible bruits or a hepatic venous hum.[9] There are no signs of encephalopathy to suggest hepatic failure.[10]*

*This patient has **tender hepatomegaly**[11]. The differential diagnosis includes:*

- (a) **infectious disease**, *(e.g. viral hepatitis)*
- (b) **alcoholic hepatitis**
- (c) **malignancy**[12]
- (d) **hepatic congestion**, *(e.g. cardiac failure)*[13]
- (e) **vascular liver disease**, *(e.g. Budd-Chiari syndrome, sickle cell disease)*

Clinical notes

1. Assessment of nutritional state is a key part of the gastrointestinal examination, and should be mentioned during presentation even if the patient is well-nourished. Formal methods include weight and anthropometry. However, a subjective assessment can be made in the examination setting (see Vol 2, Case 3 Weight Loss). Wasting of the temporalis muscle is an early sign of generalized muscle atrophy, and subjective assessment of triceps fat fold thickness gives an indication of loss of subcutaneous fat.

2. Anaemia can be present in chronic liver disease, haematological disease (i.e. sickle cell anaemia) and in malignancy. If it is not present, it is an important negative to mention in the case presentation.

3. Look for jaundice and other stigmata of chronic liver disease. Hepatomegaly, in the absence of stigmata of chronic liver disease or portal hypertension, does not necessarily mean that parenchymal liver disease or cirrhosis can be excluded. Whilst the liver is typically 'shrunken' in advanced cirrhosis, other conditions such as primary biliary cirrhosis and liver diseases characterized by fat deposition (alcoholic liver disease or non-alcoholic fatty liver disease) may present with isolated hepatomegaly.

4. Lymphadenopathy suggests infection or malignancy. Generalized lymphadenopathy can occur with infection mononucleosis, CMV, toxoplasmosis, and sarcoidosis.

5. Carefully inspect the abdomen. Look for scars (paracentesis and liver biopsy). In thin patients there may be fullness of the right upper quadrant indicating hepatomegaly. Ascites may be present in disseminated malignancy, and in portal hypertension due to chronic liver disease or vascular liver disease. The direction of flow in distended abdominal veins may differentiate inferior vena cava (IVC) obstruction due to disseminated malignancy, and portal hypertension (see Case 2 Ascites).

6. Approximately 1500mL of fluid must be present before flank dullness is present. Therefore in the absence of dullness, it is best to present the absence of flank dullness as '*there is no clinical evidence of ascites*' as opposed to '*there is no ascites*'.

7. Remember to percuss the superior and inferior borders of the liver, following palpation of the inferior margin, since hyper-expanded lungs may displace the liver inferiorly. By percussing in the mid-clavicular line, one can measure the liver span. The mean liver span in healthy subjects is 10.5cm in men and 7cm in women. It is important to comment if the liver edge is tender, as tender hepatomegaly has a specific differential diagnosis (see below). The presence of an 'irregular' liver edge is thought to suggest malignancy, although this sign is subtle and has poor sensitivity, and we therefore suggest that this description is avoided!

8. An umbilical nodule, the Sister Mary Joseph nodule, is a metastatic deposit found most commonly in gastric or colon adenocarcinoma, hepatocellular carcinoma, or lymphoma.

9. A hepatic bruit over the liver can be heard with alcoholic hepatitis or hepatic carcinoma (primary or secondary). The hepatic venous hum is a continuous murmur that is audible in portal hypertension.

10. The presence of encephalopathy with liver dysfunction raises the possibility of acute liver failure, and it is therefore an important negative to mention. Tender hepatomegaly and jaundice may suggest hepatic necrosis. These patients also have systemic vasodilatation with hypotension and tachycardia, similar to the clinical presentation of septic shock. However, the presence of hepatic encephalopathy is required for the diagnosis (see Case 1 Chronic Liver Disease for the grading of hepatic encephalopathy).

11. Tender hepatomegaly suggests stretch of the liver capsule, by a process that has caused *recent* hepatic enlargement, such as hepatitis (infectious or alcoholic), malignancy, congestion, or vascular disease. If the venous pressure is not elevated, then it is best to omit congestion, i.e. cardiac failure from the differential diagnosis list (see below).

12. If suspecting malignancy as the underlying cause, then it is important to consider both primary and secondary malignancies. Tell the examiner you would like to examine other systems to look for possible primary tumours that may metastasize to the liver. In female patients it would be important to examine for breasts lumps.

13. At the end of the examination, ask the examiner for permission to examine the venous pressure. This should be done at the end of the GI examination if the patient has ascites or hepatomegaly. Cirrhosis is typically associated with systemic vasodilatation, hence the cardiac filling pressure is

low or normal. An elevated venous pressure indicates right heart failure, and thus hepatic congestion as the cause of hepatomegaly. Look for the giant systolic waves of tricuspid regurgitation, which is associated with pulsatile hepatomegaly.

Questions commonly asked by examiners

What are the causes of hepatomegaly (without splenomegaly)?

- Malignancy—primary or secondary
- Cirrhosis
    - Alcoholic liver disease
    - Non-alcoholic fatty liver disease (NAFLD)
    - Primary biliary cirrhosis
- Hepatic congestion
    - Right heart failure
    - Constrictive pericarditis
    - Restrictive cardiomyopathy
- Alcoholic hepatitis
- Infectious disease
    - Viral hepatitis
    - Toxoplasmosis
    - Hydatid disease
    - Pyogenic liver abscess
    - Amoebic liver abscess
- Infiltration
    - Amyloidosis
    - Sarcoidosis
    - Glycogen storage disorders
- Vascular liver disease
    - Budd-Chiari syndrome
    - Sickle cell disease
- Polycystic liver disease
- Tertiary syphilis (due to syphilitic gumma)
- Obstetric liver disease*

Which tumours commonly metastasise to the liver?

Colorectal cancers account for the majority of cases of metastatic liver disease. Others include oesophageal, lung, gastric, breast, lymphatic, renal, endometrial, neuroendocrine, sarcomatous, and bone tumours.

Do you know of any benign liver tumours?

- Cavernous haemangioma—most common benign liver tumour, typically affecting women of childbearing age.
- Hepatic adenoma—associated with use of oestrogen-containing contraceptives.
- Focal nodular hyperplasia—also affects women of childbearing age, although not associated with oestrogen use.

---

* Acute fatty liver of pregnancy typically occurs in the third trimester, hence hepatomegaly is obscured by the gravid uterus.

- Nodular regenerative hyperplasia—affects elderly patients, often with systemic autoimmune disease.

What are the infective causes of acute hepatitis?

- Hepatitis A
- Hepatitis B
- Hepatitis C (until recently this was not thought to cause acute hepatitis, although outbreaks have been reported in HIV-positive men)
- Hepatitis E
- EBV
- CMV
- Toxoplasmosis
- Herpes Simplex virus

What are the causes and clinical manifestations of the Budd-Chiari syndrome?

The Budd-Chiari syndrome is characterized by obstruction to hepatic venous outflow, most commonly due to thrombosis, which may occur at the level of the hepatic venules, the hepatic vein, or the inferior vena cava. This causes venous stasis, congestion, and damage to hepatic parenchymal cells.

An underlying cause can be identified in 75% of patients, such as myeloproliferative disorders, or thrombophilias such as deficiency of protein C, protein S, or antithrombin III, the factor V Leiden mutation, the prothrombin-gene mutation, the antiphospholipid syndrome, or paroxysmal nocturnal haemoglobinuria.

Patients either present acutely with jaundice and hepatic encephalopathy, or more commonly with the subacute onset of abdominal pain and hepatomegaly. Ascites may be absent due to the development of a hepatic venous collateral circulation.

Diagnosis is usually by doppler ultrasound of the hepatic vein. Treatment involves anticoagulation and the medical management of ascites, unless encephalopathy or liver failure are present, in which case thrombolysis, angioplasty, or liver transplantation are indicated.

What are the hepatic manifestations of sickle cell anaemia?

- Gall stone disease—due to chronic haemolysis causing pigment stones.
- Sickle hepatic crisis—due to sickle thrombosis causing sinusoidal obstruction. Presents with right upper quadrant pain, jaundice, and tender hepatomegaly.
- Intrahepatic cholestasis—due to sickle thrombosis in sinusoids, causing hepatocyte swelling and intrahepatic biliary obstruction.
- Associated liver conditions—iron overload due to blood transfusion, viral hepatitis contracted through blood transfusion.

Case 4 ◆ **Splenomegaly** (with or without hepatomegaly)

Examiner's note

Splenomegaly has a large number of causes, and these include non-gastrointestinal causes. Despite the extensive list of causes, there are only a limited number that are frequently encountered in the MRCP (PACES) examination. The most common causes to appear are:

- Haematological malignancy
- Portal hypertension

Other less common causes that may be encountered include:

- Haemolytic anaemia
- Felty's syndrome

Strictly speaking this is an abdominal station, however it is important to make general observations to determine the underlying cause. Although it may be acceptable to provide a diagnosis of splenomegaly and then provide a differential diagnosis, if a clear cause can be identified, it will impress examiners and gain valuable marks. In the final presentation, mentioning important negatives demonstrates to the examiner a systematic and coherent approach to a patient with splenomegaly.

CASE PRESENTATION 1

*This patient is **anaemic**.[1] There is no evidence of icterus.[2] There are no stigmata of chronic liver disease[3] and there is no evidence of rheumatological disease.[4] There is **no lymphadenopathy**.[5] There are **excoriation marks** to suggest pruritis.[6] There is **splenomegaly** with the splenic edge palpable 8cm below the costal margin.[7] There is no hepatomegaly, ascites or peripheral oedema. There is no venous hum.[8] There are no signs of hepatic encephalopathy.*

*This patient has **anaemia** and **splenomegaly**. In the absence of stigmata of chronic liver disease and portal hypertension, the most likely cause is a **myeloproliferative disease**.[9]*

CASE PRESENTATION 2

*This patient is **anaemic**.[1] There is no evidence of icterus.[2] There are no stigmata of chronic liver disease[3] and there is no evidence of rheumatological disease.[4] There is **widespread lymphadenopathy**[5] and there are **excoriation marks** to suggest pruritis.[6] There is **hepatosplenomegaly** with the liver edge palpable 3cm below the costal margin and the splenic edge palpable 4cm below the costal margin.[7] There is no ascites or peripheral oedema. There is no venous hum.[8] There are no signs of hepatic encephalopathy.*

*This patient has **hepatosplenomegaly** with **widespread lymphadenopathy**. In the absence of stigmata of chronic liver disease and portal hypertension, the most likely cause is a **lymphoproliferative disease**.[9]*

CASE PRESENTATION 3

*This patient is **anaemic**.[1] There is no evidence of icterus.[2] There are no stigmata of chronic liver disease.[3] There is a **symmetrical deforming arthropathy** affecting the small joints of the hands, with ulnar deviation and nodules on the forearms.[4] There is also a **vascultic rash**.[4] There is splenomegaly with the* *splenic edge palpable 4cm below the costal margin.[7] There is no hepatomegaly, ascites or peripheral oedema. There is no venous hum.[8] There are no signs of hepatic encephalopathy.*

*This patient has **rheumatoid arthritis**. The presence of **splenomegaly** in the absence of stigmata of chronic liver disease and portal hypertension makes **Felty's syndrome** the most likely diagnosis. I would like to see evidence of neutropenia on the blood count to confirm the diagnosis.*

Clinical notes

1. Anaemia is most reliably demonstrated by looking for conjunctival pallor. This is thought to be more sensitive than looking for pallor of skin creases, nails, or other mucosal membranes. If there is no evidence of anaemia, it is an important negative to mention in the final case presentation.

2. In the absence of stigmata of chronic liver disease, the presence of jaundice with splenomegaly should raise the suspicion of haemolysis in the context of haematological malignancy, in particular 'cold' autoimmune haemolytic anaemia associated with chronic lymphocytic leukaemia.

3. Look carefully for the stigmata of chronic liver disease (see Case 1 Chronic Liver Disease). The presence of stigmata of chronic liver disease lends support to portal hypertension as the cause of splenomegaly.

4. Look for signs of rheumatological disease, in particular rheumatoid arthritis. In the context of splenomegaly this would support a diagnosis of Felty's syndrome, which occurs in 5% of patients with long-standing rheumatoid arthritis. Hyperuricaemia due to haematological malignancy may also occur, causing acute gout, although signs of chronic tophaceous gout are unlikely to be present.

5. Lymphadenopathy must be carefully sought if splenomegaly or hepatosplenomegaly is found, since haematological disease is an important differential. Many tutors favour examining the cervical lymph nodes with the patient supine, prior to abdominal palpation. However, an alternative approach is to examine for lymphadenopathy at the *end* of the routine, with the patient sitting upright. Not only does this facilitate examination of all cervical lymph nodes, rather than just supraclavicular nodes, but the candidate also has knowledge of the findings of abdominal palpation, and may therefore proceed to examine the axillary, inguinal, and epitrochlear lymph nodes if haematological disease is suspected. Lympahdenopathy can also occur in Felty's syndrome.

6. Pruritis occurs with cholestatic liver or biliary disease, but may also be a feature of haematological malignancies.

7. The spleen is typically 12cm in length, and lies in the left upper quadrant. In healthy states, the spleen cannot be palpated since it lies beneath the rib cage, but as it enlarges it becomes palpable below the costal margin and towards the right iliac fossa. However, the spleen is only palpable below the costal margin once it is greater than 15cm in length. Subtle splenic enlargement is therefore missed by palpation. Percussion over *Traube's space* may detect subtle splenic enlargement. This involves percussion over the area between the left sixth rib, and the left costal margin, in the mid-axillary line. The stomach, which is resonant to percussion, normally occupies this area, however the percussion note becomes dull in the presence of splenomegaly. This technique may be more sensitive than palpation for subtle splenomegaly.

9. A venous hum is best appreciated over the epigastrium and indicates portal hypertension. This is an important negative to mention in a patient with hepatosplenomegaly.

10. In the setting of haematological malignancy, there are two general patterns of presentation to be aware of:

    (a) Splenomegaly **without** lymphadenopathy is most likely to be a **myeloproliferative** condition such as **chronic myeloid leukaemia** (CML). The spleen is more likely to be markedly enlarged (see below) and anaemia is more common. Remember that lymphadenopathy cannot be completely excluded by the bedside, and adequate imaging will be required.

(b) Splenomegaly **and** lymphadenopathy is most likely to be a **lymphoproliferative** condition such as **lymphoma** or **chronic lymphocytic leukaemia**. The spleen is not typically as large as in myeloproliferative disorders, and the patients are less likely to be anaemic. However, hepatomegaly is more common.

Questions commonly asked by examiners

What are the characteristics of the spleen on palpation?

- Enlarges towards the right iliac fossa
- Possesses a medial notch
- Is dull to percussion (unlike a kidney, which is resonant due to overlying colon)
- One cannot palpate 'above' a spleen—between the spleen and the costal margin
- The spleen is not ballotable (unlike a kidney)

What are the causes of splenomegaly?

In order of frequency:*

- Portal hypertension—33%
- Haematological malignancy—27%
- Infection (e.g. HIV, endocarditis)—23%
- Congestion or inflammation (e.g. cardiac failure)—8%
- Primary splenic disease (e.g. splenic vein thrombosis)—4%
- Other—5%

By degree of splenic enlargement:

- *Massive splenomegaly (crossing the midline)*
  - CML
  - Myelofibrosis
  - Kala-azar (visceral leishmaniaisis)
  - Malaria
  - AIDS with Mycobacterium avium complex
- *Moderate splenomegaly*
  - Portal hypertension
  - Lymphoma
  - Leukaemia (acute or chronic)
  - Thalassaemia
  - Glycogen and lipid storage diseases (e.g. Gaucher's disease)
- *Mild splenomegaly*
  - Other myeloproliferative diseases (e.g. polycythaemia rubra vera)
  - Haemolysis
  - Infection (e.g. EBV, infective endocarditis)
  - Autoimmune disease (e.g. rheumatoid arthritis, SLE)
  - Infiltrative conditions (e.g. amyloid, sarcoid)

Which of these conditions cause isolated splenomegaly without hepatomegaly?

This distinction is often over-emphasized, since all haematological causes of splenomegaly may also cause hepatomegaly, due to extramedullary haematopoiesis. The infective and infiltrative

---

* From series of 449 patients attending a single medical centre in San Francisco, USA. West J Med 1998; 169(2):88–97.

causes of splenomegaly may also cause hepatomegaly. The conditions which are most likely to cause isolated splenomegaly are autoimmune diseases, and primary splenic diseases such splenic vein thrombosis or splenic abscess.

How would you evaluate this patient?

- History
  - Ask about constitutional symptoms—fever, night sweats, malaise, weight loss. These suggest an underlying infective, malignant, or autoimmune condition. They also represent 'B symptoms' in non-Hodgkin's lymphoma (NHL).
  - Ask specifically about risk factors for HIV infection.
  - Ask about risk factors for lymphoma, particularly family history of lymphoma, use of radiation therapy, immunosuppressive therapy, chemotherapy, or organ transplantation.
  - Ask about bone and joint pain. This may occur in myeloproliferative disease due to increased haematopoiesis, or due to secondary hyperuricaemia causing acute gout.
  - Ask about symptoms of pancytopaenia, such as bruising (thrombocytopaenia), or fatigue (anaemia). These are unusual in myeloproliferative disease, but may signify the transformation of CML to acute myeloid leukaemia (AML) (blast crisis).
  - Ask about a history of autoimmune disease.
  - Ask about a history of liver disease.
  - Take a thorough travel history, including malaria risk and prophylaxis.
- Investigations
  - FBC, blood film, LFTs, serum LDH, beta-2 microglobulin, and autoimmune profile.
  - Chest X-ray (CXR)
  - HIV testing
  - Imaging (ultrasound initially to evaluate splenomegaly, but axial imaging of the chest, abdomen and pelvis will be required to evaluate for lymphadenopathy or disseminated malignancy. Positron Emission Tomography is highly sensitive for non-Hodgkin's lymphoma, although not specific, and may also be positive in infection or metastatic malignancy.)
  - Lymph node excision biopsy (rather than fine needle aspirate, since intact tissue is required for histological assessment).
  - Bone marrow biopsy—will diagnose conditions such as lipid storage diseases, mycobacterial infection, granulomatous disease, and lymphoid or myeloid disorders. It is also required to evaluate for extra-nodal disease during staging of non-Hodgkin's lymphoma.

What is the significance of B-symptoms in non-Hodgkin's lymphoma?

Approximately 40% of patients with NHL present with B-symptoms. These have been formally defined as:

- Fever >38°C
- Weight loss >10% of body weight over 6 months
- Drenching night sweats

If one of these symptoms is present, then the patient's clinical staging is altered accordingly.

What do you know of the cytogenetics of CML?

The *Philadelphia chromosome* is present in 90–95% of patients with CML. This is a chromosomal translocation, characterized by the fusion of the oncogene *c-abl* on chromosome 9, with *bcr* on chromosome 22. This fusion leads to increased oncogene activity through tyrosine kinase signalling, and eventually leads to malignancy.

Detection of the *bcr-abl* gene product mRNA is used for the diagnosis of CML, and for monitoring disease activity. Furthermore, monoclonal antibodies to tyrosine kinases have revolutionized the treatment of CML.

What do you understand by the term 'blast crisis'?

This phase of the disease is similar to acute leukaemia, and survival is 3–6 months. Blast cells are found in the bone marrow and peripheral blood. Skin or tissue infiltration also defines blast crisis.

What are the causes of hyposplenism?

- Splenic infarction (e.g. sickle cell anaemia, vascultitis)
- Splenic artery thrombosis
- Infiltrative conditions (e.g. amyloid, sarcoid)
- Coeliac disease
- Autoimmune disease

What advice would you give a patient with hyposplenism, or following splenectomy?*

- *Vaccinations*—Pneumococcal, Haemophilus influenzae B, and Meningococcal group C. Ensure that repeat vaccinations are administered every 5–10 years.
- *Prophylactic antibiotics*—oral phenoxymethylpenicillin or erythromycin for at least two years, and may be continued lifelong.
- Patients who develop infection despite these measures should attend hospital urgently, for consideration of parenteral antibiotics.
- Patients should be counselled regarding malaria prophylaxis and travel advice.
- Patients should carry an information card, or wear a medic-alert bracelet, to inform healthcare practitioners of their condition.

What do you understand by Felty's syndrome?

Felty's syndrome was originally described as seropositive rheumatoid arthritis complicated by neutropenia and splenomegaly. However, since splenomegaly may occur in rheumatoid arthritis in the absence of neutropenia, and splenomegaly is not always clinically detectable, splenomegaly is no longer considered an absolute diagnostic requirement.

Case 5 ◆ Haemochromatosis

CASE PRESENTATION

*This patient is not icteric.[1] There is evidence of **skin pigmentation**[2] and **koilonychia**.[3] There is* **gynaecomastia** and **decreased body hair**.[4] *There is **hepatomegaly** with the liver edge palpable 4cm below the costal margin.[5] There is no evidence of splenomegaly, ascites, or peripheral oedema. There are no hepatic bruits and there is no hepatic venous hum.[6] There are no signs of hepatic encephalopathy.*

*The walking aid suggests the presence of **arthropathy**.[7] Furthermore, the blood glucose meter and finger-prick marks suggest the presence of **diabetes mellitus**.[8]*

*The diagnosis is **haemochromatosis**.[9]*

---

* From British Committee for Standards in Haematology guidelines, 2002.

Clinical notes

The classical description of 'bronze diabetes' with cirrhosis, diabetes mellitus, and 'slate-grey' pigmentation is increasingly rare, due to improved diagnosis and treatment of the condition. Indeed, the combination of diabetes mellitus and cirrhosis is more likely to represent NAFLD than haemochromatosis. However, patients with advanced haemochromatosis do tend to crop up in the MRCP (PACES) examination, hence this is presented as a separate case to chronic liver disease.

1. Jaundice may or may not be present. Although liver function abnormalities occur in 75% of patients, jaundice is absent early in the course of disease.

2. Cutaneous pigmentation is seen in >90% of patients with idiopathic haemochromatosis, and is one of the earliest signs of the disease (though it may be mild). It is more evident on sun-exposed areas of the skin, i.e. the face and hands. The pigmentation can vary from bronze to slate-grey to metallic grey discoloration. Other skin changes that can occur are ichthyosiform changes and skin atrophy (particularly on the anterior surface of legs).

3. Haemochromatosis is a cause of koilonychia. Koilonychia affecting the thumb and index finger has been reported to occur in 50% of patients. Prominent koilonychia affecting all nails occurs in 25% of patients. Look for stigmata of chronic liver disease. These are absent early in the course of disease. Cirrhosis occurs in 13% of patients and occurs late.

4. Gynaecomastia and decreased body hair can be manifestations of chronic liver disease or hypogonadism. Hypogonadism occurs due to iron deposition in pituitary gland. Any pituitary deficit may be present, however hypogonadism is the most common. Visual field defects do not occur. Amenorrhoea in women is much less common than hypogonadism in men. Partial loss of body hair is seen in 60% of patients. Complete loss of body hair is seen in 12% of patients. The pubic region is the most commonly affected area.

5. Hepatomegaly is common at presentation and is firm and regular. Whilst cirrhosis only occurs in 10–15% of patients, the risk of hepatocellular carcinoma in patients with haemochromatosis and cirrhosis is greater than for other liver diseases,. Some specialists advocate increased frequency of hepatocellular carcinoma surveillance in these patients (3-monthly rather than 6-monthly).

6. A hepatic bruit in the context of haemochromatosis signifies the development of hepatocellular carcinoma, and a hepatic venous hum indicates portal hypertension.

7. Arthropathy (pseudogout) is due to calcium pyrophosphate crystal deposition. The most common distribution is a symmetrical, small-joint arthropathy, similar to rheumatoid arthritis. However, arthralgia is more common than synovitis. The most commonly affected joints are the metacarpophalangeal (MCP) and proximal interphalangeal (PIP) joints. Inspect the hips and knees for joint replacement scars when examining the legs for oedema.

8. Look at the lateral aspects of the fingertips for skin pricks, which indicate glucose testing. Furthermore, when palpating the abdomen for masses look for evidence of lipoatrophy and lipohypertrophy in the subcutaneous tissue as a clue to suggest insulin administration.

9. If the diagnosis of haemochromatosis is presented, then tell the examiner you would like to look for:

    (a) **Diabetes**: finger pricks (glucose testing), fundoscopy(retinopathy), urinalysis (glycosuria)

    (b) **Restrictive or dilated cardiomyopathy**: raised venous pressure, third or fourth heart sound

Questions commonly asked by examiners

What is the mode of inheritance of hereditary haemochromatosis?

Hereditary haemochromatosis is inherited as an autosomal recessive trait. The HFE gene has been localized to the short arm of chromosome 6 (6p21.3).

Most Caucasian patients with haemochromatosis are homozygous for the cysteine-to-tyrosine substitution at position 282 (C282Y). A smaller proportion are homozygous for the histidine-to-aspartate substitution at position 63 (H63D). A minority are compound heterozygotes for these mutations.

How does one diagnose haemochromatosis?

Diagnosis of iron overload

Iron overload is suggested by serum iron studies. A fasting transferrin saturation >60% in males, or >50% in females, has a high specificity for iron overload. In clinical practice, a transferrin saturation >45% is considered significant enough to warrant investigation. The serum ferritin is also elevated in iron overload, however since ferritin is an acute phase protein, the specificity of this test is less than for transferrin saturation.

Liver biopsy, to confirm parenchymal iron deposition, is considered if the blood tests suggest abnormal liver function.

Diagnosis of haemochromatosis

Genetic testing for the C282Y and H63D mutations will confirm the diagnosis of haemochromatosis in over 90% of cases. However, other mutations are responsible for some cases of haemochromatosis, particularly in non-Caucasian populations. First-degree relatives of patients with haemochromatosis should undergo screening with genetic testing.

What is the treatment of haemochromatosis?

Phlebotomy is the mainstay of treatment for haemochromatosis. Initially, one unit of blood should be removed once to twice weekly, until the transferrin saturation falls below 50%, or the ferritin falls below 50ng/mL. Maintenance phlebotomy should then be performed every three months.

Iron removal through phlebotomy improves insulin sensitivity, fatigue, and skin pigmentation. However, arthropathy, hypogonadism, and cirrhosis do not respond to treatment. Hepatocellular cancer (HCC) accounts for 30% of all deaths in haemochromatosis, therefore all patients with cirrhosis should undergo HCC surveillance with six-monthly ultrasound and α-fetoprotein measurement.

What are the cardiac complications of haemochromatosis?

Haemochromatosis can cause a restrictive or dilated cardiomyopathy. Cardiac MRI (magnetic resonance imaging) is a sensitive modality for detecting myocardial iron deposition.

Do you know any other causes of iron overload?

Conditions requiring regular blood transfusion (haemoglobinopathy or refractory anaemia) are a cause of transfusional iron overload. If phlebotomy cannot be used to treat these patients, iron chelators such as desferrioxamine are used to decrease body iron. Porphyria cutanea tarda, most commonly associated with hepatitis C infection, is also associated with iron overload and abnormal liver function.

Case 6 ◆ **Primary Biliary Cirrhosis**

CASE PRESENTATION

This middle-aged lady[1] *is* **icteric**,[2] *with* **generalised hyperpigmentation**.[3] *There is no evidence of anaemia*.[4] *There is* **clubbing**, **xanthelasma**,[5] **tendon xanthomata**[5] *and multiple* **excoriation marks**.[6] *There are* multiple **petechiae** and **echymoses**.[7] Multiple **spider naevi** are present on the upper limbs, trunk, and face. There is **hepatosplenomegaly** with the liver edge palpable 3cm below the costal margin[8] and the splenic edge palpable 3cm below the costal margin.[9] There are no hepatic bruits but there is a **hepatic venous hum**.[10] There is no ascites, peripheral oedema, or signs of hepatic encephalopathy.

This patient has kyphosis and there is evidence of old fractures, suggestive of **metabolic bone disease**. There is **proximal muscle wasting and weakness**. There are features to suggest **autoimmune disease**.[11]

The diagnosis is **primary biliary cirrhosis** with portal hypertension.

Clinical notes

1. A middle-aged female patient with chronic liver disease is highly suggestive of primary biliary cirrhosis. It is important to remember that approximately 75—90% of patients are female, although males can be affected.

2. Jaundice is a late feature of the disease.

3. Pigmentation is due to melanin deposition rather than jaundice.

4. The causes of anaemia in primary biliary cirrhosis include GI blood loss (oesophageal varices and peptic ulcers) and those related to additional underlying autoimmune disorders (pernicious anaemia, atrophic gastritis, and Coeliac's disease). It is important to remember that there is an increased incidence of peptic ulcer disease in patients with primary biliary cirrhosis.

5. Xanthalesma occur in 10% of patients, and often occur late in the disease. Tendon xanthomata can occur, but are uncommon. Both are a consequence of hypercholesterolaemia.

6. Pruritis is a common presenting symptom, even in the absence of advanced liver disease. Dermatological manifestations are the presenting feature in a third of patients. These include xerosis, dermographism, and fungal nail infection. Be aware of skin findings that would relate to additional underlying autoimmune diseases (see below).

7. Coagulopathy and thrombocytopenia are features of chronic liver disease and portal hypertension (see Case 1 Chronic Liver Disease). However, primary biliary cirrhosis is also associated with malabsorption of fat-soluble vitamins (A, D, E, and K). Therefore, vitamin K malabsorption contributes to the coagulopathy seen in primary biliary cirrhosis.

8. Hepatomegaly occurs in 70% of patients and is often smooth and non-tender. It is important to note that in 10% of patients there is unexplained right upper quadrant discomfort, thus one should be especially careful to avoid causing discomfort when examining these patients!

9. Splenomegaly and ascites are late features of the disease and indicate portal hypertension. Of note, patients with primary biliary cirrhosis may develop oesophageal varices and variceal haemorrhage early in the course of disease, even in the absence of established cirrhosis.

10. Hepatic bruits would signify malignancy, which is a complication of the disease. A venous hum would signify portal hypertension.

11. Although this case is similar to other cases of chronic liver disease, the successful detection of additional clinical features will enable the candidate to make the correct diagnosis of primary biliary cirrhosis. If additional features are not present, then it would be best to present the diagnosis as 'chronic liver disease' or 'isolated hepatomegaly/splenomegaly' and provide a differential diagnosis. Throughout your examination look for the following features:

    (a) Kyphosis and evidence of old fractures (osteopenia and osteoporosis)

    (b) Proximal myopathy (osteomalacia)

    (c) Features of other autoimmune diseases:

    • **Graves disease**: goitre (?thyroidectomy scar), eye signs, thyroid acropachy, pretibial myxoedema, features of hypo- or hyperthyroidism

    • **Sjogren's syndrome**: dry mouth, dry eyes

    • **Rheumatoid arthritis**: symmetrical deforming arthropathy, eye signs

- **Scleroderma**: telangiectasia, tight shiny skin, sclerodactyly, calcinosis, dystrophic nails
- **Dermatomyositis**: heliotrope rash, Gottron papules
- **Idiopathic pulmonary fibrosis**: bibasal crepitations
- **Myasthenia gravis**: myasthenic facies, ptosis, diplopia, proximal weakness, and fatigability
- **Vitiligo**: hypopigmented patches
- **Atrophic gastritis**: pallor, koilonychia-iron deficiency anaemia

Questions commonly asked by examiners

What are the clinical features of primary biliary cirrhosis?

Fatigue, pruritis, and hypercholesterolaemia occur at all stages. Liver disease occurs late, and is rarely a presenting feature, particularly with recent advances in diagnosis and treatment.

How does one diagnose primary biliary cirrhosis?

Serum anti-mitochondrial (M2) antibodies are present in 95%. In the presence of cholestasis and positive antibodies, liver biopsy may not be required. The histological lesion is portal tract granuloma, progressing to cirrhosis. Ultrasound and ERCP/MRCP (endoscopic retrograde cholangiopancreatography/magnetic resonance cholangiopancreatography) are often performed to exclude extra-hepatic cholestasis.

Which drugs can cause cholestasis?

- Phenothiazines
- Sulphonamides
- Penicillins
- Rifampicin
- Macrolides
- Carbamazepine
- Synthetic androgenic steroids
- Diclofenac

What is the prognosis of primary biliary cirrhosis?

It is associated with increased mortality, however less than half of deaths are liver-related. Fatigued patients have a worse outcome, and are more likely to have a non-liver related death.

What is the management of primary biliary cirrhosis?

Supplementation of fat soluble vitamins

Due to fat malabsorption, and subsequent loss of fat-soluble vitamins, vitamins A, D, E, and K should be supplemented.

Treatment of bone disease

Patients should also undergo bone densitometry to screen for metabolic bone disease. Osteoporosis occurs in up to a third of patients. Severe bone disease that resulted in multiple fractures is now uncommon. There is no proven treatment for bone disease associated with primary biliary cirrhosis except liver transplantation. Vitamin D and calcium supplementation should be given. Bisphosphonates may increase bone density. Oestrogen replacement may improve osteoporosis in post-menopausal women.

Treatment of hypercholesterolaemia

The serum cholesterol may be markedly elevated in patients with primary biliary cirrhosis. Interestingly, patients with primary biliary cirrhosis do not appear to have an increased mortality secondary to atherosclerosis. Cholesterol lowering agents (statins) may be used if the LFTs are monitored appropriately.

Treatment of liver disease

Ursodeoxycholic acid has been shown to improve liver biochemistry and possibly retard disease progression. It is the only drug approved by the US Food and Drug Administration (FDA) in the treatment of primary biliary cirrhosis. However, a convincing effect on histology or transplant-free survival has not been demonstrated.

Management of pruritis

Pruritis is thought not to be a result of bile acid deposition in the skin but rather a consequence of bile acids on sensory nerve fibres. Biliary obstruction must be excluded. Colestyramine has limited data on efficacy, but it is safe and frequently used. However, it will prevent absorption of other drugs taken simultaneously, such as ursodeoxycholic acid. Rifampicin has been shown to be effective in four placebo-controlled trials. Naltrexone has also been demonstrated to be effective in three trials, although the anti-opioid mechanism of action often exacerbates chronic pain. Anti-histamines do not work, and may worsen encephalopathy.

Management of fatigue

Fatigue is not a consequence of co-morbid depression. Co-existent hypothyroidism or anaemia must be excluded. Naltrexone may be of some benefit.

Referral for transplantation

Patients are referred for transplant consideration when the serum bilirubin >50µmol/L, or in the presence of refractory fatigue or pruritis. Recurrence in the graft may occur (15% at 3 years and 30% at 10 years).

Case 7 ♦ A 'Renal' Abdomen

Examiner's note

A 'renal' abdomen is a common case at the abdomen station in the MRCP(PACES) clinical examination. These patients are often stable on their renal replacement therapy and have many clinical signs, and thus are good for clinical examinations. The method of renal replacement therapy is often very clear or, otherwise, can be easily deduced. To obtain a 'pass' at this station is straightforward, but these patients display many clinical signs that relate to previous methods of renal replacement therapy; previous complications of renal replacement therapy; complications of immunosuppressive therapy; and possibly underlying aetiology of renal disease. Therefore, many additional marks can be gained, and transforming a 'pass' into a 'clear pass' is very simple. Candidates are often poorly prepared for this station, and it is important to be aware of the different methods of renal replacement therapy and the multiple clinical signs one must look for when examining such patients.

When presenting a case at the abdomen station, a generic approach that has been adopted in this book and one that is commonly favoured by examiners starts peripherally from the hands to the face and ending on the abdomen. However, in a renal abdomen, the approach to presentation is different, and the following structured framework should be used:

1. Current mode of renal replacement therapy
2. Previous modes of renal replacement therapy (old scars)
3. Adequacy of renal replacement therapy (uraemia and volume status)

4. Complications of renal failure, i.e. anaemia
5. Complications immunosuppressive therapy (often with renal transplantation)
6. Aetiology of renal disease (this may not be possible)

CASE PRESENTATION 1

This patient has a **tunnelled central venous catheter** in the right subclavian vein, with no evidence of catheter-site infection.[1] There are also **scars on the chest wall** from previous sites of vascular access for haemodialysis, and there is a functioning and immature arteriovenous fistula in the left arm.[2]

There is no asterixis of the out-stretched hands and there are **no signs of uraemia**. The venous pressure is not elevated, there is no peripheral oedema, and the patient is **euvolaemic**.[3]

There is no clinical evidence of anaemia.[4] There are **pinpricks at the lateral aspects of the fingertips**, indicating frequent glucose testing. There is **lipohypertrophy** of the subcutaneous tissues indicating subcutaneous insulin use.[6]

This patient has end-stage renal failure and receives renal replacement therapy through **haemodialysis**. The patient currently receives haemodialysis through a tunnelled venous catheter whilst the arteriovenous fistula matures. The most likely aetiology of renal disease is **diabetes**.[7]

CASE PRESENTATION 2

This patient has a **peritoneal dialysis catheter** in the abdomen, with no evidence of catheter-site infection. The abdomen is distended, soft, and non-tender. There is a midline laparotomy scar. There is flank dullness that shifts with rotation of the patient, consistent with dialysis fluid within the peritoneal cavity. There are no abdominal wall herniae.[1] There are also scars from previous sites of vascular access for haemodialysis.[2]

There is no asterixis of the out-stretched hands and there are **no signs of uraemia**. The venous pressure is not elevated, there is no peripheral oedema, and the patient is **euvolaemic**.[3]

There is no clinical evidence of anaemia.[4] There are no peripheral stigmata of systemic disease.[6]

This patient has end-stage renal failure and receives renal replacement therapy through peritoneal dialysis. The aetiology or renal disease is not clear (but has a differential diagnosis).[7]

CASE PRESENTATION 3

This patient has a **scar in the right iliac fossa**. This overlies a **smooth, firm, and non-tender mass**.[1] It has a dull percussion note. There is no associated bruit. There are **scars on the chest wall** from previous sites of vascular access for haemodialysis. There is a **non-functioning arteriovenous fistula** in the right arm.[2]

There is no asterixis of the out-stretched hands and there are **no signs of uraemia**. The venous pressure is not elevated, there is no peripheral oedema, and the patient is **euvolaemic**.[3]

There is no clinical evidence of anaemia.[4] There is evidence of **gum hypertrophy**. There are no stigmata of active infection.[5] There is an **erythematous, maculopapular rash** in a **butterfly distribution** over the cheeks and the bridge of the nose, sparing the nasolabial folds, with scaling and **follicular plugging**. There is also a symmetrical **arthropathy** of the small joints of the hands.[6]

*This patient has end-stage renal failure and has a **renal transplant**. Given the patient is euvolaemic and in the absence of other signs of active renal replacement therapy, the renal transplant is functioning. The patient is currently on **cyclosporin** immunosuppressive therapy. The most likely aetiology of renal disease is **systemic lupus erythematosus**.*[7]

Clinical notes

1. **Current mode of renal replacement therapy.** This should be obvious from the end of the bed, or otherwise can easily be deduced.

    (a) *Tunnelled central venous catheter.* These are usually sited in the left or right subclavicular area through the subclavian vein. Tunnelled lines are typically silastic, double-lumen catheters that allow intermediate-duration haemodialysis whilst an arteriovenous fistula matures. It is important to comment on the absence or presence of catheter-site infection.

    (b) *Arteriovenous fistula.* Arteriovenous fistulae are the preferred form of vascular access for haemodialysis, and are typically placed in the non-dominant upper limb. The fistula requires months to mature, hence referral for haemodialysis must be made well in advance of clinical need, and temporary haemodialysis through a venous catheter may be necessary. The absence of a palpable thrill suggests non-function.

    (c) *Peritoneal dialysis.* A peritoneal dialysis catheter should be obvious during examination of the abdomen and provides long-term access to the peritoneal cavity. It is important to comment on the absence and presence of catheter site infection. Clinical examination may indicate fluid in the peritoneal cavity. Look for abdominal wall and inguinal herniae.

    (d) *Renal transplant.* Look carefully for scars in the right iliac fossa (Ruiterford-Morrison Scar), and carefully feel for the presence of a smooth mass below the scar. Occasionally there may be an additional scar in the left iliac fossa with a palpable mass. This will baffle candidates, and the most likely explanation for this would be a repeat transplantation following failure of the old renal transplant. Remember, a scar in the right iliac fossa DOES NOT ALWAYS imply the presence of a renal transplant, as patients may have previously had an appendicectomy! It is therefore important to fell carefully for fullness or a mass below the scar. Once the mass is identified:

    - Palpate the margins (often smooth)
    - Estimate the size (this can vary, but usually 8cm × 5cm)
    - Comment on whether it is tender or non-tender
    - Comment on the consistency (often a firm mass)
    - Percuss over the mass (usually a dull percussion note)
    - Auscultate for bruits

2. **Previous modes of renal replacement therapy.** Look carefully for scars in the subclavicular areas for previous tunnelled lines scars. Look carefully on the arms for arteriovenous fistulae. Look carefully for scars on the abdominal wall indicating previous peritoneal dialysis. Make particular note of the presence of laparotomy scars that may indicate previous surgery for peritonitis, an established complication of peritoneal dialysis.

3. **Adequacy of renal replacement therapy.** Assessing fluid status is important. Clinical signs of uraemia include:

    (a) Altered mental status
    (b) Asterixis (metabolic encephalopathy)
    (c) Excoriation marks (secondary to pruritis)
    (d) Tachypnoea (metabolic acidosis with respiratory compensation)
    (e) Pericardial rub (uraemic pericarditis)

4. **Complications of renal replacement therapy.** The absence or presence of anaemia should be included in the final presentation. The absence of anaemia is an important negative.

5. **Complications of immunosuppressive therapy.** This is relevant in patients with renal transplantation although it could be argued that end-stage renal failure itself is an 'immunocompromised' state. Complications for immunosupression should be sought for in the following manner:

(a)   Stigmata of infection

(b)   Presence of skin lesions (benign and malignant)

(c)   Complications relating to specific drugs:
   - *Cyclosporin*: gum hypertrophy, hirsutism, coarse tremor, hypertension, diabetes mellitus
   - *Steroids*: purpura, cushingoid features, diabetes mellitus
   - *Tacrolimus*: diabetes mellitus

6. **Aetiology of renal failure.** This may not be clear, but look for common causes:

(a)   *Diabetes*: fingertips for pinpricks (glucose testing), lipodystrophy, diabetic retinopathy

(b)   *Hypertension*: ask for the blood pressure

(c)   *Vasculitis*: skin lesions, stigmata of rheumatological disease

(d)   *Polycystic kidney disease*: palpable kidneys, look for *nephrectomy scars*
and rarities:

(e)   *Alport's syndrome*: hearing aid

(f)   *Tuberous sclerosis*: subungal fibromas sebacuous aderomas

(g)   membranoproliferative glomerulonephritis type 2 lipodystrophy (face/upper trunk/arms)

7. **Final presentation.** This is important, and should summarize your clinical findings. If the aetiology of renal disease is not clear, then provide a differential diagnosis for renal failure (given below). Tell the examiner you would like to

(a)   Measure the blood pressure

(b)   Check a urinalysis (glycosuria, haematuria, and proteinuria)

(c)   Auscultate the heart for a pericardial rub (uraemic pericarditis)

Questions commonly asked by examiners

What are the major causes of chronic renal disease in developed countries?
Diabetes mellitus 34%
Glomerulonephritis 21%
Hypertension 12%
Miscellaneous 10%

(including drugs, paraproteinaemia, obstructive uropathy)
Polycystic kidney disease 6%
Reflux nephropathy 6%
Analgesic nephropathy 6%
Uncertain 5%

What are the principles of the management of chronic renal disease?
- **Treatment of reversible causes of renal dysfunction**
  - Diagnosis of treatable glomerular disease (e.g. vasculitis, glomerulonephritis)—renal biopsy is indicated unless both kidneys are small (suggesting irreversible disease), or there is a specific contraindication.
  - Cessation of nephrotoxic drugs (e.g. diuretics, nonsteroidal anti-inflammatory drugs (NSAIDs), antibiotics).
  - Exclusion of obstructive uropathy and renovascular disease—ultrasound of the renal tract +/– MR angiography.

- **Slowing disease progression**
    - Treatment of hypertension—the target blood pressure for patients with proteinuria is 130/80mmHg. The first line agents should be ACE (angiotensin converting enzyme) inhibitors or angiotensin-II receptor antagonists (in the absence of significant renovascular disease).
    - Treatment of cardiovascular risk factors—Consider cardiovascular protection with aspirin and lipid lowering therapy if 10 year risk of CHD is >20%. Advise about smoking cessation.
- **Treatment of the complications of chronic renal disease**
    - Volume overload—dietary sodium restriction and loop diuretics.
    - Hyperkalaemia—dietary potassium restriction, loop diuretics, and oral sodium bicarbonate.
    - Hyperphosphataemia—phosphate binders, such as calcium carbonate, limit the development of renal osteodystrophy. Patients with hypercalcaemia due to hyperparathyroidism should receive alternative phosphate binders.
    - Metabolic acidosis—treatment of acidosis with oral sodium bicarbonate limits renal osteodystrophy and symptomatic uraemia.
    - Renal osteodystrophy—treatment of hyperphosphataemia, and the administration of vitamin D analogues, limit the development of secondary hyperparathyroidism, which predisposes to renal osteodystrophy. Parathyroidectomy should be considered if the patient develops symptomatic hypercalcaemia due to hyperparathyroidism, refractory to medical therapy.
    - Anaemia—normochromic, normocytic anaemia occurs due to reduced production of erythropoietin by the kidney. Following the adequate treatment of concomitant iron-deficiency, almost invakbly with intravenous iron if necessary, regular administration of erythropoietin improves symptoms and cardiovascular morbidity.

What are the indications for renal replacement therapy?

Preparation for renal replacement should begin when the glomerular filtration rate decreases to 30mL/min, or between 30 and 40mL/min in diabetics. The clinical indications for acute haemodialysis are:

- Pericarditis or pleuritis due to uraemia
- Uraemic bleeding diathesis (due to platelet dysfunction)
- Volume overload refractory to diuretics
- Hypertension refractory to antihypertensive drugs
- Refractory hyperkalaemia
- Refractory acidosis
- Encephalopathy or decline in mental status due to uraemia
- Removal of toxins (lithium, salicylates etc.)

Can you think of any problems associated with dialysis?

Haemodialysis

- **Dialysis washout**—due to removal of too much fluid (excessive ultrafiltration), or too rapid fluid removal. This may cause hypotension, fatigue, chest pain, leg cramps, nausea, and headache.
- **Bacteraemia**—particularly associated with tunnelled or non-tunnelled venous catheters. Metastatic infection may occur, especially with *staphylococcus aureus* infection, causing osteomyelitis, endocarditis, endopthalmitis, or hepatic and splenic abscesses. These complications must be actively sought and excluded in the presence of *staphylococcus aureus* bacteraemia.
- **Bleeding**—may occur due to the use of heparin as an anticoagulant during haemodialysis. inor bleeding is generally self-limiting with the cessation of anticoagulation. Rarely, protamine

sulphate may be required to reverse anticoagulation in the context of major bleeding. Haemodialysis can be performed without anticoagulation in patients at high risk of bleeding.

- **Dialysis related amyloidosis**—occurs due to decreased clearance of β_2-microglobulin. The musculoskeletal manifestations include carpal tunnel syndrome, scapulohumeral arthropathy, spondyloarthropathy, bone cysts, and pathological fractures. Systemic manifestations are less common, but are characterized by amyloid deposits around blood vessels in the mucosa of the gastrointestinal tract, heart, lungs, and urinary tract. Rarely, gastrointestinal haemorrhage, cardiac arrhthymias and renal vein thrombosis have been described.

Peritoneal dialysis

- **Bacterial peritonitis**—is a common complication of peritoneal peritonitis, occurring approximately once every patient year. The typical presentation is with abdominal pain, which may be mild, or with cloudy dialysates. Fever is frequently absent. Treatment is typically with intraperitoneal antibiotics, although occasionally removal of the dialysis catheter and a change in dialysis modality may be necessary.
- **Solute clearance or ultrafiltration failure**—as a consequence of peritoneal sclerosis, may necessitate a change in dialysis modality.
- **Diabetes mellitus**—may occur due to systemic absorption of glucose from the peritoneal dialysate.
- **Local complications**—such as abdominal wall hernias, fluid leakage into surrounding soft tissue, or catheter exit site infections.

What are the manifestations of renal osteodystrophy?

- **Osteitis fibrosa**—increased bone turnover, due to secondary hyperparathyroidism. This is usually asymptomatic, although bone pain and tenderness may occur, and bone cysts may develop which are termed 'brown tumours'.
- **Osteomalacia**—decreased mineralization of bone, predominantly due to aluminium deposition in bone, from aluminium-containing phosphate binders.
- **Adynamic bone disease**—is the most common bone lesion in haemodialysis and peritoneal dialysis patients. Bone turnover is markedly reduced, although there is no defect in

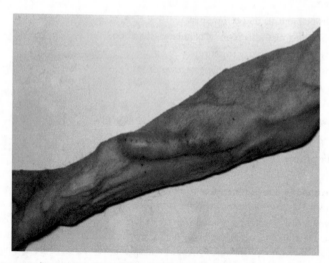

Figure 7.1 A mature radio-cephalic arteriovenous fistula for haemodialysis.
Reproduced from Barratt et al. Oxford Desk Reference Nephrology. 2009, with permission from Oxford University Press.

mineralization as in osteomalacia. Patients have decreased serum parathyroid hormone (PTH), due to the use of phosphate binders and vitamin D analogues.

What is the differential diagnosis of bone pain in patients with renal disease?

- Osteitis fibrosa
- Osteomalacia
- Dialysis-related amyloid
- Myeloma or skeletal metastases
- Osteomyelitis due to bacteraemia from infected vascular access
- Neuropathic pain from nerve compression by arteriovenous fistulae

Case 8 ◆ Nephrotic Syndrome

Examiner's notes

Nephrotic syndrome is an uncommon case in the MRCP (PACES) examination, however it has been reported to appear and candidates should therefore be prepared for this case. The key clinical pointers to the diagnosis are features of **hypoalbuminaemia** and **evidence of fluid overload** (ascites, pleural effusions, and oedema). The case presentation below is similar to the case presentation for ascites (see Case 2 Ascites), and should therefore be read in conjunction with the ascites clinical notes.

Throughout your examination, look for clues for the underlying aetiology and evidence of underlying systemic disease. Often in the examination, the patient will have ascites, and it is important to look thoroughly for signs and complications of chronic liver disease (as this is the most common cause for ascites). The following case presentation is typical for a patient with nephrotic syndrome and has been adapted from the case presentation for ascites. When preparing for this case, please read in conjunction with the case presentation and clinical notes for ascites (see page).

CASE PRESENTATION

*This patient has marked **peripheral oedema** and **periorbital oedema**.[1] There is **leuconychia** and **Muehrcke's lines** are visible across the nail beds.[2] There are no splinter haemorrhages, nail-fold infarcts or rash.[3] There are no stigmata of chronic liver disease.[4] There is no evidence of lymphadenopathy.[5] The **venous pressure is elevated**.[6] The **abdomen is distended**, with clinical evidence of **ascites**. There is no evidence of hepatosplenomegaly. There are no signs of hepatic encephalopathy.*

*This patient demonstrates features of **hypoalbuminaemia** with **fluid retention** and **ascites**. The unifying diagnosis is **nephrotic syndrome**.[7]*

Clinical notes

1. Peripheral oedema in renal disease is first seen in tissues with low resistance, such as the periorbital region or the scrotum and labia. This is unlike right-sided heart failure, where the peripheral oedema is more generalized.

2. Examine the hands carefully, looking for signs of hypoalbuminaemia. Look for Muehrcke's lines, which are pairs of transverse lines extending all the way across the nail bed, and occurring in more than one digit. This sign is specific for hypoalbuminaemia, as a consequence of the nephrotic syndrome, liver disease, or enteropathy. These should not be confused with Mee's lines, which are also transverse lines across the nail, associated with heart failure, Hodgkin's lymphoma, chemotherapeutic agents, and arsenic poisoning. Muehrcke's lines affect the nail bed, and hence do not move with nail growth, unlike Mee's lines, which are defects in the nail matrix. Leukonychia is non-specific finding associated with hypoalbuminaemia as well as other systemic conditions such as heart failure, liver disease, renal disease, Hodgkin's lymphoma, and diabetes mellitus.

3. Also look for signs of underlying vasculitis or rheumatological disease as a cause of glomerular disease (membranous glomerulonephritis).

4. Look carefully for signs of chronic liver disease. Hypoalbuminaeia occurs in chronic liver disease, and thus it may be more appropriate to state 'there are no *other* stigmata of chronic liver disease', as opposed to 'there are no stigmata of chronic liver disease'.

5. Lymphadenopathy indicates infection or haematological malignancy as causes of nephrotic syndrome.

6. Assessment of the JVP is essential in patients with peripheral oedema or ascites. In patients with significant oedema, assessment of the volume status and distribution of oedema can aid differential diagnosis. The venous pressure will be elevated in nephrotic syndrome only with marked fluid overload (as in patients with renal failure). Such patients are unlikely to appear in the MRCP (PACES) examination.

	JVP	Peripheral Oedema/Ascites
Right heart failure	Elevated	+
Renal failure	Variable	+
Nephrotic syndrome	Variable	+
Liver disease	Not elevated	+
Venous insufficiency	Not elevated	+
		Peripheral oedema may be asymmetrical

7. After having presented a unifying diagnosis of nephrotic syndrome, tell the examiner you would like to:
    (a) Confirm the presence of proteinuria*
    (b) Measure the blood pressure
    (c) Look for evidence of underlying aetiology (see below for causes)
    (d) Examine the chest for pleural effusions

If the venous pressure were elevated (unlikely in the MRCP (PACES) examination), then another important differential would be right heart failure. In such cases, tell the examiner you would like to examine the cardiovascular system.

Questions commonly asked by examiners

What is the definition of the nephrotic syndrome?

The nephrotic syndrome is a clinical syndrome, characterized by heavy proteinuria (>3g/24 hours), hypoalbuminaemia (<30g/L), and oedema. Hyperlipidaemia and thrombotic disease is frequently observed, but are not essential for the diagnosis.

What is the difference between proteinuria and the nephrotic syndrome?

Proteinuria is a manifestation of glomerular disease. Urinary protein excretion in the normal adult should be less than 150mg per day, of which 30mg is albumin. An alternative to 24-hour urine

---

* Proteinuria is required for the diagnosis of the nephrotic syndrome, although non-nephrotic range proteinuria may occur in other conditions. Urinalysis is a useful bedside test to demonstrate proteinuria, but will not reliably quantify proteinuria. The demonstration of heavy proteinuria, greater than 3g in 24 hours, is required for the diagnosis.

collection is the estimation of the total protein:creatinine ratio (normal <15mg/mmol). This correlates with daily protein excretion, and is less cumbersome than a 24-hour collection, although the limitations of the tests include variations with time of day, with race, and with body mass.

Any condition causing glomerular disease can cause a spectrum ranging from asymptomatic proteinuria, to heavy proteinuria without symptoms, or to the nephrotic syndrome. Patients with the nephrotic syndrome are at greater risk of complications such as thrombotic disease or infection, than those with isolated proteinuria.

What are the ways in which glomerular disease may present?

- *Focal nephritic disease*—This is characterized by inflammatory lesions in less than one-half of glomeruli on light microscopy. Urinalysis reveals haematuria, mild proteinuria, and occasionally red cell casts. Findings of advanced disease, such as oedema, hypertension, and renal insufficiency, are absent. These patients typically present with asymptomatic haematuria.
- *Diffuse nephritic disease*—Diffuse glomerulonephritis affects most, or all, of the glomeruli. These patients may present with features of advanced disease, such as oedema, hypertension, renal insufficiency, or the nephrotic syndrome.
- *Nephrotic syndrome.*

What is the differential diagnosis of the nephrotic syndrome?

In adults, approximately 30% have a systemic disorder, such as *diabetes mellitus, amyloidosis,* or SLE. The remainder are due to intrinsic renal disease, such as minimal change disease, focal glomerulosclerosis, and membranous glomerulonephritis. Minimal change disease accounts for the vast majority of nephrotic syndrome in children.

- *Minimal change disease*—This has typically normal light microscopic appearances, with no evidence of immune complex deposition on immunofluorescence. The disorder is most common in children, but may also occur in adults as either an idiopathic condition, or associated with diabetes, IgA nephropathy, NSAIDs, HIV infection, or as a paraneoplastic effect of malignancy most commonly Hodgkin's lymphoma.
- *Focal segmental glomeruloscerosis*—This is characterized by segmental glomerular mesangial collapse and sclerosis on light microscopy. It accounts for over 35% of cases of nephrotic syndrome in developed countries, and over 50% amongst Afro-Caribbean populations. The disorder can be idiopathic, but is also associated with HIV infection, NSAID use, and massive obesity.
- *Membranous glomerulonephritis*—This disorder is characterized by basement membrane thickening on light microscopy, with little cellular infiltration. Causes include infection (hepatitis B and C, malaria, schistosomiasis, and syphilis), autoimmune disease (SLE, rheumatoid arthritis, dermatomyositis, and Sjogren's syndrome), paraneoplastic syndrome to a solid organ malignancy (lung, colon, stomach, breast, and lymphoma), and drugs (gold, penicillamine, and NSAIDs).
- *Mesangiocapillary glomerulonephritis*—This is characterized by proliferation of mesangial and endothelial cells and expansion of the mesangial matrix and a double-contour or tram-track appearance on light microscopy. It can be divided into primary (idiopathic) and secondary types. The secondary types are more common than the idiopathic types. In idiopathic type, immune complex deposition occurs within the glomerulus and can be further sub-categorized as type 1 (subendothelial deposits) or type 2 (basement membrane deposits). Causes include infection (chronic hepatitis B and C, leprosy, endocarditis), cryoglobulinaemia, and autoimmune disease (SLE, rheumatoid arthritis, scleroderma, and Sjogren's syndrome).

How would you assess a patient with proteinuria?

- *Confirm presence of proteinuria*—Urinalysis should be performed on at least two separate occasions to exclude proteinuria due to intercurrent illness.

- *Look for other signs of glomerular disease*—The urine sediment should be examined for haematuria and red cell casts. Also look for hypertension, diabetes mellitus, and impaired renal function. Ask about symptoms suggestive of an underlying systemic vasculitis, or about a family history of renal disease. (see Vol 2, Station 2 History taking skills).
- *Exclude orthostatic proteinuria*—This is a benign condition, typically affecting young adults under 30 years of age. In this condition, an overnight urine collection shows normal protein excretion (i.e. <50mg during an 8 hour period).
- *Establish degree of proteinuria*—Protein excretion can be measured with a 24-hour urine collection. However, the protein:creatinine ratio from a single urine specimen is the most commonly used screening test for proteinuria. The albumin:creatinine ratio should be used to detect microalbuminuria.
  - *Microalbuminuria*—This describes pathological albuminuria, which is not detectable by dipstick urinalysis. It is defined as a 24-hour urine albumin excretion of 30–300mg, or a urinary albumin:creatinine ratio >2.5mg/mmol (men), and >3.5mg/mmol (women).
  - *Proteinuria*—This is defined as between 300mg and 3g of proteinuria in 24 hours, or a protein:creatinine ratio >30mg/mmol.
  - *Nephrotic range proteinuria*—This is defined as proteinuria >3g/day, or a protein:creatinine ratio >300mg/mmol. The nephrotic syndrome is diagnosed if hypoalbuminaemia and oedema are also present.
- *Look for treatable causes of glomerular disease:*
  - *Autoimmune profile*—including antinuclear antibodies (ANAs), anti-DNA antibodies, complement levels, and cryoglobulins.
  - *Viral serology*—including hepatitis B, hepatitis C, and HIV.
  - *Urine and plasma protein electrophoreisis.*
  - *Antistreptococcal antibodies.*
  - *Renal biopsy*—is usually indicated to guide specific therapy if nephrotic syndrome is present, and the kidneys are not small on imaging (suggesting irreversible renal disease).

What are the complications of the nephrotic syndrome?

- *Oedema*—controlled by salt restriction and diuretics
- *Hypertension*—should be treated to a target of 125/75, using ACE inhibitors and angiotensin-II receptor antagonists in the first instance.
- *Hypercholesterolaemia*—usually requires lipid lowering therapy.
- *Thrombosis*—routine prophylactic anticoagulation is not recommended, however immobile patients should receive heparin prophylaxis.
- *Infection*—patients should receive *Pneumococcal* and *Meningococcal* vaccinations. Penicillin prophylaxis has not been shown to be beneficial.

How would you initiate treatment in a patient with significant oedema?

- High doses of loop diuretics are often required, since patients with nephrotic syndrome are often relatively resistant to diuretics. Thiazide diuretics, such as bendroflumethiazide or metolazone, may be added for synergistic diuresis.
- Monitor diuresis by measuring weight and postural blood pressure. Aim for weight loss of between 0.5–1 kg/day. Over-diuresis is signalled by excess weight loss, or the presence of postural hypotension >20mmHg.

Case 9 ◆ Polycystic Kidneys

CASE PRESENTATION

*This patient has no stigmata of chronic liver disease.[1] There is no evidence of anaemia.[2] The venous pressure is not elevated.[3] The abdomen is distended with fullness in the flanks.[4] There is an **irregular, non-tender liver edge** palpable 3cm below the costal margin.[5] There is no evidence of splenomegaly.[6] There are **bilateral flank masses**. These masses are **ballotable**; it is possible to **palpate above** these masses, and the **overlying percussion note is resonant**.[7] There are no signs of uraemia or encephalopathy.[8] There is **no evidence of renal replacement therapy**.[9]*

*The diagnosis is **polycystic kidney disease**.[10]*

Clinical notes

1. Look for stigmata of chronic liver disease. Although hepatic cysts and hepatomegaly is common in polycystic kidney disease, the liver function is usually normal and cirrhosis is rare.

2. Mention the presence or absence of anaemia. Anaemia is a complication of chronic renal disease. Also look for plethoric facies that would suggest polycythaemia. Polycystic kidney disease is associated with increased erythropoietin production and is therefore an important secondary cause of polycythaemia.

3. It is important to comment on volume status in a patient with chronic renal disease.

4. When inspecting the abdomen look carefully for nephrectomy scars. Nephrectomy scars can be unilateral or bilateral. Nephrectomy is often necessary in the context of trauma and haemorrhage, as polycystic kidneys are very prone to traumatic injury. Other indications include pain, recurrent infections, and cyst rupture. Nephrectomy is frequently undertaken at the time of renal transplantation. Also look carefully in the right and left iliac fossae for scars suggesting a renal transplant.

5. Hepatic cysts occur in up to 70% of patients, but this may not always result in palpable hepatomegaly. If hepatomegaly is present, the liver will have an irregular nodular edge. It is common for hepatomegaly to be missed in patients with large polycystic kidneys. When palpating the liver, start from the left iliac fossa with the hand placed firmly flat over the abdomen, aiming to feel the liver edge with the radial border of the index finger as it descends with inspiration. Continue to do this as you successively move up to the right costal margin. By placing the hand firmly on the abdomen, the renal mass is displaced posteriorly, and attention can be paid to feeling for the descent of the liver edge. A common error is where the lower border of the enlarged kidney is mistaken for the liver edge in thin patients. In such cases it is important to remember that the kidney will not descend with inspiration.

6. Splenic cysts can also occur (5% of patients), but are less common than hepatic cysts.

7. The liver and spleen can be differentiated clinically from renal masses by the following general rules:

	Liver and spleen	Renal mass
Percussion note	Dull	Usually resonant
Movement with respiration	Yes	No
Palpate above	No	Yes
Ballotable	No	Yes

Although these are taught as golden rules for differentiating kidneys from liver and spleen, there are some exceptions and the following clinical points should be noted:

◆ In patients with hepatomegaly AND a large right renal mass, it may be difficult to palpate above the renal mass. This may falsely indicate the presence of a single large renal mass.

However, detecting the presence of a descending liver edge in inspiration, the resonant percussion note over the mass BELOW the liver edge and the ballotable nature of the mass will help diagnose both hepatomegaly AND a renal mass.

♦ In thin patients with large kidneys, especially in cases where the kidneys are visible during inspection (flank fullness) and easily palpable during light palpation of the abdomen, the percussion note can be dull (as opposed to resonant)!

8. Asterixis of the out-stretched hands indicates a metabolic encephalopathy. Metabolic encephalopathies, especially hepatic and renal, are the most common causes of bilateral asterixis. Other causes of asterixis include hypercapnoea, electrolyte abnormalities (hypoglycaemia, hypokalaemia, and hypomagnesaemia) and drug intoxication (barbiturate, phenytoin, and primidone).

9. Throughout your examination look carefully for evidence of previous or current renal replacement therapy. Patients may have stable polycystic kidney disease, and may not have reached end-stage renal failure. Mentioning the absence or presence of renal replacement therapy is an important negative.

10. The above case presentation is appropriate when presenting a patient with polycystic kidney disease who has not reached end-stage renal failure. In patients with evidence of renal replacement therapy, we suggest using the presentation framework for a renal abdomen (see Case 7 Renal Abdomen).

Polycystic kidney disease is a multi-system disorder. Tell the examiner you would like to look for other features and associations of the disease, and proceed as follows:

• **Measure the blood pressure** (hypertension predates the onset of renal failure)
• **Examine the cardiovascular system** (mitral valve prolapse, aortic regurgitation, left ventricular heave [hypertension])
• **Examine the neurological system**: (evidence of old stroke; third nerve palsy [Berry aneurysm])

Questions commonly asked by examiners

What other diseases cause bilateral renal cysts?
• Multiple simple cysts
• Tuberous sclerosis
• Von Hippel Lindau syndrome
• Meckel-Gruber syndrome
• Laurence-Moon-Bardet-Biedl syndrome
• Trisomies 13 (Patau syndrome), 18 (Edward syndrome), and 21 (Down syndrome)

What is the differential diagnosis of a single palpable kidney?
• Polycystic kidney disease (with only one palpable kidney)
• Hydronephrosis
• Hypertrophy of a single functioning kidney
• Renal cell carcinoma

What is the differential diagnosis for bilateral palpable kidneys?
• Bilateral renal cysts (see above)
• Bilateral hydronephrosis
• Amyloidosis
• Bilateral renal cell carcinoma (occurs in von Hippel-Lindau syndrome)

What do you know about the genetics of adult polycystic kidney disease?
• Polycystic kidney disease is typically autosomal dominant (ADPKD). A variety of genetic defects have been described. ADPKD1 accounts for 90% of cases, and has been mapped to

chromosome 16. Most of the remainder of cases are ADPKD2, which has been mapped to chromosome 4, and has a less severe phenotype. In 10% of patients, the disease arises from a spontaneous mutation.

- Autosomal recessive kidney disease (ARPKD) is a rare disease, presenting in infancy and frequently causing severe liver and renal disease.

What are the features of ADPKD?

- Flank and abdominal pain is common, caused by stretching of the capsule or traction of the renal pedicle.
- Acute pain suggests haemorrhage, infection, or torsion of a cyst. Kidney stones also occur in 20%, and may cause obstructive uropathy.
- Nocturia occurs due to impaired ability to concentrate urine
- Renal call carcinoma is *not* more common in ADPKD. However, the tumours are more likely to be bilateral, and are more difficult to diagnose.

What are the extra-renal manifestations of ADPKD?

Cerebral aneurysms

- Subarachnoid haemorrhage as a consequence of a ruptured cerebral aneurysm is the most serious complication of ADPKD. Aneurysms occur in 4% of younger patients, and up to 10% of older patients.
- The role of magnetic resonance angiography has not been settled, and is probably only desirable for high risk patients with a family history of haemorrhage. This is because of the dilemma of treating small aneurysms (<7mm) whose risk of rupture may be less than the risk from neurosurgical treatment.

Liver cysts

- Liver cysts occur later than kidney cysts in ADPKD, and are present in up to 70% of cases. They rarely cause symptoms, although local symptoms, cholestasis, portal hypertension, and venous obstruction have been described.
- Autosomal dominant polycystic liver disease is a *separate* disorder, not associated with kidney cysts or cerebral aneurysms.

Other extra-renal cysts

- Pancreatic cysts occur in 9% and splenic cysts occur in 5% of patients. Cysts have also been reported in the thyroid, parathyroid, lung, pituitary gland, ovary, uterus, testis, seminal vesicles, epididymis, bladder, and peritoneum.

Valvular heart disease

- Mitral valve prolapse and aortic regurgitation are more common in this population, although the clinical significance of these lesions is uncertain.

What are the principles of management of ADPKD?

Management of acute flank pain

- Distinguishing infection, haemorrhage or renal stones may be difficult. Infection rarely causes a positive urine culture, since the cysts are not in continuity with the collecting system. Imaging may not distinguish infection or haemorrhage, but will exclude renal stones.
- Infected cysts must be treated with lipid-soluble antimicrobials that penetrate the cyst, since they are not in contact with the glomerular system. Aminoglycosides and penicillins should not be used, but quinolones and vancomycin are suitable.
- Cyst aspiration is rarely performed, since it does not improve renal function, and the lesions are multiple.

Management of renal failure

- Control hypertension.
- Ensure adequate nutrition—there is no evidence for protein restriction.
- Treat anaemia. Replenish iron stores, and consider erythropoietin only after controlling hypertension.
- Phosphate binders if the serum phosphate is elevated.
- Vitamin D supplementation if the serum PTH is elevated.
- For persistent hyperparathyroidism, consider calcimimetics or parathyroidectomy.
- Early specialist referral for renal replacement therapy.

Screening for ADPKD

- Cysts are present in infancy, and increase in size with age. However, onset of clinical disease is rare in children, and cysts may be missed radiologically when small. Therefore, screening in those with a family history occurs after the age of 20.

What do you know about Von-Hippel-Lindau syndrome?

- Autosomal dominant condition (chromosome 3) with 80–90% penetrance
- Cerebellar, retinal, and spinal haemangioblastomas
- Cysts occur in the kidneys, liver, spleen, and epididymis
- Increased risk of renal cell carcinoma (bilateral in 40% of cases) and phaechromocytoma

Case 10 ◆ Abdominal Mass

CASE PRESENTATION 1

This patient is **cachectic**.[1] There is evidence of **anaemia**. There is no evidence of clubbing[2] and there are no stigmata of chronic liver disease. There is a palpable **left supraclavicular lymph node**.[3] The abdomen is soft and non-tender. There is no organomegaly. There is a palpable **mass in the left upper quadrant**. It is non-tender, firm, and ill-defined. It does not move with respiration, and is not fixed to the abdominal wall. The mass is not pulsatile, and is not ballotable. The overlying percussion note is dull. It is possible to palpate between the mass and the left costal margin. On auscultation of the mass, there are no bowel sounds, bruits, or rubs.[4]

This patient has a **left upper quadrant mass**—most likely **colonic** or **gastric** in origin. The presence of cachexia and lymphadenopathy raises the suspicion of **malignancy**.[5]

CASE PRESENTATION 2

This patient is **cachectic**.[1] There is evidence of **anaemia**. On examination of the hands there is **clubbing**[2] and **leuconychia**. There is **oral ulceration**. There is no lymphadenopathy.[3] There is a **midline laparotomy scar**. The abdomen is soft but tender in the right lower quadrant. There is no organomegaly. There is a palpable **mass in the right lower quadrant**. It is tender, firm, and ill-defined. It does not move with respiration,[4] and is not fixed to the abdominal wall. The mass is not pulsatile, and is not *ballotable.[4] The overlying percussion note is dull. It is possible to palpate between the mass and the left costal margin. On auscultation of the mass, bowel sounds are audible, but there are no bruits, or rubs.[4]*

*This patient has a **right lower quadrant mass**—most likely **colonic** in origin. The presence of clubbing, oral ulceration, and abdominal tenderness suggests an **inflammatory mass due to Crohn's disease**.[5]*

Clinical notes

1. Cachexia may be noticeable from standing at the end of the bed. Otherwise, a cachectic state may be demonstrated by a poor nutritional status from a reduced tricep fat fold thickness that can be easily assessed during the examination. Wasting of the temporalis muscle is an early sign of generalized muscle atrophy.

2. Gastrointestinal causes of clubbing include chronic liver disease, inflammatory bowel disease, gastrointestinal lymphoma, coeliac disease, tropical sprue, parasitosis, Whipple's disease, and achalasia.

3. In the context of an abdominal mass, lymphadenopathy suggests malignancy. Virchow's node (or signal node) is an enlarged, hard, left supraclavicular lymph node which can contain metastasis of visceral (abdominal) malignancy. Malignancies of the internal organs can reach an advanced stage before giving symptoms. The left supraclavicular node, or Virchow's node, is an early site of metastatic GI cancer because it is on the left side of the neck where the lymphatic drainage of most of the body (from the thoracic duct) enters the venous circulation via the left subclavian vein. The differential diagnosis of an enlarged Virchow's node includes lymphoma, other intra-abdominal malignancies, breat cancer, lung cancer, and infection (e.g. of the arm). An enlarged Virchow's node is also referred to as Troisier's sign.

4. Look below for differential diagnoses for masses in the four quadrants of the abdomen. Having established the presence of an abdominal mass it is important to look for the following features:

FEATURE	CLINICAL NOTES
Size	Comment on the size. This need not be accurate, and a rough estimate will suffice.
Consistency	Is it soft or firm?
Border	Well-defined or ill (poorly)-defined? Ensure to define the contour of the mass by inspection, percussion, and palpation. A well-defined mass may be an intra-abdominal organ (e.g. liver, spleen), whilst an ill-defined mass may be matted loops of bowel or mesentery, or a neoplastic mass.
Tender	Tender or non-tender
Attached to abdominal wall	This suggests either an abdominal wall mass (e.g. lipoma or rectus sheath haematoma), or an inflammatory or neoplastic mass that is fixed to the abdominal wall.
Movement with respiration	A mobile intra-abdominal mass will move with respiration (e.g. liver, spleen), whilst retroperitoneal structures (e.g. aorta, kidney) or an abdominal wall mass will not.
Pulsatile	A pulsatile mass is suggestive of a vascular lesion, such as an aneurysm or arterio-venous fistula.
Ballotable	The kidneys are the only ballotable masses in the abdomen.
Percussion note	Solid masses with a firm consistency will give a dull percussion note.
Auscultatory findings	The presence of bowel sounds suggests that the mass is intestinal in origin. The presence of a bruit suggests a vascular origin, whilst a rub suggests an inflammatory or neoplastic origin.

Remember with right/left upper quadrant masses, it is important to establish if it is possible to palpate above the mass. This will differentiate the mass from a liver/spleen (not possible to palpate above the liver or spleen).

5. When presenting the final diagnosis, try to establish the location of the mass. Use other clinical signs to make a diagnosis. If this is not possible, then provide a differential diagnosis based on the four quadrants in which the mass lies (see below).

Questions commonly asked by examiners

What are the causes of:

A right upper quadrant mass

- Liver—moves with respiration.
- Right kidney—retroperitoneal and ballotable, but does not move with respiration.
- Riedel's lobe of liver—this is a sessile projection of the right lobe of the liver, which descends to the right of the gallbladder. It is considered a normal variant.
- Gallbladder—moves with respiration.
- Colon—does not move with respiration. High-pitched bowel sounds suggest obstruction.

A left upper quadrant mass

- Spleen—moves with respiration. Possesses a medial notch, and enlarges towards the right iliac fossa.
- Left kidney—distinguished from the spleen by being ballotable and resonant to percussion.
- Colon/pancreas/stomach—these are impossible to differentiate by clinical examination. Pancreatic masses include cystic neoplasms, pseudocysts, and solid tumours.

A right lower quadrant mass

- Colon/small intestine/appendix—inflammatory masses may be tender, although neoplastic masses are usually painless.
- Pelvic mass—bimanual palpation may distinguish an intestinal and pelvic mass.

A left lower quadrant mass

- Sigmoid colon—an inflammatory mass may be due to diverticular disease or inflammatory bowel disease. Neoplastic lesions are more common in the left colon than the right colon.
- Pelvic mass

Do you know of any inherited conditions predisposing to colorectal cancer?

- *Hereditary Nonpolyposis Colorectal Cancer (HNPCC) or Lynch syndrome*—An autosomal dominant disorder with high penetrance, caused by mutations in one of several DNA mismatch repair genes. Lynch syndrome accounts for 1–3% of colonic adenocarcinomas, and is also associated with extra-colonic tumours such as endometrium, ovary, stomach, small intestine, hepatobiliary, and urogenital. The Amsterdam Criteria have been proposed for the clinical diagnosis of HNPCC:
  - ≥3 relatives with colorectal cancer, one of whom is a first-degree relative of the other two.
  - Involvement of at least two generations
  - One or more cancers diagnosed before the age of 50

A problem with this approach is the low sensitivity, so a significant number of patients with hereditary syndromes may be missed. An alternative approach is to use molecular methods to detect microsatellite instability, or mutation of DNA repair genes, in tumours of patients with colorectal cancer. Relatives can then be screened for these mutations from blood tests. However, the cost-effectiveness of this approach remains to be assessed.

- *Familial Adenomatous Polyposis (FAP)*—An autosomal dominant disorder, caused by mutation in the adenomatous polyposis coli (APC) gene. Approximately one-third of patients with FAP have no family history of the disease, and probably represent new mutations. The diagnosis of FAP is based upon the presence of more than 100 adenomatous colorectal polyps. Almost all patients develop colorectal cancer by the age of 45, unless colectomy is performed. Patients remain at risk of extra-colonic tumours, including duodenal ampullary cancer, gastric cancer, follicular or papillary thyroid cancer, and CNS tumours. *Gardner's syndrome* is a variant of FAP with extraintestinal lesions such as desmoid tumours, sebaceous cysts, lipomas, osteomas, and supernumerary teeth. *Turcot's syndrome* is a rare FAP variant, associated with medulloblastoma.

- *Peutz-Jeghers Syndrome*—An autosomal dominant condition, characterized by multiple hamartomatous polyps in the small intestine, colon, and stomach. Clinically, patients develop numerous pigmented lesions on the lips and buccal mucosa. The overall cancer risk is increased 9-fold for both gastrointestinal, and non-gastrointestinal sites, including breast, lung, uterus, and ovary. (See volume 1, case Family History of Cancer)

What are the most common small intestinal tumours?

Small intestine tumours are rare, accounting for less than 2% of all gastrointestinal cancers. In order of frequency, the most common small intestinal tumours are:

- **Neuroendocrine tumour**—Often termed carcinoid tumours, although they represent a heterogenous group of cell types. These tumours typically present late due to a lack of specific symptoms, and may present with intestinal perforation or obstruction. Secretory tumours may cause the carcinoid syndrome if liver metastases are present, due to bioactive products bypassing hepatic inactivation.

- **Lymphoma**—These are usually non-Hodgkin's lymphomas. Presentation with abdominal pain is common, although an abdominal mass is rare. T-cell lymphomas may occur as a consequence of celiac disease.

- **Adenocarcinoma**—These occur most commonly in the duodenum. Coeliac disease, Crohn's disease, and polyposis syndromes are risk factors.

- **Sarcoma and gastrointestinal stromal tumour**—These originate from interstitial cells of the intestine, and were previously referred to as smooth muscle tumours. They typically express the *kit* oncogene, which encodes a tyrosine kinase. Biological drugs, which inhibit this tyrosine kinase (e.g. Imatinib), have revolutionized the treatment of these tumours.

Respiratory System

Case 11 ◆ Interstitial Lung Disease

CASE PRESENTATION 1

This patient is (is not) breathless at rest.[1] There is evidence of **peripheral cyanosis**.[2] The **fingers are clubbed**.[3] There are no stigmata of rheumatological disease.[4] There is no evidence of nicotine staining.[5] There is **steroid purpura** peripherally.[6] There are no palpable lymph nodes.[7] On examination of the chest, there are no scars.[8] The trachea is central and the cricoid-notch distance is not reduced.[9] **Chest expansion** is **equal** but **reduced bilaterally**.[10] The **percussion note is dull** and **vocal fremitus is reduced** at both bases.[11] On auscultation, there are **fine end-inspiratory crackles at both bases**.[12] There are no audible squawks and there is no wheeze.[13] There is no peripheral oedema and there are no signs of pulmonary hypertension.[14]

The diagnosis is **interstitial lung disease**. The patient is on **steroid therapy**.[15]

CASE PRESENTATION 2

This patient is (is not) breathless at rest.[1] There is evidence of **peripheral** and **central cyanosis**.[2] The **fingers are clubbed**.[3] The skin over the fingers and face is smooth, shiny, and tight. There is sclerodactyly, atrophic nails, and evidence of Raynaud's phenomenon.[4] There is no evidence of nicotine staining.[5] There is **steroid purpura** peripherally.[6] There are no palpable lymph nodes.[7] On examination of the chest, there are no scars.[8] The trachea is central and the cricoid-notch distance is not reduced.[9] **Chest expansion** is **equal** but **reduced bilaterally**.[10] The **percussion note is dull** and **vocal fremitus is reduced** at both bases.[11] On auscultation, there are **fine end-inspiratory crackles at both bases**.[12] There are no audible squawks and there is no wheeze.[13]

In addition, the **venous pressure is elevated**. There is a **prominent parasternal heave**, and a **loud pulmonary component to the second heart sound**. There is **peripheral oedema**.[14]

The diagnosis is advanced **interstitial lung disease** most likely secondary to **systemic sclerosis**, with evidence of **pulmonary hypertension**. The patient is on **steroid therapy**.[15]

Clinical notes

Interstitial lung disease is a common case for the respiratory section of the MRCP PACES examination. Quite often they are cases of idiopathic pulmonary fibrosis (cryptogenic fibrosing alveolitis) or in the context of systemic (commonly rheumatological) disease. The above cases reflect these common scenarios. To make the diagnosis of interstitial lung disease is relatively straightforward, but presenting other physical signs of underlying aetiologies, mentioning important negatives, and appreciating and recognizing complications of therapy and the disease will impress examiners, not to mention gain considerable extra marks.

1. In approaching a respiratory patient, it is often useful in starting to present the case with a comment on functional status. They may be breathless at rest. They may be on oxygen therapy. Ask the patient to cough. The presence of a non-productive or a productive cough should give clues to underlying

diagnosis. Patients with interstitial lung disease often have a non-productive cough, unless this has been complicated by infection.

2. Patients often have peripheral cyanosis. Central cyanosis may be present in advanced disease.

3. Clubbing may not always be present in cases of interstitial lung disease. If present, don't miss it!

4. Spend a little extra time when examining hands and making general observations. There are many systemic disorders that are associated with pulmonary fibrosis. The presence of peripheral stigmata of systemic disease, usually connective tissue or rheumatological disease, will provide an important clue to the respiratory diagnosis. Look for

   - **rheumatoid arthritis** (symmetrical deforming arthropathy of the hands, rheumatoid nodules)
   - **systemic sclerosis** (tight and shiny skin, telangiectasia, sclerodactyly, calcinosis, atrophic nails, and Raynaud's phenomenon)
   - **SLE** (petechial rash, livedo reticularis, purpura, arthropathy, butterfly skin rash)
   - **dermatomyositis** (Gottron's papules, heliotrope rash of eyelids/periorbital areas, proximal myopathy)
   - **ankylosing spondylitis** (loss of lumber lordosis, fixed kyphosis, stooped posture)
   - **neurofibromatoisis** (neurofibromata, café au lait patches)
   - **sarcoidosis** (erythema nodosum, maculopapular skin lesions, lupus pernio, lympahdenopathy)
   - **drugs**, i.e. amiodarone (grey slate skin pigmentation—the irregular pulse of atrial fibrillation (AF) may be a clue)
   - **radiation therapy** (erythema and/or field markings on chest wall)

5. Cigarette smoking is not necessarily associated with interstitial lung disease. However, it is associated with chronic obstructive airways disease, and in long-standing cases pulmonary fibrosis can occur.

6. Steroid purpura reflects steroid immunosuppressive therapy. Look for other features of steroid use: cushingoid appearance and proximal myopathy—if correctly identified and presented, this will impress examiners. In some cases, other steroid sparing drugs may be used: azathioprine, methotrexate, and cyclophosphamide. In specific cases, other immunosuppressive or anti-fibrotic drugs may be used: colchicine, cyclosporin, and D-penicillamine. Look for gingival hyperplasia—a sign of ciclosporin use.

7. Lymphadenopathy may be present in sarcoidosis, a cause of pulmonary fibrosis.

8. Look for scars suggesting previous mediastinoscopy (scar at the level of suprasternal notch), thoracoscopy (often multiple scars over the right or left thorax), lymph node biopsy (scar in the supraclavicular fossa), or lung biopsies (scars over the right or left thorax).

9. Usually, there is symmetrical involvement of the lungs, thus trachea is central. In cases of asymmetrical involvement, the trachea may be pulled to the affected side (especially in cases of apical fibrosis). A reduced cricoid-notch distance (usually less than 3 fingerbreadths) is a sign of hyperinflation, suggestive of obstructive airways disease.

10. In idiopathic pulmonary fibrosis and in the context of rheumatological disease, it is common for lung volumes to be reduced globally, hence equal and reduced chest expansion. In cases, where the fibrosis is predominantly unilateral or apical, the reduction in chest expansion will be localized.

11. The bases are often associated with a dull percussion note, reduced vocal or tactile fremitus and reduced air entry. In cases of apical fibrosis, these findings are predominantly apical, and the trachea may be pulled to one side if asymmetrical apical fibrosis is present. Bronchial breathing may be present in cases of apical fibrosis, especially over a deviated trachea.

12. In cases of basal pulmonary fibrosis, fine end-inspiratory crackles are present at the bases (which can extend up to mid-zones). Sometimes, it may be difficult to auscultate very fine crackles, and these need to be sought for carefully. On the other hand, with predominant apical involvement, the crackles are localized to the apices.

13. Inspiratory squawks may be present with the involvement of smaller airways (bronchiolitis) or in hypersensitivity pneumonitis. Wheeze is not a feature of idiopathic pulmonary fibrosis (cryptogenic fibrosing alveolitis). The presence of wheeze signifies airways obstruction, as in obstructive airways disease, or in sarcoidosis.

14. It should be routine, at the end of a respiratory examination to look for signs of pulmonary hypertension— this will be particularly important in interstitial lung disease for which pulmonary hypertension is a

recognized complication. Look for an elevated venous pressure (prominent a waves, or systolic v waves if tricuspid regurgitation is present), parasternal heave and thrill, right ventricular third and fourth heart sounds, widely split second heart sound with a loud pulmonary component, and peripheral oedema.

15.   When presenting the final diagnosis, try to mention the possible aetiology, complications, i.e. pulmonary hypertension, and signs of immunosuppressive therapy, namely steroids and rarely ciclosporin. Picking up interstitial lung disease is relatively straightforward, but presenting other physical signs of underlying aetiologies, mentioning important negatives, and appreciating and recognizing complications of therapy and the disease will impress examiners and gain extra marks.

Questions commonly asked by examiners

What are the causes of chronic interstitial lung disease?

- **Idiopathic pulmonary fibrosis (cryptogenic fibrosing alveolitis)**
- **Rheumatological diseasen**
    - ◆   Rheumatoid arthritis
    - ◆   Systemic sclerosis
    - ◆   SLE
    - ◆   Polymyositis
    - ◆   Dermatomyositis
    - ◆   Sjogren's syndrome
    - ◆   Mixed connective tissue disease
    - ◆   Ankylosing spondylitis
    - ◆   Psoriasis
- **Eosinophilic lung disease**
    - ◆   Drugs (nitrofurantoin, imipramine, and sulphasalazine)
    - ◆   Aspergillosis
- **Other respiratory disease**
    - ◆   Sarcoidosis
    - ◆   Tuberculosis
- **Vasculitis**
    - ◆   Polyarteritis nodosa
    - ◆   Wegner's granulomatosis
    - ◆   Churg-Strauss syndrome
    - ◆   Goodpasture's syndrome
- **Inhaled agents**
    - ◆   Extrinsic allergic alveolitis
    - ◆   Asbestosis
    - ◆   Silicosis
    - ◆   Beryliosis
- **Drugs**
    - ◆   Amiodarone
    - ◆   Nitrofurantoin
    - ◆   Busulphan
    - ◆   Bleomycin
    - ◆   Gold
    - ◆   Methotrexate

- **Radiation fibrosis**
- **Other rare causes**
  - Neurofibromatosis
  - Tuberous sclerosis
  - Lymphangiomyelomatosis
  - Niemann-Pick disease
  - Gaucher's disease

What are the respiratory causes of clubbing?

- Interstitial lung disease
- Carcinoma of the lung
- Mesothelioma
- Bronchiectasis
- Cystic fibrosis
- Lung abscess
- Empyema
- Tuberculosis

What do you know about 'idiopathic pulmonary fibrosis'?

This is a chronic progressive lung disease of unknown aetiology and is characterized by inflammation and fibrosis of the lung parenchyma. Although idiopathic pulmonary fibrosis is a general term, it is also known as cryptogenic fibrosing alveolitis. Idiopathic pulmonary fibrosis is diagnosed when other causes of interstitial lung disease have been excluded. These idiopathic interstitial pneumonias are a group of diffuse infiltrative pulmonary diseases with similar clinical presentation, characterized by dyspnoea, restrictive physiology and bilateral interstitial infiltrates on chest radiograph. From a pathological perspective, these diseases have characteristic patterns of tissue injury with chronic inflammation and varying amounts of fibrosis. The latest ATS/ERS (American Thoracic Society/ European Respiratory Society) classification system lists seven different types (see below). Using this classification system for idiopathic pulmonary fibrosis, treatment can be selected and a general prognosis can be provided. The most common histological diagnosis is 'usual interstitial pneumonia' (UIP).

How would you investigate a patient with interstitial lung disease?

Blood tests

- FBC*
- Inflammatory markers (including ESR (erythrocyte sedimentation rate))
- Immunoglobulins
- Autoimmune profile (ANA, ENA (extractable nuclear antigen), ANCA (anti-neutrophil cytoplasmic antibody), anti-GBM (anti-glomerular basement membrane antibody))
- Creatine kinase**
- Rheumatoid factor
- Precipitins***
- Serum ACE****

---

* Anaemia may be present in vasculitis; polycythemia may indicate hypoxia in long-standing disease; leucocytosis can suggest acute hypersensitivity pneumonitis

** An elevated CK is present in polymyositis and dermatomyositis

*** Precipitating antibodies to various antigens may help diagnose hypersensitivity pneumonitis

**** Serum ACE is often elevated in sarcoidosis, but this has poor specificity

Arterial blood gas sampling
- Type 1 respiratory failure

CXR
- Bilateral basal reticulonodular infiltrates (advance upwards as the disease progresses)
- In advanced cases, marked destruction of the lung parenchyma gives a 'honeycombing' appearance
- Bilateral hilar lymphadenopathy may be present in sarcoidosis
- Calcified pleural plaques in asbestos exposure

Lung function tests
- Reduction in lung volumes (total lung capacity (TLC), functional residual capacity (FRC), and right ventricle (RV))
- Restrictive pattern of defect (forced expiratory volume/forced vital capacity (FEV1/FVC) ≥70%)[a]
- Reduced gas transfer factor and gas transfer coefficient

HRCT
- This is useful in assessing the pattern and distribution of disease.
- A pattern of coarse, reticular, linear opacities, and cystic air spaces suggest a fibrotic histopathological process.
- A pattern of ground-glass opacities is highly predictive of cellular inflammatory process, which responds well to steroids or immunosuppressive agents.

MRI
- Better for imaging in upper lobe lesions.
- Generally better than CT for evaluation near the lung apex, spine, and thoracoabdominal junction.

Broncho-alveolar lavage
- Lymphocytosis indicates steroid responsiveness and a better prognosis.
- Malignant cells, asbestos bodies, and eosinophils, if present, may help in making a diagnosis.

Lung biopsy
- Fibre-optic bronchoscopy with trans-bronchial lung biopsy (Berylliosis, silicosis, sarcoidosis, hypersensitivity pneumonitis, lymphangitis carcinomatosa).
- Video-assisted thoracoscopic lung biopsy/open lung biopsy (idiopathic pulmonary fibrosis, connective tissue disease, vasculitis, histiocytosis X).

Which conditions cause a predominant (a) apical and (b) basal distribution of fibrosis?

Apical fibrosis
- **B**erylliosis*
- **R**adiation
- **E**xtrinsic allergic alveolitis (hypersensitivity pneumonitis)*
- **A**llergic bronchopulmonary aspergillosis
- **S**arcoidosis (upper to mid-zones)

---

[a] In certain cases, e.g. sarcoidosis, histiocytosis X, hypersensitivity pneumonitis(extrinsic allergic alveolitis), or co-existent obstructive airways disease, there may be a mixed obstructive and restrictive pattern.

- **T**uberculosis
- **S**ilicosis*

- **C**oal worker's pneumoconiosis*
- **L**angerhans cell histiocytosis (Histiocytosis X)
- **A**nkylosing spondylitis
- **P**soriasis

Pneumonic to remember: BREASTS CLAP

Basal fibrosis

- Idiopathic pulmonary fibrosis
- Rheumatological disease (except ankylosing spondylitis and psoriasis)
- Connective tissue disease
- Drugs
- Asbestosis*

What are the complications of interstitial lung disease?

- Respiratory failure
- Chest infection
- Pulmonary hypertension
- Cor pulmonale
- Carcinoma of the lung

What do you know about the ATS/ERS classification for idiopathic pulmonary fibrosis?

- Acute interstitial pneumonia (AIP)
- Usual interstitial pneumonia (UIP)
- Non-specific interstitial pneumonia (NSIP)
- Desquamative interstitial pneumonia (DIP)
- Lymphoid interstitial pneumonia (LIP)
- Cryptogenic organizing pneumonia (COP)
- Respiratory bronchiolitis-interstitial lung disease (RB-ILD)

How do would you manage this patient?

General measures

- Smoking cessation
- Discontinuation of toxic medication
- If aetiology is inhalational exposure, then remove exposure
- Treat respiratory infections promptly
- Long-term oxygen therapy

Immunosuppressive therapy

- All patients should receive a course of oral steroids if no contraindications exist (prednisolone 40mg OD for 6 weeks)
- If the response is good, then continue. Optimal duration of therapy is not known, but treatment for 1–2 years is suggested.

---

* Remember, ALL inhaled agents except asbestos cause APICAL fibrosis.

- If response to steroids is not good, then discontinue and taper over 1 week
- In steroid non-responders, azathioprine, methotrexate, or cyclophosphamide may be used.

Anti-fibrotic therapy
- Colchicine and D-penicillamine may be used in specific cases including idiopathic pulmonary fibrosis.

Surgery
- Single or double lung transplantation in advanced disease.
- Survival rates for single lung transplantation are 74% at 1 year, 58% at 3 years, 47% at 5 years, and 24% at 10 years.

What is the prognosis?
The clinical course is unpredictable—some may have a rapidly progressive fatal course; others demonstrate a deterioration in lung function over a longer period. The median survival is 3–5 years from the onset of symptoms. The 5-year survival rate is 50%: 65% in steroid responders and 25% in steroid non-responders.

Case 12 ◆ Chronic Obstructive Pulmonary Disease

CASE PRESENTATION

*This patient is breathless at rest and audible wheeze can be heard with the unaided ear.[1] There is **pursed lip breathing** during **prolonged expiration**.[2] There is **nicotine staining** of the fingers.[3] The fingers are not clubbed.[4] There is no flapping tremor of the outstretched hands.[5] The venous pressure is not elevated[6]. The trachea is central with a **reduced cricoid-notch distance**.[7] There is a **tracheal tug**.[8] The patient uses the **accessory muscles of respiration**[9] and there is **indrawing of the lower intercostal muscles** on inspiration.[10] The chest is **hyper-inflated** and chest expansion is primarily vertical with reduced horizontal chest expansion.[11] The percussion note is **hyper-resonant** throughout both lung fields, obliterating the cardiac and hepatic dullness. The **breath sounds are quiet**, particularly at the bases.[12] The **expiratory phase is prolonged** with widespread **expiratory wheeze**.[13] The **forced expiratory time (FET) is greater than 6 seconds** in keeping with a diagnosis of airflow obstruction.[14] There is no peripheral oedema. There are no signs of pulmonary hypertension.[15]*

*The diagnosis is **chronic obstructive pulmonary disease (COPD)**.*

Clinical notes

1. In certain cases, wheeze can be heard from the end of the bed. Often the patients are receiving oxygen therapy and it is important to look for this. Ask the patient to cough—patients often have a chronic productive cough. Look for the sputum pot by the bedside.
2. Obstructive airways disease is characterized by airflow limitation and the expiration phase of the respiratory cycle is prolonged. Pursed lip breathing provides a mechanism of splinting the airways open during expiration.

3. Smoking is associated with COPD. Look for nicotine staining of the fingers. Always look for the steroid purpura of chronic steroid use in patients with long-standing COPD. If present, look for other features of steroid use: cushingoid appearance and proximal myopathy—if correctly identified and presented, this will impress examiners.

4. Often these patients have a strong smoking history, and thus are at high risk of developing carcinoma of the lung. Therefore, if clubbing is not present, it is an important negative to mention when presenting the clinical findings.

7. In advanced cases, or those with acute exacerbation, there is severe hypercapnoea, which may manifest as a flapping tremor of the outstretched hands. In chronic severe hypercapnoea, there may be papilloedema.

6. Long-standing COPD is an important cause of pulmonary hypertension. Look for an elevated venous pressure, and if present, the other signs of pulmonary hypertension must be sought.

7. COPD is characterized by a hyper-inflated chest, thus the cricoid-notch distance is reduced (less than 3cm).

8. As chest expansions are primarily vertical, a tracheal tug may be present.

9. In severe cases, on in states of exacerbation, there is exaggerated use of the accessory muscles of respiration. These include the sternocleidomastoid, scalene, pectoralis major, trapezius, intercostal, and abdominal muscles.

10. With a hyper-inflated rib cage, there is visible indrawing of the lower intercostal muscles. This easier to spot in thin patients.

11. As the rib cage is hyper-inflated, the horizontal chest expansions are often reduced, and the chest expansion is mainly in a vertical direction. This forms the basis of the tracheal tug.

12. There is a hyper-resonant percussion note throughout the hyper-inflated lung fields. The hyper-inflated lungs displace the liver caudally, obliterating the hepatic dullness. The cardiac dullness may be obliterated, and often the apex beat is difficult to palpate in these patients. Breath sounds are often reduced globally, in particular over bullae. In COPD, with a centri-acinar pattern of involvement, the upper lobes and apices are more affected; bullae and therefore a greater reduction in breath sounds will be noted in the upper zones. On the other hand, with a pan-acinar pattern of involvement, the lower lobes are more affected; bullae and therefore a greater reduction in breath sounds will be in the lower zones. Occasionally breath sounds are extremely quiet, giving the impression of absent breath sounds.

13. COPD is characterized by airflow limitation and obstruction that manifests as expiratory wheeze. This can be diffuse and marked. In severe advanced cases, there may be a marked reduction in breath sounds and there may be no audible wheeze.

14. Forced expiratory time (FET) is a simple bedside respiratory function test, and if performed correctly, will impress the examiners. Ask the patient to take a deep breath in and then breathe out as hard and fast as he/she can until the lungs are empty. Normally, a person should be able to empty the lungs in less than 6 seconds. **An FET > 6 seconds demonstrates airflow obstruction.**

15. Look for signs of pulmonary hypertension and cor pulmonale. Even if not present, they are important negatives to mention.

Questions commonly asked by examiners

How do you define (a) COPD, (b) chronic bronchitis, (c) emphysema and (d) airflow obstruction?

(a) **COPD**: Progressive and irreversible (or partially reversible)* airflow obstruction due to chronic bronchitis or emphysema.

(b) **Chronic bronchitis**: Cough productive of sputum on most days for 3 months during 2 consecutive years (*a clinical diagnosis*).

---

* There may be an element of reversibility in airflow obstruction owing to some degree of airway hyper-reactivity.

(c) **Emphysema:** Abnormal and permanent enlargement of air spaces distal to the terminal bronchioles associated with destruction of their walls without obvious fibrosis (*a pathological diagnosis*).

(d) **Airflow obstruction:** FEV_1 < 80% predicted *and* FEV_1:FVC < 70%.

What are the differences between chronic bronchitis and emphysema?

Feature	Chronic bronchitis	Emphysema
Diagnosis	A clinical diagnosis	A pathological diagnosis
Appearance	'Blue bloater'	'Pink puffer'
Cyanosis	Prominent	Absent
Hyper-inflation	+	++
Dyspnoea	+	++
Cor pulmonale	++	+
Inspiratory drive	Reduced	Present

What is the pathophysiology of COPD?

The pathological changes of COPD occur in the large central airways, small peripheral bronchioles, and lung parenchyma. Activated neutrophils and macrophages release elastases, which cannot be effectively counteracted by the anti-proteases. This imbalance between protease and anti-protease activity results in lung destruction. Smoking induces macrophages to release neutrophil chemotactic factors and elastases. Additionally, smoking results in increased oxidative stress due to free radicals that leads to apoptosis and necrosis.

Chronic bronchitis

Mucosal gland hypertrophy is the histological hallmark. The primary changes occur within the bronchiolar walls with hyperplasia of the smooth muscle, inflammation, bronchial wall thickening, ciliary abnormalities and focal squamous metaplasia. The respiratory bronchioles show an inflammatory process with lumen occlusion by mucous plugging, goblet cell metaplasia, smooth muscle hyperplasia and fibrosis. These changes combined with loss of alveolar attachments, cause airflow limitation.

Emphysema

There are two common morphological patterns:

	Airway involvement	Pattern of damage
CENTRI-ACINAR	Limited to respiratory bronchioles and central portions of acinus. More distal alveolar ducts and alveoli are well preserved.	Upper lobes and apex > lower lobes
PAN-ACINAR	The whole acinus with the entire alveolus distal to the terminal bronchiole.	Lower lobe > upper lobes and apex

A combination of emphysema and bronchitis are found in patients with COPD. When emphysema is more predominant, loss of elastic recoil rather than bronchiolar inflammation is the mechanism of airflow limitation. When bronchitis is more predominant, bronchiolar inflammation is more responsible for airflow limitation.

• Is airflow obstruction reversible in COPD? Airflow obstruction in emphysema is irreversible. However, there is some degree of bronchial hyper-reactivity with bronchoconstriction due to inflammation in chronic bronchitis. This accounts for some degree of airflow obstruction reversibility in COPD. In patients with COPD, 30% of demonstrate an increase in FEV1 by 15% or more after bronchodilator therapy.

- What are the causes of COPD?
  - **Common causes**
    - Smoking   mixed centri-acinar and pan-acinar pattern
    - α_1 antitrypsin deficiency   pan-acinar pattern
    - Coal dust   centri-acinar pattern
  - **Rarer causes**
    - Swyer-James syndrome   a cause of unilateral emphysema (see page)
- How would you investigate this patient?
  - Bloods
    - FBC ($\uparrow$ white cell count (WCC) in infective exacerbations or may reflect chronic steroid use (neutrophilia); $\uparrow$ haemoglobin (Hb) in secondary polycythaemia)
    - Urea and electrolytes (U&E) (important to know K^+, especially with bronchodilator therapy, which will lower it)
    - LFT (hepatic involvement in α_1 antitrypsin deficiency)
    - Inflammatory markers (acute infective exacerbations)
    - Serum α_1 antitrypsin assay (for α_1 antitrypsin deficiency)*
  - CXR
    - Hyper-inflated lung fields with flattened hemidiaphrgams
    - Long narrow heart shadow
    - Hyperlucency of lung fields
    - Bullae
    - Increased retrosternal airspace in lateral films
    - Prominent hilar pulmonary vasculature (if pulmonary hypertension is present)
  - ECG
    Right ventricular hypertrophy +/− strain
    - Right atrial hypertrophy (P pulmonale)
    - Multifocal atrial tachycardia*
  - ABG
    - Type 2 respiratory failure (p_aO_2<8 and p_aCO_2>6)
    - Elevated HCO_3^- in chronic compensated respiratory acidosis in stable patients
    - Respiratory acidosis in acute exacerbations
    - Useful for deciding suitability for long-term oxygen therapy
  - Sputum
    - Microscopy culture and sensitivity
  - Lung function tests
    - FEV_1 < 80% predicted AND FEV_1:FVC < 70% (airflow obstruction)
    - $\uparrow$ TLC, FRC, and RV
    - $\downarrow$ vital capacity (VC)

---

* Always measure serum α_1 antitrypsin assay in patients aged < 40years, or those with a family history.

* This tachycardia is characterized by HR >100bpm, at least 3 different P wave morphologies with varying PR intervals. This is a benign arrhythmia and can be seen during acute exacerbations.

- $\downarrow T_LCO$ (carbon monoxide transfer factor) (decreased in proportion to severity of COPD)
- HRCT
  - The most sensitive technique for diagnosing emphysema, as sometimes bullae may not be seen on a chest radiograph.

What are the most common pathogens in acute infective exacerbations?
- *Streptococcus pneumoniae*
- *Haemophilus influenzae*
- *Moraxella catarrhalis*

How would you manage an acute infective exacerbation of COPD?
- 24% oxygen[a]
- Nebulized bronchodilators
- Antibiotics
- Steroids[b]
- Consider intravenous theophylline if poor response to nebulized bronchodilators
- Non-invasive ventilation for severe hypercapnoeic respiratory failure (pH<7.35)[c]
- Consider respiratory stimulants, i.e. doxapram if non-invasive ventilation is not available

What are the requirements for long-term oxygen therapy in patients with COPD?
Inappropriate oxygen therapy in patients with COPD may cause respiratory depression; therefore patients are selected carefully using the following criteria:

- Patients who have stopped smoking (carboxyhaemoglobin < 3%)

AND

- p_aO_2 < 7.3 when stable

OR

- p_aO_2 = 7.3–8.0 when stable and one of
  (a) secondary polycythaemia
  (b) pulmonary hypertension
  (c) peripheral oedema (cor pulmonale)
  (d) nocturnal hypoxaemia (S_aO_2<90% for >30% of the time)

Arterial blood gases should be measured when the patient is clinically stable and on two occasions which are at least 3 weeks apart. Oxygen should be given via a concentrator for at least 15 hours per day.

What do you know about α1 antitrypsin deficiency?
This is an autosomal dominant condition. The genetic defect is on chromosome 14, which encodes α_1 antitrypsin. The primary function of this enzyme is to inhibit neutrophils elastases.

---

[a] The aim of providing supplemental oxygen is to keep SaO_2 > 90% without worsening the hypercapnoea and precipitating respiratory acidosis.

[b] Intravenous hydrocortisone may be given initially, however oral prednisolone is used thereafter. In patients with acute exacerbations, the course of steroids should be continued for 7–14 days.

[c] Non-invasive ventilation is an alternative to endotracheal intubation, and avoids the complications of intubation. Non-invasive ventilation has been shown to reduce the need for endotracheal intubation, length of hospital stay, and in-hospital mortality.

There are three main phenotypes of this enzyme, which can be characterized by their electrophoretic mobility: M (medium), S (slow) and Z (very slow).

Phenotype	% normal serum α_1 antitrypsin levels
MM	100% (20–53mmol/L)
MS	80%
SS	60%
MZ	60%
SZ	40%
ZZ	10% (3–7mmol/L)

Serum levels >11mmol/L appear to be protective, and emphysema usually develops with serum levels <9mmol/L. The phenotypes ZZ and SZ are associated with severe deficiency. The hepatocytes synthesize α_1 antitrypsin. After its release, it circulates and diffuses into interstitial and alveolar fluids. The genetic defect results in alteration of the configuration of the α_1 antitrypsin molecule, which prevents its release from hepatocytes. As a result, the serum and alveolar concentrations of α_1 antitrypsin is low leading to destruction of lung tissue by the neutrophils elastases. The pattern of lung damage is pan-acinar with a predilection for the lower lobes. Furthermore, the accumulation of α_1 antitrypsin in the hepatocytes leads to destruction of these cells manifesting as chronic liver disease. Cigarette smoking accelerates the progression of emphysema in patients with α_1 antitrypsin deficiency (symptoms may develop 10 years earlier in smokers).

Treatment consists of smoking cessation, enzyme replacement therapy (if levels <11mmol/L), management of emphysema, lung transplantation (for severe emphysema), and liver transplantation (severe liver disease). Liver transplantation results in conversion to the genotype of the donor.

What is the general management of COPD?

These management guidelines are based on the NICE guidelines (2004):

- **General measures**
  - Stop smoking (may require pharmacological treatment)
  - Immunizations for influenza and pneumococcal pneumonia
  - Prompt treatment of respiratory infections (antibiotics and steroids)
- **Bronchodilator therapy**
  - Short-acting bronchodilator (β_2-agonist or anti-cholinergic)
  - If still symptomatic combine short-acting bronchodilators (β_2-agonist and anti-cholinergic)
  - If still symptomatic use long-acting bronchodilator (β_2-agonist or anti-cholinergic)
  - If still symptomatic combine long-acting bronchodilator (β_2-agonist or anti-cholinergic) and inhaled corticosteroids (discontinue steroids if no benefit after 4 weeks)
  - If still symptomatic consider adding theophylline
- **Anti-inflammatory therapy**
  - Use inhaled corticosteroids (as above)
  - Inhaled corticosteroids should be prescribed to patients with FEV_1 <50% predicted AND ≥2 infective exacerbations (requiring antibiotics and oral steroids) in a 12-month period
  - Long-term oral steroids are not usually recommended in COPD. Some patients with advanced COPD may require maintenance oral steroids when they cannot be withdrawn following an exacerbation.*

---

* An increase in FEV_1 ≥20% has been used as a surrogate marker for steroid response.

- *Mucolytic therapy*
    - Consider a trial in patients with chronic productive cough
    - Continue if symptomatic improvement
- *Long-term oxygen therapy*
    - See above for patient selection
    - Supplementary oxygen should be used for >15 hours/day (greater benefit if >20hours/day)
- *Treatment of cor pulmonale*
    - Diuretics for congestive symptoms
    - Appropriate treatment of pulmonary hypertension (see page)
- *Pulmonary rehabilitation (multidisciplinary programme)*
    - Patient education
    - Nutritional advice
    - Psychological support
    - Physcial training

What is the role of surgery in COPD?

Procedure	Notes
Bullectomy	Bullae can range from 1–4cm in size. Giant bullae can occupy 33% of the hemithorax. These can compress adjacent lung tissue, reducing blood flow and ventilation to healthier lung tissue. Bullectomy results in expansion of the compressed lung and improved function. Patients who have an FEV_1 <50% predicted have better outcomes after bullectomy.
Lung volume reduction surgery	Involves resection of 20–30% of each lung (most diseased areas, often in the upper zones). This results in ↑ FEV_1 (+82%), ↑ FVC (+27%), ↓ TLC, improved 6-minute walk distance and quality of life.
Lung transplantation	Criteria for patient selection are not yet established, but patients should have a life expectancy ≤ 2years due to COPD. Lung transplantation does not improve survival but improves quality of life.

Case 13 ◆ **Pleural Effusion**

CASE PRESENTATION

*This patient is not breathless at rest.[1] The patient does not appear cachectic and the nutritional status is good.[2] The fingers are not clubbed.[3] There is no evidence of nicotine staining.[4] There are no peripheral stigmata of rheumatological disease.[5] The venous pressure is not elevated.[6] There are no palpable lymph nodes.[7] The trachea is central.[8] On examination of the chest, there are no scars.[9] There is **reduced chest expansion** on the right. The **percussion note is stony dull** at the right base extending up to the right mid-zone, with **reduced vocal fremitus**. On auscultation the **breath sounds are diminished** in this area, with an area of **bronchial breathing above the area of dullness**.[10] There is no peripheral oedema.[11].*

*The diagnosis is a right **pleural effusion**.[12]*

Clinical notes

1. In approaching a respiratory patient, it is often useful in starting to present the case with a comment on functional status. They may be breathless at rest. They may be on oxygen therapy. Ask the patient to cough. The presence of a non-productive or a productive cough should give clues to underlying diagnosis. A productive cough may suggest underlying infection, bronchiectasis, or malignancy.

2. Cachexia may be present in a patient with malignancy. In the context of a pleural effusion, nutritional status is important to mention, as hypoalbuminaemia is an important cause of pleural effusions (often bilateral).

3. If the fingers are clubbed, then this provides a list of possible respiratory causes that should be looked for. Most importantly, one would need to consider malignancy as a cause of pleural effusion.

4. Nicotine staining would suggest possible underlying obstructive airways disease or malignancy.

5. Spend a little extra time when examining hands and making general observations. Rheumatological disease is an important cause of pleural effusions. If not present it is an important negative to mention.

6. An elevated venous pressure may reflect underlying pulmonary hypertension secondary to respiratory disease, or congestive cardiac failure as a cause of pleural effusion (often bilateral).

7. Palpable lymph nodes may suggest underlying infection or malignancy. Sarcoidosis is associated with lymphadenopathy.

8. The trachea is usually central, unless the pleural effusion is large, and the trachea is displaced to the opposite side. If the trachea is central in the context of a large pleural effusion, then this suggests underlying collapse.

9. Look carefully for scars for previous biopsies and intercostal drainage. Look for radiation burns, which would support an underlying malignancy.

10. The classical findings of a pleural effusion include: reduced chest expansion, stony dull percussion note, reduced vocal fremitus and reduced breath sounds with area of bronchial breathing above the effusion.

11. Peripheral oedema may be present in hypoalbuminaemic states or congestive cardiac failure.

12. If possible, try to determine the aetiology and present this in your findings. Common causes of pleural effusions in examinations include:

    *   **Carcinoma of the lung** (nicotine staining, clubbing, lymph nodes, radiation burns)
    *   **Lymphoma** (lymph nodes, radiation burns, hepatosplenomegaly)
    *   **Carcinoma of the breast** (breast lump, nipple changes, lymphadenopathy, previous mastectomy/lumpectomy)
    *   **Rheumatoid arthritis** (symmetrical deforming arthropathy of the hands, rheumatoid nodules)
    *   **SLE** (petechial rash, livedo reticularis, purpura, arthropathy, butterfly skin rash)
    *   **Chronic liver disease** (jaundice, ascites, peripheral oedema, and other stigmata of chronic liver disease)
    *   **Hypoalbuminaemia** (Cachexia, poor nutritional status, peripheral oedema)
    *   **Congestive cardiac failure** (raised venous pressure, third and fourth heart sound, peripheral oedema)

Questions commonly asked by examiners

What are the causes of a pleural effusion?

A pleural effusion can be broadly classified into a transudate (protein <30g/L) or an exudate (protein <30g/L).

Exudate (protein >30g/L)

- *Neoplasia*
  - ◆ Carcinoma of the lung
  - ◆ Secondary malignancy (breast, ovarian, pancreatic, and gastrointestinal)
  - ◆ Mesothelioma
  - ◆ Lymphoma
  - ◆ Meig's syndrome (ovarian fibroma)
- *Connective tissue disease*
  - ◆ Rheumatoid arthritis
  - ◆ SLE
- *Infection*
  - ◆ Pneumonia
  - ◆ Tuberculosis
- *Pulmonary infarction*
- *Sub-diaphragmatic*
  - ◆ Pancreatitis
  - ◆ Sub-phrenic abscess
  - ◆ Hepatic abscess
- *Drugs*
  - ◆ Practolol
  - ◆ Procarbazine
  - ◆ Methysergide
  - ◆ Bromocriptine
  - ◆ Methotrexate
  - ◆ Nitrofurantoin
- *Other*
  - ◆ Asbestosis
  - ◆ Sarcoidosis
  - ◆ Dressler's syndrome
  - ◆ Trauma
  - ◆ Oesophageal rupture (Borehave's syndrome)
  - ◆ Yellow nail syndrome
  - ◆ Chylothorax

Transudate (protein <30g/L)

- Congestive cardiac failure
- Constrictive pericarditis
- Hypoalbuminaemia
- Nephrotic syndrome
- Cirrhosis
- Peritoneal dialysis
- Uraemia
- Hypothyroidism

What volume of pleural fluid can be detected as a pleural effusion on a chest radiograph?

Standard chest radiographs can detect pleural fluid in excess of 180mL. The earliest sign is loss of costophrenic angle on the anterio-posterior (AP) view or loss of clear definition of the diaphragm posteriorly on the lateral view.

How could you confirm the suspicion of a small pleural effusion?

- Use a lateral decubitus view (fluid accumulates as a layer along dependent chest wall, unless loculated). If layering of fluid is 1cm thick, it indicates a pleural effusion greater than 200mLs
- Use ultrasonography (useful if loculated)

How is ultrasound useful in the context of pleural effusions?

- Detection of small pleural effusions
- Diagnosis of loculated pleural effusions
- Guiding pleural fluid aspiration or drainage
- Guiding pleural biopsy
- Differentiating pleural fluid from pleural thickening

What is the appearance and composition of normal pleural fluid?

- A clear ultrafiltrate of plasma
- pH = 7.60–7.64
- protein <1–2g/L (<2%)
- WCC <1000/mm^3
- Lactate dehydrogenase (LDH) <50% of plasma concentration
- Glucose similar to plasma concentration

What is the pathophysiology of a pleural effusion?

Normal pleural space contains approximately 1mL of fluid representing the balance between

- hydrostatic and oncotic forces in the visceral and parietal pleural vessels and
- extensive lymphatic drainage.

Pleural effusions result from disruption of this balance. The following mechanisms play a role in formation of a pleural effusion:

Mechanism	Examples
Altered permeability of pleural membranes	Inflammation, neoplasia, pulmonary embolism (PE)
Reduced intravascular oncotic pressure	Hypoalbuminaemia, cirrhosis, nephrotic syndrome
Increased capillary permeability or vascular disruption	Trauma, inflammation, neoplasia, infection, PE, uraemia, pancreatitis, drug hypersensitivity
Increased capillary hydrostatic pressure	Congestive cardiac failure, superior vena cava (SVC) obstruction
Decreased lymphatic drainage	Trauma, malignancy
Increased fluid in peritoneal cavity and migration across the diaphragm via lymphatics	Peritoneal dialysis, cirrhosis

What are Light's criteria for an exudate?

- Pleural fluid protein: serum protein >0.5
- Pleural fluid LDH: serum LDH >0.6
- Pleural fluid LDH >2/3 of the upper limit of normal serum value

In patients receiving chronic diuretic therapy, what precautions must be taken when interpreting pleural fluid results?

Chronic diuretic therapy increases the concentration of protein and LDH in the pleural fluid into the exudative range. To diagnose an exudate in this situation, the serum-effusion protein gradient (serum protein—effusion protein) should be used. If this is less than 31g/L, then this more correctly identifies an exudate.

What is the differential diagnosis of dullness and dull percussion note at a lung base?

- Pleural effusion
- Pleural thickening
- Collapse
- Consolidation
- Raised hemidiaphragm
- Lower lobe lobectomy (in the presence of thoracotomy scar)

If the pleural fluid LDH level >1000IU/L, what would that suggest?

- Empyema
- Malignant effusion
- Rheumatoid effusion
- Pleural paragonimiasis*

What are the causes of a haemorrhagic pleural effusion?

- Malignancy
- Pulmonary embolus
- Tuberculosis
- Chest trauma

How would you diagnose a chylothorax?

- Milky-white appearance of pleural fluid
- Pleural fluid cholesterol >4g/L

What are the causes of a chylothorax?

- Lymphatic obstruction (lymphoma or solid tumours)
- Lymphatic damage (post cardiothoracic surgery)
- Nephrotic syndrome
- Cirrhosis

What are the causes of low glucose concentration in pleural fluid?

- Malignancy
- Empyema
- Tuberculosis
- Oesophageal rupture
- Rheumatoid arthritis
- SLE

---

* Paragonimus westermani infection is an important endemic disease in Asia, and many immigrants with paragonimiasis have been reported in the developed world. The infection is acquired through ingestion of raw freshwater crayfish or crabs. Radiographic abnormalities include segmental or diffuse infiltrates, cavities, nodules, and pleural effusions.

What are the causes of low pH of pleural fluid?

The pleural fluid pH has a strong correlation with pleural fluid glucose concentration. If the pleural fluid pH <7.3, with a normal arterial blood pH, then the causes are the same for low glucose concentration.

What are the causes of an elevated amylase in pleural fluid?

- Pancreatitis
- Malignancy
- Bacterial pneumonia
- Oesophageal rupture

What is the significance of a low pH (<7.3) in the context of a malignant pleural effusion?

- More extensive pleural involvement
- Higher yield on cytology
- Decreased success rate of pleurodesis
- Shorter life expectancy

How reliable is pleural fluid biochemistry and microbiology in the diagnosis of tuberculous pleuritis?

- As most tuberculous pleural effusions result from a hypersensitivity reaction to the mycobacterium rather than microbial invasion, acid-fast bacillus stains of pleural fluid are rarely diagnostic (<10% of cases) and pleural fluid cultures grow *Mycobacterium tuberculosis* in 65% of cases.
- The combination of histology of pleural tissue (pleural biopsy) and culture increases the diagnostic yield to 90%.
- Adenosine deaminase activity (ADA) >43U/mL supports the diagnosis of tuberculosis. However sensitivity is 78%, and thus values less than 43U/mL do not exclude tuberculous pleuritis.
- Interferon-gamma concentration in pleural fluid >140pg/mL also supports tuberculous pleuritis, but this test is not routinely available.

How would you investigate a patient with pleural effusion?

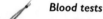

Blood tests
  - FBC
  - U&Es
  - LFTs
  - Serum albumin and lipid profiles
  - Serum LDH
  - Serum amylase
  - Thyroid function tests
  - Rheumatoid factor
  - Autoimmune profile (ANA, ENA and ANCA)
- **Chest radiograph**
- **Arterial blood gas sampling**
- **Pleural tap**
  - Protein, LDH, glucose, and pH
  - Amylase (if pancreatitis, malignancy, or oesophageal rupture suspected)

- ◆ Cholesterol (if chylothorax is suspected)
- ◆ Cytology
- ◆ Microscopy and culture
- ◆ Ziehl-Neelson staining and mycobacterial culture (if tuberculosis is suspected)
- ◆ Rheumatoid factor and ANA (if autoimmune disorder is suspected)

Other tests may be indicated for further evaluation and/or determining the cause:

- **Pleural biopsy** (if tuberculosis of malignancy suspected)
- **CT pulmonary angiography** (if pulmonary embolus suspected)
- **CT chest** (if lung malignancy or lymphoproliferative disorder is suspected)
- **Bronchoscopy** (if malignancy is suspected)
- **Echocardiogram** (if cardiac failure suspected)
- **Mammogram** (in females if a primary breast malignancy is suspected)
- **CT abdomen** (if lymphoproliferative, gastrointestinal, or renal malignancy suspected)

What are the complications of pleural fluid drainage?
- Pneumothorax
- Haemothorax
- Hypovolaemia
- Unilateral pulmonary oedema

What are the indications for pleurodesis?
- Recurrent malignant pleural effusions
- Recurrent pneumothoraces

What agents can be used for chemical pleurodesis?
- Talc (most effective sclerosing agent)
- Doxycyline
- Bleomycin
- Zinc sulphate
- Quinacrine hydrochloride

Case 14 ◆ **Bronchiectasis**

CASE PRESENTATION

This patient is (is not) breathless at rest and has a **productive cough**.[1] *There is no evidence of cyanosis.*[2] **Inspiratory clicks** *can be heard with the unaided ear.*[3] *The* **fingers are clubbed**.[4] *There is no evidence of nicotine staining.*[5] *The venous pressure is not elevated.*[6] *There are no palpable lymph nodes.*[7] *The trachea is central and the cricoid-notch distance is not reduced.*[7] *On examination of the chest there are no scars.*[8] *Chest expansion is normal.*[9] *The percussion note is resonant throughout both lung fields.*[10] *Vocal fremitus is normal.*[11] *On auscultation there are* **coarse inspiratory crepitations** *at the right base and the* **characteristics of the crackles alter with coughing**.[12] *There is widespread* **expiratory wheeze**.[13] *There is no peripheral oedema and there are no signs of pulmonary hypertension.*

The diagnosis is right basal **bronchiectasis**.[14]

Clinical notes

1. In approaching a respiratory patient, it is often useful in starting to present the case with a comment on functional status. They may be breathless at rest. They may be on oxygen therapy. Ask the patient to cough. This may help differentiate the crackles of bronchiectasis and pulmonary fibrosis. Bronchiectasis is associated with copious purulent sputum and recurrent haemoptysis. **Look for the sputum pot by the bedside.**

2. Cyanosis signifies advanced disease.

3. Inspiratory clicks may be heard from the end of the bed. If heard, they are characteristic of bronchiectasis.

4. The fingers may not always be clubbed. It is more frequent in moderate–severe bronchiectasis.

5. Look for nicotine staining. Although smoking is not always associated with bronchiectasis, it is associated with carcinoma of the lung—an important differential diagnosis for the above clinical finding (productive cough, clubbing, and coarse crackles). Most patients with bronchiectasis seen in clinics also have COPD. In up to 30% of patients with COPD, bronchiectasis is present, and can be confirmed by CT.

6. Look for pulmonary hypertension, in long-standing cases of bronchiectasis.

7. Palpable lymph nodes may be present in carcinoma of the lung—an important differential diagnosis. Lymphadenopathy is also a feature of sarcoidosis and tuberculosis, which are associated with bronchiectasis.

8. Bronchiectasis can be associated with hyperinflation (reduced cricoid-notch distance). Remember, 30% of patients with COPD have bronchiectasis. In cases of unilateral involvement, the associated fibrosis, reduction in lung volumes and presence of collapse, may lead to tracheal deviation to the affected side.

9. Chest expansion is often normal. However, in long standing cases with fibrosis and reduction in lung volumes, chest expansion may be reduced over the areas of involvement.

10. Percussion note findings are variable. It may be dull over bronchiectatic areas, especially if fibrosis, collapse, or consolidation is present.

11. Vocal fremitus findings are variable. It may be normal. It may be reduced, especially if underlying collapse is present. It may be increased if coexistent pneumonia (consolidation) is present.

12. The hallmark auscultatory findings are coarse crepitations, which alter with coughing. They may occur during late inspiration, span throughout inspiration or present during both inspiration and expiration. Bronchiectasis is more commonly a focal process involving a lobe, segment, or subsegment of the lung, and therefore the crackles are often localized to these areas. The most common sites for localized disease are the left lower lobe and the lingula. However, it may be a diffuse process and crackles may therefore be diffuse. It is important to state the extent and localization of crackles, i.e. bronchiectatic involvement.

13. Scattered wheeze may be present in up to a third of cases. This may be due to airway obstruction from secretions, masses, lymphadenopathy, granulomata; airway destruction leading to collapsibility; or presence of co-existent obstructive airways disease.

14. The presence of a productive cough, clubbing, and coarse crackles has the following differential diagnosis:

    (a) **Bronchiectasis** (inspiratory clicks)

    (b) **Carcinoma of the lung** (nicotine staining, lymphadenopathy)

    (c) **Lung abscess**

    (d) **Pulmonary fibrosis** (the crackles are usually less coarse [usually bilateral and symmetrical], non-productive cough—though productive cough may occur with super-added infection).

*   The presence of inspiratory clicks would favour bronchiectasis. In pulmonary fibrosis, the distribution and pattern of crackles is usually bilateral and symmetrical. If the crackles are localized suggesting particular area(s) of bronchiectasis, then always state the area(s) of

involvement. If inspiratory clicks are not heard, it would be better to present the clinical findings and present the above differential diagnosis list, stating the clinical signs and features favouring each diagnosis.

Questions commonly asked by examiners

What are the causes of bronchiectasis?

- **Respiratory childhood infections**
  - Pertussis
  - Measles
  - Tuberculosis
- **Bronchial obstruction**
  - Foreign body
  - Chronic aspiration
  - Endobronchial tumour
  - Lymph nodes (tuberculosis, sarcoidosis, and malignancy)
  - Granulomata (tuberculosis, sarcoidosis, Chediak-Higashi syndrome)
- **Fibrosis**
  - Long-standing pulmonary fibrosis
  - Fibrosis complicating tuberculosis and sarcoidosis
  - Fibrosis complicating unresolved or suppurative pneumonia
- **Muco-ciliary clearance defects**
  - Cystic fibrosis
  - Immotile cilia syndrome
  - Kartagener's syndrome — *Situs inversus, Chronic sinusitis, Bronchiectasis*
  - Young syndrome
- **Immunodeficiency**
  - Congenital and acquired hypogammaglobulinaemia
  - Acquired Immunodeficiency syndrome (AIDS)
- **Allergic bronchopulmonary aspergillosis** *ABPA*
- **Autoimmune disease**
  - Rheumatoid arthritis (Rheumatoid lung)
  - Sjogren syndrome
  - Inflammatory bowel disease (ulcerative colitis>Crohn's disease)
- **Congenital anatomical defects** *Congenital Bronchiectasis*
  - Bronchopulmonary sequestration
  - William-Campbell syndrome
  - Mounier-Kuhn syndrome
  - Swyer-James syndrome
  - Yellow nail syndrome *(Primary Lymphoedema)* — *Pleural effusion, Lymphoedema, Yellow Dystrophic Nails, Bronchiectasis*
- **Idiopathic**

What is the pathophysiology of bronchiectasis?

- Abnormal bronchial wall *dilatation*, *destruction*, and transmural *inflammation*.
- This abnormal dilatation of the proximal and medium sized bronchi (diameter >2mm) is caused by destruction of the muscular and elastic components of the bronchial walls. This leads to inflammation, oedema, scarring, and ulceration of bronchial walls.

- Severely impaired clearance of secretions causes colonization and infection. This results in further bronchial damage, dilatation, impaired clearance of secretions, recurrent infections, and more bronchial damage (a vicious cycle).

What do you understand by the term 'traction bronchiectasis'?

This is the distortion of airways secondary to mechanical traction on the bronchi from fibrosis of the surrounding lung parenchyma. This leads to airway dilatation and bronchiectasis. Traction bronchiectasis is seen in the setting of pulmonary fibrosis.

What are the complications of bronchiectasis?

- Pneumonia
- Pneumothorax
- Empyema
- Collapse
- Metastatic cerebral abscess
- Respiratory failure
- Pulmonary hypertension
- Amyloidosis

Is bronchiectasis associated with smoking?

Smoking per se is not associated with bronchiectasis, and most patients with bronchiectasis have never smoked (55%). However, smoking is associated with COPD, and 30% of patients with COPD have evidence of bronchiectasis on CT.

What is the cause and significance of wheeze in a patient with bronchiectasis?

The presence of wheeze often signifies airway obstruction. The causes of wheeze in bronchiectasis include:

- Airway collapsibility (destruction of muscular and elastic components in bronchial walls)
- Airway obstruction (secretions, lymph nodes, granulomata, malignancy)
- Co-existent obstructive airways disease

How can the anatomical distribution of bronchiectasis help diagnose the cause or associated condition in bronchiectasis?

Cause of bronchiectasis	Common anatomical distribution of bronchiectasis
Infection	Lower lobes, right middle lobe, and the lingula
Obstruction	Right middle lobe
Tuberculosis, chronic fungal infections	Upper lobes
Allergic bronchopulmonary aspergillosis	Upper lobes; involves central bronchi (proximal bronchiectasis) whereas most other forms of bronchiectasis involve distal bronchial segments.

What is the role of CT in diagnosing bronchiectasis?

High-resolution CT scanning (resolution is 1–2mm thickness compared to 10mm thickness in standard CT) is the gold standard for diagnosing bronchiectasis, and has replaced bronchoscopy as the defining modality of bronchiectasis. The 'signet ring sign': bronchial diameter greater than adjacent vessel diameter.

What would the spirometry findings be in this patient?

- Pulmonary function tests may be normal
- Most common abnormality is an obstructive pattern (FEV_1: FVC <70%).

- The obstruction is not always reversible with bronchodilator therapy. A small subgroup of patients may have airway hyper-reactivity that will respond to bronchdilator therapy
- In severe advanced disease, there may be a restrictive pattern (FEV_1: FVC >70%) secondary to scarring and atelectasis. A restrictive pattern may occur with underlying pulmonary fibrosis.

What are the most common respiratory pathogens in patients with bronchiectasis?

- *Staphylococcus aureus*
- *Haemophilus influenzae*
- *Pseudomonas aeruginosa*
- *Streptococcus pneumoniae*
- *Klebsiella pneumoniae*
- *Aspergillus species*

What do you know about the different conditions associated with bronchiectasis?

(a) Cystic fibrosis

An autosomal recessive condition, occurring in 1 in 2500 individuals. Characterized by defect on chromosome 7 (ΔF508 mutation in 75% of cases) that encodes the CFTR chloride channel, which plays an important role in secretory function in the nasal epithelium, lungs, salivary glands, pancreas, intestines, and bile duct.

- **Respiratory manifestations**: nasal polyps, otitis media, asthma, bronchiolitis, recurrent pneumonia, and bronchiectasis
- **Gastrointestinal manifestations**: meconium ileus (birth), rectal prolapse (neonate), malabsorption, steatorrhea, meconium ileus equivalent (adults), gallstones, and secondary biliary cirrhosis
- **Other manifestations**: non-erosive arthropathy, infertility (males)

(b) Allergic bronchopulmonary aspergillosis

This results from a hypersensitivity reaction to *Aspergillus fumigatus* in patients with asthma or cystic fibrosis. Excessive mucus production in association with impaired ciliary function leads to mucoid impaction of the airways. These plugs of insipissated mucus contain the organism and eosinophils, but the organisms remain in the bronchial lumen, characterizing this from invasive aspergillosis. Precipitating antibodies produce a type I hypersensitivity reaction with release of IgE and IgG immunoglobulins. The immune complexes and inflammatory cells are then deposited within the bronchial mucosa. This incites a type III reaction resulting in damage to the bronchial walls with subsequent development of bronchial dilatation and bronchiectasis in the proximal bronchi.

(c) Chediak-Higashi syndrome

An autosomal recessive condition. This is a granulation disorder of lysosomes with reduced myeloperoxidase secretion. This leads to a chronic granulomatous disease of the lungs. Death usually occurs by 10 years of age.

(d) Yellow nail syndrome

A disorder characterized by slow growing, excessively curved (both longitudinal and transverse), and thickened yellow nails. Other features include exudative pleural effusions, bronchiectasis, sinusitis, and lymphoedema.

(e) William-Campbell syndrome

Congenital absence of cartilage and a cause of bronchiectasis in the young.

(f) Immotile cilia syndrome (Primary ciliary dyskinesia)

This is an autosomal recessive disorder. Characterized by recurrent chronic sinusitis, recurrent otitis media, nasal polyps, hypoplastic frontal sinuses, chronic bronchitis, obstructive airways disease, immotile cilia, bronchiectasis (lower lobes), and infertility. The underlying cause is a defect in the cilia (axonemal dynein heavy chain protein-DNAH5) making them unable to beat.

(g) Kartagener's syndrome

This is an autosomal recessive disorder, being a variant of immotile cilia syndrome. It has all the features of immotile cilia syndrome *plus* dextrocardia and situs invertus (50% of cases).

(h) Young syndrome

This disorder is characterized by excessively thick mucous, but ciliary activity is normal. This is characterized by a triad of bronchiectasis, rhino-sinusitis, and male infertility.

(i) Mounier-Kuhn syndrome

This is also known as tracheobronchmegaly. This disorder is characterized by multiple tracheal diverticulae associated with marked dilatation of the trachea and main bronchi, bronchiectasis, and recurrent respiratory infections.

(j) Swyer-James Syndrome (MacLeod syndrome)

A manifestation of post-infectious bronchiolitis, resulting in diminished vascualrity, arrest of progressive growth and alveolarization of the affected lung. This results in a resultant hypoplastic lung. Radiologically, there is pulmonary hyperlucency caused by over-distended alveoli and diminished arterial flow characteristics. Organisms causing the infection include respiratory synctial virus, mycoplasma, influenza virus, staphylococcal, and streptococcal infections. Remember, the lung grows by progressive alveolarization in the first 2–8 years of life, after which growth is by hyper-expansion of existing alveoli.

How would you manage this patient?

- **General measures**
  - Stop smoking
  - Adequate nutritional intake and supplementation if necessary
  - Immunizations for influenza and pneumococcal pneumonia
  - Confirm immunity to measles, pertussis, and rubella
  - Long-term oxygen therapy in advanced cases
  - Multi-disciplinary management addressing all aspects of disease in cystic fibrosis
- **Antibiotics**
  - Oral, parenteral, or nebulized antibiotics (depending on clinical situation)
  - Nebulized tobramycin for pseudomonas infections in cystic fibrosis
- **Postural drainage and physiotherapy**
  - Postural drainage with percussion and vibration
  - Other devices to help with mucous clearance include flutter devices and pneumatic compression devices
  - Nebulized saline and mucolytics
  - Maintaining good hydration reduces the viscosity of secretions
  - Nebulized recombinant DNase in patients with cystic fibrosis
- **Bronchodilator therapy**
- **Anti-inflammatory medication**
  - Inhaled or oral corticosteroids

- **Surgery**
  - ◆ Surgical resection for localized bronchiectasis (poorly controlled by antibiotics)
  - ◆ Bronchial artery embolization for massive haemoptysis
  - ◆ Foreign body or tumour removal
  - ◆ Lung transplantation in patients with cystic fibrosis.

Case 15 ◆ **Carcinoma of the Lung**

Examiner's notes

Carcinoma of the lung can present in many ways in the examination, with a wide spectrum of clinical signs. The presentations often include:

- pleural effusion
- collapse/consolidation
- Pancoast tumour

Sometimes, there may be no respiratory signs, and the only positive clinical findings may be cachexia, finger clubbing, nicotine staining, and possibly lymphadenopathy. Look carefully for the sputum pot by the bedside. There may be a history of weight loss from the examination instructions. The key is put all the findings together, and if the diagnosis is not clear, present a differential diagnosis for the clinical findings. The presence of cachexia, productive cough, finger clubbing, and nicotine staining would put carcinoma of the lung high on the differential diagnosis list.

CASE PRESENTATION 1

This **cachectic patient** has a **productive cough** and is breathless at rest.[1] The fingers are **clubbed**.[2] There is **nicotine staining** of the fingers.[3] There is a **palpable lymph node** in the left supraclavicular fossa.[5] The venous pressure is not elevated.[6] The trachea is central and the cricoid-notch distance is not reduced.[8] On examination of the chest there are no scars.[9] There is **reduced chest expansion** on the left. The **percussion note is stony dull** at the left base extending up to the left mid-zone, with **reduced vocal fremitus**. On auscultation the **breath sounds are diminished** in this area, with an area of **bronchial breathing above the area of dullness**.[10] There is no peripheral oedema.

The diagnosis is a left **pleural effusion**, most likely secondary to **carcinoma of the lung**.

CASE PRESENTATION 2

This **cachectic patient** has a **productive cough** and is breathless at rest.[1] The fingers are **clubbed**.[2] There is **nicotine staining** of the fingers.[3] There is **wasting of the small muscles of the right hand** with **reduced sensation in the C8-T1 dermatomes**.[4] There are **palpable lymph nodes** in the right axilla and supraclavicular fossa.[5] The venous pressure is not elevated.[6] There is right partial ptosis, miosis, and anhidrosis, constituting a **right Horner's syndrome**[7]. The **trachea is deviated to the right** and the cricoid-notch distance is not reduced.[8] On examination of the chest there is a **radiation burn** on the right upper chest wall.[9] There is **reduced chest expansion** of the right upper chest, where the **percussion note is dull** and the **vocal fremitus is increased**. On auscultation there is **bronchial breathing** over this area.[10] There is no peripheral oedema.

The diagnosis is a right **Pancoast syndrome** due to a right **apical carcinoma of the lung**, with associated **collapse and consolidation**. This patient has had **radiotherapy**.

Clinical notes

1. Comment on the general appearance of the patient. Cachexia may be noticeable from standing at the end of the bed. Otherwise, a cachectic state may be demonstrated by a poor nutritional status from a reduced tricep fat fold thickness that can be easily assessed during the examination. Don't forget to ask the patient to cough. Don't miss the sputum pot by the bedside. When introducing yourself to the patient, try to make deductions about the character of the patient's voice. Hoarseness may occur with left-sided lesions and involvement of the recurrent laryngeal nerve.

2. Carcinoma of the bronchus is an important respiratory cause of clubbing. Look for the tender swollen wrist joints suggesting hypertrophic pulmonary osteoarthropathy.

3. Smoking is strongly associated with carcinoma of the lung. In certain cases, nicotine staining may not be evident. Remember, not all forms of carcinoma are associated with smoking. Furthermore, if patients have stopped smoking for many years, nicotine staining may gradually disappear.

4. With Pancoast tumours, involvement of the C8-T1 nerve roots will give rise to wasting of small muscles of the hands. There may be sensory loss associated with these dermatomes.

5. Feel carefully for cervical, supraclavicular, and axillary lymph nodes. There may be scars in the supraclavicular fossa, suggesting previous lymph node biopsy.

6. Fixed engorged neck veins would suggest SVC obstruction.

7. With Pancoast tumours, involvement of the cervical sympathetic chain will lead to an ipsilateral Horner's syndrome: miosis, partial ptosis, and anhidrosis. Look carefully for this with apical lesions.

8. The trachea may be deviated to the opposite side with large pleural effusions, unless there is underlying collapse. The trachea may be deviated to the ipsilateral side with collapse. Ipsilateral tracheal deviation is often more pronounced with apical carcinomas. Often patients with respiratory malignancy have a smoking history, and it is not uncommon to have coexistent COPD, in which case the cricoid-notch distance will be reduced.

9. Don't miss scars (previous lobectomy, pneumonectomy, lung biopsy, or thoracocentesis) or radiation burns on the chest wall.

10. Findings on examination will reflect the underlying pathological process. This could be a pleural effusion, lung collapse, or consolidation. There may be signs of underlying COPD: hyper-expanded lung fields, intercostal recession, prolonged expiratory phase of the respiratory cycle and expiratory wheeze.

Questions commonly asked by examiners

How are bronchial carcinomas classified?
There are 2 broad classifications:

Small cell carcinoma (SCLC)
Account for 20% of lung cancers and are the most aggressive and rapidly growing of all lung cancers. Also known at **oat cell carcinoma**. They arise from Kulchitsy cells (members of amine precursor uptake and decarboxylation (APUD) system) and secrete many polypeptide hormones. Often considered a systemic disease. About 60–70% of patients have disseminated disease at presentation.

Non-small cell carcinoma (NSCLC)

Most common, and account for 80%, of all lung cancers. They can be further classified based on the cells that make up the tumour:

Adenocarcinoma	Most common type, accounting for 50% of NSCLC; occurs in non-smokers as well as smokers; often in outer or peripheral lung areas
Bronchoalveolar carcinoma	A subtype of adenocarcinoma that develops at multiple sites; spreads along the pre-existing alveolar walls.
Squamous cell carcinoma	Account for 30% of NSCLC; also known as **epidermoid carcinomas**. Often cavitating lesions.
Large cell carcinoma	The least common type to NSCLC; also known as **undifferentiated carcinomas**.

What are the risk factors for lung cancers?

- Smoking
- Interstitial lung disease
- Radon (radioactive gases released by granite; occupants of houses)*
- Asbestos*
- Arsenic*
- Chromium*
- Iron Oxide*
- Coal tar*
- Radiation

Which lung cancers have the strongest link with smoking?

Although smoking is a strong risk factor for all lung cancers, SCLC and squamous cell carcinoma have the strongest correlation with smoking.

What do you know about the TNM classification system for lung cancers?

The TNM classification system takes into account the degree of spread of primary tumour (T); extent of lymph node involvment (N); and presence or absence of metastases (M).

Primary tumour (T)

Tx	Positive malignant cytology findings, but no identifiable lesion
Tis	Carcinoma in situ
T1	Diameter <3cm and surrounded by lung tissue
T2	Diameter >3cm, invasion of the pleura, involvement of main bronchus (>2cm from carina), lung atelectasis
T3	Extrapulmonary extension with limited involvement of parietal or mediastinal pleura, fat, pericardium, and diaphragm; involvement of main bronchus (<2cm from carina)
T4	Extrapulmonary extension with involvement of mediastinal structures, great vessels or vertebral bodies; SVC obstruction; recurrent laryngeal or phrenic nerve involvement; malignant pleural or pericardial effusion.

---

* These occupational exposures are associated with adenocarcinomas, which are less related to smoking

Lymph nodes (N)

N0	No nodal involvement
N1	Ipsilateral intrapulmonary nodal involvement
N2	Ipsilateral mediastinal of hilar nodal involvement
N3	Contralateral nodal involvement or any scalene or supraclavicular nodal involvement

Metastases (M)

M0	No metastases
M1	Metastases present

What do you know about staging of lung cancers?

The TNM classification can be incorporated into a staging system. This aims to highlight candidates suitable for surgical resection and provide prognosis. Generally:

* **STAGE I**   confined to the lung
* **STAGES II and III**   confined to the chest (larger and more invasive tumours classed as III)
* **STAGE IV**   spread beyond the chest involving other parts of the body

Stage	TNM Classification			5-year survival (%)
	T	N	M	
IA	1	0	0	75
IB	2	0	0	55
IIA	1	1	0	50
IIB	2	1	0	40
IIIA	3	any	0	10–35% (technically resectable)
	any	2	0	
IIIB	any	3	0	5% (technically not resectable)
	4	any	0	
IV	any	any	1	<1%

How would you investigate this patient?

Blood tests

* FBC: anaemia of chronic disease, thrombocytopaenia
* Clotting profile: disseminated intravascular coagulation (DIC)
* U&E: hyponatraemia (syndrome of inappropriate anti-diuretic hormone—SIADH), hypokalaemic alkalosis (ectopic adrenocorticotrophic hormone (ACTH) production)
* Calcium: hypercalcaemia (bony metastases or PTHrP production)
* LFT: may be deranged with hepatic metastases, raised ALP with bony metastases

CXR

* May identify location and size of tumour
* May present with collapse, consolidation, or pleural effusion
* Raised hemidiaphragm with phrenic nerve involvement

Urinalysis

* Proteinuria (membranous glomerulonephritis)

Sputum cytology

- Good yield for endobronchial tumours, i.e. squamous cell carcinoma and SCLC, and poor yield for peripheral tumours, i.e. adenocarcinoma

Pleural fluid

- Haemorrhagic pleural fluid aspirate
- Exudate
- Low pH (<7.3)
- Low glucose
- Raised amylase
- Cytology

Computed tomography (CT)

- Contrast-enhanced helical CT of the thorax, abdomen (includes liver and adrenals) is the standard investigation for staging lung tumours.

Pulmonary function tests

- An FEV_1 <1.5 is contraindication for surgical resection

Bronchoscopy

- Brushings, washings, and biopsies may be obtained

Positron emission tomography (PET)

- PET is superior to CT in the assessment of mediastinal nodal metastases

Bone scan

- If bone metastases are suspected

What do you know of the paraneoplastic manifestations of lung cancers?

paraneoplastic syndromes are clinical syndromes involving non-metastatic systemic effects that accompany malignant disease. They commonly occur with SCLCs.

Endocrine

- SIADH (ectopic ADH hormone production)
- Cushing syndrome (ectopic ACTH production)
- Hypercalcaemia (ectopic PTH-related peptide production)*
- Hyperthyroidism (ectopic thyroid stimulating hormone (TSH) production)
- Hypoglycaemia (ectopic insulin-like growth factor production)

Neurological

- Lambert-Eaten myasthenic syndrome (pre-synaptic V-gated Ca^{2+} channel antibodies)
- Subacute cerebellar degeneration (anti-Yo or anti-purkinje cell antibody, APCA-1)
- Sensory neuropathy (anti-Hu antibody)
- Limbic encephalopathy (anti-Hu and anti-Yo antibodies)

Musculoskeletal

- Polymyositis/Dermatomyositis
- Clubbing
- Hypertrophic pulmonary osteoarthropathy*

---

* Occurs most frequently with squamous cell carcinomas
* Occurs most frequently with adenocarcinomas and squamous cell carcinomas

Cutaneous

- Acanthosis nigricans
- Gynaecomastia (ectopic HCG production)*
- Thrombophlebitis
- Thrombosis (Trousseau syndrome)**
- Ichthyosis
- Hypertrichosis
- Herpes zoster

What do you know about Pancoast tumours?

These are apical lung tumours that erode the ribs and involve the lower part of the brachial plexus (C8–T1), cervical sympathetic nerves, and ganglion. This results in ipsilateral wasting of the small muscles of the hand, ipsilateral sensory disturbances in the C8–T1 dermatomes and an ipsilateral Horner's syndrome.

What is the general management of lung cancer?

Surgery

- This is the treatment of choice for NSCLC
- Patients with SCLC often have disseminated disease at presentation, thus not suitable for surgical resection

Chemotherapy

- This is the treatment of choice for SCLC
- It can be used in NSCLC
- Can be given alone, adjuvant to surgical therapy, or in combination with radiotherapy

Radiotherapy

- Can be used for both SCLC and NSCLC
- Can be administered by external beam radiotherapy or endobronchial therapy (brachytherapy)
- Indications for radiotherapy include: bone pain, bronchial obstruction, dysphagia, haemoptysis, SVC obstruction, and Pancoast's tumour.

What treatment modalities are available for palliative care?

- Analgesia (may necessitate regular opioids)
- Steroids (increase appetite)
- Antidepressants
- Anxiolytics
- Palliative radiotherapy (bone pain, intractable cough, or haemoptysis)
- Thoracocentesis and pleurodesis (recurrent malignant pleural effusions)
- Endobronchial laser therapy (inoperable intraluminal tumours)
- Tracheobronchial stents

---

* Occurs most commonly with squamous cell carcinomas.

** Trousseau syndrome is vascular thrombosis occurring at, at least, 2 different sites. This is due to hypercaogulability, and occurs more frequently with adenocarcinomas.

Case 16 ◆ Lobectomy and Pneumonectomy

CASE PRESENTATION 1

*This patient is not breathless at rest. The fingers are not clubbed.[1] There is no evidence of nicotine staining.[2] The venous pressure is not elevated. There are no palpable lymph nodes.[3] The **trachea is deviated to the right**.[4] On inspection of the chest, there is a **thoracotomy scar on the right** and the **right lower ribs are pulled in**.[5] The **apex beat is displaced to the right**.[6] Chest expansion is reduced in the right lower zone.[7] The **percussion note is dull** and **breath sounds are reduced** in this area.[8] There is no peripheral oedema.*

*The diagnosis is **right-sided lobectomy** (lower or middle lobe).[10]*

CASE PRESENTATION 2

*This patient is not breathless at rest. The fingers are not clubbed.[1] There is no evidence of nicotine staining.[2] The venous pressure is not elevated. There are no palpable lymph nodes.[3] The **trachea is deviated to the left**.[4] On inspection of the chest, there is a **thoracotomy scar on the left** and the **left upper ribs are pulled in**.[5] The **apex beat is displaced to the left**.[6] Chest expansion is reduced in the left upper zone.[7] The **percussion note is dull** and **breath sounds are reduced** in this area.[8] There is **bronchial breathing in the left upper zone** over the deviated trachea.[9] There is no peripheral oedema.*

*The diagnosis is **left-sided lobectomy** (upper lobe).[10]*

CASE PRESENTATION 3

*This patient is not breathless at rest. The fingers are not clubbed.[1] There is no evidence of nicotine staining.[2] The venous pressure is not elevated. There are no palpable lymph nodes.[3] The **trachea is grossly deviated to the left**.[4] On inspection of the chest, there is a **thoracotomy scar on the left** with **flattening of the left chest wall**.[5] The **apex beat is displaced to the left**.[6] Chest expansion is reduced on the left.[7] The **percussion note is dull throughout the left hemithorax** and where the breath sounds are absent.[8] There is **bronchial breathing in the left upper zone** over the grossly deviated trachea.[9] There is no peripheral oedema.*

*The diagnosis is a **left pneumonectomy**.[10]*

Clinical notes

1. Look for finger clubbing, as it can provide a clue to the indication for lobectomy or pneumonectomy. Fingers may be clubbed in patients with a history of bronchiectasis, interstitial lung disease, or malignancy.
2. Nicotine staining may suggest a previous history of malignancy.
3. Palpable lymph nodes may suggest underlying malignancy.
4. In patients with a pneumonectomy, the trachea will be deviated (often grossly) to the affected side. Tracheal deviation is a variable finding in a patient with previous lobectomy. In patients with upper

lobectomy, the trachea is often deviated to the affected side. However, the trachea may or may not be deviated in a patient with right and left lower lobectomy, or right middle lobectomy.

5. Always take extra time inspecting the chest. A lot can be deduced from the scars and deformity of the chest wall. In a patient with pneumonectomy, there is flattening of the whole affected side with absent visible chest expansion on that side. In a patient with lobectomy, the signs are often localized. Ribs may be pulled in corresponding to the site of lobectomy.

6. The apex beat may be impalpable in some patients, but is displaced to the affected side, reflecting mediastinal shift.

7. Chest expansion is reduced (absent) throughout the hemithorax in a patient with pneumonectomy. Chest expansion will be reduced locally corresponding to the site in a patient with lobectomy: upper zones (upper lobectomy), lower zones (middle and lower lobectomy).

8. The key feature differentiating pneumonectomy and lobectomy is ABSENT breath sounds throughout the hemithorax in a patient with pneumonectomy. In a patient with lobectomy, the breath sounds are only reduced, often locally corresponding to the site of lobectomy. The percussion note will be dull in the affected areas. Look for signs in the other lung field, providing clues to the underlying diagnosis and possible indication for lobectomy/pneumonectomy, i.e. the fine end-inspiratory crackles of interstitial lung disease, the coarse crackles of bronchiectasis, or the expiratory wheeze of obstructive airways disease.

9. Bronchial breathing is heard over the deviated trachea. Remember the trachea will always be deviated in a patient with pneumonectomy. This may not always be the case with a lobectomy.

10. When presenting the diagnosis, it may be possible to provide an indication for the lobectomy/ pneumonectomy, if clinical signs of the underlying condition are present. The affected side in a patient with lobectomy/pneumonectomy is straightforward. Given the localized signs associated with lobectomy, it is often possible to comment on which lobe has been removed. Sometimes this may not be possible, and it is best to present it simply as a 'right/left-sided lobectomy'. In cases where signs are clearly localized, upper zone signs would signify an upper lobectomy. In cases with localized lower zone signs on the left, then a diagnosis of left lower lobectomy can be made. However, in cases with localized lower zone signs on the right, this may reflect a right middle or lower lobectomy.

In the case of a thorocotomy scar on one side with a healthy sounding lung on the side of the scar and unhealthy lung on the opposite side—consider single lung transplant.

The clinical signs associated with lobectomy and pneumonectomy can often confuse candidates, especially when trying to localize involvement in lobectomy cases. The following table summarizes the key clinical findings:

Sign	Pneumonectomy	Left lobectomy		Right lobectomy	
		LUL	LLL	RUL	RML/RLL
Chest wall	Flattening of the affected side	Upper ribs pulled in	Lower ribs pulled in	Upper ribs pulled in	Lower ribs pulled in
Tracheal deviation*	Grossly deviated to the affected side	Deviated to affected side	Central (may be deviated to the affected side)	Deviated to affected side	Central (may be deviated to the affected side)
Expansion	Reduced (absent) throughout affected side	Reduced (LUZ)	Reduced (LLZ)	Reduced (RUZ)	Reduced (RLZ)
Breath sounds	Absent throughout affected side	Reduced (LUZ)	Reduced (LLZ)	Reduced (RUZ)	Reduced (RLZ)

* Bronchial breathing is often heard over the deviated trachea.

Questions commonly asked by examiners

What are the possible indications for a lobectomy?

- Bronchiectasis (uncontrolled symptoms, i.e. recurrent haemoptysis)
- Malignancy (NSCLC)
- Solitary pulmonary nodule (unknown cause)
- Cystic fibrosis
- Tuberculosis
- Lung abscess

What the possible indications for pneumonectomy?

- Bronchiectasis
- Malignancy
- Tuberculosis

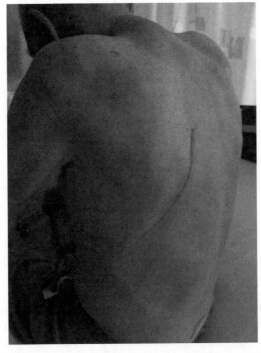

Figure 16.1 Left thoracotomy scar. Note that these scars can be very posterior and can initially be missed. This is common especially with left thoracotomy scars, when approaching and examining patients from the right side.

Case 17 ◆ **Old Tuberculosis**

Examiner's note

Before the advent of effective chemotherapy, tuberculosis was treated in many ways. Although these methods are now obsolete, there are patients who are still alive and well today that were treated by such methods. They are stable whilst displaying many clinical signs and thus commonly appear in MRCP (PACES) examinations. The clinical presentations for old tuberculosis in examinations (some of which are presented below) include:

- Apical fibrosis
- Thoracoplasty
- Pneumonectomy
- Lobectomy
- Plombage therapy (may be difficult to clinically differentiate from lobectomy)
- Phrenic nerve crush
- Recurrent pneumothoraces (manifesting as pleural thickening)

CASE PRESENTATION 1

This patient is not breathless at rest. The fingers are not clubbed. There is no evidence of nicotine staining. The venous pressure is not elevated. There are no palpable lymph nodes. The **trachea is deviated to the right***. On inspection of the chest, there is* **right apical flattening***. There are no scars.* **Chest expansion is reduced in the right upper zone***. The* **percussion note is dull; vocal fremitus is increased; breath sounds are reduced** *with* **inspiratory crepitations at the right apex***. There is* **bronchial breathing** *over the deviated trachea.*

The diagnosis is **apical fibrosis***, of which* **old tuberculosis** *is an important cause.*

Clinical notes

The above clinical findings would suggest an apical pathology. This could represent malignancy, consolidation, collapse, or fibrosis.

- **Malignancy**: look for clubbing, cachexia, nicotine staining, and lymphadenopathy; there may be features of a Pancoast syndrome (C8–T1 sensory disturbance and Horner's syndrome); clubbing and lymphadenopathy may also be features of tuberculosis.
- **Consolidation**: dull percussion note, increased vocal fremitus, and bronchial breathing (although bronchial breathing would be expected over a deviated trachea).
- **Collapse**: dull percussion note, reduced vocal fremitus, and breath sounds. Although bronchial breathing is not associated with collapse, it can be heard over the deviated trachea.
- **Fibrosis:** The presence of crackles should differentiate this from the above, although crackles may be present in the context of malignancy and possibly consolidation. Crackles may be present in the context of infection. Fibrosis is often associated with a non-productive cough,

and thus the crackles of fibrosis may be differentiated from that of infection by asking the patient to cough.

The differential diagnosis of apical fibrosis (mnemonic: BREASTS CLAP):

*   **B**erylliosis
*   **R**adiation
*   **E**xtrinsic allergic alveolitis (hypersensitivity pneumonitis)
*   **A**llergic bronchopulmonary aspergillosis
*   **S**arcoidosis (upper to mid zones)
*   **T**uberculosis
*   **S**ilicosis

*   **C**oal worker's pneumoconiosis
*   **L**angerhans cell histiocytosis (Histiocytosis X)
*   **A**nkylosing spondylitis
*   **P**soriasis (very rare)

CASE PRESENTATION 2

*This patient is not breathless at rest. The fingers are not clubbed. There is no evidence of nicotine staining. The venous pressure is not elevated. There are no palpable lymph nodes. The **trachea is grossly deviated to the right**. On inspection of the chest, there is a **left thoracotomy scar posteriorly** with evidence of **rib resections superiorly** on the left. **Chest expansion is reduced**; the **percussion note is dull**; **vocal fremitus is reduced** and there are **crepitations at the left upper zone**. There is **bronchial breathing over the deviated trachea**.*

*This patient has had a **left thoracoplasty** for the treatment of tuberculous before the days of anti-tuberculosis therapy.*

Clinical notes

A patient with a thoracoplasty for old TB can cause some confusion in examinations, and is often confused with a pneumonectomy. Both present as chest deformities, however the deformity is more marked with a thoracoplasty. Differentiating clinical features include:

Clinical feature	Thoracoplasty	Pneumonectomy
Deformity	More prominent with evidence of rib resections superiorly	Present, but less marked
Chest expansion	Reduced in the upper zone, corresponding to the area of rib resections	Reduced throughout the affected hemithorax
Percussion note	Dull in the upper zone	Dull throughout the affected hemithorax
Breath sounds	Reduced in the upper zone, but present in the lower zones	Absent throughout the affected hemithorax

CASE PRESENTATION 3

This patient is not breathless at rest. The fingers are not clubbed. There is no evidence of nicotine staining. The venous pressure is not elevated. There are no palpable lymph nodes. The trachea is not deviated. On inspection of the chest, there is a **left supraclavicular scar. Chest expansion is reduced on the left**. *The* **percussion note is dull** *and* **vocal fremitus is reduced** *and* **breath sounds are reduced at the left base**.

This patient has had a **left phrenic nerve crush** *for the treatment of tuberculosis before the days of anti-tuberculosis therapy.*

Clinical notes

The differential diagnosis for the above chest findings would include pleural effusion, collapse, pleural thickening, and raised hemidiaphragm. In case of a phrenic nerve crush, the underlying pathology accounting for the clinical signs is a raised hemidiaphragm due to diagrammatic paralysis. The key clinical feature pinpointing previous phrenic nerve crush as the diagnosis is the presence of a left supraclavicular scar. This is often missed and needs to be carefully looked for. If there is no supraclavicular scar, but there are numerous scars suggesting previous recurrent thoracocentesis of the affected side, then in the context of old TB the diagnosis may be pleural thickening resulting from recurrent pneumothoraces (another method of treatment before the days of chemotherapy).

Questions commonly asked by examiners

What is the prevalence of TB?

The prevalence worldwide is 2 billion individuals, with 8 million cases diagnosed every year. 95% of all cases occur in developing countries.

Which patients are at increased risk of developing tuberculosis?

*   Immigrant population (from countries with a high incidence of TB)
*   Immunocompromised individuals (malignancy, HIV/AIDS, immunosuppressive drugs)
*   Elderly patients
*   Alcoholics
*   Malnutrition
*   Homeless individuals
*   Occupational exposure (doctors, nurses, and chest physiotherapists)

How do you manage a patient with old TB?

Old TB does not require any specific anti-tuberculosis treatment. Treatment is required if there is reactivation of tuberculosis or associated long-term complications, e.g. bronchiectasis.

What are the complications of tuberculosis?

Acute complications

*   Pneumothorax
*   Pleural effusion
*   Empyema
*   Collapse*
*   Tubulointerstitial nephritis

---

* Right middle lobe collapse can occur due to hilar node involvement by tuberculosis (Brock's syndrome)

- Laryngitis
- Enteritis
- Respiratory failure
- Acute respiratory distress syndrome (ARDS) (rare)
- Tuberculous meningitis
- Miliary TB (widespread dissemination via bloodstream)

Chronic complications

- Pulmonary fibrosis
- Bronchiectasis*
- Cor pulmonale (secondary to extensive disease and fibrosis)
- Aspergilloma (*A.fumigatus* in a healed open cavity)
- Reactivation

How do you investigate a patient with suspected TB?

Blood tests

- FBC
- U&E
- LFT
- Inflammatory markers
- Blood cultures
- HIV serology (all newly diagnosed patients with active TB)

Chest radiograph

- Upper lobe involvement is most common
- Cavitating lesion is indicative of advanced infection
- Primary infection: hilar/mediastinal lymphadenopathy and radiological findings similar to a community acquired pneumonia
- Reactivation: classically upper lobe involvement (posterior segment of right upper lobe, apicoposterior segment of left upper lobe and apical segment of lower lobes)
- Tuberculomas are homogeneously calcified nodules (5–20mm) that represent old infection
- Uniform miliary shadows are seen in miliary TB (tubercles are 1–2mm in diameter)

Sputum

- Three sputum samples are required (early morning on 3 consecutive days)
- Smear using Ziehl-Neilson staining for acid-alcohol fast bacilli (AAFB)
- Culture in Dover's or Lowenstein-Jensen medium for 4–8 weeks (to determine sensitivity takes another 3–4 weeks)
- For rapid diagnosis, polymerase chain reaction (PCR) using radiolabelled DNA probes can identify organisms in 48 hours.

Computed tomography

- May help to better define abnormalities in patients with vague findings on chest radiographs

Fibre-optic bronchoscopy

- Washings from affected lobes, if no sputum is available
- Transbronchial biopsies can be obtained

---

* Right middle lobe bronchiectasis is a typical outcome of hilar node involvement by tuberculosis in childhood (Brock's syndrome)

Does a negative smear exclude a diagnosis of active tuberculosis?

The absence of a positive smear does not exclude active infection. Approximately 35% of culture-positive specimens are associated with negative smear results.

When would you isolate a patient with active pulmonary tuberculosis?

Isolation for 2 weeks is recommended for patients with smear positive TB. Those with smear-negative or non-pulmonary TB do not require isolation.

What is the role of tuberculin testing in active tuberculosis?

- Tuberculin testing indicates exposure to mycobacteria, and is not a sensitive test for active infection. It is most valuable as a screening test and for contact cases.
- In cases where sputum is negative on direct smear or culture, tuberculin testing is useful. In a patient who has not previously had tuberculosis or BCG vaccination, a strongly positive tuberculin test ranks tuberculosis high among the differential diagnoses, and increases the probability that active tuberculosis is the diagnosis.

What do you know about the different tuberculin tests available?

Mantoux Test

- Intradermal injection of 0.1mL of purified protein derivative (PPD)
- The diameter of the induration (rather than the erythema) is measured at 72 hours
- Diameter > 10mm or >15mm (if previously received BCG vaccination) is positive

Heaf Test

- More suitable for large scale screening
- A small amount of PPD is placed on the skin and 6 needle puncture is made through it with a heaf gun.
- After 3–7 days, the heaf reaction is graded as follows:
    - **Grade 1**: 4–6 small, indurated papules
    - **Grade 2**: indurated ring formed by confluent papules
    - **Grade 3**: solid induration with a diameter of 5–10mm
    - **Grade 4**: induration > 10mm
- Grade 2–3 reaction indicates previous infection in those without prior BCG vaccination
- Grade 3–4 reaction indicates previous infection in those with prior BCG vaccination
- An anergic response is seen in sarcoidosis, lymphoma, advanced malignancy, HIV, immunosupression, and some weeks after measles and EBV infection.

What is the role of interferon gamma testing in tuberculosis?

This is an expensive test. However, in patients who have previously received BCG vaccination and have a strongly positive tuberculin test, an interferon gamma test will differentiate that and active tuberculosis as the cause of the strongly positive tuberculin test.

What do you know about contact testing?

All close contacts of those with active TB infection should be assessed with inquiry into previous BCG vaccination, Heaf testing and chest X-ray.

What are the indications for chemoprophylaxis in tuberculosis?

- All children aged less than 5 years who are close contacts with smear-positive individuals irrespective of tuberculin test result.
- All patients with previous history of tuberculosis or radiological evidence of previous tuberculosis who are receiving immunosuppressive therapy (including renal dialysis)

How was tuberculosis treated in the days prior to effective chemotherapy?

The most common treatments were rest, isolation, fresh air, good nutrition, and medical supervision. By the late 1800s it was thought that intentional collapsing of the affected lung would allow the lung to rest and heal. However, this usually did nothing except to worsen the condition of the patient. Numerous methods were developed for iatrogenic lung collapse that were practised up until the advent of anti-tuberculosis chemotherapy in the mid-1940s.

(a) Thoracoplasty

This was the surgical removal of several upper ribs in order to collapse the lung (predominantly upper lobes). An average patient required the removal of 7–8 ribs, and most surgeons preferred to remove only 2–3 ribs at a time. Thus patients had to endure several procedures before the entire thoracoplasty was completed.

(b) Plombage therapy

This involved the insertion of a 'plombe' into the extra-pleural space to collapse the upper lobes. They included fat (taken from elsewhere in the body), solid paraffin wax, lucite spheres, plastic ping pong balls, sponges of inert plastic material, and oleothorax (oil in the pleural cavity). Patients often have a thoracotomy scar and clinical findings resemble that of a patient with previous lobectomy.

(c) Artificial pneumothoraces

Air was introduced into the pleural cavity on the affected side causing collapse of the affected lung. The result of recurrent pneumothoraces often resulted in pleural thickening and a reduced volume of lung on the affected side.

(d) Phrenicotomy (phrenic nerve crush)

This led to unilateral diaphragmatic paralysis and the lung remained in a relaxed phase higher in the chest.

(e) Postural rest

The patient lies on the affected side, which restricted lung movement thus inducing partial rest.

(f) 'Shot bag' method

A bag containing one pound of shot was placed on the clavicle of the patient on the affected side. The weight would be increased by 5 ounces each week until the patient would be carrying 5 pounds of weight on the upper part of the lung. This restricted lung movement and induced partial rest, allowing it to heal.

What is the definition of multi-drug resistant tuberculosis (MDR TB)?

This refers to *M. tuberculosis* that is resistant to at least two different drugs, usually isoniazid and rifampicin.

How would you treat pulmonary tuberculosis?

- All newly diagnosed cases of tuberculosis should be treated with rifampicin, isoniazid, pyrizinamide, and ethambutol for 2 months followed by rifampicin and isoniazid (4 months).
- The principles for treating MDR TB are to use bactericidal drugs not previously used and to which the organism is sensitive. The duration of treatment depends on the response. In general, treatment with at least 3 different drugs should be continued until the sputum culture becomes negative, and then a regimen of at least 2 different drugs should be continued for 12–24 months.

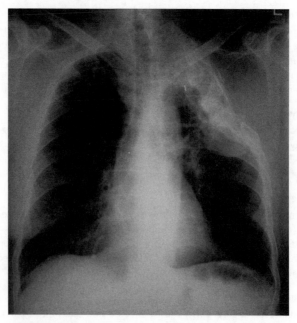

Figure 17.1 An X-ray of a patient with previous left thoracoplasty. Note the rib resections superiorly resulting in marked chest deformity.

In the current era, what is the role of surgery in the treatment of tuberculosis?
Surgical resection of the infected lung is only considered in the context of MDR TB to reduce the bacillary burden. Procedures used include segmentectomy, lobectomy, and pneumonectomy.

Case 18 ◆ **Lung Consolidation**

CASE PRESENTATION 1

*This patient is breathless at rest and has a **productive cough** with purulent sputum.[1] The fingers are not clubbed. There is no evidence of nicotine staining.[2] The venous pressure is not elevated.[3] There are no palpable lymph nodes.[4] The trachea is central and the cricoid-notch distance is not reduced.[5] There is **reduced chest expansion** in the **left lower zone**. The **percussion note is dull** at the left base where there is **increased vocal resonance, coarse crepitations, bronchial breathing**, and a **pleural rub**. There is no peripheral oedema.[7] There are no signs of pulmonary hypertension.[8]*

*The clinical signs suggest **left basal consolidation**. The presence of a productive cough with purulent sputum would suggest an underlying **bacterial pneumonia**.[9]*

CASE PRESENTATION 2

This **cachectic patient** has a **productive cough** and is breathless at rest.[1] The fingers are **clubbed**. There is **nicotine staining** of the fingers.[2] The venous pressure is not elevated.[3] There is a **palpable lymph node** in the right supraclavicular fossa.[4] The trachea is central and the cricoid-notch distance is not reduced.[5] There is **reduced chest expansion** in the **right lower zone**. The **percussion note is dull** at the right base where there is **increased vocal resonance, coarse crepitations, bronchial breathing,** and a **pleural rub**.[6] There is no peripheral oedema.[7] There are no signs of pulmonary hypertension.[8]

The clinical signs suggest **right basal consolidation**. The presence of cachexia, finger clubbing, nicotine staining, lymphadenopathy, and a productive cough would suggest underlying **malignancy**.[9]

CASE PRESENTATION 3

This patient is breathless at rest.[1] The fingers are not **clubbed**. There is no evidence of nicotine staining.[2] The **venous pressure is elevated**.[3] There are no palpable lymph nodes.[4] The trachea is central and the cricoid-notch distance is not reduced.[5] There is **reduced chest expansion** in the **left lower zone**. The **percussion note is dull** at the left base where there is **increased vocal resonance, coarse crepitations, bronchial breathing,** and a **pleural rub**.[6] The right calf is swollen and tender (suggesting venous thrombosis).[7] There are signs of pulmonary hypertension.[8]

The clinical signs suggest **left basal consolidation**. The presence of pulmonary hypertension and clinical evidence of venous thrombosis suggests **pulmonary infarction (embolism)** as the underlying cause.[9]

Clinical notes

When considering lung consolidation, it is important to remember the 3 principal causes: pneumonia, malignancy, and infarction. Once having established a diagnosis of consolidation, use other clinical signs, to find the underlying cause.

1. Assess functional status. Patients with consolidation in the examination setting will often be breathless. Those with bacterial pneumonia may have pyrexia. Ask for a cough. Bacterial pneumonia or malignancy is associated with purulent sputum +/– haemoptysis. Examine the sputum pot if present. In patients with pulmonary infarction, fever is less prominent, and occasionally there may be a productive cough with mucoid sputum and haemoptysis.

2. Examine the hands carefully. The presence of clubbing will suggest underlying malignancy. Nicotine staining will suggest smoking, which is a strong risk factor for malignancy.

3. An elevated venous pressure has many causes, but if present in the context of consolidation, should suspect one to consider pulmonary infarction. Other signs of pulmonary hypertension should carefully be sought for later in the examination. Look for bruising or purpura (suggests anticoagulation in pulmonary infarction).

4. Lymphadenopathy would suggest underlying malignancy or infection.

5. The trachea is often central, but may be pulled to the affected side if the consolidation is associated with collapse. A reduced cricoid-notch distance is a feature of hyperinflation, which may reflect underlying obstructive airways disease in a patient with nicotine staining.

6. These are the constellation of clinical signs associated with consolidation. A pleural rub suggests associated involvement and inflammation of the overlying pleura.

7. When examining the legs for oedema, look for discrepancy in calf size and/or swelling, suggesting underlying venous thrombosis. This would support a diagnosis of pulmonary infarction.

8. Signs of pulmonary hypertension include parasternal heave and thrill, right ventricular third or fourth heart sound, widely split S_2 with a loud P_2.

9. When making a diagnosis of consolidation, use other signs to provide an underlying cause. Sometimes this may not be possible, and the best thing is to provide a list of differential diagnoses for consolidation:

   (a) Pneumonia (pyrexia, purulent sputum, haemoptysis)

   (b) Malignancy (cachexia, clubbing, nicotine staining, lympahdenopathy, productive cough)

   (c) Infarction (signs of pulmonary hypertension, deep venous thrombosis, bruising-suggesting anticoagulation)*

Questions commonly asked by examiners

What are the causes of lung consolidation?

- Bacterial pneumonia
- Malignancy
- Pulmonary infarction (embolism)

How would you investigate a patient with consolidation?

The tests profile will reflect the history, and suspected underlying diagnosis:

- Bloods
  - FBC
  - Inflammatory markers
  - U&Es
  - LFTs
  - Arterial blood gas sampling
  - D-dimer*
  - Blood cultures
  - Serological testing for Mycoplasma and Legionella
- Chest radiograph
- ECG
  - Features of PE (see below)
- Sputum
  - Culture
  - Cytology (for malignant cells)
- Urine
  - Urinalysis (proteinuria and haematuria)
  - Legionella antigen
  - Pneumococcal antigen
- Ventilation-perfusion (V-Q) scan
  - If suspecting PE**

---

* Patients with lung malignancy may present with PE, as malignancy is a thrombotic risk factor. In these cases, both features of malignancy and infarction will be present.

* The D-dimer may be elevated in infection or with underlying malignancy. However, a negative D-dimer reliably excludes PE if there is a low pretest probability. However, a low d-dimer doesn't exclude PE if the pretest probability is moderate or high.

** V-Q scan should only be considered as a first-line investigation for PE, if the CXR is normal and there is no significant cardiopulmonary disease. A normal V-Q scan reliably excludes a PE, but an intermediate scan should be followed up by CT pulmonary angiography (which remains the gold standard).

- Computed tomography
  - If suspecting underlying malignancy
  - Pulmonary angiography if suspecting PE

What are the causes of community acquired pneumonia?

Typical organisms

- *Streptococcus pneumoniae* (most common, accounting for 60–70% of cases)
- *Haemophilus influenzae*
- *Staphylococcus aureus* (following influenza viral illness or in intravenous drug users)
- *Klebsiella pneumoniae* (debilitated patients, elderly, alcoholics)

Atypical organisms

- *Mycoplasma pneumoniae* (second most common, accounting for 15–20% of cases)
- *Legionella spp.*
- *Chlamydia spp.*
- *Coxiella spp.*

Viral causes

- Influenza
- CMV
- Varicella-Zoster virus
- Other respiratory viruses

What are the common causes of hospital acquired pneumonia?

This is defined as pneumonia developing ≥48 hours after hospital admission. Organisms include:

- Gram-negative organisms (most common): *Klebsiella spp, Pseudomonas spp, E. Coli, Serratia spp. Acinetobacter spp.*
- *Staphylococcus aureus*
- Anaerobes
- Fungi

What is the role of aspiration in hospital acquired pneumonia?

Aspiration may complicate dysphagia, stroke, or states of impaired consciousness. Anaerobes, arising from the oropharynx, are the principal pathogens in aspiration pneumonia.

However, aspiration plays an important role in the pathogenesis of hospital-acquired pneumonia. Approximately 45% of healthy individuals aspirate to some extent during sleep, and a greater proportion of patients who are severely ill. Depending on the virulence of the organism and host defence factors, pneumonia may develop. The oropharynx of most hospitalized patients may become colonized with aerobic gram-negative bacilli within a few days of admission. Thus gram-negatives are an important cause of hospital-acquired pneumonia.

What are the causes of a cavitating lung lesion?

Infectious causes

- *Staphylococcus aureus*
- *Klebsiella pneumonia*
- *Anaerobic infections*
- *Pseudomonas aeruginosa*
- Tuberculosis
- Aspergilloma

- Histoplasmosis
- Coccidiomycosis

Non-infectious causes
- Malignancy
- Wegners granulomatosis
- Pulmonary rheumatoid nodule
- Caplan's syndrome

What do you know about mycoplasma pneumonia?

- An important cause of atypical pneumonia
- Occurs in epidemics (every 3–4 years), and common during the winter months
- Often seen in children and young adults
- Incubation period is 2–3 weeks
- Often associated with a prolonged prodromal symptoms (fever, headache, diarrhoea, and vomiting)
- Often associated with widespread extrapulmonary involvement (see below)
- A four-fold rise in complement fixation tests between acute and convalescent specimens indicates an acute infection. Detection of IgM antibodies is more sensitive, and can give positive results on a single specimen.

What are the extrapulmonary manifestations of mycoplasma pneumonia?

Neurological
- Aseptic meningitis
- Encephalitis
- Transverse myelitis
- Guillain-Barré syndrome
- Cranial and peripheral neuropathy
- Bullous myringitis

Cardiac
- Myocarditis
- Pericarditis

Rheumatological
- Arthralgia
- Myalgia
- Myositis

Haematological
- Thrombocytopenia
- Cold autoimmune haemolytic anaemia (cold agglutinin in 50% of cases)
- Disseminated intravascular coagulation

Gastrointestinal
- Diarrhoea
- Vomiting
- Hepatitis
- Pancreatitis

Dermatological
- Erythema nodosum
- Erythema multiforme
- Steven-Johnson syndrome

Endocrine
- Syndrome of inappropriate ADH secretion (SIADH)

Renal
- Glomerulonephritis
- Interstitial nephritis

What do you know about Legionnaire's disease?

Pneumonia caused by *Legionella pneumophilia*
- Often occurs in local outbreaks, but can occur sporadically
- *Legionella pneumophilia* colonizes contaminated water-cooling systems, showers, or air-conditioning systems
- Predisposing factors: elderly, debilitated, alcoholism, smoking, COPD, immunodeficiency
- Legionella pneumonia often has a predilection for the lower lobes
- Gastrointestinal symptoms are common (50% of patients): diarrhoea, nausea, vomiting, and anorexia
- Diagnosis can be made using detection of Legionella antigen in the urine (present in 90% of cases in 48 hours) or direct immunoflorescence or PCR of respiratory specimens
- Complications include hepatitis, pancreatitis, renal failure, and SIADH

What do you know about the CURB-65 criteria for managing community-acquired pneumonia?

One point is given for any of the following:
- Confusion
- Urea >7mmol/L
- Respiratory rate ≥30/minute
- Blood pressure (systolic) <90mmHg
- Age ≥65 years

The CURB-65 score can be used to decide upon prognosis and management, i.e. oral (PO) versus intravenous (IV) antibiotics and inpatient versus outpatient treatment.

Score	Mortality	Antibiotics	Inpatient versus outpatient treatment
≤1	Low (1.5%)	PO	Outpatient
2	Intermediate	PO	Outpatient; consider short stay in hospital or hospital-supervised outpatient treatment
≥3	High (22%)	IV	Inpatient (treat as severe community acquired pneumonia)

What are the ECG features of PE?
- Sinus tachycardia
- Tall R wave in V_1
- Right ventricular strain
- Right bundle branch block

- T wave inversion in $V_1–V_3$
- $S_1S_2S_3$ (classically described but rarely seen)
- $S_1Q_3T_3$ (classically described but rarely seen)
- Inferior ST elevation (rare, but has been described)

What are the risk factors for thromboembolism?

- Recent surgery
- Malignancy
- Immobility
- Previous thromboembolism
- Oral contraceptive pill
- Pregnancy
- Thrombophilic disorders (Protein S, Protein C, and Antithrombin III deficiency)

Case 19 ◆ Pneumothorax

Examiner's note

A patient with a large pneumothorax is unlikely to present in the MRCP(PACES) examination, as it would be treated with aspiration or with a chest drain, and therefore clinical signs would disappear. It is important to look for chest drains and scars indicating pleural aspiration. Patients with small pneumothoraces may be stable and display some clinical signs, and thus may appear in clinical examinations.

CASE PRESENTATION

This patient is not breathless at rest. The fingers are not clubbed.[1] There is no evidence of nicotine staining.[2] The venous pressure is not elevated.[3] There are no palpable lymph nodes. The trachea is central and the cricoid-notch distance is not reduced.[4] On examination of the chest, there are no scars.[5] There is **reduced chest expansion** *on the right. The apex beat is palpable and undisplaced.[6] The* **percussion note is hyper-resonant**, **vocal fremitus**, *and* **breath sounds are reduced** *on the right.[7]*

The diagnosis is right **pneumothorax**.

Clinical notes

1. Look for underlying respiratory disease, an important cause of secondary pneumothoraces. Finger clubbing will provide a differential diagnosis of underlying respiratory disease (bronchiectasis, cystic fibrosis, malignancy, and interstitial lung disease).
2. Nicotine staining would indicate COPD, the most common cause of secondary pneumothorax. Furthermore, smoking increases the risk of first spontaneous pneumothorax by 20-fold in men and 10-fold in women. The increased risk of pneumothorax and recurrence is approximately proportional to the number of cigarettes smoked.

3. A raised venous pressure is a hallmark of tension pneumothorax.

4. The trachea will be deviated to the opposite side in a large pneumothorax or in cases of tension pneumothorax. Therefore mentioning the presence or absence of tracheal deviation is important. A reduce cricoid-notch distance is a sign of hyperinflation, suggesting underling COPD.

5. Look for signs of previous intercostal drain scars. Recurrence of pneumothorax is common (15–40%). Up to 15% of recurrences can be on the contralateral side. Secondary pneumothoraces are more likely to recur, with cystic fibrosis carrying the highest recurrence rates (70–80%). Look for other potential iatrogenic causes: recent pleural aspiration/biopsy, recent pacemaker insertion, and recent central venous access.

6. The apex beat will be displaced to the opposite side in large pneumothoraces, demonstrating mediastinal shift.

7. The above signs are classical findings of a pneumothorax. It is also important to look for other signs of underlying respiratory disease: prolonged expiration, expiratory wheeze in COPD; coarse crepitations in bronchiectasis; fine crepitations in interstitial lung disease.

Questions commonly asked by examiners

What are the causes of a pneumothorax?

Primary pneumothorax

Secondary pneumothorax

- *Respiratory disease*
    - COPD
    - Asthma
    - Cystic fibrosis
    - Interstitial lung disease
    - Tuberculosis
    - Malignancy
    - Pneumonia
    - Lung abscess
    - Pneumoconiosis
    - Sarcoidosis
- *Connective tissue disease*
    - Marfan's syndrome
    - Ehlers-Danlos syndrome
    - Pseudoxanthoma elasticum
- *Lung cysts*
    - Lymphangioleiomyomatosis
    - Langerhans cell histiocytosis X
    - Tuberous sclerosis
    - Neurofibromatosis
- *Iatrogenic*
    - Pleural aspiration
    - Pleural biopsy
    - Thoracocentesis
    - Central venous access (internal jugular or subclavian vein puncture)
    - Pacemaker insertion
    - Cardiopulmonary resuscitation
- *Trauma*

What are the clinical signs of a tension pneumothorax?
- Tracheal deviation (to the opposite side)
- Mediastinal shift (apex beat displaced to the opposite side)
- Raised venous pressure

What are the BTS guidelines on the management of a spontaneous primary pneumothorax?
NB. Patients who have minimal symptoms and have a rim of air <2cm on CXR can be allowed home with a repeat CXR in 7–10 days. They should be given clear written advice to return if they develop breathlessness.

What would you do if the clinical suspicion of a pneumothorax is high, but the pulmonary artery (PA) chest radiograph is normal?
Request a lateral chest or lateral decubitus film. Although small pneumothoraces in patients without respiratory disease have little clinical significance, in patients with suspected secondary pneumothoraces, even small pneumothoraces have significant implications, and therefore the lateral chest and lateral decubitus films are valuable.

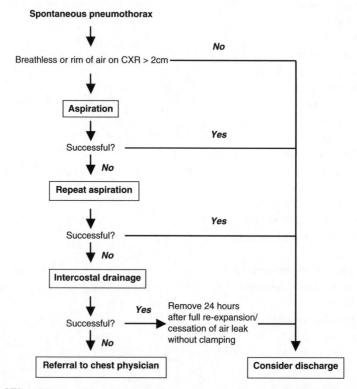

Figure 19.1 BTS guidelines on the management of a spontaneous primary pneumothorax.

Reproduced from M Henry, T Arnold and J Harvey, BTS Guidelines for the management of spontaneous pneumothorax, 58(supplement 2):ii39–ii52 Copyright © 2003 with permission from BMJ Publishing Group Ltd & British Thoracic Society.

What is the role of CT scanning in diagnosing a pneumothorax?

CT scanning is recommended when differentiating a pneumothorax from complex bullous disease or when the plain chest radiography is obscured by surgical emphysema.

What size of tube should be used for intercostal drainage?

There is no evidence that large tubes (20–24F) are better than small tubes (10–14F) in the management of pneumothoraces. The initial use of large tubes is not recommended. Small tubes (10–14F) should be used first. The use of a catheter over a guidewire system (Seldinger technique) is becoming increasingly popular. However, a smaller tube may need to be replaced with a larger one if there is suspicion of a persistent air leak.

What is the role of chest drain suction?

- This should not be applied directly after intercostal tube insertion
- It can be added after 48 hours for persistent air leak or failure of a pneumothorax to expand
- High-volume and low-pressure systems are recommended (−10 to −20cm H2O)

How would you manage a secondary pneumothorax?

- All patients with pneumothorax and underlying respiratory disease should be hospitalized for observation
- Observation alone is only recommended with small pneumothoraces (<1cm) or isolated apical pneumothorax in asymptomatic patients.
- Generally, all patients with secondary pneumothoraces require intervention.
- If age <50 years, asymptomatic or a small pneumothorax (rim of air < 2cm), they should be aspirated. If successful, they should be observed for 24 hours prior to discharge. If unsuccessful, then they will require an intercostal drain.
- If age >50years, symptomatic or a large pneumothorax (rim of air >2cm), an intercostal drain should be inserted.

What is the management of a tension pneumothorax?

- High-flow oxygen
- Insertion of a large bore cannula into the second intercostal space mid axillary line on the affected side
- Prompt insertion of an intercostal drain (the cannula remain until the drain is positioned and secured)

What is the most important predictor of re-expansion pulmonary oedema?

The greater the length of time the lung has remained collapsed, the greater the risk of re-expansion pulmonary oedema. This occurs in patients with primary pneumothoraces, who do not seek medical advice for several days (46% of patient with symptomatic primary pneumothorax wait for 2 days with symptoms!).

What is the rate of resolution/reabsorption of a spontaneous primary pneumothorax?

There is slow absorption of air from the pleural cavity, and the rate of absorption is 1.22–1.8% of the volume of hemithorax every 24 hours.

What is the pathophysiology of primary spontaneous pneumothoraces?

These result from rupture of apical pleural blebs under the visceral pleura. They are typically observed in tall young individuals without underlying respiratory disease. 90% of patients are smokers. Smoking increases the risk of primary spontaneous pneumothorax by 20-fold in males and 10-fold in females.

Case 20 ◆ **Rheumatoid Lung**

CASE PRESENTATION

This patient has a **productive cough** and is not breathless at rest.[1] There is no evidence of cyanosis.
Inspiratory clicks can be heard with the unaided ear.[2] There is a **symmetrical deforming
arthropathy of the small joints of the hands**, inkeeping with **rheumatoid arthritis**.[3] The **fingers
are clubbed**.[4] There is no evidence of nicotine staining.[5] There is **steroid purpura** over the extremities.[6]
The venous pressure is not elevated.[7] The trachea is central and the **cricoid-notch distance is reduced**.[8]
On examination of the chest there are no scars.[9] Chest expansion is symmetrical but reduced bilaterally.[10]
The percussion note is dull at both bases.[11] Vocal fremitus is normal.[12] On auscultation of the lung fields
there are **fine end-inspiratory crackles at both lung bases, extending up to mid zones, which do
not alter with coughing**.[13] In addition, there are **coarse inspiratory crepitations** at the right base and
the **characteristics of the crackles alter with coughing**.[14] There are **inspiratory squawks** and there
is diffuse **high-pitched expiratory wheeze**.[15] There is no peripheral oedema.[16] There are no signs of
pulmonary hypertension.[17]

This patient has evidence of **rheumatoid arthritis**. The clinical findings suggest both **interstitial lung
disease** and right basal **bronchiectasis**, which are both respiratory manifestations of rheumatoid arthritis.
The unifying diagnosis is **rheumatoid lung**.[18]

Clinical notes

Rheumatoid arthritis has many respiratory manifestations, but the most common manifestation of
rheumatoid arthritis in clinical examination settings includes pulmonary fibrosis, bronchiolitis
obliterans, pleural effusion, or bronchiectasis. Once identifying rheumatoid arthritis, it is
important to keep these in mind and focus on identifying relevant clinical signs.

1. Ask the patient to cough. This may help differentiate the crackles of bronchiectasis and pulmonary
   fibrosis (both of which can be present in a patient with rheumatoid arthritis). Bronchiectasis is associated
   with copious purulent sputum and recurrent haemoptysis. Look for the sputum pot by the bedside

2. Inspiratory clicks may be heard from the end of the bed. If heard, they are characteristic of
   bronchiectasis.

3. Although a respiratory station, examine hands looking for evidence of rheumatological disease,
   especially in patients with interstitial lung disease. Spend a little extra time when examining hands and
   making general observations. Failure to pick up rheumatoid arthritis will disable you to make a final
   unifying diagnosis!

4. Both interstitial lung disease and bronchiectasis can cause finger clubbing. It may be absent. If present
   don't miss it!

5. Nicotine staining may suggest underlying obstructive airways disease secondary to smoking.
   Rheumatoid arthritis can also cause hyperinflation with expiratory wheeze (bronchiolitis). Often
   patients may have multiple respiratory diagnoses, and it is important to keep this in mind.

6. Steroid use can manifest as steroid purpura, cushingoid appearance, and proximal myopathy.

7. If the venous pressure is elevated, then this is a sign of pulmonary hypertension. Other features of
   pulmonary hypertension should be carefully sought for.

8. Trachea is often central. It may be pulled to one side in cases of apical fibrosis. The cricoid-notch
   distance will be reduced with a hyerinflated chest. In the context of rheumatoid arthritis, hyperinflation
   is associated with bronchiolitis obliterans.

9. Look carefully for scars of previous lung biopsies, intercostal drainage (pleural effusions), and previous lobectomy (for bronchiectasis)

10. Rheumatoid arthritis is often associated with a symmetrical restrictive lung defect, and chest expansion will be reduced symmetrically. In cases of localized bronchiectasis or underlying collapse, reduction in chest expansion may be more localized.

11. With basal lung fibrosis, the bases are often associated with a dull percussion note, reduced vocal or tactile fremitus and reduced air entry. In cases of apical fibrosis, these findings are predominantly apical, and the trachea may be pulled to one side if asymmetrical apical fibrosis is present.

12. Vocal fremitus findings are variable. It may be normal. It may be reduced, especially if underlying collapse is present. It may be increased if coexistent pneumonia (consolidation) is present.

13. In cases of basal pulmonary fibrosis, fine end-inspiratory crackles are present at the bases (which can extend up to mid-zones). Sometimes, it may be difficult to auscultate very fine crackles, and these need to be sought for carefully. On the other hand, with predominant apical involvement, the crackles are localized to the apices. Bronchial breathing may be present in cases of apical fibrosis, especially if the trachea is deviated.

14. The hallmark auscultatory findings in bronchiectasis are coarse crepitations, which alter with coughing. They may occur during late inspiration, span throughout inspiration, or present during both inspiration and expiration. Bronchiectasis is more commonly a focal process involving a lobe, segment, or subsegment of the lung, and therefore the crackles are often localized. Scattered wheeze may be present in up to a third of cases of bronchiectasis. This may be due to airway obstruction from secretions, airway destruction leading to collapsibility, bronchiolitis obliterans, or co-existent obstructive airways disease.

15. Causes of peripheral oedema in rheumatoid arthritis include pulmonary hypertension (cor pulmonale), membranous glomerulonephritis secondary to rheumatoid arthritis, gold, or penicillamine. Furthermore, amyloidosis is a complication of long-standing bronchiectasis, which can also result in nephrotic syndrome.

16. Scattered wheeze may be present in up to a third of cases of bronchiectasis. This may be due to airway obstruction from secretions, airway destruction leading to collapsibility, bronchiolitis obliterans, or co-existent obstructive airways disease. Bronchiolitis obliterans is associated with hyperinflation, high-pitched expiratory wheeze, and inspiratory squawks.

17. Pulmonary hypertension is a recognized complication of rheumatoid lung. The most common cause of pulmonary hypertension is lung parenchymal disease (interstitial lung disease or bronchiectasis).

18. Rheumatoid arthritis has numerous respiratory manifestations (see questions below). On making a diagnosis of rheumatoid arthritis and presenting separate respiratory diagnoses, a unifying diagnosis will impress examiners. Most common manifestation of rheumatoid arthritis in clinical examination settings include
    (a) basal pulmonary fibrosis (basal crackles and signs)
    (b) apical pulmonary fibrosis (apical crackles and signs)
    (c) bronchiolitis obliterans (hyperinflation, inspiratory squawks, high pitched expiratory wheeze)
    (d) pleural effusion
    (e) bronchiectasis

Questions commonly asked by examiners

What are respiratory manifestations of rheumatoid arthritis?

- Pleural effusion
- Basal pulmonary fibrosis (rheumatoid arthritis, gold, methotrexate)
- Apical pulmonary fibrosis (rheumatoid arthritis)
- Pneumonitis
- Bronchiolitis obliterans (rheumatoid arthritis, gold, penicillamine)

- Pleural effusion
- Pleural thickening
- Pulmonary nodules
- Bronchiectasis
- Caplan's syndrome
- Apical fibrobullous disease
- Pulmonary arteritis (and pulmonary hypertension)
- Bronchial carcinoma (rare complication)

What is the most common respiratory manifestation of rheumatoid arthritis?

The most common manifestation is pleural disease, which can occur with or without a pleural effusion. This is often asymptomatic, and may be associated with pericardial disease. Approximately 50% of patients have pleural disease at autopsy.

How common is interstitial lung disease in rheumatoid arthritis?

A classical picture of idiopathic pulmonary fibrosis is present in 2% of patients. However, many patients have findings of interstitial lung disease at autopsy, and thus subclinical interstitial lung disease is more common. Up to 25% of patients with rheumatoid arthritis have changes of interstitial lung disease, and up to 50% of patients have reduced diffusion capacity.

Can rheumatoid interstitial lung disease be present in the absence of arthritis?

Interstitial lung disease often occurs in patients with known rheumatoid disease. However, in some cases, it may precede the onset of arthritis by months or even years.

What do you know about pulmonary nodules in rheumatoid arthritis?

Histologically, they are similar to subcutaneous nodules. They may appear as a single nodule or they may be multiple. They may be present in the pleura or lung parenchyma, and often have a predilection for the upper lobes. The size is variable, ranging from few millimetres to 6cm in diameter. They may increase or decrease often in proportion to severity of systemic disease. If present, they are usually associated with other respiratory manifestations of rheumatoid arthritis. Approximately a third of patients with pleural disease have co-existing pulmonary nodules. Often the nodules do not compromise respiratory function, but complications include secondary infection, cavitation, and development bronchopulmonary fistula.

What are the causes of pulmonary hypertension in patients with rheumatoid arthritis?

The most common cause of pulmonary hypertension is lung parenchymal disease (interstitial lung disease or bronchiectasis). Rarely, the disease is primarily in the vasculature and interstitial lung disease is not present. This is a rare cause of pulmonary hypertension, and the lung pathology is almost identical to that of primary pulmonary hypertension.

What would be the features of a rheumatoid pleural effusion?

- Never blood stained
- Exudate
- High protein and LDH (LDH > 1000 IU/L)
- Low glucose and complement (C3 and C4)
- High rheumatoid factor (often higher than blood concentrations)

What is Caplan's syndrome?

This is the presence of pneumoconiosis (pulmonary massive fibrosis, PMF) in a patient with rheumatoid arthritis. It was originally described occuring in coal miners, but has also been associated with other occupations that result in silica exposure, i.e. boiler scaling, roof tile manufacturing, asbestos mining, and aluminium production. It is characterized by single or multiple nodules (0.5–5.0cm in diameter) developing in the lung periphery. The nodules do not require specific treatment. Patients may become symptomatic, and this is often secondary to smoking or associated pneumoconiosis.

Is there a link between rheumatoid arthritis and bronchial carcinoma?

Bronchial carcinoma has more recently been recognized as a complication of rheumatoid interstitial lung disease. Although the risk is highest in smokers, there is also an increased risk in non-smokers.

Case 21 ◆ **Lung Collapse**

CASE PRESENTATION

This **cachectic patient** is breathless at rest.[1] The **fingers are clubbed**. There is **nicotine staining** of the fingers.[2] The venous pressure is not elevated. There is a **palpable lymph node** in the left supraclavicular fossa.[3] The trachea is deviated to the left.[4] There is **reduced chest expansion** in the **left lower zone**. The **percussion note is dull** at the **left base** where there are **decreased breath sounds** and **vocal resonance**.[5] There is no peripheral oedema. There are no signs of pulmonary hypertension.

The clinical signs suggest **left basal collapse**. The presence of cachexia, finger clubbing, nicotine staining, lymphadenopathy, and a productive cough would suggest underlying **malignancy**.[6]

Clinical notes

1. Assess functional and nutritional status. Patients with collapse in the examination setting will often be breathless. Ask for a cough. Malignancy is associated with a productive cough and cachexia. Examine the sputum pot if present. Cachexia would suggest underlying malignancy.
2. Examine the hands carefully. The presence of clubbing will suggest underlying malignancy. Nicotine staining will suggest smoking, a strong risk factor for malignancy.
3. Lymphadenopathy would suggest underlying malignancy or infection.
4. The trachea is deviated to the affected side.
5. These are the classical features of collapse. These clinical signs may be seen with a pleural effusion, but the trachea will not be deviated to the affected side (often central, or deviated to the opposite side with large pleural effusions). However, tracheal deviation to the affected side may be seen if the pleural effusion is associated with underlying collapse. If there is underlying consolidation present, then bronchial breathing will be present, and the vocal resonance may be increased.

6. When presenting the diagnosis, try to establish the possible cause of collapse:
   (a) **Malignancy** (cachexia, clubbing, nicotine staining, lymphadenopathy)
   (b) **Tuberculosis** (apical signs, lymphadenopathy)
   (c) **Hilar lymphadenopathy, i.e. sarcoidosis** (erythema nodosum, maculopapular skin lesions, lupus pernio, lympahdenopathy)
   (d) **Mucus plugs** (features of asthma, COPD, or bronchiectasis)

Questions commonly asked by examiners

What is the pathophysiology of collapse?

Collapse (atelectasis) can be physiologically divided into obstructive (most common) and non-obstructive atelectasis.

(a) Obstructive atelectasis

This results from the absorption of gas from the alveoli when communication between the alveoli and the trachea is obstructed. Obstruction can occur at occur at the level of small or large bronchus. Common causes include:

- Malignancy
- Extrinsic compression by hilar lymphadenopathy (sarcoidosis, tuberculosis)
- Tuberculosis
- Mucus plugs (asthma, COPD, bronchiectasis)
- Foreign body
- Malpositioned endotracheal tube

(b) Non-obstructive atelectasis

There are many causes, which can be divided as follows:

Non-obstructive atelectasis	Mechanism	Example
Relaxation (passive) atelectasis	Loss of contact between visceral and parietal pleura. This leads to a reduction in lung volume forcing air out of alveoli.	Pleural effusion (LL>UL)* Pneumothorax (UL>LL) Large emphysematous bulla
Compression atelectasis	Space occupying lesion compresses, thus forcing air out of alveoli	Malignancy Loculated pleural effusion
Adhesive atelectasis	Surfactant deficiency (surfactant decreases surface tension of alveoli and decreases collapsibility)	ARDS Radiation pneumonitis Blunt chest trauma PE Pneumonia Post-operative Smoke inhalation
Cicatrization atelectasis	Severe parenchymal scarring leading to a reduction of lung volume	Interstitial lung disease Granulomatous lung disease Necrotizing pneumonia
Rounded atelectasis	Folded lung tissue with adhesions to visceral pleura	Asbestos pleural plaques

* LL = lower lobe; UL = upper lobe

Case 22 ◆ **Superior Vena Cava Obstruction**

CASE PRESENTATION

*This cachectic patient is breathless at rest.[1] The pulse is regular.[2] The fingers are clubbed. There is nicotine staining of the fingers.[3] The **upper limbs and face are oedematous, plethoric**, and **cyanosed**. There is **conjunctival suffusion**. There are multiple **venous angiomata on the undersurface of the tongue**. There are **prominent and dilated superficial veins over the upper limbs, neck and anterior chest wall superior to the nipples**.[4] The **venous pressure is elevated and fixed**.[5] There are no scars on the neck.[6] There are no palpable lymph nodes.[7] On examination of the chest there are radiation burns on the anterior chest wall.[8] There is reduced chest expansion on the right. The percussion note is stony dull at the right base extending up to the right mid-zone, with reduced vocal fremitus. On auscultation the breath sounds are diminished in this area, with an area of bronchial breathing above the area of dullness.[9] There is no peripheral (lower limb) oedema.[10]*

*The diagnosis is **superior vena cava obstruction**. This is most likely due to bronchial carcinoma, and the patient has received **radiotherapy**. This patient also has a **right pleural effusion**.[11]*

Clinical notes

1. Assess functional and nutritional status. Cachexia suggests underlying malignancy.
2. It is important to determine if the patient is in sinus rhythm or not. This will help in assessing the venous pressure waveform (although in superior vena cava (SVC) obstruction, there is fixed elevation of the venous pressure). In the absence of SVC obstruction, sinus rhythm is associated with a double JVP waveform (a and v waves), whereas a waves are absent in AF.
3. Examine the hands carefully. The presence of clubbing will suggest underlying malignancy. Nicotine staining will suggest smoking, a strong risk factor for malignancy. There may be wasting of the small muscles of the hand and sensory disturbance in the C8–T1 dermatomal distribution (Pancoast syndrome).
4. The SVC drains blood from head, neck, upper limbs, and upper thorax (above the nipples). With obstruction, these become oedematous, plethoric, and cyanosed. The conjunctivae are suffused, and venous angiomata may be prominent on the face and more notably under the tongue.
5. SVC obstruction is characterized by FIXED engorgement of neck veins, and loss of the classical JVP waveform.
6. Look carefully for scars of recent central venous access, as thrombosis is a recognized complication, resulting in obstruction.
7. Look carefully for cervical, supraclavicular, infraclavicular ,and axillary lymph nodes. Causes include malignancy and lymphoproliferative disorders.
8. Patients with SVC obstruction in examination settings have often received treatment. Look carefully for radiotherapy burns or radiotherapy ink marks.
9. Chest findings can be variable. There may be none. An example of a right pleural effusion is given in the above case.
10. Lower limb oedema is not usually a feature of SVC obstruction, and is often seen with inferior vena cava obstruction. In certain cases of right atrial masses or tumours and central venous thrombosis, the obstruction may involve both superior and inferior vena cava. Peripheral oedema may be present in patients with malignancy and cachexia, reflecting poor nutritional state, hypoalbuminaemia state, or nephrotic syndrome (membranous glomerulonephritis).

11. Once confirming the diagnosis, try to give a possible cause. The diagnosis of malignancy is quite clear in this example. Don't forget to provided additional diagnoses if present, i.e. pleural effusion, Pancoast syndrome, collapse, or consolidation.

Questions commonly asked by examiners

What are the symptoms of SVC obstruction?

- Dyspnoea
- Headache
- Nasal stuffiness
- Head, facial, and arm swelling
- Visual disturbance
- Dysphagia
- Dizziness

NB. Symptoms increase on bending forward, lying down, or coughing.

What are the causes of SVC obstruction?

- Malignancy
  - Lymphoma (NHL>HL; especially large cell type)
  - Bronchial carcinoma (especially SCLC)
  - Leiomyosarcoma of mediastinal vessels
  - Plasmacytoma
- Mediastinal goitre
- Thoracic aortic aneurysm
- Mediastinal fibrosis
- Benign mediastinal masses
  - Teratoma
  - Thymoma
  - Cystic hygroma
  - Dermoid cyst
- Infections
  - Histoplasmosis
  - Syphilis
  - Tuberculosis
  - Actinomycosis
- Vasculitis
- Central venous thrombosis
  - Thrombophilic disorders
  - Complication of central venous catheters
- Right atrial tumours (i.e. myxoma)

What is the management?

The aims are to relieve symptoms and treat primary pathology, i.e. malignant tumour.

- *Conservative treatment*
  - Elevation of head
- *Specific treatment*
  - Steroids and diuretics if cerebral or laryngeal oedema

- ◆ Radiotherapy (NSCLC or lymphoma)*
- ◆ Chemotherapy (SCLC)*
- ◆ Thrombolysis or anticoagulant therapy (central venous thrombosis)
- ◆ Percutaneous SVC stenting**

What is the prognosis in these patients?

- Benign SVC obstruction: no effect on prognosis
- Malignant SVC obstruction: survival correlates with tumour histology

Case 23 ◆ **Stridor**

CASE PRESENTATION

*This **cachectic patient** is not breathless at rest.[1] There are loud, **high-pitched sounds with each inspiration** that can be heard from the end of the bed.[2] There is no evidence of cyanosis. The fingers are **clubbed**. There is **nicotine staining** of the fingers.[3] The venous pressure is not elevated. There are **palpable lymph nodes** in the **right supraclavicular fossa**.[4] There are no neck masses or scars.[5] Examination of the oropharynx is unremarkable.[6] The trachea is central and the cricoid-notch distance is not reduced.[7] On examination of the chest there are no scars. Percussion note and vocal resonance is normal. Auscultation reveals vesicular breath sounds and no added breath sounds.[8] There is no peripheral oedema.*

*This patient has **inspiratory stridor**, which implies **extrathoracic upper airways obstruction**. The presence of cachexia, clubbing, and lymphadenopathy would suggest underlying **malignancy** as the cause.[9]*

Clinical notes

1. Assess functional status. Cachexia suggests malignancy. In the context of stridor, other malignancies outside the lungs are important and should be considered: trachea, larynx, lymphoid tumours, thyroid, and oesophagus.

2. Stridor is a high-pitched crowing sound that is often heard from the end of the bed, without the need of a stethoscope. It can be present during inspiration and expiration. Wheezing is high-pitched, musical, varying sounds with breathing, most prominent during expiration. In extreme cases, it may be audible from the end of the bed, but is often only heard on auscultation. Stridor is typically shorter, however, it is louder and longer during inspiration. It is important to differentiate stridor from wheeze (see below).

3. Finger clubbing suggests malignancy. Nicotine staining will suggest smoking, thus possible obstructive airways disease, and is a strong risk factor for malignancy.

4. Lymphadenopathy suggests infection, tuberculosis, sarcoidosis, or malignancy.

5. Look carefully for neck masses, i.e. goitre and if present, assess for retrosternal extension. Look for old tracheostomy scars. Look for signs of central venous access and invasive haemodynamic monitoring,

---

* Radiotherapy or chemotherapy should only be used when the histological diagnosis of tumour is known.

** Can provide relief of severe symptoms while the histological diagnosis is being pursued.

suggesting recent intensive care admission, as prolonged endotracheal intubation can result in tracheal stenosis. Look for other scars suggestive of old trauma or burns to the neck.

6. The trachea may be deviated secondary to neck or thyroid swellings. The reduced cricoid-notch distance suggests hyperinflation, i.e. obstructive airways disease.

7. Look carefully in the oral cavity for infections. Inspect the tonsils and peri-tonsillar areas for infections, swellings or masses.

8. Examination of the chest may be normal. The findings may be variable depending on the underlying pathology. Expiratory stridor may be confused with expiratory wheeze. Look carefully for signs of obstructive airways disease, the most important cause of expiratory wheeze. Look carefully for signs of old tuberculosis, an important cause of tracheal stenosis.

9. Remember, stridor is a symptom and NOT a diagnosis. The underlying cause must be determined. Use other clinical signs or pointers in the given history to establish a possible cause. If this is not possible, then present a differential diagnosis to the examiner (see below).

Questions commonly asked by examiners

What are the causes of stridor?

Stridor can be divided into inspiratory (most common) and expiratory stridor:

Inspiratory stridor (extrathoracic airway obstruction)

- Acute epiglottitis
- Croup (laryngotracheobronchitis)
- Vocal cord dysfunction
- Foreign body
- Neck surgery
- Trauma (eg. due to relapsing polychondritis)
- Pharyngeal muscle weakness
  - Bulbar/Pseudobulbar palsy
- Tracheal pathology
  - Tracheal tumour
  - Tracheal web
  - Tracheomalacia
  - Endotracheal intubation
  - Tracheostomy
- Laryngeal pathology
  - Acute or chronic laryngitis
  - Laryngeal tumour
  - Laryngeal web
  - Laryngeal cyst
- Pharyngeal pathology
  - Retropharyngeal abscess
  - Tonsillar or adenoid hypertrophy
  - Peri-tonsillar abscess
- Angiooedema
- Anaphylaxis
- Burns

- Smoke inhalation
- Goitre
- Lymphadenopathy
  - Malignancy
  - Sarcoidosis
  - Lymphoproliferative disorders
- Wegners granulomatosis
- Aortic arch aneurysm

Expiratory stridor (intrathoracic airway obstruction)
- Foreign body
- Bronchial carcinoma
- Bronchial stenosis
  - Tuberculous stricture
  - Stricture secondary to sarcoidosis
- Lymphadenopathy
  - Lymphoproliferative disorders
  - Tuberculosis
  - Sarcoidosis

What are the difference between wheeze and stridor?

Wheeze	Stridor
Turbulent air flow through constricted smaller airways (bronchioles)	Turbulent airflow through narrowed segments of larger airways
Predominantly during expiration	Predominantly during inspiration, although it can occur during inspiration and expiration
Usually heard with a stethoscope, but in extreme cases, may be heard with the unaided ear	Readily heard without a stethoscope
Longer	Often shorter, but is louder and longer during inspiration
Common causes are asthma and COPD. Other causes include bronchiolitis, bronchiectasis, vasculitis, and pulmonary eosinophilic syndromes	Many causes (see above). Inspiratory stridor is more common

How would you investigate a patient with stridor?

- AP and lateral chest and neck X-rays
- Lung function tests (respiratory flow loop curves)
- Direct laryngoscopy and bronchoscopy
- CT chest (to demonstrate mediastinal pathology)

NB. Investigations will reflect history and working clinical diagnosis

What would changes you expect to see on respiratory flow loop curves in (a) extrathoracic and (b) intrathoracic airways obstruction?

(a) Extrathoracic obstruction

Extrathoracic obstruction can be *variable* (upper airway malignancy, lymphadenopathy, vocal cord dysfunction, and pharyngeal muscle weakness) or *fixed* (tracheal stenosis).

In *variable extrathoracic obstruction*, the inspiratory flow loop is blunted, whilst the expiratory flow loop is preserved:

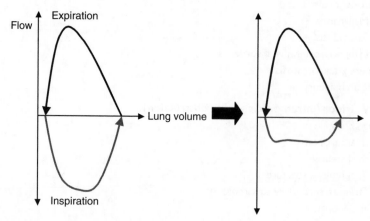

Figure 23.1 Variable extrathoracic obstruction.

In *fixed extrathoracic obstruction*, both the inspiratory and expiratory flow loops are blunted, with the inspiratory loop being more affected:

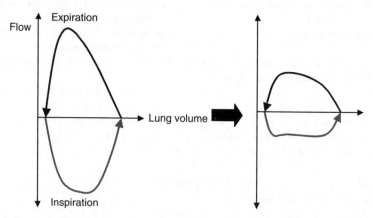

Figure 23.2 Fixed extrathoracic obstruction.

(b) Intrathoracic obstruction

The inspiratory flow loop is unaffected, whilst the expiratory flow loop is reduced:

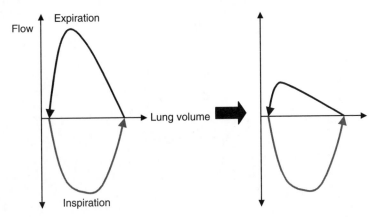

Figure 23.3 Intrathoracic obstruction.

Station 3 ◆ **Cardiovascular System**

Central Nervous System

Cardiovascular System

Case 24 ◆ **Aortic Stenosis**

CASE PRESENTATION

*There are no peripheral stigmata of endocarditis.[1] The pulse rate is …beats/min, regular/irregular, of **low volume** and exhibits a **slow-rising character**.[2] The blood pressure is …/…mmHg with a **narrow pulse pressure**.[3] The venous pressure is not elevated.[4] On examination of the precordium, the **apex beat is undisplaced**[5] with a **presystolic impulse**[6] (if in sinus rhythm) and has a **heaving character**.[5] There is a **systolic thrill** palpable in the aortic area.[7] On auscultation, the first heart sound is normal, but the **second heart sound is soft** with a **soft aortic component** and **reversed splitting**.[8] There is a **fourth heart sound** (if in sinus rhythm).[9] There is a harsh **ejection systolic murmur**,[10] heard throughout the precordium but loudest in the aortic area,[11] which is **louder in expiration**, and **radiates to the carotids**.[12] The lung fields are clear to auscultation and there is no peripheral oedema.[13]*

*The diagnosis is **severe aortic stenosis**.[14]*

Clinical notes

1. Always mention presence/absence of signs of endocarditis in any patient with physical signs of valvular heart disease. More than often, they are absent—but this is an important negative finding.

2. Both a low volume and a slow-rising pulse are signs of severe aortic stenosis. If the patient is in atrial fibrillation (AF), then the pulse usually has a variable volume, and some examiners believe that one cannot fully conclusively comment on pulse volume in AF. In patients with aortic stenosis and AF, the pulse exhbits a variable but diminished volume. It would be more appropriate in this setting to say, '*the pulse is of variable but diminished volume*'.

3. A narrow pulse pressure signifies a low cardiac output state, thus a sign of severe aortic stenosis. Other causes of a narrow pulse pressure include severe mitral stenosis or a hypovolaemic state.

4. If venous pressure is elevated, then look for signs of pulmonary hypertension (usually with giant systolic 'v' waves of tricuspid regurgitation, parasternal heave and thrill, and a loud pulmonary component to the second heart sound) or pulmonary congestion/cardiac failure (bibasal crepitations). The presence of pulmonary hypertension and pulmonary congestion are markers of severe aortic stenosis.

5. The left ventricle (LV) is hypertrophied, and is minimally displaced with a heaving character. A displaced apex beat indicates a dilated left ventricle, i.e. left ventricular failure. In the late stages of severe aortic stenosis, the left ventricle dilates and heart failure develops. However, the character of the apex beat remains the same. If the apex is displaced, in the absence of signs of severe aortic stenosis, then consider other causes of heart failure.

6. The presystolic impulse is transmission of atrial contraction just before closure of the mitral valve, as a result of forceful atrial contraction against a highly non-compliant and hypertrophied left ventricle. This is often accompanied by a fourth heart sound, and would be a marker of severe aortic stenosis. These signs would not be present in AF. A presystolic impulse is seen in other conditions with marked left ventricular hypertrophy, i.e. hypertensive heart disease or hypertrophic cardiomyopathy (giving a double apical impulse).

7. A systolic thrill is a marker of severe aortic stenosis.

8. These signs are both markers of severe aortic stenosis. Sometimes it can be difficult to appreciate the reversed splitting of the second heart sound (especially if the aortic component is diminished), thus don't say it if you cannot appreciate it! Sometimes, it may not be possible to hear the separate components of the second heart sound, and it may just be soft. The aortic component may be absent. If the physical signs are suggestive of severe aortic stenosis, but the second heart sound is loud, then you are most likely hearing a loud pulmonary component, then make sure that you have not missed other signs of pulmonary hypertension!

9. A fourth heart sound is a low frequency sound heard before the first heart sound. It results from forceful atrial contraction, at the end of diastole to fill a hypertrophied non-compliant left ventricle. It is a sign of severe aortic stenosis.

10. The intensity of the murmur does not correlate with severity. However, late peaking of a long systolic murmur is a marker of severe aortic stenosis. In advanced aortic stenosis the murmur may diminish, especially if the left ventricular function is compromised with a low cardiac output as cardiac failure supervenes.

11. Sometimes the murmur may not be loudest in the aortic area. It may be loudest at the apex, due to the Gallavardin phenomenon (see below). The successful candidate should be able to appreciate the quality of the murmur and in combination with other physical signs be able to make the correct diagnosis of aortic stenosis.

12. Sometimes the murmur may not radiate to the carotids, even in severe aortic stenosis.

13. Bibasal crepitations would be suggestive of pulmonary congestion, a marker of severe aortic stenosis. Look for a raised venous pressure and/or signs of pulmonary hypertension.

14. Having given the diagnosis of aortic stenosis, it is important to determine the severity. Remember the 11 clinical markers of severe aortic stenosis (see below).

Questions commonly asked by examiners

What are the causes of aortic stenosis?

Common causes

- Bicuspid aortic valve (most common cause in the young)
- Degenerative calcification (most common cause in the elderly)
- Rheumatic valve disease (this has declined dramatically)
- Congenital

Rarer causes

- Infective endocarditis
- Hyperuricaemia
- Alkaptonuria
- Paget's disease of the bone

What do you understand by the term 'ejection systolic murmur'?

It is a crescendo--decrescendo murmur after the first heart sound, or after an ejection click (in patients with a bicuspid aortic valve). The murmur peaks in mid to late systole, and ends before the second heart sound. An increased length of the murmur with late systolic peaking is a marker of severe aortic stenosis.

What would be the differential diagnosis of an ejection systolic murmur louder in expiration?

- Aortic stenosis
- Hypertrophic obstructive cardiomyopathy
- Supravalvular aortic stenosis (William's Syndrome, see below)

How do you classify the severity of aortic stenosis?

Using aortic valve area

The normal aortic valve orifice is 3–4 cm^2 in area, and the ACC/AHA guidelines have graded aortic stenosis as mild (valve area >1.5cm^2), moderate (valve area: 1.5–1.0cm^2) and severe (valve area <1.0cm^2).

Using pressure gradient

The mean gradient across the aortic valve is calculated by the Gorlin formula. This incorporates the aortic valve area, cardiac output, and heart rate (HR). The reduction in valve area to 1.5cm^2 is associated with little haemodynamic disturbance. Beyond this, any further decrement in aortic valve area produces a steep rise in left ventricular outflow obstruction. As a general rule, severe aortic stenosis is defined as a mean gradient >50mmHg.

What is aortic sclerosis?

This is characterized by mild thickening and/or calcification of a trileaflet aortic valve, and can be distinguished from aortic stenosis by the absence of outflow obstruction. It affects over a quarter of people aged over 65 years. Studies suggest that aortic sclerosis is a progressive disease, and over time increasing calcification and thickening results in outflow obstruction producing aortic stenosis. In one study, one third of patients with aortic sclerosis developed aortic stenosis over a mean follow-up period of 4 years. A recent study has shown that aortic sclerosis is associated with 50% increased risk of cardiovascular mortality and risk of myocardial infarction, even in the absence of haemodynamically significant aortic stenosis. As atherosclerosis and aortic sclerosis have been shown to share a common aetiology, suggesting an atherosclerosis-like process affecting the aortic valve, the findings of this study suggest that aortic sclerosis may be a novel marker for silent coronary artery disease.

How would you clinically differentiate aortic sclerosis from aortic stenosis?

Compared to aortic stenosis, in aortic sclerosis, the pulse volume and character will be normal. The apex beat will be undisplaced and with a normal character. The aortic component of the second hard sound will not be diminished. The murmur is often localized to the aortic area. In most, but not all, cases the murmur does not radiate to the carotids.

What are the clinical signs of severe aortic stenosis?

- Low volume pulse
- Slow-rising pulse
- Narrow pulse pressure
- Heaving apex
- Systolic thrill
- Reversed splitting of the second heart sound
- Soft or absent aortic component of the second heart sound
- Fourth heart sound
- Late systolic peaking of a long murmur
- Signs of pulmonary hypertension
- Signs of pulmonary congestion (or cardiac failure)

What are the other causes of reversed splitting of the second heart sound?

- Left bundle branch block
- Hypertrophic obstructive cardiomyopathy
- Patent ductus arteriosus
- Wolf-Parkinson-White Syndrome (Type B)

What are the complications of aortic stenosis?

- Left ventricular failure
- Sudden death (predominantly in symptomatic aortic stenosis)
- Pulmonary hypertension
- Arrhythmias (AF and ventricular tachycardia)
- Heart block (calcification of the conduction system)
- Infective endocarditis
- Systemic embolic complications (disintegration of aortic valve apparatus)
- Haemolytic anaemia
- Iron deficient anaemia (Heyde's syndrome)

This patient is asymptomatic, what would you tell the patient?

- Advise endocarditis prophylaxis.
- Report symptoms of angina, palpitations, syncope, and breathlessness.

Patients with severe aortic stenosis should be regularly screened for these symptoms. Sudden death predominantly occurs in symptomatic patients and these patients warrant aortic valve replacement. If the aortic valve is not replaced, then the onset of angina, syncope, and dyspnoea has been shown to correlate with an average time to death of 5, 3, and 2 years.

This patient has a normal coronary angiogram. What is the mechanism of angina in aortic stenosis?

With the development of aortic valve stenosis and progressive pressure overload, the left ventricle undergoes adaptive and maladaptive changes. The compensatory left ventricular hypertrophy allows the left ventricle to counter the outflow obstruction, maintaining the ejection fraction. However, hypertrophied hearts have decreased coronary blood flow reserve, even in the absence of coronary artery disease. Such hearts have been shown to exhibit increased sensitivity to ischaemic injury and usually have larger infarcts.

What is mechanism of syncope in aortic stenosis?

- A low cardiac output state
- Transient electro-mechanical dissociation (left ventricle unable to contract against a stenosed aortic valve)
- Presence of arrhthymias (AF or ventricular tachycardia)
- After exercise, when peripheral vasodilatation is not accompanied by an increase in cardiac output
- Vasodilator drugs (contraindicated in severe aortic stenosis, see below)

How would you investigate this patient?

Electrocardiogram (ECG)

- Left ventricular hypertrophy
- Left ventricular strain pattern
- Left atrial hypertrophy (bifid P waves in lead II)
- Left atrial dilatation (inverted of biphasic P waves in V_1–V_2)
- Left axis deviation
- Conduction abnormalities (left bundle branch block, first degree heart block)

CXR

- Post-stenotic dilatation of proximal ascending aorta (marked in bicuspid aortic valve)
- Rib notching (sign of coarctation of the aorta, frequently seen with bicuspid aortic valve)
- Calcification of aortic valve

- Cardiomegaly (late stages)
- Pulmonary congestion
- Prominent pulmonary arteries (pulmonary hypertension)

Echocardiogram
- Left ventricular size and function
- Aortic valve area

Coronary angiography
- To exclude coronary artery disease as a cause for symptoms.
- All patients having valve replacement should have coronary angiography to exclude significant coronary stenoses that would require bypass grafting at the time of valve replacement.

What are the indications for aortic valve replacement?

Symptomatic patients
- Symptomatic severe aortic stenosis (mean gradient >50mmHg)

Asymptomatic patients
- Moderate/severe aortic stenosis undergoing other cardiac surgery, i.e. coronary artery bypass surgery, aortic surgery or other valve surgery
- Severe aortic stenosis AND any of the following:
  - Left ventricular systolic dysfunction (mean gradient >40mmHg)
  - Abnormal blood pressure (BP) response to exercise (on SUPERVISED exercise treadmill testing)
  - Ventricular tachycardia
  - Valve area <0.6cm^2

Is the murmur of aortic stenosis always heard in the aortic area?

The murmur of aortic stenosis can frequently be heard throughout the precordium, but is usually loudest in the aortic area. In elderly patients, the *Gallavardin Phenomenon* is recognized. The high-frequency components of the ejection systolic murmur may reflect of the calcified ascending aorta, and the murmur is heard loudest over the apex. This may falsely suggest mitral regurgitation. It is the quality of the murmur (ejection systolic versus pansystolic) that helps differentiate the two murmurs, and make the correct diagnosis.

What do you know about Williams Syndrome?

This is a rare genetic condition whose clinical manifestations include a distinct facial appearance (elfin facies), cardiovascular anomalies, mental retardation, sensorineural hearing deficit, and hypercalcemia. Most common cardiac anomalies include supravalvular aortic stenosis, but pulmonary stenosis and mitral valve regurgitation can also occur. It is caused by a deletion at chromosome band 7q11.23 involving the elastin gene.

What is the role of statins in patients with aortic stenosis?

As calcific aortic stenosis resembles an atherosclerosis-like process, the use of statins was thought to slow the progression of aortic stenosis. Initial retrospective studies showed statin therapy to limit the progression of aortic stenosis. However, a recent prospective study (SALTIRE trial) did not show statin therapy to significantly reduce the progression of calcific aortic stenosis. Currently, statins are not routinely recommended for the management of aortic stenosis.

What do you know about Heyde's syndrome?

In 1958, Heyde first described the association between aortic stenosis and occult gastrointestinal bleeding (usually from colonic angiodysplastic lesions). The mechanisms underlying Heyde's syndrome have been the subject of debate, but recent evidence suggests that this bleeding is caused by an acquired defect in von Willebrand factor-an acquired type 2A von Willebrand syndrome.

High shear forces, as blood passes through the stenotic aortic valve, increase the susceptibility of von Willebrand factor to proteolysis. This results in loss of the largest multimers of von Willebrand factor, which are the most effective in platelet-mediated haemostasis. In these patients, aortic valve replacement restores von Willebrand multimers profiles, and eliminates haemorrhagic complications.

Case 25 ◆ Mitral Stenosis

CASE PRESENTATION 1

*There are no peripheral stigmata of endocarditis.[1] The pulse rate is …beats/min, **irregular**, normal volume and character.[2] The blood pressure is …/…mmHg. The venous pressure is not elevated.[3] There is no malar flush.[4] On examination of the precordium, there are no scars.[5] The apex beat is undisplaced and has a **tapping quality**.[6] There are no heaves or thrills.[7] On auscultation, the **first heart sound is loud**,[8] and the second heart sound is normal.[9] There is an **opening snap**[10] in early diastole followed by a **mid-diastolic rumbling murmur** at the apex, heard best in **expiration** with the patient in the **left lateral position**.[11] The lung fields are clear to auscultation and there is no peripheral oedema.[12]*

*The diagnosis is **mitral stenosis**. There are no signs of pulmonary hypertension.[15]*

CASE PRESENTATION 2

*There are no peripheral stigmata of endocarditis.[1] The pulse rate is …beats/min, **irregular, low volume**, and normal character.[2] The blood pressure is …/…mmHg. The **venous pressure is elevated** with systolic 'v' waves.[3] There is a **malar flush**.[4] On examination of the precordium, there is a **lateral thoracotomy scar**.[5] The apex beat is undisplaced and has a **tapping quality**.[6] There is a **parasternal heave** and a **parasternal thrill**.[7] On auscultation, the **first heart sound is loud**,[8] and there is a **loud pulmonary component** to the second heart sound.[9] There is an **opening snap**[10] in early diastole followed by a **mid-diastolic rumbling murmur** at the apex, heard best in **expiration** with the patient in the **left lateral position**.[11] In addition, there a **pansystolic murmur at the lower left sternal edge**, which is **louder in inspiration**,[13] and a short **early diastolic murmur in the pulmonary area**, radiating down the left sternal edge, **louder in inspiration**.[14] On auscultation of the lung fields, there are **bibasal crepitations**, and there is **peripheral oedema**.[12]*

*This patient has previously had **mitral valvotomy**, and now has **severe mitral stenosis** with signs of **pulmonary hypertension, pulmonary congestion**, and **right-sided cardiac failure**.[15]*

Clinical notes

1. Always mention presence/absence of signs of endocarditis in any patient with physical signs of valvular heart disease. More than often, they are absent—but this is an important negative finding.
2. Patients with mitral stenosis are usually in AF. Sometimes an irregular pulse may be difficult to ascertain, especially if bradycardic. The pulse volume is often variable in AF. The pulse volume can be low in severe

mitral stenosis, as this is a low cardiac output state, and you may expect a narrow pulse pressure in this situation.

3. Look for a raised venous pressure. This would suggest cardiac failure and/or pulmonary hypertension. The presence of systolic 'v' waves should prompt you to look for other signs of pulmonary hypertension: parasternal heave, parasternal thrill (tricuspid regurgitation), loud pulmonary component of the second heart sound, the pansystolic murmur of tricuspid regurgitation, Graham-Steell murmur of pulmonary regurgitation).

4. This may not always be present. A malar flush signifies a low cardiac output state with pulmonary hypertension and is often seen in patients with severe mitral stenosis. Remember, there are other causes of appearances that may resemble a malar flush (see below). A malar flush should always be looked for in a cardiovascular examination, but its absence or presence should be commented on in the final presentation in the presence of mitral valve disease.

5. Look carefully for previous mitral valvotomy scar on the left lateral chest wall.

6. A tapping apex beat is a palpable first heart sound, and in this setting the first heart sound will be loud. In cases where the first heart sound is not loud (see below), the first heart sound will not be palpable and thus the apex beat will not demonstrate a tapping quality.

7. With a raised venous pressure, you will expect to find signs of pulmonary hypertension and right-sided cardiac failure. A parasternal heave signifies right ventricular pressure overload. A parasternal thrill signifies underlying 'functional' tricuspid regurgitation (if present, don't miss the systolic 'v' waves in the venous pressure).

8. A loud first heart sound is usually heard, that reflects mobile and pliable valve leaflets. However, if the mitral valve leaflets themselves are calcified and immobile, then the first heart sound will be soft and the opening snap will be lost. Calcification of valve leaflets DOES NOT indicate severity, thus a soft first heart sound and absence of an opening snap cannot be used as markers of severe mitral stenosis.

9. The pulmonary component of the second heart sound will be loud with pulmonary hypertension. If present do not miss other signs of pulmonary hypertension.

10. The opening snap will be heard with a loud first heart sound, and indicates the mitral valve leaflets are mobile and pliable. This will be lost if the leaflets are calcified. The opening snap follows the second heart sound and occurs in early diastole. The earlier the opening snap, the greater the left atrial pressure, thus the greater the severity of mitral stenosis. As a general rule if time to opening snap is <0.1s, left atrial pressure >20mmHg. If time to opening snap is >0.1s, left atrial pressure <15mmHg. It is virtually impossible to comment on time delays in heart sounds (especially in the examination settings); however, it is important to know the implications of an early opening snap and the underlying pathophysiology.

11. The murmur of mitral stenosis can be difficult to hear. It is a low-frequency murmur, and is heard best in expiration with the patient in the left lateral position, using the bell of the stethoscope. If unsure of the murmur, it can be accentuated with exercise. Ask the patient to touch the toes and recline back and forth 10 times, or ask the patient to hop on one foot 10 times (this will usually not be expected in the examination, but is important to know for discussion). If the patient is in sinus rhythm, the murmur has pre-systolic accentuation, i.e. increases in intensity before the first heart sound is heard.

12. Mitral stenosis will initially lead to pulmonary venous hypertension, pulmonary congestion and then pulmonary arterial hypertension, and right-sided cardiac failure. In the presence of signs of pulmonary hypertension, look carefully for bibasal crepitations (pulmonary congestion) and peripheral oedema. The lung fields can be clear, and peripheral oedema can be minimal especially if the patient is on diuretics.

13. This is the murmur of 'functional ' tricuspid regurgitation and is associated with systolic 'v' waves in the venous pressure and a parasternal thrill. The murmur is louder in inspiration (Carvallo's sign). If present, look carefully for other signs of pulmonary hypertension.

14. This is the Graham-Steell murmur of pulmonary regurgitation. This signifies elevated pulmonary arterial pressures, and is a marker of severe mitral stenosis. This is often a very short murmur in early diastole, usually in the pulmonary area, and only radiates a few intercostal spaces down the left sternal edge. It is differentiated from aortic regurgitation by being much shorter and louder in inspiration. This murmur is almost always associated with a loud and often palpable pulmonary component of the second heart sound. Look for other signs of pulmonary hypertension.

15. Once having given a diagnosis of mitral stenosis, it is important to assess severity. Remember the markers of severe mitral stenosis (see below).

Questions commonly asked by examiners

What are the causes of mitral stenosis?
- **Rheumatic fever** (most common, the others are rare)
- Congenital mitral stenosis
- Rheumatoid arthritis
- Systemic lupus erythematosus (SLE)
- Carcinoid Syndrome
- Mucopolysaccharidoses
- Fabry's disease
- Methysergide therapy
- Whipples disease

What other conditions could give a mid-diastolic rumbling murmur?
- Left atrial mass (typically myxomas)
- Left atrial thrombus
- Cor triatriatum[*]
- Severe mitral regurgitation (increased forward flow across the mitral valve)

What is the pathophysiology of mitral stenosis?
- The normal area of the mitral valve orifice is 4–6cm². Narrowing of the valve area to less than 2.5cm² impedes the free flow of blood between the left atrium (LA) and left ventricle and increases left atrial pressure. This is required to maintain transmitral flow volume.
- Critical mitral stenosis occurs when the opening is reduced to 1cm². At this stage, a left atrial pressure of 25mmHg is required to maintain a normal cardiac output. With progressive stenosis, critical flow restriction reduces cardiac output. The left atrium enlarges and pulmonary venous and capillary pressures increase. The resulting pulmonary congestion and reduced cardiac output can mimic primary left ventricular failure, but left ventricular contractility is normal in most cases of mitral stenosis.
- As the disease evolves, chronic elevation of left atrial pressures leads to pulmonary hypertension, tricuspid and pulmonary valve incompetence, and secondary right heart failure.

How do you classify the severity of mitral stenosis?
The severity can be classified according to mitral valve area:
- Mild: >1.5 cm²
- Moderate: 1–1.5 cm²
- Severe: <1.0 cm²

What are the clinical markers of severe mitral stenosis?
- Early opening snap (lost with calcified leaflets)
- Increasing length of murmur[a]

---

[*] A congenital anomaly where the heart has 3 atria—either the left or right atrium (RA) is divided into 2 by a fibromuscular band.

[a] Sometimes the murmur in severe mitral stenosis may be inaudible, and the only clinical findings are of pulmonary hypertension

- Signs of pulmonary hypertension[b]
- Signs of pulmonary congestion
- Graham-Steell murmur (pulmonary regurgitation)
- Low pulse pressure[c]

What are the complications of mitral stenosis?

- Left atrial enlargement
- Atrial fibrillation
- Left atrial thrombus formation
- Pulmonary hypertension
- Pulmonary oedema
- Right heart failure

What is the pathology underlying the malar flush?

A malar flush is seen in mitral stenosis with the development of severe pulmonary hypertension, leading to a low cardiac output state.

What is the differential diagnosis of a malar flush?

- Mitral stenosis
- Hypothyroidism
- Cold weather
- Carcinoid syndrome
- SLE
- Systemic Sclerosis
- Irradiation
- Polycythaemia

How would you investigate this patient?

ECG

- Atrial fibrillation is common. Some patients may be in sinus rhythm
- Left atrial hypertrophy (bifid P waves in lead II) if in sinus rhythm
- Left atrial dilatation (inverted or biphasic P waves in V_1–V_2) if in sinus rhythm

CXR

- Double right heart border (left atrial enlargement)
- Splaying of the carina (an old sign used to demonstrate a grossly dilated left atrium)
- Pulmonary congestion
- Prominent pulmonary arteries (pulmonary hypertension)

Coronary angiography

- To exclude coronary artery disease as a cause for symptoms.
- All patients having mitral valve replacement should have coronary angiography to exclude significant coronary stenoses that would require bypass grafting at the time of valve replacement.

---

[b] Raised venous pressure (systolic v waves), parasternal heave, loud and palpable P_2, tricuspid and pulmonary regurgitation

[c] Signifies a low cardiac output state

How would you manage a patient with mitral stenosis?

Asymptomatic patients in sinus rhythm:
- Endocarditis prophylaxis
- Regular follow-up with echocardiography

Management of AF
- Adopt a rhythm control or rate control strategy[a,b]
- Patients with mitral valve disease should be anticoagulated with warfarin if no contra-indications exist.

Management of symptomatic patients:
- Diuretics reduce left atrial pressure and relieve mild symptoms
- As symptoms worsen, and pulmonary hypertension begins to develop, these patients should be referred for surgery.

What procedures can be used to treat mitral stenosis?

Closed commisurotomy

This can be achieved by closed mitral valvotomy (not done nowadays) or mitral valvuloplasty.

Open commisurotomy

Requires open heart surgery with cardiopulmonary bypass and valve repair under direct vision.

Mitral valve replacement

Requires open heart surgery with cardiopulmonary bypass.

What are the indications for surgery?
- Pulmonary congestion
- Pulmonary hypertension
- Haemoptysis
- Recurrent thromboembolic events despite therapeutic anticoagulation

What are the criteria for using valvuloplasty?
- Mobile valve (loud first heart sound and opening snap)
- Minimal calcification of the valve and subvalvular apparatus
- Absence of mitral regurgitation
- Absence of left atrial thrombus (on transoesophageal echocardiography)

If this patient developed a hoarse voice, what would you be thinking?

An enlarged left atrium in mitral stenosis may compress the left recurrent laryngeal nerve, leading to left vocal cord paralysis. This is called *Ortner's Syndrome*. Another possibility could be hypothyroidism secondary to amiodarone therapy (used to treat AF which is strongly associated with mitral valve disease).

---

[a] Recent evidence suggests rate control is not inferior to rhythm control. Rate control can be achieved with digoxin, beta blockers or calcium antagonists. Rhythm control can be achieved with class I and III drugs (flecainide, amiodarone, and sotalol).

[b] Rhythm control is unlikely if left atrial diameter is greater than 5cm, as these patients have a high chance of recurrence of AF. Patients with mitral stenosis have a dilated left atrium, that acts as a substrate for AF, thus a rate-control strategy is often used.

Case 26 ◆ **Prosthetic Aortic Valve**

Examiner's note

Patients with prosthetic valves are very common in the examination. They are usually stable following their valve replacements, and easy to bring in for MRCP (PACES) examinations. There are many different types of prosthetic aortic valves, but on clinical grounds, they can be separated primarily into those that produce one audible click or those that produce two audible clicks (Starr-Edwards prosthesis). The case presentations below reflect this.

A prosthetic aortic valve is relatively easy to pick up, but considerable extra marks can be gained in these cases, that may make the difference between a 'pass' and a 'clear pass', and more importantly between an overall pass or fail. It is important to be able to demonstrate to the examiner that you are aware of the complications of prosthetic valves and mention the absence or presence of these in your final presentation:

(a) Are there any signs of infective endocarditis?
(b) Is the prosthesis functioning well?
(c) Are there any complications of anticoagulation?

CASE PRESENTATION 1

There are no peripheral stigmata of endocarditis.[1] The pulse rate is …beats/min, regular/irregular, …volume, and …character.[2] The blood pressure is …/…mmHg.[3] There is no evidence of anaemia.[4] The venous pressure is not elevated.[5] A **prosthetic click can be heard** with the unaided ear.[6] On examination of the precordium there is a **mid-line sternotomy scar**.[7] The apex beat is displaced/undisplaced with a …character.[8] There are no heaves or thrills.[9] On auscultation the first heart sound is normal followed by an **ejection systolic murmur**[10] and a **prosthetic click at the second heart sound**.[11] The lung fields are clear to auscultation and there is no peripheral oedema.

This patient has had an **aortic valve replacement**, which appears to be functioning well.[12]

CASE PRESENTATION 2

There are no peripheral stigmata of endocarditis.[1] The pulse rate is …beats/min, regular/irregular, …volume, and …character.[2] The blood pressure is …/…mmHg.[3] There is no evidence of anaemia.[4] The venous pressure is not elevated.[5] **Prosthetic clicks can be heard** with the unaided ear.[6] On examination of the precordium there is a **mid-line sternotomy scar**.[7] The apex beat is displaced/undisplaced with a …character.[8] There are no heaves or thrills.[9] On auscultation the first heart sound is normal followed by a **prosthetic click**, an **ejection systolic murmur**[10] and a **prosthetic click at the second heart sound**.[11] The lung fields are clear to auscultation and there is no peripheral oedema.

This patient has had an **aortic valve replacement**, which appears to be functioning well. The opening and closing clicks would suggest a **Starr-Edwards (Ball and Cage)** prosthesis.[12]

Clinical notes

1. Always mention presence/absence of signs of endocarditis in any patient with a prosthetic valve. More than often, they are absent—but this is an important negative finding.

2. Assess the pulse for low volume and slow-rising character, which would signify a stenotic prosthetic aortic valve. Starr-Edwards prosthesis can give a slow-rising pulse, even in the absence of haemodynamically significant aortic stenosis. On the other hand, a large volume and collapsing pulse would suggest aortic regurgitation, i.e. a malfunctioning aortic prosthesis.

3. A narrow pulse pressure would suggest aortic stenosis. A large pulse pressure would suggest aortic regurgitation.

4. Anaemia is an important complication to look for in patients with prosthetic valves. This can occur secondary to blood loss (anticoagulation), haemolysis (look for jaundice), and endocarditis. Look for evidence of purpura, suggesting anticoagulant use—that would suggest the patient has (a) AF (look for an irregular pulse) or (b) mechanical prosthesis (especially if the pulse is regular, suggestive of sinus rhythm).

5. If venous pressure is elevated, then look for signs of pulmonary hypertension (usually with giant systolic 'v' waves of tricuspid regurgitation, parasternal heave and thrill and a loud pulmonary component to the second heart sound) or pulmonary congestion (bibasal crepitations). Pulmonary hypertension may be present in patients after aortic valve replacements, as it may persist after surgery. Pulmonary hypertension is initially reversible and can reverse following surgery with afterload reduction. However, if pulmonary hypertension had been present for some time prior to surgery, then this can lead to permanent changes to the pulmonary vasculature, thus the pulmonary hypertension will persist even after corrective surgery. It is more common to see pulmonary hypertension persisting after corrective valve surgery in patients with mitral valve replacements, who have often had longstanding pulmonary hypertension prior to valve replacement.

6. Prosthetic valves can click when they open or close. Often, the CLOSING CLICKS ARE LOUDER THAN THE OPENING CLICKS, hence only closing clicks are often heard and more easily appreciated. Thus it is the timing of the closing click that is the key to making the diagnosis. Clicks may be heard without the stethoscope, and in some cases even at the end of the bed. Timing these clicks with the pulse may provide useful clues to the position of the prosthesis, even before auscultation. Remembering, the carotid pulse occurs at the first heart sound, then a closing click that coincides with and occurs at the carotid pulse would suggest mitral valve prosthesis. Similarly, a click that occurs shortly after the carotid pulse would suggest the closing click coincides with the second heart sound, and is likely to represent an aortic valve prosthesis. However, the older Starr-Edwards (ball and cage) prostheses often produce two equally loud opening and closing clicks and this technique may be used, but the multiple clicks can be difficult to time and is best avoided in such cases. This technique of timing the audible clicks with the carotid impulse requires considerable practice, and is best appreciated in less tachycardic states (HR <80bpm). With increasing pulse rate, the timing of audible clicks with the carotid impulse becomes more difficult.

7. Most patients with previous valve surgery have mid-line sternotomy scars. Look carefully at the legs and arms for signs of saphenous vein or radial artery harvest scars, as this would suggest previous or concurrent coronary artery bypass graft (CABG) surgery.

8. The apex position and character will assess the presence of aortic stenosis and regurgitation. An undisplaced heaving impulse would suggest aortic stenosis. In patients who previously had aortic stenosis and who have had a successful aortic valve replacement, the heaving character to the apex beat may persist. This is because although aortic valve replacement results in afterload reduction and some degree of regression of left ventricular hypertrophy, some degree of left ventricular hypertrophy may persist. Additionally, patients may have hypertension, which is an important cause for left ventricular hypertrophy. A displaced thrusting impulse would indicate aortic regurgitation, i.e. a regurgitant prosthesis.

9. A parasternal heave or thrill would suggest pulmonary hypertension. A parasternal heave signifies right ventricular pressure overload. A parasternal thrill signifies underlying 'functional' tricuspid regurgitation (if present, don't miss the systolic 'v' waves in the venous pressure).

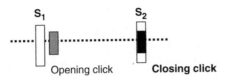

Figure 26.1

10. All aortic valve replacements will produce an ejection systolic murmur. Other physical signs, i.e. pulse volume and character, pulse pressure, quality of the second heart sound, will help decide if there is any haemodynamically significant aortic stenosis. Listen carefully for the murmur of aortic regurgitation, which signifies valve dysfunction. Occasionally, some patients may have some degree of paraprosthetic or transprosthetic aortic regurgitation that is usually demonstrated on echocardiography, and does not represent valve dysfunction. In certain patients, this may be heard with a stethoscope. In the setting of a clinical examination, any prosthetic valve regurgitant murmur should be regarded as valvular dysfunction until proven otherwise.

11. Remember, CLOSING CLICKS ARE LOUDER THAN THE OPENING CLICKS. Starr-Edwards (ball and cage) prostheses often produce two equally loud opening and closing clicks. **All aortic valve prostheses produce a prosthetic (closing) click at the second heart sound**. In addition, the Starr-Edwards aortic prostheses produce an additional ejection click shortly after the first heart sound. Differentiating this ejection click from the first heart sound requires practice.

12. When presenting the diagnosis, it is important to state the absence or presence of complications and if the prosthesis is functioning well.

Questions commonly asked by examiners

What are the indications for aortic valve replacement?

A Aortic stenosis

- *Symptomatic*
    - ♦ Severe aortic stenosis (mean gradient >50mmHg)
- *Asymptomatic*
    - ♦ Moderate/severe aortic stenosis undergoing other cardiac surgery, i.e. coronary artery bypass surgery, aortic surgery, or other valve surgery
    - ♦ Severe aortic stenosis AND any of the following:
        - – Left ventricular systolic dysfunction (gradient >40mmHg)
        - – Abnormal BP response to exercise
        - – Ventricular tachycardia
        - – Valve area <0.6cm^2

B Aortic regurgitation

- *Symptomatic*
    - ♦ Severe aortic regurgitation with angina or dyspnoea
- *Asymptomatic*
    - ♦ Moderate/severe aortic regurgitation undergoing other cardiac surgery, i.e. coronary artery bypass surgery, aortic surgery, or other valve surgery
    - ♦ Left ventricular dysfunction (ejection fraction <50%)
    - ♦ Dilated left ventricle (end-systolic diameter ≥55mm)

C Other

- Infective endocarditis with failed medical therapy
- Enlarging aortic root diameter (≥50mm) irrespective of degree of aortic regurgitation
- Acute severe aortic regurgitation (infective endocarditis and ruptured sinus of valsalva aneurysm)

What are the different kinds of prosthetic valves?

Mechanical prostheses

- *Starr-Edwards valve*: a ball and cage device, with blood flowing around the ball, thus a high incidence of haemolysis. The silastic ball is cured to prevent lipid accumulation
- *Medtronic-Hall valve*: a titling disc valve, made of pyrolytic carbon
- *Bjork-Shiley valve*: a single tilting disc valve with laminar flow, thus low incidence of haemolysis.
- *St Judes valve*: a double-tilting disc valve (bileaflet)

Xenografts

- *Porcine valve*
- *Pericardial valve*

Homografts

- These are cadaveric aortic or pulmonary valves (do not produce clicks)

Which patients should receive a bioprosthetic valve?

- In patients where anticoagulation would be contraindicated
- Life expectancy shorter than the predicted lifespan of prosthesis
- Patient age >70years, as rate of degeneration is slow in these patients

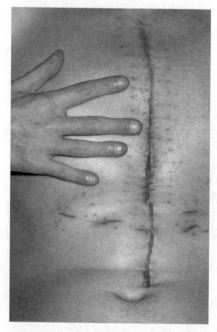

Figure 26.2 A prominent midline sternotomy scar. These scars can be very prominent especially in patients with keloid scar formation. In some patients, these scars can be very faint, and the key is to look carefully and not miss them. Note the small scars below the central midline scar. These represent drain sites inserted at the end of the cardiac surgical procedure.

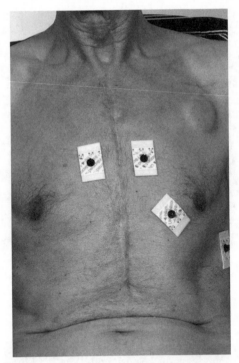

Figure 26.3 Midline sternotomy scar and a left infraclavicular scar (pacemaker scar). Note the prominence below the scar—this is the pacemaker generator box. This is often visible in thin patients.

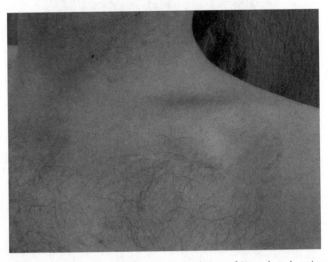

Figure 26.4 Left infraclavicular pacemaker scar. These scars can be very faint and can be missed. Look for this scar particularly in patients with aortic valve replacement, as conduction disease is common in aortic valve disease. It is not uncommon for patients to require a permanent pacemaker following aortic valve replacement.

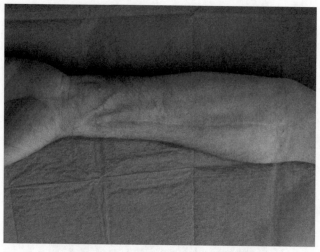

Figure 26.5 Left radial artery harvest scar. The radial artery can be used for conduits in CABG surgery. If present, do not miss this scar!

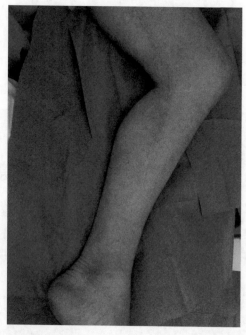

Figure 26.6 Left saphenous vein harvest scar.

What are the complications of prosthetic valves?

- Thromboembolism
- Complications of anticoagulation, i.e. bleeding
- Valve dysfunction, i.e. leakage, dehiscence, and obstruction due to thrombosis, fibrosis, and clogging
- Endocarditis
- Haemolysis

What are advantages and disadvantages of porcine heart valves?

- 8Advantages: No need for warfarin anticoagulation, thus safer in women of child-bearing age and in the elderly.
- Disadvantages: Reduced lifespan of prosthesis compared to mechanical valves, due to degeneration and calcification.

When are homograft valves used?

In young patients, they are considered the valve of first choice. Commonly used for replacing infected valves in infective endocarditis, as they are more resistant to re-infection.

What are the causes of anaemia in a patient with a prosthetic valve?

- Blood loss secondary to anticoagulation
- Haemolysis (commonly aortic prostheses)
- Endocarditis

Case 27 ◆ Prosthetic Mitral Valve

Examiner's note

Patients with mitral valve replacements are potentially more complicated than those with aortic valve replacements. They may have previously had mitral valvotomy (don't miss the scar) and most patients are left with permanent pulmonary hypertension. Depending on the type of prosthetic valve, prosthetic valves may produce 1 or 2 audible clicks. Therefore, mitral valve replacements can occur within a broad spectrum of clinical and examination findings. The case presentations below reflect this variety encountered in the MRCP (PACES) examination.

A prosthetic mitral valve is relatively easy to pick up, but considerable extra marks can be gained in these cases, that may make the difference between a 'pass' and a 'clear pass', and more importantly between an overall pass or fail. It is important to be able to demonstrate to the examiner that you are aware of the complications of prosthetic valves and mention the absence or presence of these in your final presentation.

CASE PRESENTATION 1

There are no peripheral stigmata of endocarditis.[1] The pulse rate is …beats/min, regular/irregular, … volume, and …character.[2] The blood pressure is …/…mmHg. There is no evidence of anaemia.[3] The venous pressure is not elevated.[4] A **prosthetic click can be heard** *with the unaided ear, which* coincides with the first heart sound.[5] On examination of the precordium there is a **mid-line sternotomy scar**.[6] The apex beat is undisplaced.[7] There are no heaves or thrills.[8] On auscultation, there is a **prosthetic click at the first heart sound** and the second heart sound is normal.[9,10] The lung fields are clear to auscultation and there is no peripheral oedema.

This patient has had a **mitral valve replacement**, which appears to be functioning well.[12]

CASE PRESENTATION 2

There are no peripheral stigmata of endocarditis.[1] The pulse rate is …beats/min, regular/irregular, … volume, and …character.[2] The blood pressure is …/…mmHg. There is no evidence of anaemia.[3] The **venous pressure is elevated** with systolic 'v' waves.[4] **Prosthetic clicks can be heard** with the unaided ear.[5] On examination of the precordium there is a **mid-line sternotomy scar** and **a left lateral thoracotomy scar**.[6] The apex beat is displaced.[7] There is a **parasternal heave** and a **parasternal thrill**.[8] On auscultation, there is a **prosthetic click at the first heart sound**, and a **prosthetic click after the second heart sound** (in early diastole), followed by a **mid-diastolic flow murmur at the apex**, heard best in **expiration** in the **left lateral position**. The **pulmonary component of the second heart sound is loud**.[9,10] There is a **pansystolic murmur** at the lower left sternal edge, **louder in inspiration**.[11] The lung fields are clear to auscultation and there is **peripheral oedema**.

This patient has had a **mitral valvotomy for mitral stenosis** in the past followed by **mitral valve replacement**, which appears to be functioning well. The opening and closing clicks would suggest this is a **Starr-Edwards (Ball and Cage)** prosthesis. There are signs of **pulmonary hypertension**.[12]

CASE PRESENTATION 3

There are no peripheral stigmata of endocarditis.[1] The pulse rate is …beats/min, regular/irregular, … volume, and …character.[2] The blood pressure is …/…mmHg. There is no evidence of anaemia.[3] The **venous pressure is elevated** with systolic 'v' waves.[4] A **prosthetic click can be heard** with the unaided ear, which **coincides with the first heart sound**.[5] On examination of the precordium there is a **mid-line sternotomy scar**.[6] The apex beat is displaced.[7] There is a **parasternal heave** and a **parasternal thrill**.[8] On auscultation, there is a **prosthetic click at the first heart sound** and the **pulmonary component of the second heart sound is loud**.[9,10] There is a **pansystolic murmur** at the lower left sternal edge, **louder in inspiration**.[11] The lung fields are clear to auscultation and there is **peripheral oedema**.

This patient has had a **mitral valve replacement**, which appears to be functioning well. There are signs of **pulmonary hypertension**.[12]

CASE PRESENTATION 4

There are no peripheral stigmata of endocarditis.[1] The pulse rate is …beats/min, regular/irregular, … volume, and …character.[2] The blood pressure is …/…mmHg. There is no evidence of anaemia.[3] The venous pressure is not elevated.[4] A **prosthetic click can be heard** with the unaided ear, which **coincides with the first heart sound**.[5] On examination of the precordium there is a **mid-line sternotomy scar**.[6] The apex beat is displaced with a thrusting character.[7] There is a **parasternal heave** but no thrills.[8] On auscultation, there is a **prosthetic click at the first heart sound** and the **pulmonary component of the second heart sound is loud**.[9,10] There is a **pansystolic murmur** at the **apex**, which is **louder in expiration,** and **radiates to the axilla**.[11] On auscultation of the lung fields, there are **bibasal crepitations**. There is **peripheral oedema**.

*This patient has had a **mitral valve replacement**, and the murmur of **mitral regurgitation** suggests it is leaking. There are signs of **pulmonary congestion** and **pulmonary hypertension**.[1,2]*

Clinical notes

1. Always mention presence/absence of signs of endocarditis in any patient with a prosthetic valve. More than often, they are absent—but this is an important negative finding.

2. Patients with mitral valve disease are more likely to be in AF. Look for an irregular pulse. Sometimes an irregular pulse may be difficult to ascertain, especially if bradycardic. The pulse volume is often variable in AF.

3. Anaemia is an important complication to look for in patients with prosthetic valves. This can occur secondary to blood loss (anticoagulation), haemolysis (look for jaundice) and endocarditis. Look for evidence of purpura, suggesting anticoagulant use. Most patients with mitral valve disease have AF, and therefore will be on warfarin therapy. Patients with mechanical valve require anticoagulation with warfarin.

4. If venous pressure is elevated, then look for signs of pulmonary hypertension (usually with giant systolic 'v' waves of tricuspid regurgitation, parasternal heave and thrill, and a loud pulmonary component to the second heart sound) or pulmonary congestion (bibasal crepitations). In a patient with mitral valve replacement, it is not uncommon for them to have signs of pulmonary hypertension, which may persist after successful valve replacement (commonly seen in patients with previous mitral stenosis and mitral valvotomy scars).

5. Prosthetic valves can click when they open or close. Often, the CLOSING CLICKS ARE LOUDER THAN THE OPENING CLICKS, hence only closing clicks are often heard and more easily appreciated. Thus it is the timing of the closing click that is the key to making the diagnosis. Clicks may be heard without the stethoscope, and in some cases even at the end of the bed. Timing these clicks with the pulse may provide useful clues to the position of the prosthesis, even before auscultation. Remember, the carotid pulse occurs at the first heart sound, then a closing click that coincides with and occurs at the carotid pulse would suggest mitral valve prosthesis. Similarly, a click that occurs shortly after the carotid pulse would suggest the closing click coincides with the second heart sound, and is likely to represent aortic valve prosthesis. However, the older Starr-Edwards (ball and cage) prostheses often produce two equally loud opening and closing clicks and this technique may be used, but the multiple clicks can be difficult to time and is best avoided in such cases. This technique of timing the audible clicks with the carotid impulse requires considerable practice, and is best appreciated in less tachycardic states (HR <80bpm). With increasing pulse rate, the timing of audible clicks with the carotid impulse becomes more difficult.

6. Always spend a little extra time looking for scars. Patients with previous valve surgery have mid-line sternotomy scars. Look carefully at the legs and arms for signs of saphenous vein or radial artery harvest scars, as this would suggest previous or concurrent CABG surgery. Don't miss the left lateral mitral valvotomy scar.

7. A displaced and thrusting apex in a patient with mitral valve prosthesis suggests prosthesis dysfunction with mitral regurgitation. The closing click at the first heard sound may be palpable in some patients. This is analogous to a palpable first heart sound in mitral stenosis, and this may be associated with a tapping apex beat!

8. A parasternal heave or thrill would suggest pulmonary hypertension. A parasternal heave signifies right ventricular pressure overload. A parasternal thrill signifies underlying 'functional' tricuspid regurgitation (if present, don't miss the systolic 'v' waves in the venous pressure).

9. Remember, prosthetic valves can only click when they open or close, and that CLOSING CLICKS ARE LOUDER THAN THE OPENING CLICKS. Starr-Edwards (ball and cage) prostheses often produce two equally loud opening and closing clicks. **All mitral valve prostheses produce a prosthetic (closing) click at the first heart sound.** In addition, Starr-Edwards mitral prostheses produce an additional

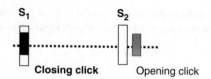

Figure 27.1

opening click shortly after the second heart sound (in early diastole). Differentiating this ejection click from the second heart sound requires practice.

10. Mitral valve prostheses may be associated with a flow murmur across them. This is more commonly heard with Starr-Edwards prostheses, and manifests as a short low-frequency mid-diastolic murmur at the apex. This is best heard in expiration in the left lateral position using the bell of the stethoscope (as in mitral stenosis).

11. If you see systolic 'v' waves in the venous pressure, then listen carefully for the pansystolic murmur of tricuspid regurgitation, at the lower left sternal edge. It becomes louder in inspiration (Carvallo's sign). If mitral regurgitation is also present, then differentiating the two murmurs can be difficult. It is important to be able to distinguish mitral regurgitation from tricuspid regurgitation, as incorrect diagnosis of mitral regurgitation in a patient with mitral valve prosthesis will incorrectly imply prosthesis dysfunction (see Case 28 Mitral Regurgitation).

12. When presenting the diagnosis, it is important to state the absence or presence of complications and if the prosthesis is functioning well.

Questions commonly asked by examiners

The questions commonly asked for prosthetic mitral valves are similar to those asked for prosthetic aortic valves. Please refer to the questions for prosthetic aortic valve (Case 26 Prosthetic Aortic Valve). You will be expected to know the indications for mitral valve replacement.

What are the indications for mitral valve replacement?
Mitral stenosis
- Signs of pulmonary congestion
- Pulmonary hypertension
- Haemoptysis
- Recurrent thromboembolic episodes despite therapeutic anticoagulation

Mitral regurgitation
- Signs of left ventricular dysfunction
- Ejection fraction ≤60% (even in the absence of symptoms)
- Left ventricular end-systolic diameter ≥45mm (even in the absence of symptoms)

Case 28 ◆ **Mitral Regurgitation**

CASE PRESENTATION 1

*There are no peripheral stigmata of endocarditis.[1] The pulse rate is …beats/min, **irregular**, normal volume and character.[2] The blood pressure is …/…mmHg. The venous pressure is not elevated.[3] On examination of the precordium, there are no scars.[4] The apex beat is **displaced** and has a **thrusting quality**.[5]*

There are no heaves but there is an **apical thrill**.[6] On auscultation, the **first heart sound is soft**,[7] and the second heart sound is normal.[8] There is a **pansystolic murmur** at the apex, loudest in **expiration**, which **radiates to the axilla**.[10] The lung fields are clear to auscultation and there is no peripheral oedema.[12]

The diagnosis is **mitral regurgitation**. There are no signs of pulmonary hypertension.[13]

CASE PRESENTATION 2

There are no peripheral stigmata of endocarditis.[1] The pulse rate is …beats/min, **irregular**, normal volume and character.[2] The blood pressure is …/…mmHg. The **venous pressure is elevated** with **systolic 'v' waves**.[3] On examination of the precordium, there is a **lateral thoracotomy scar**.[4] The apex beat is **displaced** and has a **thrusting quality**.[5] There is a **parasternal heave** and a **precordial thrill**.[6] On auscultation, the **first heart sound is soft**,[7] there is a **loud pulmonary component of the second heart sound**[8] and a **third heart sound**.[9] There is a **pansystolic murmur** at the apex, loudest in **expiration**, which **radiates to the axilla**.[10] In addition, there a **pansystolic murmur at the lower left sternal edge**, which is **louder in inspiration**.[11] On auscultation of the lung fields, there are **bibasal crepitations**, and there is **peripheral oedema**.[12]

This patient has previously had **mitral valvotomy**, and now has **severe mitral regurgitation** with signs of **pulmonary hypertension** and **pulmonary congestion**.[13]

Clinical notes

1. Always mention presence/absence of signs of endocarditis in any patient with physical signs of valvular heart disease. More than often, they are absent—but this is an important negative finding.
2. Patients with mitral regurgitation are usually in AF. Sometimes an irregular pulse may be difficult to ascertain, especially if bradycardic. The pulse volume is often variable in AF.
3. If venous pressure is elevated, then look for signs of pulmonary hypertension (usually with giant systolic 'v' waves of tricuspid regurgitation, parasternal heave and thrill, and a loud pulmonary component to the second heart sound) or pulmonary congestion (bibasal crepitations). The presence of systolic 'v' waves should prompt you to look for other signs of pulmonary hypertension.
4. Look carefully for previous mitral valvotomy scars on the left lateral chest wall. Patients with previous valvotomy for mitral stenosis may either develop re-stenosis, mitral regurgitation, or a combination of both. Mitral regurgitation was a common complication of mitral valvotomy.
5. Mitral regurgitation is associated with a volume overloaded left ventricle, thus a hyperdynamic and thrusting apex beat. Over time, the left ventricle compensates for the volume overload, with resultant increase in left ventricular dimension, i.e. a displaced apex beat.
6. A systolic thrill is a sign of severe mitral regurgitation. This is usually felt over the apex, but may be felt throughout the precordium. Pulmonary hypertension is associated with functional tricuspid regurgitation, which is associated with a parasternal thrill. Differentiating both thrills is clinically difficult. In examination settings, if a thrill is palpated and there are signs of mitral and tricuspid regurgitation, then it is best to refer to it as 'a precordial thrill'. Trying to differentiate between thrills of mitral and tricuspid regurgitation can cause confusion, and is best avoided in the examination.
7. A soft first heart sound is a marker of severe mitral regurgitation.
8. The pulmonary component of the second heart sound will be loud in the presence of pulmonary hypertension. If present, then make sure other signs of pulmonary hypertension are sought for. Severe mitral regurgitation is associated with wide splitting of the second heart sound. This is due to a high proportion of the stroke volume (the regurgitant volume—can be up to 60% of the stroke volume in severe mitral regurgitation) being emptied into the left atrium as opposed to aorta, thus a reduced ejection time with the aortic valve closing earlier.

9. A third heart sound occurs in mitral regurgitation due to rapid ventricular filling (increased left ventricular preload secondary to the mitral regurgitant volume from the previous cardiac cycle), and does not necessarily signify left ventricular dysfunction. A third heart sound can be used as a sign of severe mitral regurgitation, but it must be interpreted with other signs of severity. A third heart sound alone in the absence of other signs of severity does not itself imply severe mitral regurgitation. A fourth heart sound (if in sinus rhythm) is also a marker of severe mitral regurgitation.

10. The murmur of mitral regurgitation is pansystolic. In severe mitral regurgitation, one can often hear a soft and short mid-diastolic flow murmur at the apex, i.e. increased flow across the mitral valve. This signifies increased left ventricular filling secondary to increased left ventricular preload secondary to the mitral regurgitant volume from the previous cardiac cycle. When mitral regurgitation is functional, i.e. secondary to left ventricular dilatation as a result of impaired left ventricular function, the murmur may be mid, late, or pansystolic. Other causes of short systolic murmurs at the apex include mitral valve prolapse and papillary muscle dysfunction. These murmurs may not radiate to the axilla, but often radiate up the left sternal edge.

11. This is the murmur of 'functional' tricuspid regurgitation. This murmur is louder in inspiration (Carvallo's sign) and may be associated with a parasternal thrill. There will be systolic 'v' waves in the venous pressure, as would other signs of pulmonary hypertension. Mitral regurgitation will initially lead to pulmonary venous hypertension, pulmonary congestion, and then pulmonary arterial hypertension, and right-sided cardiac failure. In the presence of signs of pulmonary hypertension, look carefully for bibasal crepitations (pulmonary congestion) and peripheral oedema. The lung fields can be clear, and peripheral oedema can be minimal especially if the patient is on diuretics. Listen carefully for the Graham-Steell murmur of pulmonary regurgitation if other signs of pulmonary hypertension are present.

12. In the context of severe mitral regurgitation, one would usually expect pulmonary congestion and peripheral oedema. It is important to remember that such patients can have clear lung fields and may appear euvolaemic if on diuretic therapy. Thus, the absence of pulmonary congestion and peripheral oedema in the presence of other signs of severity should not preclude one from making the diagnosis of severe mitral regurgitation.

13. Having given a diagnosis of mitral regurgitation, it is important to comment on evidence of previous mitral valvotomy, the absence or presence of pulmonary hypertension and the severity of mitral regurgitation (see below).

Questions commonly asked by examiners

What are the causes of mitral regurgitation?

Chronic mitral regurgitation

- Rheumatic fever
- Mitral valve prolapse
- Infective endocarditis
- Left ventricular dilatation (functional mitral regurgitation)
- Marfan's syndrome
- Ehlers Danlos Syndrome
- Pseudoxanthoma elasticum
- Osteogenesis imperfecta
- Rheumatoid arthritis
- SLE (Libman-Sachs endocarditis)
- Papillary muscle dysfunction (ischaemia or degenerative diseases of the chordae)
- Mitral annular calcification
- Cardiomyopathies (restrictive, hypertrophic, and dilated)

Acute mitral regurgitation

- Infective endocarditis
- Rupture of chordae tendinae (infective endocarditis, acute rheumatic fever, and ischaemia)
- Trauma

What is the mechanism of 'functional' mitral regurgitation?

Functional mitral regurgitation refers to mitral regurgitation as a result of left ventricular dilatation secondary to impaired left ventricular systolic function. Left ventricular dilatation can lead to dilatation of the mitral valve annulus and lateral displacement of papillary muscles, which give rise to a regurgitant mitral valve.

What are the clinical signs of severe mitral regurgitation?

- Soft first heart sound
- Third heart sound
- Fourth heart sound (if in sinus rhythm)
- Displaced apex beat (sign of left ventricular enlargement)
- Precordial thrill
- Mid-diastolic flow murmur
- Widely split second heart sound
- Signs of pulmonary hypertension
- Signs of pulmonary congestion

Does the presence of a third heart sound always signify severe mitral regurgitation?

When assessing the severity of mitral regurgitation, all clinical signs must be taken into account. In patients with mitral regurgitation, a third heart sound is due to rapid ventricular filling due to the increased blood volume in the left atrium due the regurgitant volume in the previous cardiac cycle. Thus it does not necessarily signify left ventricular systolic dysfunction. A third heart sound alone in the absence of other signs of severity (see above) does not itself imply severe mitral regurgitation.

What is the differential diagnosis of a precordial pansystolic murmur?

- **Mitral regurgitation**—can be heard throughout the precordium, but usually loudest at the apex; radiates to axilla; loudest in expiration.
- **Tricuspid regurgitation**—best heard at the left lower parasternal edge; louder in inspiration (Carvallo's sign).
- **Ventricular septal defect**—can be heard throughout the precordium, but usually loudest at the left lower parasternal edge; small restrictive defects are associated with a louder murmur.

How can you differentiate mitral and tricuspid regurgitation clinically?

Clinical sign(s)	Mitral regurgitation	Tricuspid regurgitation
Pulse	Normal or jerky (if severe)	Normal
Jugular venous pressure (JVP)	No specific association	Systolic 'v' waves
Palpation	Apical systolic thrill	Parasternal systolic thrill
	Thrusting displaced apex	Parasternal heave
Auscultation	Pansystolic murmur loudest in expiration; radiating to axilla	Pansystolic murmur loudest in inspiration; no radiation to axilla
Hepatomegaly	No specific association	Pulsatile hepatomegaly

How would you investigate this patient?

ECG

- Atrial fibrillation is common. Some patients may be in sinus rhythm
- Left atrial hypertrophy (bifid P waves in lead II) if in sinus rhythm
- Left atrial dilatation (inverted or biphasic P waves in V_1–V_2) if in sinus rhythm

CXR

- Double right heart border (left atrial enlargement)
- Left atrial appendage
- Splaying of the carina (an old sign used to demonstrate a grossly dilated left atrium)
- Cardiomegaly (increasing left ventricular dimensions)
- Pulmonary congestion
- Prominent pulmonary arteries (pulmonary hypertension)

Echocardiogram

- Determine anatomy of mitral valve and subvalvular apparatus
- Establish mechanism of mitral regurgitation (endocarditis, unileaflet/bileaflet prolapse, functional, ischaemic)
- Assess severity of mitral regurgitation
- Assess left ventricular systolic function
- Assess right heart function
- Estimate pulmonary artery systolic pressure

Coronary angiography

- To exclude coronary artery disease as a cause for symptoms
- To exclude coronary artery disease as a cause for mitral regurgitation, i.e. functional mitral regurgitation in ischaemic cardiomyopathy or ischaemic mitral regurgitation.
- Right heart catherization will provide estimates for pulmonary artery systolic pressures, if these are not available from echocardiography. Large 'v' waves can be seen on wedge tracings, which signify severe mitral regurgitation.

All patients having valve surgery should have coronary angiography to exclude significant coronary stenoses that would require bypass grafting at the time of valve replacement.

What do you understand by the terms 'right' and 'left heart catherization'?

- **Left heart catherization** involves the introduction of catheters through an arterial route (femoral/radial/brachial) to the aortic root, i.e. the left heart. This allows us to perform a coronary angiogram and a left ventriculogram (by crossing the aortic valve into the left ventricular cavity).
- **Right heart catheterization** involves the introduction of catheters through the deep venous system (usually femoral vein route) to the right heart. This allows us to measure pressures in the RA, RV, PA, and PCWP.* Furthermore, blood samples can be obtained to measure oxygen saturations, if considering intracardiac shunts. Haemodynamic measurements such cardiac output can be calculated.

---

* RA = right atrium, RV = right ventricle, PA = pulmonary artery, PCWP = pulmonary capillary wedge pressure

When would you expect the murmur of mitral regurgitation to radiate up the parasternal edge as opposed to the axilla?

This can occur where mitral regurgitation is due to posterior mitral leaflet prolapse. The anteriorly directed regurgitant jet impinges upon the left atrial wall adjacent to aortic root. Thus the murmur appears to radiate up the parasternal edge and into the neck.

How would you manage a patient with mitral regurgitation?

Asymptomatic patients

- Advise antibiotics for endocarditis prophylaxis.
- Annual echocardiography to assess progression of mitral regurgitation.

Management of AF

- Rate control: digoxin, beta blockers, or calcium antagonists[*]
- Rhythm control: amiodarone, sotalol, or flecainide (if no contra-indications)
- Antithrombotic therapy: warfarin should be used in patients with mitral valve disease (if no contra-indications)

Heart failure

- Diuretics for congestive symptoms
- angiotensin converting enzyme (ACE) inhibitors/angiotensin-2 receptor blockers, beta blockers, spironolactone, and digoxin (if in sinus rhythm) in accordance with heart failure therapy guidelines
- Patients with heart failure should be considered for surgery

What are the indications for mitral valve surgery?

- Patients who are symptomatic, i.e. New York Heart Association (NYHA) functional class III or IV, despite optimum medical therapy.
- Asymptomatic patients should be followed up every 6 months with echocardiography or radionuclide assessment of left ventricular size and function. When the left ventricular ejection fraction falls to 60% or when the left ventricular end-systolic diameter is greater than 45mm, mitral valve surgery should be considered.

Case 29 ◆ **Aortic Regurgitation**

CASE PRESENTATION

*There are no peripheral stigmata of endocarditis.[1] The pulse rate is …beats/min, regular, **large volume**, and with a **collapsing** character.[2] The blood pressure is …/…mmHg.[3] There are **visible carotid pulsations** in the neck.[4] The venous pressure is not elevated.[5] On examination of the precordium, there are no scars. There are no heaves or thrills.[6] The apex beat is **displaced** and has a **thrusting quality**.[7]*

---

[*] Patients with mitral regurgitation have a dilated left atrium that acts as a substrate for AF, thus a rate-control strategy is often used

On auscultation, the first and second heart sounds are normal.[8] There is an **early diastolic murmur** at the **left sternal edge**, loudest with the **patient sitting forward** in **expiration**.[9] The lung fields are clear to auscultation and there is no peripheral oedema.

The diagnosis is **aortic regurgitation**.[10]

Clinical notes

1. Always mention presence/absence of signs of endocarditis in any patient with physical signs of valvular heart disease. More often than not, they are absent—but this is an important negative finding.

2. The pulse in aortic regurgitation is often of large volume, and with its rapid fall with low diastolic pressures, results in a collapsing character. The collapsing character is characterized by the 'water-hammer' pulse felt at the radial artery with the arm raised. Find the most proximal aspect of the radial pulse which is palpable and then place your fingers just below. If the pulse becomes stronger when you lift the arm (the column of blood is felt against the fingers) then this is referred to as a 'water-hammer' pulsation. The collapsing character can also be confirmed by palpation of the carotid pulse. Remember, there are other causes of a collapsing pulse, and this can be seen in any hyperdynamic circulation with a marked increase in stroke volume (see below).

3. Aortic regurgitation is associated with low diastolic blood pressures, hence a wide pulse pressure.

4. There are many eponymous signs and associations with aortic regurgitation, which may not always be present but can often be asked by examiners. In total, there are 11 eponymous signs (see below), and should not be routinely looked for, as it takes time and can cause confusion. However, the following selected eponymous signs can be looked for easily, and if present and correctly identified, they will impress.

    (a) **Corrigan's sign**: visible carotid pulsations in the neck

    (b) **Quinke's sign**: capillary pulsations in fingernails

    (c) **De Musset's sign**: head nodding with each heart beat

    (d) **Muller's sign**: systolic pulsations of the uvula

    Vigorous neck pulsations in the neck may be confused with the JVP. There are important differences between arterial and venous pulsations in the neck (see below).

5. If venous pressure is elevated, then look for signs of pulmonary hypertension (usually with giant systolic 'v' waves of tricuspid regurgitation, parasternal heave and thrill and a loud pulmonary component to the second heart sound) or pulmonary congestion (bibasal crepitations). The presence of systolic 'v' waves should prompt you to look for other signs of pulmonary hypertension.

6. A parasternal (right ventricular) heave would suggest pulmonary hypertension. If present, look for other signs of pulmonary hypertension.

7. Chronic aortic regurgitation is characterized by a volume-overloaded left ventricle. With time, the left ventricle compensates with increasing left ventricular dimensions, thus the apex is displaced. A thrusting apex beat reflects a hyperdynamic circulation.

8. Listen carefully, and be sure not to miss prosthetic heart sounds in the presence of old surgical scars. The pulmonary component of the second heart sound will be loud in the presence of pulmonary hypertension. If present, then make sure other signs of pulmonary hypertension are sought for. Often the aortic component of the second heart sound is diminished in patients with aortic regurgitation, but unlike aortic stenosis, this finding is not a marker of severe aortic regurgitation.

9. The murmur of aortic regurgitation is a high-pitched, early diastolic decrescendo murmur. It is usually heard at the mid-sternal region or at the lower left sternal edge. It is heard best with the patient sitting

forward and with breath held in end-expiration. The murmur of aortic regurgitation secondary to syphilitic aortitis is usually louder in the aortic area. There is often an accompanying ejection systolic flow murmur due to increased flow across the aortic valve as a result of the regurgitant volume from the previous cardiac cycle, and doesn't necessarily indicate co-existent aortic stenosis. Sometimes, in severe aortic regurgitation a separate low-pitched mid diastolic murmur is heard at the apex (similar to mitral stenosis, but without the opening snap). This is caused by the aortic regurgitation jet impinging on the anterior mitral valve leaflet, resulting in functional mitral stenosis. This is known as the **'Austin Flint' murmur**, and is a marker of severe aortic regurgitation. The longer the murmur the more severe is the aortic regurgitation. In its extreme form, severe torrential aortic regurgitation can be assocataed with a murmur spanning throughout diastole (referred to as a holo-diastolic murmur). It is common to hear a soft ejection systolic flow murmur across the aortic valve in aortic regurgitation. This represents increased forward flow, i.e. stroke volume plus regurgitant volume from preceding cardiac cycle.

10. When presenting the diagnosis of aortic regurgitation, try to look for the underlying aetiology. This may not always be present, but if present and correctly identified and presented to the examiners, it will definitely impress:

- **Bicuspid aortic valve**: ejection click in early systole (look for this in a young patient with aortic regurgitation)
- **Syphilitc aortitis**: Argyll Robertson pupil
- **Marfan's Syndrome**: Tall, high-arched palate, arm span>height
- **Ankylosing spondylitis**: loss of lumber lordosis, fixed kyphosis, stooped posture
- **Rheumatoid arthritis**: symmetrical deforming arthropathy of the small joints of the hands
- **SLE**: butterfly rash over the face, arthropathy
- **Osteogenesis imperfecta**: blue sclerae, hearing aids, evidence of old fractures
- **Pseudoxanthoma elasticum**: plucked chicken skin appearance, loose skins over neck and axillae
- **Ehlers-Danlos**: blue sclera, hyperextensible skin and joints, evidence of poor skin healing, purpura

Questions commonly asked by examiners

What are the causes of chronic aortic regurgitation?

- Bicuspid aortic valve
- Hypertension
- Rheumatic fever
- Aortitis (syphilis, Takayasu's arteritis, ankylosing spondylitis, Reiter's syndrome, psoriatic arthropathy)
- Rheumatoid arthritis
- SLE
- Connective tissue disorders (Marfan's syndrome, pseudoxanthoma elasticum, Ehlers-Danlos syndrome, osteogenesis imperfecta)
- Perimembranous VSD with prolapse of right coronary cusp

What are the causes of acute aortic regurgitation?

- Aortic dissection
- Infective endocarditis
- Ruptured sinus of Valsalva aneurysm

How can you differentiate clinically between vigorous arterial pulsations in the neck and venous pulsations of the JVP?

Clinical feature	Arterial pulsations	Venous pulsations
Waveform	Single waveform	Double waveform (in sinus rhythm)[a]
Respiratory variation	No effect	Inspiration cause in reduction in the waveform
Patient position	No effect	Lying the patient supine will raise the waveform, making if more visible
Hepato-jugular reflux[b]	No effect	Will raise the JVP waveform
Palpation	Palpable	Not palpable
Compression[c]	Doesn't abolish arterial pulsations	Usually abolishes JVP waveform

[a] If the patient is in AF, there is only one prominent wave of the JVP making differentiation from the single arterial pulsation difficult using this method. However other features outlined above should overcome this problem.

[b] Confirm patient has no right upper abdominal discomfort, and gently press under the right costal margin. This will transiently increase venous return, thus elevating the JVP waveform.

[c] Apply gentle compression a few centimetres above the clavicle. This will abolish venous pulsations on the same side. Arterial pulsations will not be affected.

What are the clinical signs of severe aortic regurgitation?

* Wide pulse pressure
* Long duration of the decrescendo diastolic murmur*
* Third heart sound
* Austin Flint murmur
* Signs of pulmonary hypertension
* Signs of left ventricular failure

What is the Austin Flint murmur?

This is a low-frequency mid diastolic murmur heard at the apex caused by (a) the aortic regurgitant jet impinging on the anterior mitral valve leaflet leading to functional mitral stenosis; (b) the left ventricular diastolic pressure rising more rapidly than the left atrial pressure.

Clinically the Austin Flint murmur mimics that of mitral stenosis. Mitral stenosis can be differentiated by the presence of an opening snap and loud first heart sound. However, the first heart sound may be loud in aortic regurgitation (reflecting a hyperdynamic circulation), but is not palpable (as it would be in mitral stenosis, which would give a tapping apex beat).

What eponymous clinical signs are associated with aortic regurgitation?

These are a result of hyperdynamic circulation and include:

* **Corrigan's sign**: visible carotid pulsations in the neck
* **Quinke's sign**: capillary pulsations in fingernails
* **De Musset's sign**: head nodding with each heart beat
* **Muller's sign**: systolic pulsations of the uvula

---

* The length of the murmur correlates with severity. In mild aortic regurgitation, the murmur is often short. The greater the severity, the longer the duration of the murmur. In severe aortic regurgitation, the murmur may extend throughout diastole (a holodiastolic murmur).

- **Traube's sign**: (pistol shot femorals): booming sound heard over the femoral artery
- **Duroziez's sign**: to and fro systolic and diastolic murmur produced by compression of the femoral artery and auscultating proximally (a diastolic murmur implies retrograde flow and implies at least moderate aortic regurgitation)
- **Becker's sign**: visible pulsations in the retinal arteries and pupils
- **Rosenbach's sign**: systolic pulsations of the liver
- **Gerhard's sign**: systolic pulsations in the spleen
- **Hill's sign**: popliteal systolic pressure > brachial systolic pressure by greater than 60mmHg. This usually signifies at least moderate aortic regurgitation
- **Mayne's sign**: more than 15mmHg drop in diastolic pressure with arm elevation

What are other causes of a collapsing or bounding pulse?

Exaggerated or bounding pulses are not specific to aortic regurgitation. They can be seen in any hyperdynamic circulation with a marked increase in stroke volume. They include:

- Anaemia
- Fever
- Pregnancy
- Thyrotoxicosis
- Patent ductus arteriosus
- Arterio-venous fistula
- Severe bradycardia
- Severe mitral regurgitation*

What is the natural history of chronic aortic regurgitation?

Asymptomatic patients have a favourable long-term prognosis. Chronic aortic regurgitation evolves slowly, with very low morbidity during a long asymptomatic phase (compensated stage). Some patients with mild aortic regurgitation remain asymptomatic for decades, and rarely require treatment.

The transition from a 'compensated' to a 'decompensated' stage is poorly understood. The prognosis of patients with aortic regurgitation is determined by symptoms (primarily dyspnoea), left ventricular size (left ventricular end-systolic diameter >55mm) and left ventricular systolic dysfunction (an ejection fraction less than 50% that indicates serious depression of left ventricular systolic function).

Why is chronic aortic regurgitation well tolerated in the asymptomatic (compensated) stage?

Chronic aortic regurgitation is well tolerated as a result of the compensatory myocardial and haemodynamic adaptations. The increased left ventricular end-diastolic volume causes an increase in wall stress. The heart responds to this by compensatory left ventricular hypertrophy, which normalizes wall stress. The combination of left ventricular hypertrophy and enlargement increases the total stroke volume and thus cardiac output is maintained despite the regurgitant lesion. Although left ventricular volume is increased, the end-diastolic pressure is normal due to increase in left ventricular compliance. Thus the heart adapts well to chronic aortic regurgitation. This is the compensated stage.

---

* Can cause rapid rising arterial pulse, which is often short and abbreviated. They can give an impression of a collapsing pulse. However, pulse pressure is normal.

How would you investigate this patient?

ECG

- Usually no specific findings in relation to aortic regurgitation
- Left ventricular hypertrophy +/– strain pattern (especially if co-existent aortic stenosis)

CXR

- There may be valvular calcification
- Cardiomegaly (increasing left ventricular dimensions)
- Pulmonary congestion
- Prominent pulmonary arteries (pulmonary hypertension)

Echocardiography

- Assess valve morphology (bicuspid or tricuspid valve)
- Assess aortic root size and dilatation
- Establish aetiology of aortic regurgitation
- Determine severity of aortic regurgitation
- Assess left ventricular size (in particular left ventricular end-systolic diameter)
- Assess left ventricular systolic function.

Computerized axial tomography (CT)/Magnetic resonance imaging (MRI)

- Assess aortic root and ascending aorta.[*]

Cardiac catherization

- To exclude coronary artery disease as a cause for symptoms.
- All patients having aortic valve replacement should have coronary angiography to exclude significant coronary stenoses that would require bypass grafting at the time of valve replacement.
- An aortogram can provide information on the degree of regurgitation and assess aortic root size.

What is the role of vasodilators in aortic regurgitation?

- The role of vasodilator therapy is to reduce systolic blood pressure. Hypertension can increase wall stress and reduce the forward stroke volume.
- Current trial data exist for vasodilator therapy with nifedipine and ACE inhibitors/angiotensin-2 receptor blockers in patients with severe aortic regurgitation.
- Vasodilator therapy is recommended for patients with asymptomatic severe aortic regurgitation and left ventricular dilatation. Patients with severe aortic regurgitation without left ventricular dilatation and who have normal blood pressures should not be on long-term vasodilator therapy.
- Vasodilator therapy is not recommended for asymptomatic patients with mild to moderate aortic regurgitation and normal blood pressure with normal left ventricular size and function.
- Vasodilator therapy is recommended for patients with hypertension and any degree of aortic regurgitation.

---

[*] The proximal 3–4cm of the aortic root is easily visualized on echocardiography. The mid-portion of the ascending aorta may not be seen on echocardiography, and thus a CT or MRI are needed for evaluation. Yearly evaluation is required if the aortic root or ascending aorta is greater than 40mm.

What are the indications for surgery?

Symptomatic patients

- Severe aortic regurgitation and symptoms of heart failure
- Severe aortic regurgitation with angina

Asymptomatic patients*

- Left ventricular systolic dysfunction (ejection fraction <50%)
- Left ventricular dilatation (left ventricular end-systolic diameter >55mm or end-diastolic diameter>75mm)
- Aortic root dilatation ≥50mm (irrespective of the degree of aortic regurgitation)

Why would a patient with severe aortic regurgitation experience angina, even if coronary angiography did not demonstrate occlusive coronary disease?

- In aortic regurgitation, there is lowering of diastolic blood pressure. Coronary perfusion occurs during diastole. Therefore, by lowering diastolic pressure, coronary perfusion pressure is compromised, hence resulting in angina. The presence of angina with severe aortic regurgitation is an indication for surgery.
- Sometimes angina may occur at night when the heart rate slows and diastolic blood pressure falls to very low levels, thus compromising coronary perfusion.
- Marked compensatory left ventricular hypertrophy may result in angina.

Case 30 ◆ Mixed Aortic Valve Disease

CASE PRESENTATION 1

*There are no peripheral stigmata of endocarditis. The pulse rate is …beats/min, regular/irregular, of **low volume** and exhibits a **slow-rising character** (may have a **bisferiens character**). The blood pressure is…/…mmHg with a **narrow pulse pressure**. The venous pressure is not elevated. On examination of the precordium, the **apex beat is minimally displaced** with a **presystolic impulse** (if in sinus rhythm) and has a **heaving character**. There is a **systolic thrill** palpable in the aortic area. On auscultation, the first heart sound is normal, but the second heart sound has a **soft aortic component**. There is a harsh ejection systolic murmur, heard throughout the precordium but loudest in the aortic area, which is louder in expiration, and radiates to the carotids. There is also an early diastolic murmur heard at the lower left sternal edge, heard best with the patient sitting forward and in expiration. The lung fields are clear to auscultation and there is no peripheral oedema.*

*The diagnosis is **mixed aortic valve disease**. The clinical signs favour **aortic stenosis** being the **predominant valvular lesion**.*

---

* Waiting for patients to develop symptoms may result in some degree of irreversible left ventricular dysfunction. The symptoms of left ventricular dysfunction may preclude optimal surgical results. Therefore the AHA/ACC (American Heart Association/American College of Cardiology) recommend aortic valve replacement in asymptomatic individuals with evidence of left ventricular dysfunction or dilatation. A left ventricular end-systolic dimension of 55mm represents the limit of surgically reversible dilatation of the left ventricle.

CASE PRESENTATION 2

There are no peripheral stigmata of endocarditis. The pulse rate is …beats/min, regular/irregular, of **large volume** *and exhibits a* **collapsing** *character (may have a* **bisferiens character**). *The blood pressure is …/…mmHg with a* **wide pulse pressure**. *The venous pressure is not elevated. On examination of the precordium, there are no heaves or thrills. The apex beat is* **displaced** *and has a* **thrusting quality**. *There is an ejection systolic murmur, heard throughout the precordium but loudest in the aortic area, which is louder in expiration, and radiates to the carotids. There is also an early diastolic murmur heard at the lower left sternal edge, heard best with the patient sitting forward and in expiration. The lung fields are clear to auscultation and there is no peripheral oedema.*

The diagnosis is **mixed aortic valve disease.** *The clinical signs favour* **aortic regurgitation** *being the predominant valvular lesion.*

Clinical notes

A. Patients with mixed aortic valve disease are common. Patients with bicuspid aortic valves frequently have mixed aortic valve disease. Patients with aortic stenosis commonly have some degree of aortic regurgitation. Similarly, patients with aortic regurgitation may have some degree of aortic stenosis. It is quite common for an ejection systolic (flow) murmur to be heard in addition to the early diastolic murmur in aortic regurgitation in the absence of aortic stenosis. This represents increased forward flow across the aortic valve, but can cause confusion. Examiners will expect you to identify the predominant lesion. Using the following clinical features one can determine whether aortic stenosis or regurgitation is predominant:

Clinical sign	Predominant aortic stenosis	Predominant aortic regurgitation
Pulse volume	Low	Large
Pulse character	Slow-rising	Collapsing
Apex beat	Minimally displaced, heaving	Displaced, thrusting
Systolic thrill	Present	Not present
Systolic murmur	Harsh/loud long murmur, with late systolic peaking	May be harsh/loud but is usually short, peaking early in systole
Systolic blood pressure	Low	High
Pulse pressure	Narrow	Wide

B. Sometimes in the examination setting, it is not clear as to which lesion is predominant. It would be appropriate in this setting to point out the clinical signs that favour either aortic stenosis or regurgitation to being the predominant lesion. It is important to state that in such cases the use of echocardiography and/or cardiac catheterization +/– an aortogram will be useful to provide a better assessment and indicate which lesion is predominant.

Case 31 ◆ Mixed Mitral Valve Disease

CASE PRESENTATION 1

There are no peripheral stigmata of endocarditis. The pulse rate is …beats/min, irregular, normal volume and character. The blood pressure is …/…mmHg. The venous pressure is not elevated. On examination of the precordium, there are no scars. The apex beat is **undisplaced** *and has a* **tapping quality**. *There are* no heaves or thrills. On auscultation, the **first heart sound is loud**, and the second heart sound is normal. There is an opening snap in early diastole followed by a mid-diastolic rumbling murmur at the apex, heard best in expiration with the patient in the left lateral position. There is also a pansystolic murmur at the apex, louder in expiration, and radiates to the axilla. The lung fields are clear to auscultation and there is no sacral or pedal oedema.

The diagnosis is **mixed mitral valve disease.** The clinical signs favour **mitral stenosis** as being the predominant valvular lesion.

CASE PRESENTATION 2

There are no peripheral stigmata of endocarditis. The pulse rate is …beats/min, irregularly irregular, normal volume and character. The blood pressure is …/…mmHg. The venous pressure is not elevated. On examination of the precordium, there are no scars. The apex beat is **displaced** and has a **thrusting quality**. There are no heaves but there is an apical **systolic thrill**. On auscultation, the **first heart sound is soft**, and the second heart sound is normal. There is a mid-diastolic rumbling murmur at the apex, heard best in expiration with the patient in the left lateral position. There is also a pansystolic murmur at the apex, loudest in expiration, which radiates to the axilla. The lung fields are clear to auscultation and there is no sacral or pedal oedema.

The diagnosis is **mixed mitral valve disease**. The clinical signs favour **mitral regurgitation** as being the predominant valvular lesion.

Clinical notes

A. Patients with mixed mitral valve disease are common in the examination. Occasionally they can be difficult to diagnose. If the high-pitched pansystolic murmur of mitral regurgitation is loud, often a soft low-frequency mid-diastolic murmur of mitral stenosis can be missed.

B. In severe mitral regurgitation without mitral stenosis there can often be a mid-diastolic flow murmur resulting from increased forward flow across the mitral valve. In such cases, how can you tell if this represents underlying mitral stenosis or if this truly is a flow murmur? Generally, the absence of an opening snap and the presence of a third heart sound would suggest that this is severe mitral regurgitation only. Remember, a third heart sound signifies rapid ventricular filling, and therefore, the presence of a third heart sound is incompatible with any significant degree of mitral stenosis.

C. Examiners will expect you to identify the predominant lesion. Using the following clinical features one can determine whether mitral stenosis or regurgitation is predominant:

Clinical feature	Predominant mitral stenosis	Predominant mitral regurgitation
Pulse	Small volume	Sharp and abbreviated
Apex beat position	Undisplaced	Displaced
Apex beat quality	Tapping	Thrusting
First heart sound	Loud (if leaflets are mobile)	Soft
Third heart sound	Not present	Present

D. Sometimes, in the examination setting, it is not clear as to which lesion is predominant, e.g. loud first heart sound and displaced apex beat. It would be appropriate in this setting to point out the clinical signs that favour either mitral stenosis or regurgitation being the predominant lesion. It is important to state that in such cases the use of echocardiography and/or cardiac catheterization will be useful to provide a better assessment and indicate which lesion is predominant.

Case 32 ◆ **Mitral Valve Prolapse**

CASE PRESENTATION

There are no peripheral stigmata of endocarditis.[1] The pulse rate is …beats/min, regular/irregular, normal volume and character.[2] The blood pressure is…/…mmHg. The venous pressure is not elevated.[3] On examination of the precordium, there are no scars. The apex beat is undisplaced.[4] There are no heaves or thrills.[5] On auscultation, the first and second heart sounds are normal.[6] There is a **mid-systolic click**[7] *followed by a* **late systolic crescendo–decrescendo murmur** *loudest at the* **lower left sternal edge.**[8] *The lung fields are clear to auscultation.[9] There is no peripheral oedema.*

The diagnosis is **mitral valve prolapse.**[10]

Clinical notes

Mitral valve prolapse is a cause of mitral regurgitation. Although mitral valve prolapse is associated with specific signs, as the degree of mitral regurgitation increases, the clinical signs resemble those for mitral regurgitation. Candidates are advised to revise this case whilst referring to the mitral regurgitation case (Case 28, page…).

1. Always mention presence/absence of signs of endocarditis in any patient with physical signs of valvular heart disease. More than often, they are absent—but this is an important negative finding.

2. With increasing severity and resultant mitral regurgitation, there is an increased likelihood of AF. Look specifically for an (irregularly) irregular pulse. Patients with mitral valve prolapse may have frequent ventricular ectopy, which can give an irregular pulse. Mitral valve prolapse can be associated with autonomic dysfunction and there may be a resting bradycardia (increased parasympathetic tone) and postural hypotension.

3. Increasing severity of mitral valve prolapse and resultant mitral regurgitation can lead to pulmonary hypertension. If the venous pressure is elevated, then be sure to look for other signs of pulmonary hypertension in the remainder of the examination.

4. The apex beat will become displaced with a thrusting quality as the mitral valve prolapse increases in severity with increasing mitral regurgitation.

5. Systolic thrills will be palpable with severe mitral regurgitation. A parasternal heave and thrill will be felt in pulmonary hypertension.

6. Severe mitral regurgitation is associated with a soft first heart sound and a third heart sound. The pulmonary component to the second heart sound will be loud in pulmonary hypertension.

7. A mid systolic click is characteristic of mitral valve prolapse. They are heard at the apex and can be single (most common) or multiple clicks. They result from sudden tensing of the mitral valve apparatus as the leaflet prolapses into the left atrium. Clicks can often be missed, and should be sought for carefully. Anything that decreases cardiac volume, i.e. standing position and Valsalva manoeuvre, will result in an earlier click. Anything that increases cardiac volume, i.e. squatting or beta blockers, will result in a click occurring later in systole. To remember, reduced LV volume → click closer to S_1 and increased LV volume → click closer to S_2.

8. Sometimes the murmur is not present. If present, if follows the mid-systolic click. It is often heard at the lower left sternal edge, but can sometimes be heard at the apex. Remember, the click and the murmur change as the position changes. Anything that decreases cardiac volume, i.e. standing position and Valsalva manoeuvre, will prolong the murmur. Anything that increases cardiac volume, i.e. squatting or beta blockers, will result in a shorter murmur. In the supine position, the click is late (closer to S_2) and

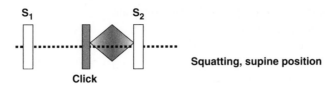

Squatting, supine position

Figure 32.1

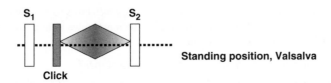

Standing position, Valsalva

Figure 32.2

the murmur is short. In the standing position, the click is earlier (closer to S$_1$) and the murmur is longer. This may identify a murmur that was not previously noted. Isometric handgrip exercise increases the intensity of the murmur (louder) without affecting position. As mitral valve prolapse increases in severity, the murmur develops into the pansystolic murmur of mitral regurgitation.

In mitral valve prolapse involving the posterior leaflet (most commonly affected), the mitral regurgitant jet hits the left atrial wall adjacent to the aortic root, and murmur appears to radiate up the sternal edge.

9. Look for signs of pulmonary congestion, a marker of severe mitral regurgitation.

10. Mitral valve prolapse can be primary (most common) and secondary (associated with other conditions). It is important to be aware of some associations and to look for these conditions. If correctly identified, and presented as a possible association, it will impress.

- **Marfan's syndrome**: high-arched palate, arm span>height, arachnodactyly, scoliosis, pectus excavatum
- **Ehlers-Danlos syndrome**: blue sclera, hyperextensible skin and joints, evidence of poor skin healing, purpura
- **Pseudoxanthoma elasticum**: plucked chicken skin appearance, loose skin over neck and axillae
- **Osteogenesis imperfecta**: blue sclerae, hearing aids
- **Polycystic kidney disease**: renal replacement therapy (renal transplant scars, dialysis lines, uraemia)
- **SLE**: butterfly rash over the face, arthropathy

Questions commonly asked by examiners

How common is mitral valve prolapse?

This occurs in 5–10% of the population, more commonly in females (female:male ratio = 3:1)

What symptoms are associated with mitral valve prolapse?

Often asymptomatic, but can be associated with palpitations (most common, 40% of cases), atypical chest pains, fatigue, dyspnoea, and anxiety.

What are the complications of mitral valve prolapse?

- Stroke (embolic phenomena)
- Chordal rupture
- Endocarditis
- Arrhythmias (prolonged QTc interval)
- Sudden death
- Progression to severe mitral regurgitation
- Cardiac neurosis

What is the pathophysiology of mitral valve prolapse?

Collagen dissolution results in myxomatous degeneration, which leads to deposition of mucopolysaccharides in the middle spongiosa layer of the mitral valve leaflets. This results in stretching of the leaflets and the chordae tendinae.

Is there any genetic predisposition to mitral valve prolapse?

Mitral valve prolapse most commonly occurs in a familial form with autosomal dominant inheritance that exhibits both sex- and age-dependent penetrance (primary mitral valve prolapse). The abnormalities of the elastic fibres in floppy mitral valves are related to genetic variants in fibrillin, elastin, and collagen I and II.

What is the differential diagnosis of a mitral valve prolapse murmur, and how would you differentiate them?

- Aortic stenosis (early systolic, usually at the upper sternal edge)
- Pulmonary stenosis (short, early systolic, louder in inspiration, diminishes with Valsalva manoeuvre
- Hypertrophic cardiomyopathy (diminishes with squatting and intensifies with standing and Valsalva manoeuvre)
- Trivial mitral regurgitation (short murmur that may not be pansystolic, but no click)

Do these patients need endocarditis prophylaxis?

Patients who have an audible click or murmur should receive antibiotic prophylaxis. Those with only echocardiographic evidence of mitral valve prolapse don't require prophylaxis.

Do you know of a reversible form of mitral valve prolapse?

Mitral valve prolapse occurs when the left ventricular size is small in comparison to an enlarged mitral annulus, leaflets, or chordae tendinae. It can be induced in healthy women with typical body habitus following dehydration that is reversed with rehydration. Mitral valve prolapse often resolves during pregnancy and following weight gain in anorexic patients.

How would you manage this patient?

- Re-assure asymptomatic patients
- Endocarditis prophylaxis in those with an audible click or murmur
- Treat atrial and ventricular arrhythmias as appropriate
- Treat atypical chest pains with simple analgesics or beta blocker

Case 33 ◆ **Pulmonary Hypertension**

CASE PRESENTATION 1

*There are no peripheral stigmata of endocarditis. The pulse rate is ...beats/min, regular/irregular, of normal volume and character.[1] The blood pressure is.../...mmHg. The venous pressure visible to angle of the jaw, with **prominent 'a' waves** and **giant systolic 'v' waves**.[2] On examination of the precordium, the apex beat is undisplaced.[3] There is a **parasternal heave**[4] and a **parasternal thrill**[5] palpable at the lower left sternal edge, and a **palpable pulmonary component to the second heart sound** (**P₂**).[6] On auscultation, the first heart sound is normal and there is a **loud pulmonary component to the second heart sound**.[7] There is a **pansystolic murmur**, at the lower left sternal edge, **louder during inspiration**.[8] There is also an **early diastolic murmur** heard at the **upper left sternal edge** (pulmonary area), **louder during inspiration**.[9] The lung fields are clear to auscultation.[10] There is **sacral and pedal oedema**.[11]*

*The diagnosis is **pulmonary hypertension** with **functional tricuspid regurgitation**, and **pulmonary regurgitation**.[12]*

CASE PRESENTATION 2

*There are no peripheral stigmata of endocarditis. The pulse rate is ...beats/min, regular/irregular, of normal volume and character.[1] The blood pressure is.../...mmHg. The venous pressure is elevated, with **prominent 'a' and 'v' waves**.[2] On examination of the precordium, the apex beat is undisplaced.[3] There is a **parasternal heave**.[4] There are no thrills.[5] On auscultation, the first heart sound is normal and there is a **loud pulmonary component to the second heart sound** (**P₂**).[6] There are no audible murmurs. The lung fields are clear to auscultation.[10] There is **sacral and pedal oedema**.[11]*

*The diagnosis is **pulmonary hypertension**.[12]*

Clinical notes

These cases illustrate how pulmonary hypertension can present as either a case with all the clinical signs and associated murmurs or with only a few clinical signs. Sometimes the only clinical signs may be a parasternal heave and loud P₂. Listen carefully for underlying murmurs (left-sided valvular heart disease) that may be the cause of pulmonary hypertension.

1. Take extra time to assess the rhythm! An (irregularly) irregular rhythm would signify AF. Sometimes patients can be bradycardic (often due to rate-control therapy), and ascertaining an irregular rhythm requires extra time. If a patient is in AF, then 'a' waves cannot be present on venous pressure tracing, thus you can expect to see a single waveform when assessing the venous pressure. Diagnosing AF and then commenting on 'a' waves will not impress the examiner! Look for the slow-rising or collapsing pulse hinting the presence of underlying aortic valve disease (which may be a cause for pulmonary hypertension).

2. Assessing the JVP often presents a challenge to candidates. It is important to appreciate the normal JVP waveform with some understanding of the underlying physiology. Once this is understood, with practice, examining the waveform and making diagnoses become simple. The normal JVP has the following constituents:

a wave:	Due to atrial contraction
x descent:	Atrial emptying with downward movement of the heart (results in atrial stretch and also contributes to a drop in pressure)
c wave:	A small flicker in the x descent due to transmission of right ventricular systolic pressure before the closure of the tricuspid valve
v wave:	Due to passive filling of right atrium against a closed tricuspid valve
y descent:	Opening of the tricuspid valve with passive emptying of blood from right atrium into right ventricle

3. A displaced apex beat would suggest left ventricular dilatation secondary to primary left ventricular dysfunction or secondary to valvular heart disease, which may cause pulmonary hypertension. The quality of the apex beat can be helpful in providing further clues to the cause of pulmonary hypertension. A thrusting apex beat is seen with aortic and mitral regurgitation. The heaving apex beat is seen in aortic stenosis and left ventricular hypertrophy (hypertensive heart disease) all of which are causes of pulmonary hypertension.

4. A parasternal heave is often felt at the left sternal edge. However, in long-standing pulmonary hypertension and right ventricular dilatation, the heave may be felt at the right parasternal edge.

5. A parasternal (systolic) thrill in the context of pulmonary hypertension is secondary to 'functional' tricuspid regurgitation.

6. Sometimes a palpable P_2 can be difficult to confirm. It is best felt over pulmonary area, and coincides with the second heart sound. This can be confirmed using one hand to palpate the carotid and the other to feel over the pulmonary area. Knowing that the carotid impulse coincides with the first heart sound, a palpable P_2 will occur AFTER carotid impulse.

7. A loud P_2 may be heard all over the precordium, but is loudest over the pulmonary area. Although A_2 occurs before P_2, a separate P_2 may be difficult to distinguish as often they merge as a loud second heart sound. If that is the case then present it as 'a loud second heart sound'.

8. This is the murmur of tricuspid regurgitation. It is often heard at the lower left sternal edge, and is louder in inspiration (Carvallo's sign). Occasionally in cases of severe right heart dilatation the murmur can be heard over the apex.

9. Pulmonary hypertension causes dilatation of the pulmonary artery, which results in pulmonary regurgitation. This is commonly known as the Graham-Steell murmur. Pulmonary regurgitation is best heard in the pulmonary area with the patient sitting forward, being louder in inspiration, and radiates a few intercostal spaces down the left sternal edge.

10. During a cardiovascular examination, the lung bases are auscultated to look for signs of pulmonary congestion. Whilst doing so, try to look for clues to possible respiratory causes of secondary pulmonary hypertension, i.e. wheeze would suggest obstructive airways disease and fine bibasal end-inspiratory crepitations would be suggestive of interstitial lung disease.

11. The oedema may be minimal if patient is on diuretics. Other signs of right-sided heart failure may be ascites and scrotal oedema.

12. After having provided the diagnosis of pulmonary hypertension, try to provide a possible cause. This will impress examiners. Throughout the examination, try to look for other underlying diagnoses. Some diagnoses are very easy to pick up:

    *   **Obstructive airways disease**: nicotine staining, hyper-inflated chest, prolonged expiratory time, and wheeze

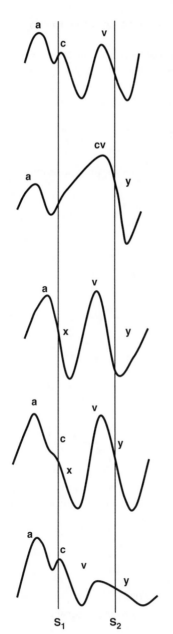

Normal JVP waveform

Tricuspid regurgitation is associated with 'cv' waves. These are also referred to 'systolic waves' or 'v' waves. It is also associated with a steep 'y descent'.

Constrictive pericarditis is associated with steep 'x'and 'y' descents.

Atrial septal defects are associated with prominent and exaggerated 'a' and 'v' waves. In atrial fibrillation, 'a' waves will be absent.

Tricuspid stenosisis associated with tall 'a' waves with a slow 'y' descent.
Tall 'a' waves are seen in pulmonary hypertension (in sinus rhythm)

Figure 33.1

- **Interstitial lung disease**: clubbing of fingers, bibasal crepitations, and stigmata of rheumatological disease
- **Systemic sclerosis**: scleroderma hands, tightening of facial skin, and telangiectasia
- **Rheumatoid arthritis**: symmetrical deforming arthropathy of the small joints of the hands
- **SLE**: butterfly rash over the face, arthropathy
- **Chronic type 2 respiratory failure**: kyphoscoliosis or obesity

Questions commonly asked by examiners

What is the definition of pulmonary hypertension?

Pulmonary hypertension is characterized by a mean pulmonary artery systolic pressure >25mmHg at rest.

What are the causes of secondary pulmonary hypertension?

(a) Increased pulmonary venous pressure

- Left ventricular systolic or diastolic dysfunction
- Mitral valve disease
- Aortic valve disease
- Veno-oclusive disease (autoimmune disease)

(b) Decreased area of pulmonary vascular bed

- Thrombo-embolic disease
- Interstitial lung disease
- Collagen vascular diseases
- Obstructive airways disease

(c) Chronic hypoxia

- Chronic airways disease
- Interstitial lung disease
- Obstructive sleep apnoea
- Obesity-hypoventilation syndrome
- High altitude
- Neuro-muscular disease (poliomyelitis, Guillian-Barré syndrome and myasthenia gravis)
- Kyphoscoliosis

(d) Left-to-right shunt

- Atrial septal defect
- Ventricular septal defect

What do you know about primary pulmonary hypertension?

- A rare disease with an incidence of 2 per million (1% of all cases of pulmonary hypertension)
- A disease of children and young adults (female:male = 2:1)
- Characterized by pulmonary hypertension in the absence of any demonstrable cause.
- One in ten cases are familial
- Associated with connective tissue disease, vasculitis, and HIV infection
- Also associated with the use of appetite suppressants, e.g. fenfluramine
- Untreated, the median survival is 3 years.

How would you investigate a patient with pulmonary hypertension?

Investigations in patients with pulmonary hypertension (a) help confirm diagnosis and severity of pulmonary hypertension, and (b) confirm the absence or presence of an underlying cause.

ECG

- Right ventricular hypertrophy
- Right ventricular strain
- Right atrial hypertrophy (P pulmonale)
- Incomplete or complete right bundle branch block

In addition, look for:

- Left atrial hypertrophy (bifid P waves in II)—suggestive of mitral valve disease
- Left atrial dilatation (biphasic P wave in V_1)—suggestive of mitral valve disease
- Left ventricular hypertrophy +/– strain—suggestive of hypertensive heart disease or aortic valve disease
- Myocardial ischaemia[*]—suggestive of left ventricular systolic dysfunction

Arterial blood gas sampling

- Type 1 respiratory failure ($pO_2 < 8.0$ and $pCO_2 < 6.0$)
- Type 2 respiratory failure ($pO_2 < 8.0$ and $pCO_2 > 6.0$)

CXR

Classical findings of pulmonary hypertension are:

- Prominent pulmonary vasculature (enlargement of central pulmonary arteries)
- Attenuation of peripheral vessels
- Oligaemic lung fields

In addition, look for:

- Cardiomegaly and/or pulmonary congestion—suggestive of left ventricular dysfunction
- Hyper-inflated chest and bullae—suggestive of obstructive airways disease
- Reticulo-nodular shadowing and honeycomb appearance—suggestive of interstitial lung disease

Echocardiogram

- Signs of chronic right ventricular pressure overload (right ventricular hypertrophy and paradoxical systolic bulging of septum into left ventricle on short axis views)
- Signs of chronic volume overload (right ventricular dilatation with diastolic splinting of septum, giving the impression of D-shaped left ventricle on short axis views)
- Right ventricular size and function (right ventricular hypertrophy or dilatation)
- Degree of tricuspid regurgitation[*]
- Pulmonary artery systolic pressure

---

[*] T wave inversion, ST depression, biphasic T waves, poor R wave progression, Q waves, and left bundle branch block.

[*] Tricuspid regurgitation is present in more than 90% of patients with severe pulmonary hypertension, and can be used to estimate pulmonary artery pressures (greater than 95% correlation with pressures measured using cardiac catheterization). Pulmonary artery systolic pressures can be estimated from the velocities of even the smallest tricuspid regurgitation jets).

In addition look for:

- Left ventricular systolic and diastolic function
- Valvular heart disease
- Intracardiac shunts

CT pulmonary angiogram/V-Q (ventilation-perfusion) scan

- To demonstrate chronic thromboembolic disease
- Diffuse mottled perfusion can be seen in primary pulmonary hypertension (as opposed to segmental or sub-segmental mismatched defects observed in secondary pulmonary hypertension)

Lung function tests

- May demonstrate obstructive or restrictive patterns in chronic respiratory disease
- Diffusion capacity is universally reduced in pulmonary hypertension

High resolution CT chest

- To demonstrate interstitial lung disease

Right and left heart catheterization

- Right heart catheterization is the standard test for diagnosis, quantification, and characterization of pulmonary hypertension
- Can be used to further assess right heart and pulmonary artery pressures (especially if difficult to measure from echocardiography)
- Can measure cardiac output and pulmonary vascular resistance
- Can conduct vasodilator trials to assess acute response to short-acting vasodilators[*]
- Can measure saturations of blood in the right and left heart, thus detection of shunts

How do you treat secondary pulmonary hypertension?

- Treat underlying cause
- Diuretics for congestive symptoms
- Long-term oxygen therapy
- Anticoagulation[*]
- Vasodilator therapy (see below)

How do you treat primary pulmonary hypertension?
Diuretics

- Help with congestive symptoms
- Reduce preload in patients with right heart failure.

Anticoagulation

Warfarin is the oral anticoagulant of choice, to achieve and INR = 2–3. Anticoagulation nearly doubles the 3-year survival rate.

---

[*] Prostacyclin, inhaled nitric oxide and adenosine. An acute response often predicts a beneficial effect from oral vasodilator therapy.

[*] The role of anticoagulation is not established in secondary pulmonary hypertension, unless there is thrombo-embolic or pulmonary veno-occlusive disease.

Vasodilator therapy

(a) *Calcium channel blockers.* Nifedipine and diltiazem are used. Those who respond to calcium channel blockers have a 5-year survival rate of 95%. They should not be used in patients with overt right heart failure.

(b) *Prostacyclin analogues.* Short acting vasodilators and inhibitors of platelet aggregation. Can be administered intravenously, subcutaneously or in a nebulized formulation. Due to its short half-life, infusions have to be given continuously through a tunnelled central venous line. Epoprostenol (Flolan) and Treprostinil (Remodulin) are intravenous preparations. Iloprost (Ventavis) is a nebulized inhalation.

(c) *Adenosine infusion*

(d) *Nitric oxide inhalation*

(e) *Nitrate infusions*

(f) *Phosphodiesterase-5 inhibitors*, e.g. sildenafil

(g) *Endothelin antagonists.* Oral endothelin antagonists include bosentan and ambrisentan.

Surgery

(a) *Atrial septostomy.* A palliative procedure by creation of right-to-left shunt. This has been shown to improve forward output and alleviate right heart failure. Atrial septostomy provides a low-resistance channel, thereby decompressing the right atrium and improving filling of the left side of the heart. Although the blood delivered to tissues has a lower overall saturation, the oxygen content delivered to tissues is increased.

(b) *Transplantation.* Lung transplantation and combined heart-lung transplantation are associated with similar survival rates. Lung transplantation can comprise single or double lung transplantation. Even a markedly depressed right ventricle improves considerably after single or double lung transplantation.

Case 34 ◆ **Ventricular Septal Defect**

CASE PRESENTATION

*There are no peripheral stigmata of endocarditis. There is no evidence of clubbing or cyanosis.[1] The pulse rate is …beats/min, regular/irregular, of normal volume and character.[2] The blood pressure is …/… mmHg.[3] The venous pressure is not elevated.[4] On examination of the precordium, there are no scars. There are no heaves.[5] There is a **parasternal thrill**.[6] The apex beat is undisplaced.[7] On auscultation the first and second heart sounds are normal.[8] There is a loud (harsh) **pansystolic murmur** heard throughout the precordium, loudest at the **lower left sternal edge**.[9] The lung fields are clear to auscultation and there is no sacral or pedal oedema.[10]*

*The diagnosis is a **ventricular septal defect** with a **left-to-right shunt**. The absence of clinical signs of pulmonary hypertension and left ventricular enlargement would suggest that this is a haemodynamically insignificant shunt.[11]*

Clinical notes

1. These are important negatives. Endocarditis is a recognized complication of ventricular septal defect (VSD). A VSD is associated with a left-to-right shunt. As the shunt becomes haemodynamically significant, pulmonary hypertension develops. In advanced cases, with increasing pulmonary artery pressures, the left-to-right shunt will reverse resulting in an Eisenmenger's syndrome. This would then be associated with cyanosis and clubbing.

2. The pulse is usually of normal volume and character.

3. The blood pressure is usually normal with a normal pulse pressure.

4. Look for signs of pulmonary hypertension, as the presence of pulmonary hypertension would place a VSD in the haemodynamically significant category. If venous pressure is elevated, then be sure to look for and not to miss other signs of pulmonary hypertension: parasternal heave and thrill and a loud pulmonary component to the second heart sound.

5. Do not miss signs of pulmonary hypertension. A parasternal heave reflects right ventricular pressure overload. A parasternal thrill reflects 'functional' tricuspid regurgitation.

6. A prominent systolic parasternal thrill is felt with a left-to-right shunt. With the development of pulmonary hypertension, shunt reversal and Eisenmenger's syndrome, if a parasternal thrill is felt, it is unlikely to represent the right-to-left shunt flow across the VSD and is more likely to represent 'functional' tricuspid regurgitation secondary to pulmonary hypertension. In this situation, you would expect to see systolic 'v' waves in the venous pressure waveform.

7. With a haemodynamically significant VSD, left ventricular volume overload will result in left ventricular dilatation and a displaced and thrusting apex beat.

8. With pulmonary hypertension, you would expect a loud pulmonary component to the second heart sound.

9. With small, restrictive, and haemodynamically insignificant defects, the heart sounds are normal and the murmur is often very loud and can be heard all over the precordium, being loudest at the lower left sternal edge. The second heart sound is normal with small defects. Occasionally, a defect may close during contraction in systole and the resulting murmur may not span the entire of systole. With the development of pulmonary hypertension, shunt reversal, and Eisenmenger's syndrome, the murmur diminishes and disappears as pressures in the left and right ventricles equalize. In this case, a single (and often loud) second heart sound indicates equalization of ventricular pressures. At this stage, a pansystolic murmur at the lower left sternal edge is likely to represent functional tricuspid regurgitation secondary to pulmonary hypertension. This murmur will be louder in inspiration (Carvallo's sign). In large defects, a large left-to-right shunting will be associated with increased pulmonary blood flow into the left atrium resulting in increased flow across the mitral valve. This can often produce short mid-diastolic flow murmurs at the apex. Such mitral diastolic flow murmur would suggest pulmonary:systemic flow ≥ 2 (see below for significance).

10. The presence of pulmonary congestion would signify impaired left ventricular function secondary to volume overload. The presence of peripheral oedema would signify pulmonary hypertension and right-sided cardiac failure.

11. It is important not only to state the diagnosis, but also to (a) establish the direction of shunt and (b) haemodynamic significance. The presence of cyanosis will suggest a right-to-left shunt. The presence of pulmonary hypertension, left ventricular enlargement/dysfunction or increased flow across the mitral valve (mid-diastolic flow murmur at the apex) will suggest a VSD is haemodynamically significant.

The following table summarizes the signs associated with haemodynamically insignificant and haemodynamically significant VSDs. A haemodynamically significant VSD in its extreme form is associated with shunt reversal, i.e. Eisenmenger's syndrome (right column in table).

	Haemodynamic significance of VSD		
	Insignificant	Significant	Significant
Defect	Samll(L→R)	Large (L→R)	Large (R→L)
Clubbing	No	No	Yes
Cyanosis	No	No	Yes
VSD murmur	Loud	Less loud	No
Apex	Normal	Displaced and thrusting	Displaced and thrusting
Pulmonary hypertension	No	Yes	Yes
S_2	A_2–P_2	A_2–P_2 (loud P_2)*	Single loud S_2

* In larger left-to-right shunts, there is increased blood passing into the right heart across the VSD and less blood crossing the aortic valve into the aorta. Thus RV emptying occurs later and LV empty-ing occurs earlier. This may give rise to a widely split second heart sound. In practice, due to the loud nature of the murmur throughout the precordium, this may not be easy to detect and appreciate.

Questions commonly asked by examiners

What are the causes of a ventricular septal defect?

Congenital

- Maternal factors
  - ♦ Maternal diabetes
  - ♦ Maternal phenylketonuria
  - ♦ Maternal alcohol consumption (fetal alcohol syndrome)
- Aneuploid syndromes
  - ♦ Down's syndrome (Trisomy 21)
  - ♦ Edward's syndrome (Trisomy 18)
  - ♦ Patau's syndrome (Trisomy 13)
  - ♦ Di George syndrome (Deletion 22q11)
  - ♦ Deletions 4q, 5p, 21, and 32

Acquired

- Ischaemia (post myocardial infarction)
- Iatrogenic (RV pacing with septal puncture, complication of alcohol septal ablation)

How are such ventricular septal defects classified?

Perimembranous (infra-cristal, conoventricular)

- This is the most common type, accounting for 80% of all VSDs.
- Occur in the membranous septum, and lie in the LV outflow tract just below the aortic valve
- These can also cause LV–RA defects (Gerbode defect)
- These defects are associated with pouches or aneurysms of the septal leaflet of the tricuspid valve, which may cause partial or complete occlusion of the defect

Supra-cristal (conal septal, infundibular, subarterial, outlet)

- Account for 5–8% of all VSDs.

* The crista supraventricularis is a muscular ridge that separates the main right ventricular cavity from the infundibular or outflow portion

- Lie beneath the pulmonary valve, and communicate with RV outflow tract, above the crista supraventricularis*
- Can be associated with prolapse of right coronary cusp of the aortic valve and aortic regurgitation.

Muscular (trabecular)
- Account for 5–20% of all VSDs
- Occur in the muscular septum

Posterior (canal type, endocardial cushion type, AV septum type, inlet)
- Account for 8–10% of all VSDs
- Lie posterior to the septal leaflet of the tricuspid valve
- Although located in the same place as VSDs observed with AV septal defects, they are not associated with tricuspid or mitral valve defects.

Are ventricular septal defects always associated with ventricular-to-ventricular shunts?

Although ventricular septal defects result in a communication between the left and right ventricle, occasionally perimembranous defects can result in a left ventricle to right atrium shunt (Gerbode defect).

What are the complications of ventricular septal defects?
- Infective endocarditis
- Pulmonary hypertension
- Left ventricular dysfunction
- Aortic regurgitation (perimembranous or supra-cristal defects)
- Ventricular arrhythmias
- Eisenmenger's syndrome

Can ventricular septal defects close spontaneously?

Spontaneous closure of small defects occurs in approximately 50% of patients, often in early childhood (by 2 years of age). Closure is uncommon after 4 years of age. This is most frequently observed in muscular (80%) followed by perimembranous (35–40%) defects. Outlet defects have a low incidence of spontaneous closure and inlet defects never close spontaneously.

What is the mechanism of spontaneous closure?
- Hypertrophy of the muscular septum (most common)
- Formation of fibrous tissue
- Subaortic tags
- Apposition of septal leaflet of tricuspid valve (perimembranous defects)

How would you investigate this patient?
CXR
- *Small defects*
  - Normal heart size and pulmonary vascular markings
- *Larger defects (with development of pulmonary hypertension)*
  - Cardiomegaly
  - Increased pulmonary vascular markings with prominent main pulmonary arteries
  - Decreased pulmonary markings in outer third of lung fields (oligaemic lung fields)
  - Enlarged left atrium (left atrial appendage and double right-heart border)

ECG

- Small defects
  - No associated ECG changes
- Larger defects
  - Left ventricular hypertrophy (secondary to volume overload)
  - Combined (biventricular) hypertrophy may manifest as large equiphasic mid-precordial voltage (>50mm) in leads V_2–V_4 (Katz-Wachtel phenomenon)
  - Right ventricular hypertrophy is often demonstrated in patients with equalization of ventricular pressures (Eisenmenger's syndrome)
  - Left atrial hypertrophy (bifid P waves in II)
  - Left atrial enlargement (biphasic P waves in V_1)

Echocardiogram

- Location, size and direction of shunt
- Right ventricular size and function
- Left ventricular size and function
- Pulmonary artery systolic pressure
- Pulmonary:systemic flow (Q_p:Q_s ratio)

Cardiac catheterization

This is often unnecessary given the diagnostic accuracy of echocardiography, but can determine the magnitude and direction of shunting and determine the severity and reversibly of pulmonary hypertension.

How would you manage this patient?

Small defects with normal pulmonary artery pressure

- Re-assurance
- Endocarditis prophylaxis
- Encourage living a normal life

Larger defects with pulmonary hypertension/right ventricular failure/left ventricular failure

- Endocarditis prophylaxis
- Diuretics for congestive symptoms
- Treatment of left ventricular dysfunction
- Treatment of pulmonary hypertension
- VSD closure (surgical or percutaneous) if no contraindications

What are the indications for VSD closure?

- Increasing pulmonary:systemic blood flow (Q_p:Q_s > 2:1)
- Left ventricular dilatation
- Left ventricular dysfunction
- Recurrent endocarditis
- Development of aortic regurgitation (at least, mild) through prolapse of right coronary cusp of the aortic valve in supra-cristal defects
- Acute rupture of interventricular septum, i.e. following myocardial infarction

---

* Severe pulmonary hypertension is defined as pulmonary vascular resistance = 2/3 (systemic vascular resistance).

What are the contra-indications for VSD closure?

- Irreversible severe pulmonary hypertension[*]

Is the development of Eisenmenger's syndrome always a contra-indication for VSD closure?

The development of severe pulmonary hypertension is associated with shunt reversal and development of Eisenmenger's syndrome. If the pulmonary hypertension is *irreversible*, then closure is contraindicated. However, if one can demonstrate *reversible* pulmonary hypertension, then closure may be undertaken:

- Evidence of pulmonary reactivity with a pulmonary vasodilator challenge.
- Lung biopsy findings consist with *reversible* pulmonary arterial changes.

Case 35 ◆ Atrial Septal Defect

CASE PRESENTATION

There are no peripheral stigmata of endocarditis. There is no evidence of clubbing or cyanosis.[1] *There are no upper limb developmental deformities.*[2] *The pulse rate is …beats/min, regular/irregular, of normal volume and character.*[3] *The blood pressure is …/…mmHg.*[4] *The venous pressure is not elevated.*[5] *On examination of the precordium, there are no scars.*[6] *There are no heaves.*[7] *There is a* **systolic thrill at the upper left sternal edge** *(pulmonary area).*[8] *The apex beat is undisplaced.*[9] *On auscultation the first heart sound is normal and there is* **fixed wide splitting of the second heart sound**.[10] *There is an* **ejection click** *and an* **ejection systolic murmur at the upper left sternal edge** *(pulmonary area).*[11] *The lung fields are clear to auscultation and there is no sacral or pedal oedema.*[12]

The diagnosis is an **atrial septal defect** *with a* **left-to-right shunt.** *The absence of clinical signs of pulmonary hypertension would suggest this is a haemodynamically insignificant shunt.*[13]

Clinical notes

1. These are important negatives. Endocarditis is a recognized complication of an atrial septal defect (ASD). An ASD is associated with a left-to-right shunt. As the shunt becomes haemodynamically significant, pulmonary hypertension develops. In advanced cases, with increasing pulmonary artery pressures, the left-to-right shunt will reverse resulting in an Eisenmenger's syndrome. This would then be associated with cyanosis and clubbing.
2. Another important negative in the context of an ASD. Holt-Oram syndrome is a rare syndrome associated with absence or reduction anomalies in the upper limb (see below). If mentioned, in a patient with an ASD, it will definitely impress examiners!
3. The pulse is usually of normal volume and character.
4. The blood pressure is usually normal with a normal pulse pressure.
5. Look for signs of pulmonary hypertension, as the presence of pulmonary hypertension would place a ASD in the haemodynamically significant category. If venous pressure is elevated, then be sure to look for and not to miss other signs of pulmonary hypertension: parasternal heave and thrill and a loud pulmonary component to the second heart sound.

6. Look in particular for scars of previous mitral valvotomy suggesting previous mitral stenosis. An important cause of an iatrogenic ASD is one that occurs in the setting of balloon mitral valvuloplasty, which requires puncture of the interatrial septum to gain access to the left atrium from a central venous (femoral) route.

7. Do not miss signs of pulmonary hypertension. A parasternal heave reflects right ventricular pressure overload. A parasternal thrill reflects 'functional' tricuspid regurgitation. There may be a palpable P_2. In such cases the ASD will be associated with a right-to-left shunt and the patient will be cyanosed (Eisenmenger's syndrome).

8. A systolic thrill in the pulmonary area signifies increased flow across the pulmonary valve.

9. The apex beat is often undisplaced in the context of an ASD as shunting occurs at the level of the atria. However, with the development of shunt reversal and Eisenmenger's syndrome, there is left ventricular volume overload, and the apex becomes displaced.

10. The pulmonary component of the second heart sound will be loud in pulmonary hypertension. The hallmark of an ASD is a *fixed and widely split second heart sound*. Fixed splitting of the second heart sound implies no effect of respiration on the two-component split of the second heart sound (A_2–P_2).

11. An ejection systolic murmur in the pulmonary area signifies increased flow across the pulmonary valve. It will never be greater than grade 2–3/6. Occasionally there may be an ejection click, which results from pulmonary artery dilatation and sometimes this click may be palpable. The ejection systolic murmur in the pulmonary area may be confused with pulmonary stenosis. Remember, in pulmonary stenosis, P_2 is often soft—the murmur becomes louder with inspiration. In large haemodynamically significant shunts, there may be a short mid-diastolic flow murmur at the lower left sternal edge, representing increased flow across the tricuspid valve.

12. The presence of pulmonary congestion would signify impaired left ventricular function secondary to volume overload. The presence of peripheral oedema would signify pulmonary hypertension and right-sided cardiac failure.

13. It is important not only to state the diagnosis, but also to (a) establish the direction of the shunt and (b) haemodynamic significance. The presence of cyanosis will suggest a right-to-left shunt. The presence of pulmonary hypertension and/or increased flow across the tricuspid valve (presence of mid-diastolic flow murmur at lower left sternal edge) would suggest an ASD is haemodynamically significant.

The following table summarizes the signs associated with haemodynamically insignificant and haemodynamically significant ASDs. A haemodynamically significant ASD in its extreme form is associated with shunt reversal, i.e. Eisenmenger's syndrome (right column in table).

	Haemodynamic significance of ASD		
	Insignificant (L→R)	Significant (L→R)	Significant (R→L)
Defect	Small (L→R)	Large (L→R)	Large (R→L)
Rhythm	Regular (SR likely)	Irregular (AF more likely)	
Clubbing	No	No	Yes
Cyanosis	No	No	Yes
ESM murmur	Yes	Yes	No
Systolic thrill	No	Yes	No
TV flow murmur	No	Yes	No
Pulmonary hypertension	No	Yes	Yes
S_2	A_2—P_2 (normal P_2) fixed and widely split	A_2—P_2 (loud P_2) fixed and widely split	A_2—P_2 (loud P_2) fixed and widely split

Questions commonly asked by examiners

What are the different types of ASDs?

Type	Frequency	Characteristics of defect
Ostium secundum ASD	~70%	Defect is at site of foramen ovale
Ostium primum ASD	~15%	Defect is at the anterior and inferior aspect of septum with involvement of mitral and tricuspid valves
Sinus venosus ASD	~15%	Defect occurs at the (a) upper atrial septum, posterior to fossa ovalis, just below the entrance of superior vena cava (SVC) into right atrium ('usual type'), and (b) junction of right atrium and inferior vena cava.
Coronary sinus ASD	~1%	Defect is in the portion of atrial septum that involves the coronary sinus; with the absence of a portion of the common wall separating the coronary sinus and the left atrium leads to interatrial shunting.

What is the mechanism of a fixed widely split second heart sound?

Normally, with inspiration, the increased venous return results in prolonged duration of right heart emptying, thus a delay in P_2. Remembering that an ASD results in a left-to-right shunt at the level of the atria, the mechanism of a fixed widely split second heart sound can be explained by:

1. Increased right heart volumes, thus it takes longer for right heart to empty (P_2 occurs later)
2. Less blood in left heart, thus the left heart will empty quicker (A_2 occurs earlier)
3. With ASD, there is equalization of RA and LA pressure, thus the effect of respiration in altering right ventricular volumes is lost. This results in a FIXED WIDELY SPLIT S_2.

What are the causes of widely split second heart sound?
- Atrial septal defect
- Ventricular septal defect
- Mitral regurgitation
- Pulmonary stenosis
- Right bundle branch block

What are the complications of an ASD?
- Atrial arrhythmias (AF is the most common)
- Pulmonary hypertension
- Eisenmenger's syndrome
- Paradoxical embolism
- Infective endocarditis
- Recurrent pulmonary infections

In an asymptomatic patient what would the onset of atrial arrhythmias signify?
Usually patients remain in sinus rhythm in the first three decades. Chronic atrial dilatation provides a substrate for atrial arrhythmias. The onset of atrial arrhythmias (AF and flutter) is often accompanied by the onset of tricuspid regurgitation secondary to pulmonary hypertension.

What other condition is associated with sinus venosus defects?
These defects are associated with anomalous pulmonary venous drainage, with the right upper pulmonary vein emptying directly into the SVC. Less commonly, it may drain into the inferior vena cava.

What is a patent foramen ovale?

A patent foramen ovale (PFO) is a remnant of the fetal circulation. During fetal life, oxygenated placental blood enters the right atrium via the inferior vena cava and crosses the foramen ovale to enter the systemic circulation. At birth the pulmonary vascular resistance and right heart pressures drop, with reversal of pressure gradient and flow across the foramen ovale. This causes the flap of the foramen ovale (septum primum) to close against the atrial septum (septum secundum), with fusion usually occurring in the first two years of life. This 'fusion' is incomplete in 25–30% of people, resulting in an oblique slit-like defect. This is termed a PFO, and functions as a valve-like structure with the 'door-jam' on the left atrial side of the atrial septum.

What is the main difference between a patent foramen ovale and ASD?

Unlike an ASD, a PFO does not allow equalization of atrial pressures.

What clinical sequelae are associated with patent foramen ovale?

In the absence of cardio-respiratory disease, a PFO is usually associated with left-to-right flow across the defect. Right-to-left blood flow only occurs when right atrial pressure exceeds left atrial pressure. Causes include:

- Inspiration*
- Valsalva release manoeuvres,* e.g. coughing or straining
- Pulmonary hypertension
- Acute pulmonary embolism (PE)
- Right ventricular infarction
- Severe tricuspid regurgitation
- Acute respiratory failure

What are the clinical sequelae of patent foramen ovale?

- Paradoxical embolism
- Cryptogenic stroke
- Migraines
- Platybasia
- Atrial arrhythmias

What do you know about cryptogenic stroke and its association with atrial septal abnormalities?

Despite a thorough evaluation, the cause of stroke cannot be determined in approximately 60% of such patients, and these are referred to as 'cryptogenic stroke'. An atrial septal aneurysm (ASA) consists of redundant atrial septal tissue bulging into the right or left atrium, sometimes even oscillating between both atria. This is often associated with a PFO. Current evidence suggests that both PFO and ASA are independent risk factors for stroke, particularly if both coexist. The possible mechanisms of stroke include paradoxical embolism, thrombus formation in PFO, and/or ASA and atrial arrhythmias resulting in thrombus formation.

At what age does shunt reversal typically occur?

Usually after 20 years of age.

What is Holt-Oram syndrome?

This is an autosomal dominant condition, associated with mutations in chromosome 12q2, which results in an ostium secundum defect with absence or reduction anomalies of the upper limb (often a hypoplastic thumb with an accessory phalanx that lies in the same plane as the other digits).

---

* The right-to-left flow may often be transient.

A patient with an ASD also has mitral stenosis. What could are the possible causes?
- Lutembacher syndrome (a congenital ASD with acquired rheumatic mitral stenosis)
- Iatrogenic ASD in a patient with mitral stenosis who has had mitral valvotomy, which requires a transeptal puncture to gain access to the left heart from a central venous (femoral) route

How would you investigate this patient?
CXR
- Increased pulmonary vascular markings with prominent main pulmonary arteries
- Decreased pulmonary markings in outer third of lung fields (oligaemic lung fields)
- Enlarged left atrium (left atrial appendage and double right-heart border)

ECG
- Incomplete right bundle branch block
- Left axis deviation (Ostium primum defects)
- Right axis deviation (Ostium secundum defects)
- Inverted P waves in inferior leads (sinus venosus defects)
- Right ventricular hypertrophy
- Right atrial hypertrophy (P pulmonale)
- Left atrial enlargement (Biphasic P waves in V_1–V_2)

Echocardiogram*
- Location, size and direction of shunt
- Right ventricular size and function
- Pulmonary artery systolic pressure
- Pulmonary:Systemic flow (Q_p:Q_s ratio)

Cardiac catheterization
This is often unnecessary given the diagnostic accuracy of echocardiography, but can determine the magnitude and direction of shunting and determine the severity and reversibly of pulmonary hypertension.

How would you manage this patient?
- Small defects with normal pulmonary artery pressure
    - Re-assurance
    - Encourage living a normal life
- Larger defects with pulmonary hypertension/right ventricular failure/left ventricular failure
    - Diuretics for congestive symptoms
    - Treatment of pulmonary hypertension
    - ASD closure (surgical or percutaneous) if no contraindications

What are the indications for ASD closure?
- Increasing pulmonary:systemic blood flow (Q_p:Q_s > 2:1)

Is the development of Eisenmenger's syndrome always a contraindication for ASD closure?
The development of severe pulmonary hypertension is associated with shunt reversal and development of Eisenmenger's syndrome. If the pulmonary hypertension is *irreversible*, then

---

* Due to limitation of transthoracic echocardiography, transoesophageal echocardiography may be necessary to identify atrial defects as well as anomalous pulmonary venous drainage.

closure is contraindicated. However, if one can demonstrate *reversible* pulmonary hypertension, then closure may be undertaken:

- Evidence of pulmonary reactivity with a pulmonary vasodilator challenge
- Lung biopsy findings consist with *reversible* pulmonary arterial changes

Case 36 ♦ Coarctation of the Aorta

CASE PRESENTATION 1

On examination, the **upper torso is better developed** *than the lower torso.[1] There are no peripheral stigmata of endocarditis.[2] The* **radial pulses are equal** *bilaterally.[3] There are* **vigorous carotid pulsations** *in the neck.[4] The carotid pulse is regular, of large volume and normal character.[5] The femoral pulses are delayed with reduced volume (***radio-femoral delay***).[6] The venous pressure is not elevated.[7] The blood pressure is equal in both arms (.../...mmHg).[8] On examination of the precordium, there are no scars.[9] There are* **visible arterial pulsations** *and* **bruits are heard over collaterals** *over the scapula, anterior axilla and left sternal border.[10] The apex beat is undisplaced and has a* **heaving character.[11]** *There are* **systolic thrills at the suprasternal notch and over the collaterals.[10]** *On auscultation, there is an* **ejection click** *followed by an* **ejection systolic murmur** *in the aortic area. The aortic component of the second heart sound is not diminished.[12] There is a* **harsh ejection systolic murmur** *over* **left sternal edge** *and* **posteriorly***, over the thoracic spine.[13] The lung fields are clear to auscultation and there is no peripheral oedema.*

The diagnosis is **coarctation of the aorta***. The level of coarctation is* **distal to the origin of the left subclavian artery***. In addition, there is a* **bicuspid aortic valve***, which is often associated with this condition.[14]*

CASE PRESENTATION 2

On examination, the **upper torso is better developed** *than the lower torso.[1] There are no peripheral stigmata of endocarditis.[2] The* **left radial pulse is diminished.[3]** *There are* **vigorous carotid pulsations** *in the neck.[4] The carotid pulse is regular, of large volume, and normal character.[5] There is no radio-femoral delay.[6] The venous pressure is not elevated.[7] The blood pressure is higher in the right arm.[8] On examination of the precordium, there is left thoracotomy scar.[9] There are* **visible arterial pulsations** *and* **bruits are heard over collaterals** *over the scapula, anterior axilla, and left sternal border.[10] There are* **systolic thrills over the collaterals.[10]** *The apex beat is undisplaced and has a* **heaving character.[11]** *On auscultation, there is an* **ejection click** *followed by an* **ejection systolic murmur** *in the aortic area. The aortic component of the second heart sound is not diminished.[12] The lung fields are clear to auscultation and there is no peripheral oedema.*

The diagnosis is a surgically **repaired coarctation of the aorta***. In addition, there is a* **bicuspid aortic valve***, which is often associated with this condition.[14]*

Clinical notes

The above two cases demonstrate the variety of clinical signs associated with coarctation of the aorta. Deducing the level of coarctation causes panic and confusion amongst candidates, but in fact is very simple. Previous repair of coarctation is common in examinations. Remember, the

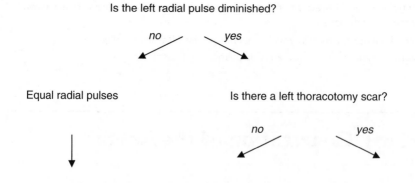

Figure 36.1 Algoritihm for tackling a reuced or absent left radial pulse.

** Consider other causes of diminished left radial pulse: left subclavian artery stenosis, atherosclerosis, arterial embolus, arterial thrombosis, and vasculitis.

radial artery may be harvested and used as a graft for CABG surgery if there is adequate collateral ulnar flow. A left radial artery harvest will result in an absent left radial pulse, and it is important to look for such scars. A simple algorithm for tackling a reduced or absent left radial pulse in examinations (in the absence of a radial harvest scar):

1. The site of coarctation is often distal to the origin of the left subclavian artery. This leads to decreased blood flow to the lower torso and limbs. With time and growth of the individual, the upper limbs and torso become better developed.

2. This condition is often associated with a bicuspid aortic valve. Always mention the absence or presence of stigmata of endocarditis.

3. When the site of the defect is distal to the origin of the left subclavian artery (in most cases), both radial pulses are of equal volume. Rarely, the defect may be proximal to the origin of the left subclavian artery, in which case the left radial pulse will be weaker. In patients who have previously had repair of coarctation, the left subclavian artery is used in the repair, thus the left radial pulse is weaker. Very rarely, the defect may be proximal to the origins of both the brachiocephalic and left subclavian arteries, in which case both radial pulses will be equal and weak. In such cases, there will be no evidence of differential development of the upper and lower body.

4. Vigorous pulsations in the neck can also be seen in aortic regurgitation.

5. The pulse is often of large volume and normal character. Coarctation of the aorta is often associated with a bicuspid aortic valve. In the presence of haemodynamic aortic regurgitation, the pulse will have a collapsing character. In the presence of haemodynamic significant aortic stenosis, the pulse will be of reduced volume and slow-rising character.

6. Palpate the right radial pulse with one hand, and the right femoral pulse with the other. In coarctation of the aorta, the femoral pulse is delayed, leading to radio-femoral delay. An important fact is that in normal individuals, the femoral pulse is felt just before the radial pulse and, therefore, if both radial and femoral pulses occur at the same time, then this should hint at a delayed femoral pulse and lead one to suspect radio-femoral delay.

7. The venous pressure will be elevated in pulmonary hypertension.

8. When the site of the defect is distal to the origin of the left subclavian artery (in most cases), blood pressure will be equal in both arms. Rarely, the defect may be proximal to origin of the left subclavian artery, in which case the blood pressure will be higher in the right arm.

9. Be sure not to miss the left thoracotomy scar of previous coarctation repair. You should have suspected this, earlier in the examination, if the left radial pulse was diminished or absent.

10. Collateral vessels develop in severe long-standing cases. In thin individuals, arterial pulsations may be seen. Often thrills may be palpated and bruits may be auscultated over these collateral arteries. In cases where coarctation has been repaired, these collaterals often persist, as do the associated clinical signs.

11. Coarctation of the aorta is associated with left ventricular pressure overload, thus compensatory left ventricular hypertrophy occurs. This gives rise to a forceful, heaving apex beat. After repair of the defect, there is afterload reduction, and there is often some degree of regression of left ventricular hypertrophy. Nevertheless, left ventricular hypertrophy often persists, especially as these patients are hypertensive, and the apex may still demonstrate a heaving character. In cases where there is a bicuspid aortic valve with aortic regurgitation, the apex will be displaced with a thrusting character.

12. A bicuspid aortic valve has an ejection click. This may not always be associated with en ejection systolic murmur (in cases without aortic stenosis). If a murmur of aortic stenosis is identified, be sure to interpret all other signs on physical examination to provide a clinical estimate of severity of aortic stenosis. Likewise, if an early diastolic murmur of aortic regurgitation is present, then comment on severity.

13. The murmur of coarctation is often heard over the coarctation. As most defects are distal to the origin of the left subclavian artery, the murmur is loudest posteriorly over the thoracic spine.

14. Although the primary diagnosis is coarctation of the aorta, comment on the presence or absence of a bicuspid aortic valve, as it is present in 50% of cases. If aortic stenosis or regurgitation is present, comment on severity. Other features to look for in the general examination of the patient are conditions associated with coarctation of the aorta. If correctly identified and presented, it will impress:

   - **Turner's syndrome**: female, short stature, wide carrying angle at elbows, webbed neck, and high-arched palate
   - **Berry aneurysms**: presence of a third nerve palsy (look for underlying polycystic kidney disease)

Questions commonly asked by examiners

How common is this condition?
Coarctation of the aorta accounts for 5–8% of congenital heart defects.

How are different types of coarctation of aorta classified?
- Infantile type (Preductal)—proximal to the origin of the left subclavian artery; presents with heart failure in infancy
- Adult type (Postductal/Juxtaductal)—distal to origin of left subclavian artery; presents between 15 and 30 years of age

What other cardiac conditions are associated with this condition?
- Bicuspid aortic valve (50% of cases)
- Patent ductus arteriosus
- Ventricular septal defect
- Mitral valve anomalies
- Transposition of the great vessels
- Tricuspid atresia
- Hypoplastic left heart syndrome
- Aortic arch hypoplasia

What other non-cardiac conditions are associated with this condition?
- Turner's syndrome (35% have coarctation of the aorta)
- Berry aneurysms

- Haemangiomas
- Renal abnormalities

Where do collaterals arise, in long-standing coarctation of the aorta?

The large arterial collaterals develop from the upper to lower parts of the body:

- Internal mammary to external iliac arteries
- Spinal and intercostal arteries to the descending aorta

What causes rib notching on a chest radiograph in these patients?

Collaterals from dilated tortuous posterior intercostal arteries, causes notching on the undersurfaces of the posterior portions of the ribs. The anterior portions are spared, as the anterior intercostal arteries do not run in the costal grooves. They commonly occur between the 3rd and 9th rib spaces. It is unusual before the age of 5 years, and observed more in patients with significant obstruction that has been long-standing (allowing collaterals to develop).

What other conditions cause rib notching?

- Blalock-Taussig shunt
- Subclavian artery obstruction
- SVC syndrome
- Neurofibromatosis
- Arterio-venous malformation of lung and chest wall

How would you investigate this patient?

ECG

- Left ventricular hypertrophy +/− strain
- Left atrial dilatation (inverted or biphasic P waves in V_1–V_2) if in sinus rhythm

CXR

- Rib notching
- Prominent aortic knuckle
- Characteristic '3 sign': the upper bulge is formed by dilatation of the left subclavian artery (high on left mediastinal border) and the lower bulge is formed by post-stenotic dilatation of the aorta
- Cardiomegaly and pulmonary congestion (if left ventricular failure)

Echocardiogram

- To assess the aorta (often the coarctation can be visualize on 2D echocardiography)
- To assess severity by measuring pressure gradient across the defect
- Presence of other cardiac defects (bicuspid aortic valve, VSD, or patent ductus arteriosus (PDA))
- Left ventricular hypertrophy
- Left ventricular function

Cardiac catheterization

- Can confirm diagnosis if echocardiography finding are not clear
- Can measure peak–peak gradients across the defect
- Aortic angiography can demonstrate defect and presence of collaterals
- A prerequisite if balloon angioplasty and stenting is being contemplated

MRI

- Sensitive for location and extent of coarctation
- Involvement of adjacent vessels

- Presence of collaterals
- Useful for detecting and monitoring aneurysms or re-stenosis

What are the complications of coarctation of the aorta?

- Hypertension
- Hypoplastic limbs (depending on site and severity of defect)
- Endocarditis (in presence of bicuspid aortic valve)
- Left ventricular diastolic dysfunction (stiff and hypertrophied left ventricle)
- Left ventricular systolic dysfunction (long-standing untreated cases)

How would is this condition treated?

Surgical repair of defect

- Resection of segment of coarctation with end-to-end anastomosis of the aorta
- Patch aortoplasty
- Left subclavian flap angioplasty

Catheter-based intervention

- Balloon angioplasty with stent insertion

Case 37 ◆ **Patent Ductus Arteriosus**

CASE PRESENTATION

*There are no peripheral stigmata of endocarditis. There is no evidence of clubbing or cyanosis.[1] The pulse rate is …beats/min, regular/irregular, **large volume**, and with a **collapsing** character.[2] The blood pressure is …/…mmHg with a **wide pulse pressure**.[3] The venous pressure is not elevated.[4] On examination of the precordium, there are no scars. There is a **parasternal heave**.[5]and a **left subclavicular thrill**.[6] The apex beat is **displaced** and has a **thrusting quality**.[7] On auscultation there is a **continuous machinery murmur** with **systolic accentuation** in the **left subclavicular area**.[8] The lung fields are clear to auscultation and there is no sacral or pedal oedema.[9]*

*The diagnosis is a **patent ductus arteriosus** with a **left-to-right shunt**. The clinical signs of **pulmonary hypertension** and **left ventricular enlargement** would suggest that this is a haemodynamically significant shunt.[10]*

Clinical notes

1. These are important negatives. Endocarditis is a recognized complication of patent ductus arteriosus (PDA). A PDA is associated with left-to-right shunt. As the shunt becomes haemodynamically significant, pulmonary hypertension develops. In advanced cases, with increasing pulmonary artery pressures, the left-to-right shunt will reverse resulting in cyanosis and clubbing. This would constitute an Eisenmenger's syndrome. As PDA usually connect the pulmonary artery to the aorta distal to origin of the left subclavian artery, pulmonary hypertension and shunt reversal will cause *differential clubbing and cyanosis*, i.e. cyanosis and clubbing of toes NOT the fingers.

2. With a large PDA, the pulse is of large volume and collapsing character. However, this is often not the case with a small narrow PDA.

3. A large PDA is associated with a large pulse pressure.

4. Look for signs of pulmonary hypertension, as the presence of pulmonary hypertension would place a PDA in the haemodynamically significant category. If venous pressure is elevated, then be sure to look for and not to miss other signs of pulmonary hypertension: parasternal heave and thrill and a loud pulmonary component to the second heart sound

5. Do not miss signs of pulmonary hypertension. A parasternal heave reflects right ventricular pressure overload. A parasternal thrill, if present, reflects 'functional' tricuspid regurgitation.

6. This thrill is often felt best on the anterior chest wall, below the left clavicle. It reflects flow through the shunt.

7. A PDA is associated with left-to-right shunt from the aorta to the pulmonary artery. Thus there is volume overload in the pulmonary circulation and in the left heart, which receives the increased blood volume. As the PDA becomes haemodynamically significant, the left ventricular dimensions increase, with a displaced and thrusting apex beat.

8. On auscultation, the first heart sound is normal. Although the second heart sound is often obscured by the murmur, it will be loud in the presence of pulmonary hypertension (loud P_2). Large haemodynamically significant shunts are associated with reversed splitting of the second heart sound (may not be easy to appreciate as this is obscured by the murmur). The classical murmur is often referred to as a 'continuous machinery murmur', and may have systolic accentuation. This is the *Gibson murmur*. The murmur begins after the first heart sound and peaks at the second heart sound, after which it trails off. It is best heard at the upper left sternal edge or left subclavicular area. The narrower the shunt, the louder the murmur. The murmur can span the whole of systole and diastole, but may occur at the later part of systole and early part of diastole. Sometimes, in young children, it may occur as a crescendo murmur in late systole. In a large haemodynamically significant PDA, where pulmonary:aortic flow is >2:1, a low-frequency mid-diastolic flow murmur may be heard at the apex due to increased flow across the mitral valve. With pulmonary hypertension, the diastolic then the systolic component becomes shorter and softer. It is then that the reversed splitting of the second heart sound may be easier to appreciate. Sometimes the murmur of a PDA can be confused with pulmonary stenosis. It is important to remember, unlike the murmur of pulmonary stenosis, the murmur of PDA is heard equally as loud posteriorly.

9. The presence of pulmonary congestion would signify impaired left ventricular function secondary to volume overload. The presence of oedema would signify pulmonary hypertension and right-sided cardiac failure.

10. It is important not only to state the diagnosis, but also to (a) establish the direction of shunt and (b) haemodynamic significance. The presence of cyanosis will suggest a right-to-left shunt. The presence of pulmonary hypertension and/or left ventricular enlargement will suggest a PDA is haemodynamically significant.

Questions commonly asked by examiners

How common is a patent ductus arteriosus?
This represents 5–10% of all congenital heart disease. It occurs in approximately 8 in 1000 of live births.

What is the pathophysiology?
The ductus is derived from the 6th aortic arch. From the 6th week of fetal life, it is responsible for most of right ventricular outflow, diverting blood from the pulmonary arteries into the systemic circulation, thus bypassing the fetal lungs. The ductus patency is promoted by prostaglandin E_2 during fetal life. Normally, functional closure of the ductus occurs within 15 hours of birth. This occurs with the first breath, and the increased pO_2 causes abrupt muscle contraction of the ductus. After functional closure, true anatomical closure, i.e. where the ductus loses its ability to re-open can take several weeks. The presence of a ductus after 3 months is usually diagnosed as a patent ductus arteriosus.

t usually connects the main pulmonary artery to the proximal descending aorta, just after the origin of the left subclavian artery.

What are other causes of a collapsing or bounding pulse?

Exaggerated or bounding pulses are not specific to patent ductus arteriosus. They can be seen in any hyperdynamic circulation with a marked increase in stroke volume. They include:

- Anaemia
- Fever
- Pregnancy
- Thyrotoxicosis
- Aortic regurgitation
- Arterio-venous fistula
- Severe bradycardia
- Severe mitral regurgitation*

What are the causes of a continuous murmur?

- Patent ductus arteriosus
- Mitral regurgitation AND aortic regurgitation
- Ventricular septal defect AND aortic regurgitation
- Pulmonary arterio-venous fistula
- Coronary arterio-venous fistula
- Ruptured sinus of Valsalva
- Pulmonary arterio-venous shunt (Blalock Taussig shunt)
- Venous hum

What are causes of a patent ductus arteriosus?

- Prematurity
- Low-birth weight
- Maternal used of prostaglandin antagonists, i.e. NSAIDs
- Maternal rubella (first trimester)
- High altitude
- Maternal hypoxia
- Fetal alcohol syndrome
- Maternal amphetamine use
- Maternal phenytoin use

What are the main complications?

- Left ventricular dysfunction (volume overload)—most common
- Infective endocarditis
- Pulmonary hypertension
- Eisenmenger's syndrome
- Ductal aneurysm and calcification
- Ductal rupture*

---

* Can cause rapid rising arterial pulse, which are often short and abbreviated. They can give an impression of a collapsing pulse. However, pulse pressure is normal.

* Ductal aneurysm formation and calcification predispose to ductal rupture.

What is 'differential cyanosis'?

A patent ductus arteriosus usually connects the pulmonary artery to the aorta distal to origin of the left subclavian artery. Pulmonary hypertension and shunt reversal will cause differential clubbing and cyanosis, i.e. cyanosis and clubbing of toes NOT of the fingers.

How would you differentiate the ductus murmur from a venous hum?

A venous hum is often heard best at the right of the sternum. It diminishes or disappears in the supine position, expiration or compression of the right JVP (all of which reduce venous return).

How would you differentiate the ductus murmur from that of pulmonary stenosis?

The murmur of a ductus is heard loudest below the left clavicle and is equally as loud posteriorly. This is not the case for pulmonary stenosis.

What is the prognosis in untreated patent ductus arteriosus?

It is estimated that the mortality rate is 20% by age 20 years, 42% by age 45 years and 60% at age 60 years. An estimated 0.6% undergo spontaneous closure.

What is the general management of a patent ductus arteriosus?

Conservative management
- Endocarditis prophylaxis*
- Diuretics for congestive symptoms

Definitive management
- In neonates, administration of prostaglandin inhibitors (intravenous indomethacin or ibuprofen) can promote ductal closure. This is often effective if administered in the first 14 days of life.
- Percutaneous ductal closure (different occluder devices are available)**
- Surgical ductal closure**

Case 38 ◆ **Pulmonary Stenosis**

CASE PRESENTATION

*There are no peripheral stigmata of endocarditis.[1] The pulse rate is …beats/min, regular/irregular, normal volume and character.[2] The blood pressure is…/…mmHg.[3] The venous pressure is not elevated but with **prominent a waves**.[4] On examination of the precordium, the apex beat is undisplaced. There is a **parasternal heave** and a **systolic thrill palpable at the upper left sternal edge** (pulmonary area).[5] On auscultation, the first heart sound is normal, and the **second heart sound is widely split with diminished pulmonary component**.[6] There is a **fourth heart sound**.[7] There is an **ejection click**[8] with an **ejection systolic murmur loudest at the upper left sternal edge** (pulmonary area), which **radiates***

---

* The annual risk of endocarditis associated with an patent ductus is 0.45%. Given the low risk associated with percutaneous and surgical closure (mortality <0.5%), closure is recommended in even a small patent ductus arteriosus.

** Closure is contraindicated once severe pulmonary hypertension has developed with Eisenmenger's syndrome.

to the suprasternal notch,[9] *and is **louder in inspiration**.*[10] *The lung fields are clear to auscultation and there is no pedal oedema.*[11]

*The diagnosis is **pulmonary stenosis**.*

Clinical notes

1. Always mention presence/absence of signs of endocarditis in any patient with physical signs of valvular heart disease. More than often, they are absent—but this is an important negative finding.

2. The pulse is usually normal. In advanced cases, there is right heart (including right atrial) dilatation that may be associated with AF.

3. The blood pressure in normal with a normal pulse pressure.

4. In sinus rhythm, the presence of a large 'a' wave on venous pressure waveform suggests severe pulmonary stenosis.

5. A parasternal heave reflects right ventricular pressure overload, and a systolic thrill represents turbulent blood flow across the pulmonary valve. Unlike aortic stenosis, presence of a systolic thrill dose not signify severe pulmonary stenosis.

6. Due to prolonged right ventricular emptying, the pulmonary component of the second heart (P_2) sound occurs later, resulting in a widely split second heart sound. The wider the split, the greater the severity of pulmonary stenosis. A soft P_2 signifies severe pulmonary stenosis. Often in severe pulmonary stenosis, as a result of a soft (or near absent) P_2, the widely split second heart sound cannot be appreciated.

7. A fourth heart sound is a sign of severe pulmonary stenosis and reflects forceful atrial contraction.

8. The timing of the ejection click can help determine severity. In mild cases, the ejection click is clearly separated from the first heart sound. With increasing severity, the ejection click becomes closer to the first heart sound. In severe cases, the ejection click may become inseparable from the first heart sound often giving the impression of an absent ejection click.

9. The murmur of pulmonary stenosis is a crescendo–decrescendo murmur loudest in the pulmonary area and radiates to the suprasternal notch. It may radiate to the axilla or the back. The length of the murmur and the timing of the peaking of the ejection murmur correlate with severity. In mild cases, the short murmur peaks early in systole ending well before A_2. In severe cases, there is wide splitting of the second heart sound and the long murmur peaks late in systole and extends beyond A_2. As P_2 is soft in severe pulmonary stenosis, and as the murmur extends beyond A_2, it therefore appears to extend into early diastole. Sometimes, A_2 may be obscured by the long systolic murmur.

10. The murmur of pulmonary stenosis is louder in inspiration, which is an important feature distinguishing this from aortic stenosis. Therefore, it is important to correctly determine this. Ask the patient to breathe in and out slowly, and the murmur intensity will increase during inspiration. Often, candidates ask the patient to take a deep breath in and hold it. This is incorrect, as by breath holding and closure of the glottis, in fact the reverse effect happens, as by doing this there is reduced venous return, with resultant reduction of the intensity of right-sided heart murmurs!

    Sometimes an early diastolic murmur of pulmonary regurgitation may be heard in the pulmonary area (radiates a few interspaces down the sternal edge; louder in inspiration). Although pulmonary regurgitation is not a feature in cases of pulmonary stenosis, if present, it may suggest previous balloon valvuloplasty. Some cases of severe pulmonary stenosis may be associated with functional tricuspid regurgitation (systolic 'cv' waves; parasternal thrill; and pansystolic murmur at lower left sternal edge louder in inspiration).

11. In severe pulmonary stenosis, the lung fields are not congested, unless there is co-existent left ventricular dysfunction and/or significant left-sided valvular pathology. In severe pulmonary stenosis, with development of pulmonary hypertension, signs of right-sided cardiac failure are more likely, i.e. peripheral oedema.

Questions commonly asked by examiners

What are the causes of pulmonary stenosis?

Valvular pulmonary stenosis

- Congenital
- Rheumatic heart disease
- Carcinoid syndrome
- Noonan's syndrome
- Watson's syndrome
- Alagille syndrome

Supravalvular pulmonary stenosis

- Congenital rubella
- William's syndrome

Subvalvular pulmonary stenosis

- Fallot's tetralogy

How common is pulmonary stenosis?

This represents 8–12% of all congenital heart disease in children. In adults, it accounts for 15% of all congenital heart disease.

What are the clinical signs of severe pulmonary stenosis?

- Large 'a' waves (if in sinus rhythm)
- Long systolic murmur with late systolic peaking
- Early ejection click (short interval between S_1 and ejection click)
- Widely split S_2
- Diminished P_2
- Fourth heart sound
- Tricuspid regurgitation

What clinical features help differentiate the murmur of pulmonary stenosis with that of aortic stenosis?

Clinical feature	Aortic stenosis	Pulmonary stenosis
Respiratory variation	Louder in expiration	Louder in inspiration
Venous pressure	Normal, unless pulmonary hypertension	Prominent tall 'a' wave
Pulse	Low volume, slow-rising	Normal volume and character
Palpation	Left ventricular heave	Parasternal heave
S_2 characteristics	Normal split in mild cases with reversed split and diminished A_2 in severe cases	Widely split S_2 with diminished P_2 in severe cases.
Murmur characteristics	Murmur ends before A_2	Murmur can extend beyond A_2

Why does the ejection systolic murmur of severe pulmonary stenosis extend into early diastole?

The features of severe pulmonary stenosis are a long crescendo–decrescendo systolic murmur with late systolic peaking, widely split S_2 with diminished P_2. Often the P_2 is not heard and only the A_2 component is heard. The murmur of pulmonary stenosis terminates with closure of the pulmonary valve, i.e. at P_2. Therefore, the murmur of severe pulmonary stenosis will extend

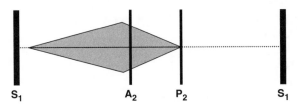

Figure 38.1 The murmur of severe pulmonary stenosis extends beyond A_2 terminating at P.

beyond A_2 terminating at P_2. As P_2 is soft, often only A_2 is appreciated; thus the murmur appears to extend into early diastole (Figure 38.1).

How do you grade pulmonary stenosis?

Pulmonary stenosis is graded using the trans-valvular gradient: mild (<50mmHg), moderate (50–79mmHg) and severe (>80mmHg). It may be graded using valvular area: mild (>1cm²), moderate (0.5–1.0cm²) and severe (<0.5cm²).

What can cause cyanosis in patients with pulmonary stenosis?

In patients with severe pulmonary stenosis, there is right ventricular hypertrophy and elevated right ventricular systolic pressures. In the presence of a shunt, i.e. ASD or VSD, this may lead to shunt reversal with right-to-left shunting resulting in cyanosis. Sometimes, in the presence of a patent foramen ovale, there may be intermittent right-to-left shunting.

What is the significance of pulmonary regurgitation in a patient with pulmonary stenosis?

Although the pulmonary regurgitation is not associated with the primary diagnosis of pulmonary stenosis, pulmonary regurgitation can result from:

* previous balloon valvuloplasty
* valvular calcification

What do you know about Noonan's syndrome?

This is an autosomal dominant condition, although sporadic cases can occur. It is considered as a male phenotypic form of Turner's syndrome. However, the karyotype is normal (XX or XY). A disease-causing gene has been identified-PTPN11, and the gene product, SHP2, plays an important role in the development of semilunar valves. Essentially, the cardiac manifestations are right-sided cardiac lesions as opposed to Turner's syndrome, which is often associated with left-sided cardiac lesions. The following features are associated with Noonan's syndrome:

* **Musculoskeletal features**
  * Short stature
  * Webbed neck
  * Wide-spaced nipples
  * Cubitus valgus
  * Pectus excavatum or carinatum
* **Cardiac features**
  * Pulmonary valvular stenosis
  * Hypertrophic cardiomyopathy
  * ASD
  * VSD
  * Branch pulmonary artery stenosis

- *Facies*
  - Triangular-shaped face
  - Ptosis
  - Strabismus
  - High nasal bridge
  - Low-set ears with thickened helices
  - Down-slanting eyes
- *Haematological features*
  - Coagulation defects (factor X, XII, and VIII)
  - Von Willebrand's disease
- *Other features*
  - Small genitalia
  - Undescended testes in boys
  - Mental retardation (30%)

What do you know about Watson's syndrome?

This is a syndrome characterized by neurofibromatosis and Noonan's phenotype. Features include pulmonary valve stenosis, café-au-lait spots, mental retardation, macrocephaly, and short stature. Although Lisch nodules are present in the majority of cases, neurofibomata are present only in a third of cases.

What do you know about Alagille syndrome?

This is an autosomal dominant disorder with variable expression associated with abnormalities of the liver, heart, skeleton, eye, kidneys, and characteristic facial appearance. Hepatic disease is the key feature, and patients present with cholestatic jaundice. Almost all patients have cardiac manifestations that include:

- Pulmonary valve stenosis
- Supravalvular pulmonary stenosis (stenoses within the pulmonary tree)
- Septal defects (ASD and VSD)
- Fallot's tetralogy
- Patent ductus arteriosus
- Pulmonary atresia

How would you investigate this patient?

ECG

- Right ventricular hypertrophy
- Right ventricular strain
- Right axis deviation[*]
- Right atrial hypertrophy (P pulmonale)

CXR

- Prominent main pulmonary artery segment (post-stenotic dilatation)
- Diminished pulmonary vascular markings

Echocardiogram

- Thickened pulmonary valve with restricted opening of the pulmonary valve
- Dilatation of the main pulmonary artery

---

[*] A superior QRS axis (left-axis deviation) is seen with dysplastic pulmonary valves and Noonan's syndrome.

Right ventricular hypertrophy

To assess right ventricular size and function

Presence or absence of other congenital heart defects

How would you manage these patients?

Endocarditis prophylaxis

Mild: often don't require treatment other than follow-up

Moderate: often don't require treatment other than follow-up

Severe: balloon valvuloplasty, percutaneous valve replacement or surgical valve replacement

Case 39 ◆ **Pulmonary Regurgitation**

CASE PRESENTATION 1

There are no peripheral stigmata of endocarditis.[1] There is no evidence of clubbing or cyanosis.[2] The pulse rate is …beats/min, regular/irregular, normal volume and character.[2] The blood pressure is…/…mmHg.[3] The venous pressure is not elevated.[4] On examination of the precordium, the apex beat is undisplaced.[5] There are no heaves or thrills.[6] On auscultation, the first and second heart sounds are normal. There is an **early diastolic murmur at the upper left sternal edge (pulmonary area)**, radiating down the left sternal edge, **louder in inspiration**.[7] The lung fields are clear to auscultation and there is no pedal edema.[8]

The diagnosis is **primary pulmonary regurgitation**.[9]

CASE PRESENTATION 2

There are no peripheral stigmata of endocarditis.[1] There is no evidence of clubbing or cyanosis.[2] The pulse rate is …beats/min, irregularly irregular, low volume and normal character.[2] The blood pressure is …/… mmHg.[3] The venous pressure is elevated with systolic 'v' waves.[4] There is a malar flush. On examination of the precordium, there is a lateral thoracotomy scar. The apex beat is undisplaced and has a tapping quality.[5] There is a parasternal heave, a parasternal thrill, and a palpable pulmonary component to the second heart sound (P_2).[6] On auscultation, the first heart sound is loud, and a loud pulmonary component of the second heart sound. There is an opening snap in early diastole followed by a mid-diastolic rumbling murmur at the apex, heard best in expiration with the patient in the left lateral position. In addition, there a pansystolic murmur at the lower left sternal edge, which is louder in inspiration, and a short **early diastolic murmur at the upper left sternal edge (pulmonary area)**, down the left sternal edge, **louder in inspiration**.[7] On auscultation of the lung fields, there are bibasal crepitations, and there is peripheral oedema.[8]

The primary diagnosis is **mitral stenosis with pulmonary hypertension**. There are murmurs of **functional tricuspid regurgitation** and **pulmonary regurgitation (Graham Steell murmur)** secondary to pulmonary hypertension.[9]

Clinical notes

Secondary pulmonary regurgitation commonly appears in examinations. Rarely, it may appear as the primary diagnosis. The above two case presentations reflect this. The causes of primary and secondary pulmonary regurgitation are listed below, and it is important to distinguish whether the pulmonary regurgitation is primary or secondary. As a general rule, secondary pulmonary hypertension is always secondary to pulmonary hypertension, thus one would expect to find signs of pulmonary hypertension to support this.

1. Always mention the presence/absence of signs of endocarditis in any patient with physical signs of valvular heart disease. More than often, they are absent—but this is an important negative finding. Endocarditis is an important cause of primary pulmonary regurgitation.

2. Cyanosis and clubbing would suggest underlying cyanotic congenital heart disease with right-to-left shunting as a cause for secondary pulmonary hypertension and pulmonary regurgitation.

3. In primary pulmonary regurgitation, the pulse is normal. Look for clues for other valvular heart disease as a possible cause for pulmonary hypertension, i.e. the slow-rising pulse of aortic stenosis, collapsing pulse of aortic regurgitation; and the short abbreviated pulse of severe mitral regurgitation.

4. A raised venous pressure would suggest pulmonary hypertension (and therefore secondary pulmonary regurgitation). Systolic 'v' waves will indicate 'functional' tricuspid regurgitation. If the venous pressure is not elevated, look for the prominent tall 'a' waves of pulmonary stenosis (in the context of pulmonary stenosis, valvular calcification, or previous pulmonary balloon valvuloplasty and may lead to pulmonary regurgitation). Prominent a waves may be present in severe pulmonary regurgitation.

5. In primary pulmonary regurgitation, the apex beat is normal. Look for clues for other valvular heart disease as a possible cause for pulmonary hypertension, i.e. the displaced and thrusting apex beat of aortic regurgitation, mitral regurgitation, ventricular septal defect, patent ductus arteriosus; the tapping apex beat of mitral stenosis, the heaving apex beat of aortic stenosis, hypertensive heart disease, and hypertrophic cardiomyopathy.

6. Look for signs of pulmonary hypertension. A parasternal heave reflects right ventricular pressure overload. A parasternal thrill reflects 'functional' tricuspid regurgitation. With significant pulmonary artery dilatation, there may be palpable pulmonary arterial pulsations at the left upper sternal border. With severe pulmonary hypertension, the closure of the pulmonary artery may be palpated with a palpable P_2. Secondary pulmonary regurgitation will almost always be associated with a palpable P_2.

7. In primary pulmonary regurgitation, the first heart sound is normal and the second heart sound is often split (delayed P_2 due to increased right ventricular stroke volume). In secondary pulmonary regurgitation (secondary to pulmonary hypertension), the second heart sound is also split but with a loud P_2. The P_2 is absent if there is congenital absence of the pulmonary valve.

   Auscultation should help to identify any underlying valvular heart disease that may cause pulmonary hypertension. Listen carefully for other murmurs, particularly those indicating left-sided valvular heart disease that may be the cause of pulmonary hypertension.

   The murmur of pulmonary regurgitation is an early diastolic murmur in the pulmonary area, radiating down the left sternal edge and louder in inspiration. In secondary pulmonary regurgitation, the murmur is high-pitched and longer and may span most of diastole because of the non-equalizing pulmonary-to-right ventricular pressure overload. In primary pulmonary regurgitation, the low-pressure regurgitant flow across the pulmonary valve is often heard as a short low-pitched (rougher in quality) early diastolic murmur.

   In the context of pulmonary hypertension, there is often a delayed P_2, and as the murmur of pulmonary regurgitation begins with P_2, it may appear as a mid-diastolic rather than an early diastolic murmur.

   A right ventricular 3rd or 4th heart sound may both be audible with right ventricular failure or hypertrophy. These sounds may be distinguished from left ventricular heart sounds because they are located at the left parasternal 4th intercostal space and because they become louder in inspiration.

8. Pulmonary congestion may be present in significant left sided valvular lesions that result in pulmonary hypertension. The presence of peripheral oedema would suggest right heart failure, a feature of advanced pulmonary hypertension. The presence of wheeze would signify underlying obstructive airways disease—a possible cause of secondary pulmonary hypertension. Fine bibasal end-inspiratory crepitations may indicate interstitial lund disease—a possible cause of secondary pulmonary hypertension (look for clubbing!).

9. When presenting the diagnosis, it is important to mention whether the diagnosis is primary or secondary pulmonary regurgitation. In cases of secondary pulmonary regurgitation, mention the possible cause(s) for pulmonary hypertension. Remember, that causes of secondary pulmonary hypertension are diverse and include non-cardiac causes. The following may be easily identified:

- **Obstructive airways disease**: nicotine staining, hyper-inflated chest, prolonged expiratory time, and wheeze
- **Interstitial lung disease**: clubbing of fingers, bibasal inspiratory crepitations, and rheumatological disease
- **Systemic sclerosis**: scleroderma hands, tightening of facial skin, telangiectasia
- **Rheumatoid arthritis**: symmetrical deforming arthropathy of the small joints of the hands
- **SLE**: butterfly rash over the face, arthropathy
- **Chronic type 2 respiratory failure**: kyphoscoliosis or obesity

In certain cases, there may be signs of pulmonary hypertension, but with no evidence for its cause. In such cases, the diagnosis of **primary pulmonary hypertension** may be suggested.

In cases of primary pulmonary regurgitation, often the cause may not be identified, but try to look for possible causes:

    (a)   presence of underlying pulmonary stenosis—suggesting previous **balloon valvuloplasty** as a cause.

    (b)   signs of **carcinoid syndrome** (flushed facial appearance, hepatomegaly)

    (c)   signs of intravenous drug use—suggesting right-sided **endocarditis** as the cause

Questions commonly asked by examiners

What are the causes of pulmonary regurgitation?

Primary pulmonary regurgitation

Infective endocarditis
Rheumatic heart disease
Carcinoid syndrome
Balloon valvuloplasty for pulmonary stenosis (iatrogenic)
Swan-Ganz catheter insertion (iatrogenic)
Complication Fallot's tetralogy repair
Marfan's syndrome (dilatation of the pulmonary trunk)
Syphilis
Congenital absence of pulmonary valve
Idiopathic

Secondary pulmonary regurgitation

Primary pulmonary hypertension
Secondary pulmonary hypertension

What is the mechanism of development of pulmonary regurgitation in pulmonary hypertension?

Pulmonary artery dilatation leads to dilatation of the pulmonary valve. This results in loss of coaptation of the valve leaflets leading to pulmonary regurgitation (Graham-Steell murmur).

At what stage of pulmonary hypertension would you expect secondary pulmonary regurgitation to develop?

This often occurs in the setting of severe pulmonary hypertension, usually when the pulmonary artery systolic pressures ≥60mmHg.

How would you distinguish between right ventricular 3rd or 4th heart sounds from left ventricular sounds?

Right ventricular 3rd or 4th heart sounds may both be audible with right ventricular failure or hypertrophy. As with left ventricular heart sounds, they are low frequency sounds, best heard with the bell of the stethoscope. These sounds may be distinguished from left ventricular heart sounds because they are located at the left parasternal 4th intercostal space and because they become louder in inspiration.

What do you know about the absent pulmonary valve syndrome?

This is commonly associated with Fallot's tetralogy although it can occur in isolation. This is associated with severe free pulmonary regurgitation. The pulmonary artery dilatation can often be excessive causing extrinsic bronchial compression.

Why is a severe or freely regurgitant pulmonary valve better tolerated than a severely regurgitant aortic valve?

- Forward pulmonary blood flow can be maintained indirectly by the work of the left heart, systemic venous return, and right atrial contraction.
- The pulmonary microvascular bed, compared with the systemic, is of low resistance and closer to the heart. With each right ventricular systole, blood moves readily forwards through the pulmonary microvessels whose low resistance acts as a 'watershed' into the pulmonary veins, which in turn are maintained at a low pressure due to the work of the left heart. Blood that passes forward through the alveolar capillaries in systole is unlikely to pass back again in diastole. The pulmonary vascular bed therefore has a valve-like effect in the setting of severe of free pulmonary regurgitation. In fact severe or free pulmonary regurgitation is associated with a regurgitant fraction of only 40%.

Case 40 ◆ Fallot's Tetralogy

CASE PRESENTATION

*There are no peripheral stigmata of endocarditis. There is **central cyanosis**[1] and there is **clubbing of the fingers**.[2] The **left radial pulse is diminished**. The pulse rate is …beats/min, regular/irregular, of normal volume and character.[3] The **left arm appears smaller than the right arm**. The **blood pressure is lower in the left arm** (and measures …/…mmHg).[4] The venous pressure is not elevated, with **absent 'a' waves**.[5] On examination of the precordium, there is a **thoracotomy scar**.[6] The apex beat is undisplaced with a normal character.[7] There is **parasternal heave** and a **systolic thrill at the upper left sternal edge (pulmonary area)**.[8] There is a **palpable second heart sound (A₂)**.[9]*

*On auscultation, the first heart sound is normal and there is a **single second heart sound (A₂)**.[10]. There is a loud **ejection systolic murmur at the upper left sternal edge (pulmonary area)**, louder in inspiration.[11]. There is a soft **early diastolic murmur at the upper right sternal edge (aortic area)** radiating down the sternal edge, which is louder with the patient sitting forward in expiration.[12] There is a* continuous murmur throughout systole and diastole in the left subclavicular area and can also be heard posteriorly.[13] The lung fields are clear to auscultation and there is no pedal oedema.[14]

The diagnosis is **Fallot's tetralogy** with a **Blalock-Taussig shunt**. There is also a murmur of **aortic regurgitation**, which is associated with this condition.[15]

Clinical notes

1. Central cyanosis is usually a feature of Fallot's tetralogy, as it is associated with right-to-left shunting. Cyanosis will always be present in patients with a Blalock-Taussig shunt. In patients with repaired Fallot's, cyanosis will not be present.

2. Clubbing is a common finding in patients with cyanotic congenital heart disease.

3. Patients with a Blalock-Taussig shunt (a shunt from the left subclavian artery to the pulmonary artery) will have a diminished left brachial and radial pulse. If the right subclavian artery is used, then the right brachial and radial pulses will be weaker, respectively.

4. A Blalock-Taussig shunt will also lead to a reduction in blood pressure on the associated side.

5. Patients with Fallot's will have an absent 'a' wave on the venous pressure waveform. This will also be absent if the patient is in AF.

6. Look for a thoracotomy scar. A left/right thoracotomy scar would suggest that the left/right subclavian artery was used in the Blalock shunt.

7. The left ventricle is often undisplaced and has a normal character. Sometimes, the apex beat may be displaced with enlarging right ventricular dimensions. A displaced and thrusting apex beat in a patient with Fallot's should lead you to suspect a significant degree of aortic regurgitation (prolapse of right coronary cusp), which is common in adult patients.

8. Due to right ventricular hypertrophy, right ventricular predominance is reflected by a left parasternal heave. With marked right ventricular enlargement, the heave may be felt on the right sternal border. The systolic thrill reflects turbulent blood flow across the right ventricular outflow tract (see point 11).

9. A palpable A_2 is best felt over the aortic area, and coincides with second heart sound. This can be confirmed using one hand to palpate the carotid and the other to feel over the aortic area. A palpable A_2 will occur AFTER the carotid impulse (which coincides with the first heart sound).

10. The pulmonary component of the second heart sound is diminished, and the second heart sound manifests as a single A_2.

11. The ejection systolic murmur represents turbulent blood across the right ventricular outflow tract. Both the presence of a systolic thrill and the intensity of the murmur are inversely related to the degree of right ventricular outflow obstruction (increased obstruction leads to increased shunting through the VSD, and thus reduction in flow across the right ventricular outflow tract). Remember, in Fallot's, the VSD is non-restrictive and is therefore not itself associated with a murmur.

12. Some patients may have aortic regurgitation, due to prolapse of right coronary cusp of the aortic valve.

13. Blalock-Taussig shunts are associated with to-and-fro systolic and diastolic murmurs. This is best heard over the left or right subclavicular area, depending on the position of the shunt and is often heard posteriorly. This can be differentiated form the murmur of a PDA (see below).

14. Fallot's tetralogy is not associated with left ventricular dysfunction, and if signs of pulmonary congestions are present, another aetiology of left ventricular dysfunction should be considered. Worsening aortic regurgitation (prolapsed of right coronary cusp—see above) may lead to left ventricular dysfunction and signs of pulmonary congestion. Signs of right-sided heart failure are often present. The oedema may be minimal if the patient is on an adequate diuretic regimen.

15. Although the primary diagnosis is Fallot's tetralogy with a Blalock shunt, if the murmur of aortic regurgitation is present, then this should be mentioned. Always comment on the clinical severity of the valvular lesion.

Questions commonly asked by examiners

What the components of Fallot's tetralogy?

- VSD (with a right-to-left shunt)
- Right ventricular outflow tract obstruction (infundibular stenosis)*
- Right ventricular hypertrophy
- Overriding aorta (with respect to the ventricular septum)**

What are the complications of Fallot's tetralogy?

- Cyanotic spells
- Endocarditis
- Right heart failure
- Polycythaemia
- Systemic thrombosis
- Paradoxical embolism
- Cerebral abscess

What causes are associated with Fallot's tetralogy?

- Fetal hydantoin syndrome
- Fetal carbamazepine syndrome
- Fetal alcohol syndrome
- Maternal phenylketonuria
- Alagille syndrome*
- CATCH 22 malformations**

What precipitates cyanotic spells?

- Exercise*
- Fever*
- Catecholamines, i.e. stress
- Hypoxia
- Dehydration
- Acidosis

What is the pathophysiology of cyanotic spells?

Infundibular spasm and/or decreased systemic vascular resistance increase right ventricular outflow obstruction. This increases right ventricular pressures resulting in increased

---

* The pulmonary valve is normal, and the obstruction is subvalvular. Symptoms generally progress secondary to hypertrophy of the infundibular septum, and acute cyanotic spells develop with infundibular spasms

** The aortic valve is positioned as to lie over the ventricular septum, thus overriding both the right and left ventricles

* This is an autosomal dominant disorder with variable expression associated with abnormalities of the liver, heart, skeleton, eye, kidneys, and characteristic facial appearance.

** Associated with deletions of a segment of chromosome 22q11 (DiGeorge syndrome region); spectrum of abnormalities include Cardiac defects, Abnormal facies, Thymic hypoplasia, Cleft palate and Hypocalcaemia.

* Result in reduced systemic vascular resistance.

right-to-left shunting and cyanosis. The murmur lessens in intensity as the outflow gradient increases.

How do you differentiate Fallot's tetralogy from Eisenmenger's syndrome clinically?

Clinical feature	Eisenmenger's syndrome	Fallot's tetralogy
Venous pressure	Prominent a waves (if in sinus rhythm)	Absent a waves
Apex beat	Displaced	Undisplaced
Pulmonary systolic thrill	Absent	Present
Pulmonary systolic murmur	Absent	Present
Characteristics of S_2	Loud P_2. Fixed spitting with ASD; reversed splitting with PDA; and single loud S_2 with VSD.	Single A_2 (with diminished P_2)

How do differentiate the systolic murmur from that of pulmonary stenosis?

In pulmonary stenosis, the 'a' wave will be prominent on the venous pressure waveform. In Fallot's tetralogy, the 'a' wave is absent.

What would you expect to see on the ECG?

Right ventricular hypertrophy

Right axis deviation

Right atrial enlargement

What would you expect to see on the CXR?

Boot shaped heart*

Decreased pulmonary vasculature

Right-sided aortic arch (present in 20–25% of cases)

What is the Blalock-Taussig shunt?

This is a palliative procedure not performed routinely nowadays due to total correction, which possible with cardiopulmonary bypass. However, this shunt may be performed if the anatomy unfavourable for total correction. The Blalock-Taussig shunt involves an anastomosis between the subclavian artery (usually the left) to the pulmonary artery, thus bypassing right ventricular outflow obstruction. A modified Blalock-Taussig shunt is the interposition of a tubular graft between the two arteries.

How do you differentiate the continuous murmur of Blalock-Taussig shunt from that of a patent ductus arteriosus?

The key is to identify clinical features, which would support an underlying diagnosis of Fallot's tetralogy. Alternatively, one can look for evidence of a Blalock-Taussig shunt, i.e. a thorocotomy scar and an absent left radial pulse.

---

* Due to uplifting of cardiac apex from right ventricular hypertrophy and the absence of a normal main pulmonary artery segment.

Clinical feature	Blalock-Taussig shunt	Patent ductus arteriosus
Thoracotomy scar	Present	Absent
Clubbing*	Present	Absent
Cyanosis*	Present	Absent
Venous pressure	Absent a waves	a waves present (in sinus rhythm)
Pulse**	Normal volume and character	Large volume and collapsing character
Radial pulse	Diminished left radial pulse	Equal radial pulses
Parasternal heave*	Present	Usually absent
Apex**	Undisplaced and normal character	Displaced and thrusting character
Characteristics of S$_2$	Single A$_2$	Reversed splitting

* Remember, in the context of a PDA, a continuous murmur throughout systole and diastole, is likely to reflect a mild lesion. In worsening cases, with the development of pulmonary hypertension the murmur will shorten to systolic murmur and eventually disappear with the onset of Eisenmenger's syndrome. Therefore, a murmur of patent ductus arteriosus that is comparable to that of a Blalock-Taussig shunt is likely to represent a **haemodynamically insignificant** lesion and will not be associated with signs of pulmonary hypertension and Eisenmenger's syndrome, i.e. clubbing and cyanosis.

** If Fallot's tetralogy is associated with haemodynamic significant aortic regurgitation, the pulse will also exhibit a large volume and collapsing character. The apex beat will be displaced and thrusting in quality.

What is the mechanism of aortic regurgitation in Fallot's tetralogy?

Aortic regurgitation is often present in adult survivors and results from a prolapsing right coronary cusp of the aortic valve.

What is the treatment for this condition?

- Total correction can be performed under cardiopulmonary bypass
- Blalock-Taussig shunt of modified Blalock-Taussig shunt
- Waterston shunt*
- Potts shunt**
- Glenn operation***

---

* Waterston shunt involves anastomosis of the back of the ascending aorta to the pulmonary artery. This is often performed under the age of 3 months when the subclavian artery is too small for a Blalock-Taussig shunt

** Potts shunt involves anastomosis of the descending aorta to the back of the pulmonary artery.

*** Glenn operation involves anastomosis of the SVC to the right pulmonary artery. A bi-directional Glenn procedure involves anastomosis to both pulmonary arteries.

Case 41 ◆ Eisenmenger's Syndrome

Examiner's note

Eisenmenger's syndrome often causes panic and confusion in examination settings. Remember, the hallmarks are central cyanosis and pulmonary hypertension. Clubbing of the fingers is often present. If these are present, then one can make a diagnosis of Eisenmenger's syndrome. The cases below demonstrate the spectrum of clinical signs, and you will note that all additional signs reflect those of pulmonary hypertension. Some patients will demonstrate all the signs of pulmonary hypertension including a pulmonary ejection click, pulmonary regurgitation and tricuspid regurgitation; others may only demonstrate a parasternal heave. Remembering the hallmarks of the condition, and not being flustered by all the signs of pulmonary hypertension, should help making the clinical diagnosis easy.

Having made the diagnosis of Eisenmenger's syndrome, the next step is to identify the underlying primary shunt (ASD, VSD, or PDA). This may not always be possible, in which case it is best to present a differential diagnosis of Eisenmenger's syndrome, i.e. right-to-left shunting through an ASD, VSD, or PDA. Essentially, it is the characteristics of S_2 that should help identify the underlying shunt. The presence of differential clubbing and cyanosis would suggest a PDA.

CASE PRESENTATION 1

There are no peripheral stigmata of endocarditis. There is **central cyanosis**[1] *and there is* **clubbing of the fingers**.[2] *The pulse rate is …beats/min, regular/irregular, of normal volume and character.*[3] *The blood pressure is …/…mmHg. The* **venous pressure is elevated** *with* **prominent 'a'** *and* **giant systolic 'v' waves**.[4] *On examination of the precordium, there are no scars. There is a* **left parasternal heave,**[5] *a* **parasternal thrill,**[6] *and a* **palpable pulmonary component to the second heart sound**.[7] *The apex beat is displaced.*[8] *On auscultation the first heart sound is normal and there is a* **single and loud second heart sound**.[9] *There is an* **ejection click**[10] *and an* **early diastolic murmur at the upper left sternal edge** *(pulmonary area), radiating down the left sternal edge,* **louder in inspiration**.[11] *There is a* **pansystolic murmur at the lower left sternal edge,** *which is* **louder in inspiration**.[12] *The lung fields are clear to auscultation and there is* **sacral and pedal oedema**.[13]

The presence of **central cyanosis, finger clubbing** *and the clinical signs of* **pulmonary hypertension** *would be inkeeping with a diagnosis of* **Eisenmenger's syndrome**. *The presence of a* **single loud second heart** *sound suggests the underlying shunt is a* **VSD**.[14]

CASE PRESENTATION 2

There are no peripheral stigmata of endocarditis. There is **central cyanosis**[1] *and there is* **clubbing of the fingers**.[2] *The pulse rate is …beats/min, regular/irregular, of normal volume and character.*[3] *The blood pressure is …/…mmHg. The* **venous pressure is elevated** *with* **prominent 'a'** *and* **'v' waves**.[4] *On examination of the precordium, there are no scars. There is a* **left parasternal heave**[5] *and a* **palpable pulmonary component to the second heart sound**.[7] *There are no palpable thrills. The apex beat is displaced.*[8] *On auscultation the first heart sound is normal and there is a* **single and loud second heart sound**.[9] *There are no audible murmurs. The lung fields are clear to auscultation and there is* **sacral and pedal oedema**.[13]

*The presence of **central cyanosis, finger clubbing** and the clinical signs of **pulmonary hypertension** would be in keeping with a diagnosis of **Eisenmenger's syndrome**. The presence of a **single loud second heart** sound suggests the underlying shunt is a **VSD**.[14]*

Clinical notes

1. Central cyanosis is a hallmark of Eisenmenger's syndrome. In patients with Eisenmenger's syndrome with shunt reversal through a PDA, there may be differential cyanosis, with cyanosis of lower extremities and not the face and upper extremities.

2. Clubbing is a feature of Eisenmenger's syndrome, but it may not always be present. In patients with Eisenmenger's syndrome with shunt reversal through a PDA, there may be clubbing of the toes and not the fingers.

3. Take extra time to assess the rhythm! An (irregularly) irregular rhythm would signify AF. Sometimes patients can be bradycardic due to rate-control therapy, and ascertaining an irregular rhythm requires extra time. If a patient is in AF, then 'a' waves cannot be present on venous pressure tracing, thus you can expect to see a single waveform when assessing the venous pressure. Diagnosing AF and then commenting on 'a' waves will not impress the examiner!

4. Prominent 'a' and 'v' waves are signs of pulmonary hypertension (a wave will be absent if in AF). Giant systolic 'v' or 'cv' waves will be present in tricuspid regurgitation.

5. Amongst all signs of pulmonary hypertension, a left parasternal heave will always be present. Be sure not to miss it, as its absence will dismiss the diagnosis of Eisenmenger's syndrome.

6. A systolic thrill at the lower left sternal edge signifies 'functional' tricuspid regurgitation.

7. A palpable second heart sound in the pulmonary area is a palpable P_2. Palpating a P_2 in patients with pulmonary hypertension can be difficult. Sometimes a palpable P_2 can be difficult to confirm. It is best felt over the pulmonary area, and coincides with the second heart sound. This can be confirmed using one hand to palpate the carotid and the other to feel over the pulmonary area. Knowing that the carotid impulse coincides with the first heart sound, a palpable P_2 will occur AFTER carotid impulse.

8. The apex beat is displaced due to enlarging left ventricular dimensions.

9. In Eisenmenger's syndrome, the timing and characteristics of A_2 and P_2 depend on the underlying shunt, and if correctly identified will give clues to the underlying cause.

Shunt	Characteristic of S_2	Mechanism of S_2
ASD	Fixed widely split (A_2–P_2)	Loss of respiratory effect on S_2, due to equalization of right and left atrial pressures
VSD	Single and loud S_2 (A_2 and P_2 occur simultaneously)	Equalization of right and left ventricular pressures
PDA	Reversed splitting (P_2–A_2)	Prolonged emptying of the left heart due to volume overload

In the context of a VSD (as in the above case presentations), a single second heart sound indicates equalization of ventricular pressures, thus A_2 and P_2 occur simultaneously, with a loud P_2 secondary to pulmonary hypertension, resulting in a single and loud second heart sound.

10. An ejection click is a result of pulmonary artery dilatation. This may not always be present.

11. This is the Graham-Steell murmur of pulmonary regurgitation secondary to pulmonary hypertension. It is differentiated from aortic regurgitation by being much shorter and louder in inspiration. This may not always be present.

12. This is the murmur of tricuspid regurgitation. This may be associated with a parasternal thrill and is louder in inspiration (Carvallo's sign). There will be systolic 'v' or 'cv' waves in the venous pressure waveform.

13. There are often signs of right heart failure, i.e. ascites, sacral, and lower limb oedema. These may not be present if the patient is on diuretics.

14. When presenting the diagnosis of Eisenmenger's syndrome, it is often helpful in establishing the hallmarks of the condition and then concluding with the diagnosis. The characteristics of the second heart sound should help identify the underlying shunt (see above). The presence of differential cyanosis and clubbing should lead one to suspect a PDA.

Questions commonly asked by examiners

What is the difference between 'Eisenmenger's syndrome and 'Eisenmenger's complex'?

Eisenmenger's syndrome results from pulmonary hypertension with shunt reversal, irrespective of the underlying shunt. However, when due to a VSD, it is termed Eisenmenger's complex.

What are the causes of Eisenmenger's syndrome?

- Atrial septal defect
- Ventricular septal defect
- Patent ductus arteriosus
- Aortopulmonary window

What is an Aortopulmonary window?

This is an uncommon congenital cardiac defect resulting from loss of the septum between the aorta and pulmonary artery. This gives rise to a communication between the two arteries. In half the cases, this occurs in isolation, whereas in the remaining half it occurs in conjunction with more complex heart disease.

What happens to the murmur of a VSD as Eisenmenger's complex develops?

A VSD is associated with left-to-right shunting, resulting in a loud pansystolic murmur. As pulmonary hypertension develops, there is equalization of ventricular pressures, and the pansystolic murmur of a VSD disappears. A pansystolic murmur in Eisenmenger's complex is likely to represent functional tricuspid regurgitation.

What happens to the murmur of ASD as Eisenmenger's syndrome develops?

An ASD is associated with left-to-right shunting resulting in increased flow across the tricuspid and pulmonary valves, resulting in mid-diastolic murmur across the tricuspid valve and an ejection systolic murmur across the pulmonary valve. With the development of pulmonary hypertension, left-to-right shunting decreases and these murmurs disappear.

What happens to the murmur of PDA as Eisenmenger's syndrome develops?

The murmur of PDA is a continuous to and fro systolic and diastolic murmur. With the development of pulmonary hypertension, this murmur shortens to a soft systolic murmur. As the pressures equalize in the pulmonary artery and descending aorta, the murmur disappears.

What are the complications of Eisenmenger's syndrome?

- Haemoptysis[*]
- Right ventricular failure
- Paradoxical embolism
- Infective endocarditis
- Sudden death

---

[*] Due to pulmonary hypertension and increased bleeding tendency.

- Polycythaemia[**]
- Thrombosis[***]
- Bleeding[****]

What effect does dehydration and hot/humid conditions have on patients with Eisenmenger's syndrome?

- Dehydration results in increased right-to-left shunting.
- Hot and humid conditions can lead to dehydration. Furthermore, the resulting vasodilatation results in syncope.

What are the principles underlying management of polycythemia in Eisenmenger's syndrome?

Phlebotomy is recommended if there are symptoms of hyperviscosity or if the haematocrit is greater than 65%. It is always important rule out dehydration before phlebotomy. Often, 200–250mL of blood is venesected and an equivalent volume of isotonic fluid is replaced. Repeated phlebotomy can result in iron deficient anaemia.

What is the management of Eisenmenger's syndrome?

- Avoid dehydration and hot/humid conditions
- Contraception, pregnancy, and genetic counselling
- Endocarditis prophylaxis
- Oxygen therapy
- Anticoagulation
- Diuretic therapy for right heart failure
- Phlebotomy for polycythemia and hyperviscosity symptoms
- Pulmonary vasodilator therapy
- Surgical repair of primary cardiac defect (selected cases, see below)
- Heart-lung transplantation

What is the role of surgical repair of the primary cardiac defect in Eisenmenger's syndrome?

Repair of the primary defect is contraindicated in the setting of established severe *irreversible* pulmonary hypertension. However, corrective surgery may be possible, if the pulmonary hypertension is *reversible*. If one can demonstrate *reversible* pulmonary hypertension, then repair may be undertaken:

- evidence of pulmonary reactivity with a pulmonary vasodilator challenge
- lung biopsy findings consist with *reversible* pulmonary arterial changes.

[**] Results in symptoms of hyperviscosity which include myalgia, headaches, visual disturbances, dizziness. and paraesthesias.

[***] Thrombotic events result from hyperviscosity.

[****] Due to dysfunctional platelets; bleeding complications include mucocutaneous bleeding, episatxis, menorrhagia, haemoptysis, and pulmonary haemorrhage.

Case 42 ◆ **Hypertrophic Cardiomyopathy**

CASE PRESENTATION

*There are no peripheral stigmata of endocarditis.[1] The pulse rate is ...beats/min, regular/irregular,[2] of normal volume and exhibits a **jerky character** with a **double carotid arterial impulse**.[3] The blood pressure is.../...mmHg. The venous pressure is not elevated, but has **prominent a waves**.[4] On examination of the precordium, the **apex beat is undisplaced**[5] with a marked **presystolic impulse giving the impression of a double apical impulse**[6] (if in sinus rhythm) and has a **heaving character**.[7] There is a **systolic thrill** palpable at the lower left sternal edge.[8] On auscultation, the first heart sound is normal, and the **second heart sound has reversed splitting**.[9] There is a **fourth heart sound** (if in sinus rhythm).[10] There is an **ejection systolic murmur at the lower left sternal edge**, which radiates up the sternal edge but not to the carotids, and a **pansystolic murmur at the apex**, which radiates to the axilla.[11] The lung fields are clear to auscultation.[12]*

*The diagnosis is **hypertrophic cardiomyopathy**.*

Clinical notes

1. Infective endocarditis is a recognized complication of hypertrophic cardiomyopathy.
2. Often, the patients can be in AF. Be careful not to miss this, as this will have bearing on other examination findings. A prominent a wave in the venous pressure waveform, double apical impulse and fourth heart sound only occur in sinus rhythm and not AF.
3. In severe cases, the pulse may have a jerky character with a double carotid impulse. The carotid pulse rises quickly because of increased velocity of blood through the LV outflow tract into the aorta. As the LV outflow tract gradient develops in mid-systole, the carotid pulse then declines. This is followed by a secondary rise in carotid pulsation during mid–late systole.
4. As a result of gross septal hypertrophy, there is reduced right ventricular compliance. The venous pressure waveform often shows prominent a waves.
5. The apex is often minimally displaced. In advanced stages of the disease, there may be systolic impairment with a dilated LV cavity and displaced apex beat.
6. The pre-systolic impulse is transmission of atrial contraction just before closure of the mitral valve, as a result of forceful atrial contraction against a highly non-compliant left ventricle. This results in a double apical impulse. A pre-systolic impulse is often accompanied by a fourth heart sound and would not be present in AF. A triple apical impulse, resulting from a late systolic bulge that occurs when the heart is almost empty and is performing near-isometric contraction is a highly characteristic finding in hypertrophic cardiomyopathy.
7. A forceful heaving apex reflects a pressure overloaded left ventricle.
8. A parasternal thrill is due to turbulent flow in the LV outflow tract. An apical thrill may be felt if there is mitral regurgitation due to the systolic anterior motion of the mitral valve. If mitral regurgitation is also present, then it is often difficult to differentiate the two separate thrills, and best way to present your findings would be to say, 'there is a precordial thrill'.
9. In severe cases, there is reversed splitting of the second heart sound and this reflects prolonged left ventricular ejection time.
10. Represents forceful atrial contraction, and is heard in sinus rhythm.
11. Principally, there are two murmurs in hypertrophic obstructive cardiomyopathy. The murmur resulting from LV outflow obstruction is typically an ejection crescendo–decrescendo murmur occurring after

the first heart sound or in mid-systole, and is best heard between the left sternal edge and apex. It radiates up the sternal border to the suprasternal notch, but not the carotids or the neck.

An increase in preload will diminish the LV outflow tract gradient and hence the murmur, e.g. Valsalva manoeuvre, squatting, beta blockers. A decrease in preload will increase the LV outflow tract gradient and hence the murmur, e.g. standing, nitrates, diuretics. A decrease in afterload will also increase the murmur, e.g. vasodilator therapy. In patients with systolic anterior motion of the mitral valve there will be an additional pansystolic murmur of mitral regurgitation, best heard at the apex radiating to the axilla. Often, the two systolic murmurs may merge, as a pansystolic murmur radiating up the sternal edge and axilla and it may be difficult to identify each separately.

12. Look for signs of heart failure. Hypertrophic cardiomyopathy is associated with diastolic dysfunction, due to a stiff non-compliant ventricle. In the late stages, ventricular dilatation may occur with systolic dysfunction.

Questions commonly asked by examiners

What is the difference between the terms 'hypertrophic cardiomyopathy' and 'hypertrophic obstructive cardiomyopathy'?

'Hypertrophic cardiomyopathy' is commonly used to describe this condition. In patients with evidence of left ventricular outflow tract gradient, only then is the term 'hypertrophic obstructive cardiomyopathy' appropriate. Hypertrophic cardiomyopathy is predominantly a non-obstructive disease, and 75% of patients do not have a significant resting outflow tract gradient.

How common is this condition?

The overall prevalence is low, and has been estimated to occur in up to 0.2% of the population.

What is the hallmark of this condition?

The hallmark of this condition is myocardial hypertrophy that is inappropriate, often asymmetric, and occurs in the absence of an obvious inciting hypertrophy stimulus. Any region of the left ventricle may be involved, but it frequently involves the interventricular septum, which can lead to an outflow tract gradient. Most cases, however, occur without outflow obstruction, and the right ventricle may also be involved.

What is the mechanism of left ventricular outflow obstruction?

- Marked asymmetrical septal hypertrophy
- Systolic anterior motion of the mitral valve[*] (the anterior mitral valve leaflet opposes the interventricular septum in systole)

What do you know about the genetics of hypertrophic cardiomyopathy?

This is inherited as an autosomal dominant condition. 50% of cases are familial. Sporadic forms may be due to spontaneous mutations. Over 200 distinct mutations have been identified in genes encoding for sarcomeric proteins, and provide the molecular basis of hypertrophic cardiomyopathy. These include:

- troponin T (chromosome 1)
- troponin I (chromosome 19)
- myosin binding protein C (chromosome 11)
- myosin light chains (chromosome 2 and 12)
- α tropomyosin (chromosome 15)
- β myosin heavy chain (chromosome 14)

---

[*] The most likely cause for this is a Venturi effect caused by the increased ejection velocity, thus pulling the mitral anteriorly towards the left ventricular outflow tract.

What are the complications?

- Diastolic heart failure
- Systolic heart failure (late stages)
- Atrial fibrillation
- Ventricular arrhythmias
- Sudden death
- Angina
- Endocarditis

What are the markers of poor prognosis?

- History of syncope
- Family history of sudden death
- Non-sustained VT on Holter monitoring
- Marked left ventricular wall thickness (>30mm)
- Drop in blood pressure during exercise
- Particular genetic mutations, e.g. myosin binding protein C and troponin T

This patient has normal coronary arteries, but complains of angina. What are the possible mechanisms of angina in this condition?

- Increased muscle mass
- Reduced capillarity density
- Abnormal intramural coronary arteries
- Impaired vasodilatory reserve
- Increased myocardial oxygen consumption

How would you investigate this patient?

ECG

- Left ventricular hypertrophy +/− strain
- Left axis deviation
- Left atrial dilatation (inverted or biphasic P waves in V_1–V_2)
- Presence of Q waves in II, III and aVF or V_2–V_6
- ST/T waves changes
- Atrial fibrillation

CXR

- Normal heart size (with left ventricular hypertrophy and diastolic dysfunction)
- Cardiomegaly (in late stages with systolic dysfunction)
- Left atrial dilatation (prominent left atrial appendage and double right heart border)
- Pulmonary congestion (secondary to diastolic dysfunction or systolic dysfunction)

Echocardiogram

- Left ventricular hypertrophy
- Asymmetrical septal hypertrophy
- Dynamic left ventricular outflow obstruction
- Systolic anterior motion of mitral valve
- Diastolic dysfunction
- Systolic dysfunction (late stages)

Exercise treadmill test
- Evidence of myocardial ischaemia
- Evidence of inducible arrhythmia

Holter monitoring
- Evidence of atrial or ventricular arrhythmia

Right and left heart catherization
- To assess coronary anatomy in those with a history of exertional angina
- To assess coronary anatomy where alcohol septal ablation is being considered
- In certain cases, haemodynamic measurements may be used to evaluate myocardial restriction
- In certain cases, endomyocardial biopsy may be necessary to exclude specific heart muscle disorders

What conditions are associated with hypertrophic cardiomyopathy?
- Friedrich's ataxia
- Fabry's disease
- Hereditary lentiginosis
- Wolf-Parkinson-White syndrome

How would you manage this patient?
General measures
- Endocarditis prophylaxis
- Patients and family education
- Family screening

Patients WITHOUT evidence of left ventricular outflow tract obstruction
- *No symptoms*
  - No therapy needed
- *Symptoms*
  - β-blocker or verapamil
  - Diuretics for congestive symptoms
  - ACE inhibitors, spironolactone,and digoxin in those with end-stage systolic dysfunction
  - Treatment of AF (anticoagulation with rate or rhythm control)
  - Amiodarone for ventricular arrhythmias
  - Implantable cardioverter defibrillator (ICD) for ventricular arrhythmias and those at high risk for sudden death

Patients WITH evidence of left ventricular outflow tract obstruction
- *No symptoms*
  - β-blocker
- *Symptoms*
  - β-blocker or verapamil
  - Diuretics for congestive symptoms
  - Treatment of AF (anticoagulation with rate/rhythm control)
  - Amiodarone for ventricular arrhythmias
  - ICD for ventricular arrhythmias and those at high risk for sudden death
  - Surgical myomectomy or alcohol septal ablation

What is alcohol septal ablation?

In certain patients, alcohol septal ablation provides an alternative to surgical myomectomy. The procedure induces a controlled septal myocardial infarction, by injecting alcohol into one of the sepal arteries. This procedure is analogous to surgical myomectomy aiming to reduce the septal myocardium. An alcohol-induced myocardial infarction destroys the ventricular septal myocardium, thereby reducing the left ventricular outflow obstruction. Complications include extension of infarct, heart block, and iatrogenic ventricular septal defect.

Central Nervous System

Case 43 ◆ **Parkinson's Disease**

CASE PRESENTATION

*This patient has a **mask-like**, **expressionless face**[1] with **infrequent blinking**[1] and **low-volume**, **monotonous, tremulous speech**.[2] When the eyes are gently closed, there is tremor of the eyelids (**blepharoclonus**).[3] There is a continuous **pill-rolling tremor** of the hands,[4] with **lead-pipe rigidity**[5] at the elbows and **cogwheel rigidity**[6] at the wrists. The rigidity in one arm is increased by voluntary movements of the opposite arm (**synkinesis**).[7] There is **bradykinesia**, with paucity and decreased amplitude of movements.[8] The signs demonstrate **asymmetry**,[9] with the tremor and rigidity being more marked on the ... side.*

*Voluntary movements are difficult to initiate, with difficulty in rising from a chair and starting to walk (**freezing**).[10] Once having started to walk, the patient adopts a **stooped posture**[11] and progresses with a **hesitant, shuffling, narrow-based gait** with **reduced arm swinging** (more marked on the ...side) and **accentuation of the pill-rolling tremor** of the hands.[12] There is **postural instability** with **propulsion** and **retropulsion**.[13]*

There are no cerebellar or pyramidal signs.[14] There are no gaze palsies.[15]

*The diagnosis is **Parkinson's disease**.[16]*

Clinical notes

As with all neurological patients, you will be more likely to pick up the diagnosis if you take a step back and look at the whole patient. Take some time to assess their facial expressions, speech, tremor, and posture. A common instruction at this station, with the patient seated on a chair is 'Look at this patient, and examine as appropriate'. Candidates are often baffled, when given this instruction. Often the patients with Parkinson's disease are given specific instructions to interlock the fingers of both hands, or place hands flat on their lap to mask the tremor. Picking up an expressionless face and low volume monotonous speech from the outset will provide useful clues to the diagnosis. If you are not sure at this stage, proceed to examining the gait. Once you are certain, that this is Parkinson's disease, you may proceed to demonstrate the other features.

1. Patients with Parkinson's disease have characteristic expressionless facies (hypomimia), often described as 'mask-like'. This is a manifestation of bradykinesia. There is a reduced blink rate. The glabellar tap (Myerson's sign) is an unreliable sign and is not recommended in the examination. This involves tapping the patient's forehead repeatedly. Normal subjects will stop blinking, but in Parkinson's disease, the patient will continue to blink. The patient may be drooling saliva (resulting from dysphagia and sialorrhoea-due to autonomic dysfunction)

2. Patients may have soft speech (hypophonia). This is also a manifestation of bradykinesia, and characteristically, the speech is low-volume, monotonous and tremulous (appears slurred).

3. Blepharoclonus is tremor of the eyelids. This will only be demonstrated if the eyes are gently closed, as opposed to tightly closing the eyes.

4. The classic tremor is present at rest and asymmetrical (more marked on one side). It is classically described as being 4–6Hz and is the initial symptom in 60% of cases, although 20% of patients never have a tremor. The tremor may appear as a 'pill-rolling' motion of the hand or a simple oscillation of the hand or arm. It is easier to spot a tremor if you ask the patient to rest their arms in their lap in the semi-prone position. Usually the tremor is seen in the hand, but you may notice a foot tremor, or even a jaw tremor. The tremor may be enhanced by mental activity. Ask the patient to count backwards from 20, with the hands dangling over the patients lap or armrests of the chair. The tremor can also be increased by walking and emotional stress. It disappears during sleep. Note that head tremor (titubation) is usually more associated with essential tremor and not Parkinson's disease.

5. The rigidity of Parkinson's disease is described as 'lead-pipe rigidity'. This indicates increased tone *throughout* the range of passive movement. This needs to be differentiated from spasticity, as seen in upper motor neuron lesions, where the increased tone is more marked at the onset of the movement, and decreases suddenly as passive movement is continued (clasp-knife phenomenon). Lead pipe rigidity is best felt on passive flexion and extension of the arm at the elbow and can also be demonstrated at the knee.

6. Cogwheeling is caused by a combination of rigidity and tremor. It can be demonstrated at the wrists and ankle. It is adequate to demonstrate this at the wrist, and can be done so by gently manipulating the hand in a circular motion at the wrist.

7. Synkinesis is particularly useful in cases where the rigidity and tremor is mild. You may also notice mirror movements, where involuntary movements of one limb mirror the voluntary movements on the opposite side of the body. They are especially seen in the upper limbs, but are not specific to Parkinson's disease.

8. Although hypomimia and hypophonia are manifestations of bradykinesia, it should be objectively demonstrated as it is a classical feature of Parkinson's disease. Look for any general slowing of the patient's movements, for example when they stand up. Demonstrate bradykinesia by asking the patient to open and close the hands repeatedly, to show the movements becoming slower and smaller in amplitude. You can demonstrate this in the lower limb by asking the patient to tap the foot several times and showing that the tapping becomes increasingly slow and smaller in amplitude.

9. The tremor in Parkinson's disease is unilateral at the onset. It usually begins in one upper extremity and may initially be intermittent. After several months or as much as a few years, it may be present on the opposite side, but is often more marked on one side, and asymmetry is often maintained. **The presence of asymmetrical signs supports a diagnosis of Parkinson's disease as opposed to parkinsonism.**

10. This is a manifestation of bradykinesia.

11. The characteristic posture of Parkinson's disease is forward stooping, with a lowered head and flexed knees and elbows. The lead-pipe rigidity results in an equal increase in tone in both flexors and extensors of all four limbs. However, the tone is slightly increased in the flexors resulting in a part flexed 'simian' posture.

12. The gait of Parkinson's disease is very characteristic. The patient will be stooped forward as if they were chasing their centre of gravity). They will take small shuffling steps, and the feet may scrape the ground. It has a narrow base, regardless of how advanced the disease is. If it widens, then think of alternative diagnoses such as multiple system atrophy with cerebellar degeneration. Patients have particular difficulty initiating movements and turning. Therefore, it is a good idea to walk with the patient, so you can support them if they look at all unsteady. Reduced arm swing is a very sensitive sign and may be the first sign of Parkinson's disease. Carefully watch both arms while the patient walks across the room, and look for asymmetry. The foot often scrapes the ground on the side of reduced arm swing. Walking also accentuates the hand tremor, so look carefully for this.

13. The patient may also have lost their postural reflexes, resulting in an increased tendency to fall. This is also termed propulsion (forward movements) and retropulsion (for backward movements). Postural instability can be demonstrated by the 'pull test', which is performed by standing behind the patient and pulling back on the shoulders. Instead of moving the arms forward and swaying back, patients with Parkinson's disease may take steps backward (retropulsion) or even fall back into the examiner's hands without attempting to maintain balance.

14. Look for features of Parkinson-Plus syndromes (see below). The presence of cerebellar and pyramidal signs suggests multiple systems atrophy.

15. Gaze palsies (vertical gaze palsy in particular) are seen in progressive supranuclear palsy.

16. Having presented the diagnosis of Parkinson's disease, tell the examiner you would like to:

    (a) measure postural blood pressure (autonomic dysfunction)

    (b) assess cognitive function (mini-mental test score)

    (c) assess handwriting (micrographia)

    (d) Look for seborrhoea and seborrhoeic dermatitis (abnormal sweating—a manifestation of autonomic dysfunction).

Questions commonly asked by examiners

What do you understand by the term 'Parkinsonism'?

Parkinsonism is a movement disorder characterized by bradykinesia and at least one of rest tremor, rigidity, and postural instability.

What are the causes of 'Parkinsonism'?

- Idiopathic (Parkinson's disease)—the most common cause
- Drugs:
  - Chlorpromazine
  - Metoclopramide
  - Prochlorperazine
  - Sodium valproate
  - Methyldopa
- Tumours of the basal ganglia
- Lewy body dementia
- Dementia pugilistica (chronic head injury)
- Normal pressure hydrocephalus
- Post encephalitis (encephalitis lethargica)*
- Anoxic brain damage, e.g. following a cardiac arrest
- Wilson's disease
- Toxins
  - CO
  - MPTP**
  - Manganese
- Parkinson Plus syndromes
  - Multiple system atrophy
  - Progressive supranuclear palsy (Steele-Richardson-Olzewski syndrome)
  - Corticobasal degeneration

What do you understand by the term 'Parkinson's disease'?

Parkinson's disease is a neurodegenerative disease caused by disruption of dopaminergic neurotransmission in the basal ganglia. Histologically, there is loss of melanin-containing

---

* In the early 1920s, epidemics of von Economo's encephalitis swept across Europe, and some patients developed progressive Parkinsonism.

** 1-methyl-4-phenyl-1,2,3,6-tetrahydropridine (MPTP) is an analogue of meperidine, that was manufactured in the early 1980s to produce a narcotic drug for recreational use. MPTP produced a syndrome that was indistinguishable from Parkinson's disease.

dopaminergic neurons in the substantia nigra and cytoplasmic inclusions called Lewy bodies in the surviving dopaminergic neurons. The loss of dopaminergic neurones occurs most prominently in the ventral lateral substantia nigra. Approximately 60–80% of dopaminergic neurones are lost before the motor signs of Parkinson's disease emerge.

What are Lewy bodies?

These are spherical, eosinophilic, cytoplasmic inclusions whose primary structural component is α-synuclein. There are two morphological types: classical (brainstem) Lewy body and the cortical Lewy body. The classical Lewy body consists of a dense core surrounded by a halo of radiating fibrils. A cortical Lewy body is less well defined and lacks the halo. Lewy bodies are not specific to Parkinson's disease and can also be seen in:

- Lewy body dementia
- Alzheimer's disease
- Hallervorden-Spatz disease*

How common is dementia in Parkinson's disease?

Dementia usually occurs late in the disease, and affects 15–30% of patients. Cognitive symptoms that occur earlier, i.e. within one year of onset of motor symptoms would suggest a diagnosis of Lewy Body Dementia.

What is the difference between Parkinsonism and Parkinson's disease?

Feature	Parkinsonism	Parkinson's disease
Distribution of signs	Symmetrical	Asymmetrical
Progression	Rapid	Progressive
Response to levodopa	Poor response	Good response
Parkinson-plus signs (see below)	May be present	Absent

What are the Parkinson-Plus syndromes?

Parkinson-Plus conditions are neurodegenerative conditions with Parkinsonian characteristics but with additional features that distinguish them from idiopathic Parkinson's disease. They reflect different pathological processes affecting different neuronal systems. Clinical clues that are suggestive of Parkinson-Plus syndromes include:

- Poor response to levodopa
- Marked symmetry of signs early in the disease
- Early onset of dementia
- Early onset of postural instability
- Early falls
- Early onset of hallucinations (with low doses of levodopa)
- Early onset of symptoms of autonomic dysfunction, i.e. postural hypotension
- Pyramidal signs (that cannot be explained by previous strokes or spinal cord pathology)
- Cerebellar signs
- Ocular signs, i.e. gaze palsies or nystagmus

---

* Autosomal recessive condition characterized by dementia, Parkinsonism, choreoathetosis, and retinitis pigmentosa

Multiple systems atrophy:

- Also known as olivopontocerebellar atrophy and striatonigral degeneration.
- Characterized by varying degrees of Parkinsonism, autonomic failure, cerebellar dysfunction, and pyramidal signs.
- There is progressive loss of neuronal and oligodendroglial cells at numerous sites in the central nervous system.
- Cytoplasmic inclusions in the oligodendrial cells, neuronal loss, astrocytosis and loss of myelin, occur predominantly in the substantia nigra, locus ceruleus, putamen, pontine nuclei, Purkinje cells and intermediolateral columns of the spinal cord. The globus pallidus, caudate nucleus, corticospinal tracts, anterior horn cells of the spinal cord, and vestibular nuclei are relatively spared.
- When Parkinsonian features are prominent, it is termed MSA-P (striatonigral degeneration).
- When cerebellar signs are prominent, it is termed MSA-C (olivopontocerebellar atrophy).
- When autonomic dysfunction is prominent, it is termed Shy-Drager syndrome.

Progressive supranuclear palsy (Steele-Richardson-Olzewski syndrome):

- This is the most common Parkinson-Plus syndrome.
- There is involvement of multiple neurotransmitter pathways (cholinergic, adrenergic and dopaminergic).
- Neuronal loss, gliosis, and neurofibrillary tangles in the pretectal area, substantia nigra, subthalamic nucleus, globus pallidus, superior colliculus and substantia innominata.
- Supranuclear gaze palsy manifests as abnormal vertical then horizontal saccades.
- Other features include difficulty opening the eyes, early and prominent falls, speech and swallowing difficulties, and frontal symptoms including depression, apathy, and cognitive impairment.
- Compared to Parkinson's disease, the Parkinsonian features are more symmetrical and axial rigidity is more prominent than limb. Tremor is less common, and tends to be bilateral and postural. There is often a poor response to levodopa. Progression is rapid, with survival from onset of 5–7 years.

Corticobasal degeneration:

- Characterized by frontoparietal cortical atrophy in addition to degeneration in the extrapyramidal system.
- Presents with atypical Parkinsonian features and associated higher cortical abnormalities. These include limb apraxia and cortical sensory loss. Severe limb apraxia has been described as the 'alien limb' phenomenon—independent movements of one limb.
- Myoclonus can also occur and dementia may develop later in the disease.
- Usually progresses to severe disability and death within 10 years from onset.

How would you differentiate the tremor in Parkinsonism and essential tremor?

Essential tremor is usually symmetrical and worse with voluntary movement. It is often accompanied by a voice and head tremor. In Parkinsonism, the tremor can affect the tongue, jaw, and chin, but not the head. About 50% of patients with Parkinsonism also have a postural component, leading one to incorrectly diagnose essential tremor. The two can be distinguished by asking the patient to write. In Parkinsonism, the tremor abates and the script becomes smaller (micrographia). In essential tremor, the tremor is exacerbated and the script becomes larger and irregular is large.

How would you investigate this patient?

The diagnosis of Parkinson's disease is a clinical one. There are no laboratory tests or imaging studies that can make the diagnosis. Structural imaging of the brain may be appropriate to exclude other conditions. Dopamine transporter single photon emission tomography (SPECT) can show loss of nigrostriatal dopamine transporter binding, but does not distinguish between idiopathic Parkinson disease and progressive supranuclear palsy or multiple systems atrophy. At the onset of symptoms, patients with Parkinson's disease show a 30% reduction in 18F-dopa uptake in the contralateral putamen. 18F-dopa is taken up by the dopaminergic neurones and converted to 18F dopamine.

What is the pharmacological management of Parkinson's disease?

A. Dopaminergic drugs

For example levodopa, dopamine agonists, and MAO-B inhibitors are the main therapeutic options for motor symptoms:

- **Levodopa** is the most effective for motor symptoms. It is used with peripheral dopa decarboxylase inhibitors to prevent metabolism of levodopa to dopamine peripherally, which can cause severe nausea. Side-effects include nausea, vomiting, postural hypotension, motor fluctuations, and confusion.

- **Dopamine agonists** (bromocriptine, pergolide, lisuride, cabergoline, pramipexole, ropinirole). Bromocriptine, pergolide, and lisuride have weak anti-Parkinsonian effect, and are often supplemented with levodopa. Pramipexole and ropinerole are non-ergolide agonists and are not associated with cardiac valve fibrosis (associated with ergolide agonists). Novel delivery systems have been developed, i.e. transdermal patch (rotigotine). Side-effects include nausea, vomiting, postural hypotension, and confusion.

- **MAO-B inhibitors** (selegiline, rasagline). Unlike selegiline, rasagline is not metabolized to amphetamine, and is associated with a lower risk of cognitive side-effects.

Drug class	Advantages	Disadvantages
Levodopa	Most effective for motor symptoms Low risk of cognitive side-effects	Short half-life (multiple dosing) Motor fluctuations and dyskinesias are common
Dopamine agonists	Effective in early and late disease Long half-life (reduced dosing frequency) Reduced motor fluctuations and dyskinesias	Less potent than levodopa Increased risk of cognitive side-effects Cardiac valve fibrosis with ergolide agonists
MAO-B inhibitors	Effective in early and late disease Once daily dosing Possible neuroprotection	Mild benefit Selegiline metabolizes to amphetamine (cognitive side-effects)

B. Anticholinergics

For example benzhexol, benzatropine, procyclidine, orphenadrine; anitcholinergics help reduce the tremor. Dopaminergic therapy does not help reduce tremor.

C. Catechol-O-methyl transferase (COMT) inhibitors

For example entacapone, tolcapone; COMT inhibitors decrease the gastrointestinal breakdown of levodopa (COMT is the primary metabolic pathway for levodopa outside the brain), thus increases the half-life of levodopa, and often, the levodopa dose has to be reduced. This will reduce the 'off' time and increase the 'on' time, thereby reducing the wearing off effect. However, the addition of COMT inhibitors can increase dyskinesias. Tolcapone has been associated with hepatotoxicity.

D. Apomorphine

This is given subcutaneously, and is useful in patients who cannot take oral medication, e.g. following surgery. It can help reverse off periods.

E. Amantadine

An antiviral agent that has a weak N-methyl-D-aspartic acid (NMDA) antagonist effect. It has a mild anti-Parkinsonian effect, but has demonstrated efficacy in reducing peak dose dyskinesias. It can cause confusion in the elderly.

How would you manage postural hypotension in Parkinson's disease?

This results from a combination of the disease process and pharmacotherapy. Patients may have other comorbidities and may be on anti-hypertensive medications. If the anti-Parkinsonian pharmacotherapy cannot be reduced, then patients respond to the standard treatment for postural hypotension, i.e. compressive stockings, fludrocortisone, and midodrine.

How would you manage psychosis associated with anti-Parkinsonian drugs?

All anti-Parkinsonian drugs can produce confusion and hallucinations. Levodopa is less likely to do so. Anticholinergics, amantadine, and selegiline should be withdrawn if hallucinations occur. If these persist, dopamine agonists should be reduced, then stopped. The levodopa dose should be minimized. If hallucinations persist on the lowest possible dose of levodopa, then an atypical neuroleptic agent should be considered. Clozapine is the best agent, although other agents, i.e. quetiapine and olanzapine, may be effective. Risperidone can exacerbate parkinsonism, and should be avoided. Electroconvulsive therapy is very effective in the treatment of drug-induced psychosis and also improves the motor symptoms of Parkinsonism.

What surgical therapies are available for Parkinson's disease?

With improvement in neuroimaging and stereotactic surgical techniques coupled with a better understanding of basal ganglia physiology and circuitry, surgical procedures are being used increasingly. Potential candidates should have a firm diagnosis of Parkinson's disease, have responded well to dopaminergic therapy, should be cognitively intact and have disability that is predominantly related to motor symptoms.

- **Thalmotomy** involves destruction of a portion of the thalamus (ventral intermediate nucleus) to relieve tremor on the contralateral side (>90% of patients see a significant improvement). It has little effect on bradykinesia, rigidity, motor fluctuations, and dyskinesias. Bilateral thalmotomy are not recommended, as these lesions are permanent and complications such as dysarthria and cognitive impairment are common.

- **Pallidotomy** involves destruction of a part of the globus pallidus interna (overactive in Parkinson's disease), and can provide long-term improvement in the contralateral cardinal features of Parkinson's disease (tremor, bradykinesia, and rigidity) as well as reducing dyskinesias. Bilateral pallidotomy are not recommended, as these lesions are permanent and complications such as dysphagia, dysarthria, and cognitive impairment are common.

- **Subthalmotomy** involves destruction of a part of the subthalamic nucleus (overactive in Parkinson's disease) and also improves the contralateral cardinal features of Parkinson's disease (tremor, bradykinesia and rigidity) as well as reducing dyskinesias.

- **Deep brain stimulation** has replaced lesion surgeries and does not involve a permanent lesion in the brain, making the procedure reversible. A lead is implanted into the targeted brain structure (thalamus, globus pallidus interna, or the subthalamic nucleus) and is connected to an implantable pulse generator (usually in the subclavicular area, similar to a pacemaker) that delivers a high-frequency electrical discharge. The stimulation amplitude, frequency and pulse width can be adjusted to control symptoms and reduce side-effects. Deep brain stimulation can be used to stimulate bilateral lesions, which would otherwise be avoided in lesion surgery.

- **Transplantation** is a potential treatment for Parkinson's disease, as the neuronal degeneration is specific for dopaminergic neurones. Many dopamine-producing cells (fetal nigral, sympathetic ganglia, carotid body glomus, and neuroblastoma cells) have been evaluated. Many patients have undergone transplantation worldwide, and most experience reduced motor fluctuations, with a less dramatic improvement in Parkinsonism, and younger patients show the greatest improvement. Although this technique offers considerable promise in the future, there are many ethical issues that need to be addressed before it is applied routinely.

Case 44 ◆ Charcot-Marie-Tooth Disease

Examiner's note

Charcot-Marie-Tooth disease is the most common inherited neurological disorder and frequently appears in the MRCP (PACES) examination. Classically the main findings that lead one to suspect the diagnosis are present in the lower limbs, but it must be remembered that the upper limbs are also affected. The most common instruction at this station is to 'examine the lower limbs'. Candidates often learn the presentation in the lower limbs, and are often baffled when asked to examine the upper limbs in these patients. The key is to perform a structured examination to demonstrate the features of a symmetrical distal motor and sensory neuropathy. The following case presentations cover specific examinations of the upper and lower limbs.

CASE PRESENTATION 1 (LOWER LIMBS)

*This patient has **distal wasting of the lower limbs**, especially of the anterolateral muscle compartment, with relative preservation of the thigh musculature, giving an **'inverted champagne bottle' appearance**.[1] There are no scars.[2] The lateral popliteal nerves are palpable.[3] There is **bilateral pes cavus** and **clawing of the toes**.[4] There is **symmetrical distal weakness**, with bilateral **weakness of dorsiflexion (foot drop)**.[5] The **deep tendon reflexes and plantar responses are absent**.[6] Sensation is reduced distally in a **symmetrical 'stocking distribution'**.[7] This patient has a **high-steppage gait** and is **ataxic** with a **positive Romberg test**.[8]*

*This patient has a distal motor and sensory neuropathy. The most likely diagnosis is **Charcot-Marie-Tooth disease**.[9]*

Clinical notes

Before examining the patient, try to get as many clues as you can from just looking at and around the patient. Look for walking aids and look at the patient's shoes, especially noting ankle supports or orthoses, which would suggest a foot drop. Also look for scuffing at the front of the shoes, which results from foot drop.

1. Distal wasting of the legs frequently affects the anterolateral compartment of the legs below the knees. The wasting appears to stop abruptly usually in the lower third of the thigh. The resulting appearance has many names: 'stork legs', 'spindle legs', and 'inverted champagne bottle appearance'. Fasciculations may be seen.

2. Look carefully for scars over the neck of the fibula, that would suggest previous trauma or fracture that would result in a common peroneal nerve lesion—an important differential for foot drop. The sensation of pain and temperature is often intact in these patients, but look for trophic changes in the feet. As a result of foot deformities, patients often experience painful calluses.

3. Palpable nerves, often large and excessively firm, are a feature Charcot-Marie-Tooth disease (type 1) and are present in 50% of patients. The lateral popliteal nerve is easily palpable in this situation, and this should be looked for in the lower limbs.

4. Pes cavus is a high arch of the foot that does not flatten when the patient weight bears. It is seen in only 70% of patients. It is an important clinical sign, and if present, indicates that the neuropathy is longstanding and therefore likely to be hereditary. This is your main clue for the diagnosis. Other foot deformities include high foot arches, hammertoes and contractures of the Achilles tendon.

5. Motor symptoms usually predominate over sensory symptoms. Distal weakness often manifests as weakness of dorsiflexion that results in foot drop. The plantar flexion is often preserved. Proximal weakness is rarely present, except in the most severely affected patients.

6. The deep tendon reflexes are markedly reduced or even absent. In most cases, the ankle jerks are absent. The plantar response is down-going, but is often absent.

7. Motor symptoms usually predominate, and sensation can be normal until adulthood. Some patients may deny sensory loss despite a marked loss of sensation on examination and absent sensory action potentials on nerve conduction studies. Vibration sense and proprioception are predominantly reduced, whilst the sensation of pain and temperature is often normal. Some patients may exhibit a mild distal pansensory loss, with decreased response to pain in a stocking distribution.

8. The high steppage gait reflects foot drop. Impaired proprioception results in a sensory ataxia and patients will become unsteady when they close their eyes (a positive Romberg test).

9. After demonstrating the signs of a symmetrical distal motor and sensory neuropathy, the presence of pes cavus and/or palpable nerves would favour a diagnosis of Charcot-Marie-Tooth disease.

CASE PRESENTATION 2 (UPPER LIMBS)

*This patient has **distal wasting of the upper limbs**. There is **wasting of the small muscles of the hands**, with dorsal guttering and there are hyperextension deformities at the metacarpophalangeal joints and flexion deformities at the interphalangeal joints, resulting in **claw-hands** (advanced cases).[1] There are no scars.[2] The ulnar nerves are palpable.[3] There is **symmetrical distal weakness**.[4] The **deep tendon reflexes are absent**.[5] **Sensation is reduced distally** in a **symmetrical 'glove distribution'**.[6]*

*This patient also exhibits a **postural tremor**.[7] On inspection of the lower limbs, there is **bilateral pes cavus** and **clawing of the toes**.[8]*

*This patient has a distal motor and sensory neuropathy. The most likely diagnosis is **Charcot-Marie-Tooth disease**.[9]*

Clinical notes

It is important to remember that in most patients with Charcot-Marie-Tooth disease, the lower limbs are affected earlier and more significantly than the upper limbs. There may be only mild distal motor and sensory signs in the upper limbs, and the key to making the diagnosis in this situation, would be to inspect the legs looking for the characteristic shape and foot abnormalities. Often, in the examination, the lower limbs may be deliberately covered to preclude easy diagnosis. If a symmetrical distal and sensory neuropathy is noted in the upper limbs, and the diagnosis of Charcot-Marie-Tooth disease is suspected, tell the examiner that you would like to inspect the lower limbs.

1. Distal wasting of the upper limbs will manifest wasting of the small muscle of both hands. In severe cases, the hands may resemble 'claw hands'. Fasciculations may be seen.

2. Look carefully for scars over the elbow, that would suggest ulnar nerve palsy—an important differential for wasting of the small muscles of the hand. However, this would often be associated with unilateral wasting-it would be unusual to have bilateral ulnar nerve palsies.

3. Palpable nerves, often large and excessively firm, are a feature Charcot-Marie-Tooth disease (type 1) and are present in 50% of patients. The ulnar nerve is easily palpable in this situation, and this should be looked for in the upper limbs.

4. Distal weakness will manifest as weakness of the small muscles of the hands. This may clearly be evident, although this may be difficult to test for if there are deformities.

5. Hyporeflexia usually affects the lower limbs more than the upper limbs. The reflexes in the upper limbs may be markedly reduced. In cases where they are mildly reduced, a reduction in reflexes may be demonstrated by enforcement. Ask the patient to clench his/her teeth, and test the reflexes. If the reflexes appear stronger using this reinforcement technique, one can conclude that reflexes are reduced.

6. Motor symptoms usually predominate, and sensation can be normal until adulthood. Some patients may deny sensory loss despite a marked loss of sensation on examination and absent sensory action potentials on nerve conduction studies. Vibration sense and proprioception are predominantly reduced, whilst the sensation of pain and temperature is often normal. Some patients may exhibit a mild distal pansensory loss, with decreased response to pain in a glove distribution.

7. A postural tremor is seen in 30–50% of patients with Charcot-Marie-Tooth disease. It is important to remember this, as this often leads candidates to focus on the tremor and look for other diagnoses!

8. As mentioned above, tell the examiner that you would like to inspect the lower legs to look for the 'inverted champagne bottle' appearance and pes cavus that will provide useful clues to the diagnosis. Although, the lower limbs are frequently more affected than the upper limbs, it is worth remembering that in one form of Charcot-Marie-Tooth disease (type 2D, autosomal dominant), the wasting and weakness is *greater* in the upper limbs and reflexes are absent in the upper limbs.

9. After demonstrating the signs of a symmetrical distal motor and sensory neuropathy, the presence of pes cavus and/or palpable nerves would favour a diagnosis of Charcot-Marie-Tooth disease.

Questions commonly asked by examiners

What is the pathogenesis of pes cavus in Charcot-Marie-Tooth disease?

Pes cavus is a high arch in the foot that does not flatten when the patient weight bears. The anterior tibialis and peroneus muscles become weak. The posterior tibialis and peroneus longus muscles antagonize these muscles and pull harder. This imbalance between the muscles results in the pes cavus deformity.

What are the other causes of pes cavus?

Unilateral

- Malunion of calcaneal or talar fractures
- Burns
- Sequelae of compartment syndrome
- Poliomyelitis
- Spinal trauma
- Spinal cord tumours*

---

* A patient with new-onset unilateral pes cavus deformity without a history of trauma should be evaluated for spinal cord tumours

Bilateral

• Friedreich's ataxia
• Muscular dystrophies
• Spinal muscular atrophy
• Cerebral palsy
• Syringomyelia
• Hereditary spastic paraparesis
• Spinal cord tumours

What are the different types of Charcot-Marie-Tooth Disease?

This is a heterogeneous group of chronic motor and sensory neuropathies, also known as hereditary motor and sensory neuropathies (HMSN). The classification of Charcot-Marie-Tooth disease is constantly changing as new underlying genetic mutations are identified. The following classification is based on pathology, neurophysiology, and mode of inheritance and is most useful for the clinician.

HMSN subtype	Key pathological feature(s)	Inheritance pattern	Nerve conduction velocity	Palpable nerves
Type 1	Demyelination	Autosomal dominant* Autosomal recessive X-linked dominant X-linked recessive	Reduced	Yes
Type2	Axonal degeneration	Autosomal dominant Autosomal recessive	Relatively normal	No
Type 3**	Demyelination	Autosomal recessive	Reduced	Yes

* The most common mode of inheritance in HMSN type 1 is autosomal dominant. The most common mutation is in the peripheral myelin protein-22 (PMP22) gene (chromosome 17). Another autosomal dominant form of HMSN type 1 involves mutations in the myelin protein zero (MPZ) gene (chromosome 1), and accounts for 5% of cases.
** Also known as Dejerine-Sottas disease or hypertrophic neuropathy of infancy, and is characterized by infantile onset. It results in severe demyelination, more severe than HMSN type 1.

Why are pain and temperature sensations usually unaffected in patients with Charcot-Marie-Tooth disease?

Pain and temperature sensations are carried by unmyelinated nerve fibres, and therefore not affected.

What do you understand by the term 'onion bulb appearance' of nerves in Charcot-Marie-Tooth disease type 1?

In response to demyelination, Schwann cells proliferate and form concentric arrays of remyelination. This repeated cycle of demyelination and remyelination results in a thick layer of abnormal myelin around peripheral axons. This results in an 'onion bulb appearance ' of the nerve on histological examination.

How does formes fruste of the disease present?

This is seen in family members of patients with Charcot-Marie-Tooth disease, where they display only minor signs, i.e. pes cavus and absent ankle jerks.

What do you know about hereditary neuropathy with pressure palsy (HNPP)?

This is also known as *tomaculous neuropathy* and is a hereditary neuropathy that is also associated with a mutation in PMP-22 gene (chromosome 17), and has an autosomal dominant pattern of inheritance. The most common presentation is recurrent acute mononeuropathy that results from minor nerve compression. Patients often report that resting the limb in an awkward position results in weakness and sensory disturbance for weeks and months, rather than seconds to months. Patients with frequent episodes may develop persistent neurological abnormalities.

How would you manage this patient?

Currently, there is no treatment to reverse or slow the disease process and treatment is symptomatic. It is best carried out with a multidisciplinary team including neurologists, orthopaedic surgeons, physiotherapists, and occupational therapists. The following should be considered:

- Patient education and advice
- Patient exercise to maintain function of the limbs
- Walking aids (<5% need a wheelchair)
- Ankle/foot orthoses for foot drop
- Occupational therapy
- Analgesia for musculoskeletal/neuropathic pain
- Orthopaedic surgery to correct deformities

Case 45 ◆ **Motor Neurone Disease**

CASE PRESENTATION

This patient[1] has a **dysarthria** *with a* **nasal quality speech**. *There is a* **wasted, flaccid tongue** *with prominent* **fasciculations**. *There is* **palatal paralysis**.[2] *Eye movements are normal.*[3]

The upper limbs show **proximal and distal wasting** *with prominent* **fasciculations**.[4] *There is* **wasting of the small muscles of the hands**.[5] *There is* **hypertonia** *and* **hyperreflexia**.[6] *The* **sensation is normal**.[7]

The lower limbs show **proximal and distal wasting** *with prominent* **fasciculations**.[4] *There is* **hypertonia** *and* **hyperreflexia**. *There is* **ankle clonus** *with bilateral* **extensor plantar responses**.[6] *The* **sensation is normal**.[7]

This patient demonstrates a combination of upper and lower motor neurone signs with no sensory involvement. This would be consistent with a diagnosis of **motor neurone disease (MND)**.[8,9,10]

Clinical notes

1. Look around the patient for walking aids, or a wheelchair. Look at the patient's shoes, especially noting ankle supports or orthoses, which would suggest a foot drop. Also look for scuffing at the front of the shoes, which results from foot drop.
2. Bulbar involvement can be lower motor neurone (LMN, bulbar palsy) or upper motor neurone (UMN, pseudobulbar palsy). Bulbar palsy is associated with upper and lower facial weakness, palatal paralysis, a

wasted and flaccid tongue with prominent fasciculations. The speech is indistinct and has a nasal quality, with slurring of the labial and lingual consonants. Pseudobulbar palsy is characterized by emotional lability (pathological laughing or crying), stiff (spastic) tongue with no fasciculations (although not typically wasted, in long standing cases it may appear wasted), and a brisk jaw jerk. The speech is indistinct and has a slow, grunting spastic quality. The articulatory muscles are rigid.

3. The oculomotor muscles are never involved in motor neurone disease.

4. Wasting and fasciculations represent lower motor neurone involvement. When inspecting the limbs, spend a little extra time to note the presence and absence of fasciculations in good light (fasciculations are often missed by candidates). These can be elicited or enhanced by tapping the muscles gently. The weakness is often unilateral, especially early in the course of the disease and begins in the arms, legs, or oropharyngeal muscles with equal frequency. Ultimately, the weakness becomes bilateral. In the limbs, the weakness is progressive and often starts distally and progresses proximally. In the legs, this often begins as foot drop, and in the arms as difficulty of fine hand movements.

5. Look for wasting of the small muscles of the hands. There may be dorsal guttering, hyperextension deformities at the metacarpophalangeal (MCP) joints, and flexion deformities at the interphalangeal joints. In advanced cases this may result in claw hands. Fasciculations may be prominent in the hands.

6. Hypertonia, hyperreflexia, ankle clonus, and extensor plantar responses represent upper motor neurone involvement. Demonstrate clasp knife spasticity in the upper limbs by rapidly flexing and extending the elbow (resistance at the beginning of the movement). You can also demonstrate Hoffman's sign, which is positive in upper motor neurone lesions. This involves rapidly flexing the middle finger DIP (distal interphalangeal) joint. In the presence of upper motor neurone lesions, this will cause the other fingers (the thumb in particular) to briefly flex.

7. Sensation is classically spared in motor neurone disease, but you should note that many patients have minor sensory symptoms and patients may also complain of pain. Objective sensory findings are against a diagnosis of motor neurone disease, unless they can be accounted for by neurological comorbidity.

8. In motor neurone disease, there is neuronal loss at all levels of the motor system, from the cortex to the anterior horn cells of the spinal cord. The key findings are a combination of upper and lower motor neurone signs, often with weak and wasted limbs with fasciculations occurring in combination with hypertonia and hyperreflexia. These signs may occur in various combinations.

9. It may be preferable to use the term 'anterior horn cell disease' in front of the patient.

10. Tell the examiner that you would like to assess cognitive function and respiratory function. Approximately, 2% of patients have frontal lobe dementia and cognitive impairment often occurs in those with bulbar involvement. In the later stages of the disease the muscles of respiration are affected, so assessment of respiratory function is important in the assessment of a patient with motor neurone disease. Look for breathlessness, especially on mild exertion or talking, a raised respiratory rate and a resting tachycardia. Ideally you would ask to measure the FVC supine and sitting, looking for a discrepancy that would suggest significant diaphragmatic weakness.

Questions commonly asked by examiners

What is motor neurone disease?

Motor neurone disease is a progressive disorder characterized by neuronal loss at all levels of the motor system from the cortex to the brainstem and anterior horn cells of the spinal cord. Physical signs therefore include both upper and lower motor neurone signs. There are different forms of motor neurone disease:

- **Amyotrophic lateral sclerosis**: both upper and motor neurone signs
- **Progressive muscular atrophy**: predominant lower motor neurone signs
- **Primary lateral sclerosis**: predominant upper motor neurone signs
- **Progressive bulbar palsy**: predominant bulbar involvement (bulbar or pseudobulbar palsy)

What is the pathophysiology of motor neurone disease?

The exact mechanism of neuronal loss is not clear. Two potential mechanisms exist:

Excitotoxicity hypothesis

This is a process by which amino acid neuromodulators, e.g. glutamate become toxic at supraphysiological concentrations. Other potential excitotoxins include AMPA (α-amino-hydroxy-5-methylisoxasole-4 propionic acid) and kainite. These excitotoxins trigger excessive calcium influx into motor neurones, which stimulates various intraneuronal cascades including free radical formation resulting in neuronal death. Riluzole, a glutamate release inhibitor, has shown some efficacy, thus supporting this hypothesis.

Free radical hypothesis

Both excitotoxic and free-radical hypotheses are not mutually exclusive. The potential role of free radicals directly damaging motor neurones was implicated following the discovery of the SOD1 gene (encodes copper-zinc superoxide dismutase) mutation in patients with familial motor neurone disease. However, anti-oxidant strategies have not so far demonstrated efficacy in motor neurone disease.

What do you know about the genetics of motor neurone disease?

Most cases are sporadic. Approximately 5–10% of cases are familial, which usually show an autosomal dominant pattern of inheritance. Mutations in the *SOD1* gene that encodes copper-zinc superoxide dismutase (chromosome 21) have been found in 2% of all patients and 20% of those with familial motor neurone disease. Other genes that have been linked to familial disease include:

- ALS2 gene (chromosome 2)—autosomal recessive
- SETX gene (chromosome 9)—autosomal dominant
- VAPB gene (chromosome 20)—autosomal dominant
- DCTN1 gene (chromosome 2)—autosomal dominant

Several other genetic mutations have been reported to alter the risk of developing sporadic motor neurone disease:

- Angiogenin (chromosome14)
- Vascular endothelial growth factor (chromosome 6)
- Survival motor neurone (chromosome 5)
- Neurofilament protein (chromosome 22)
- Charged multivesicular body protein 2B (chromosome 2)

What diseases mimic motor neurone disease?

Conditions mimicking motor neurone disease	Notes and differentiating features
UMN and LMN presentation	
Syringomyelia	This often presents with LMN signs in arms and UMN signs in the legs. Features supporting syringomyelia include a dissociated sensory loss and the presence of Horner's syndrome (may not always be present)
Cervical myelopathy	Look carefully for bulbar and sensory signs. Bulbar signs do not occur in cervical myelopathy and sensory signs do not occur in motor neurone disease

UMN presentation

HIV-related myelopathy	Occurs in end-stage HIV infection, often in conjunction with AIDS dementia. A slowly progressive spastic paraparesis associated with peripheral neuropathy and sensory ataxia. Upper limb involvement is rare. Sensory disturbance will differentiate this from motor neurone disease.
Spinal cord tumour	Sensory loss will help differentiate this from motor neurone disease

LMN presentation

Multifocal motor neuropathy	This is an acquired, autoimmune, demyelinating neuropathy which causes progressive distal weakness and atrophy. There is often asymmetrical limb wasting and weakness (arms>legs) It is very slowly progressive, up to a period of 30 years. Fasciculations occur in 50%. IgM anti-GM1 ganglioside antibodies are frequently positive. Responds to treatment with intravenous immunoglobulin.
Chronic inflammatory demyelinating polyneuropathy	Features that would differentiate this from motor neurone disease would be a raised cerebrospinal fluid (CSF) protein, autonomic dysfunction and possible sensory involvement.
Spinal muscular atrophy	A group of autosomal recessive disorders characterized by loss of lower motor neurones of the spinal cord and brainstem motor nuclei (V, VII, IX, and XII). This presents as a lower motor neurone syndrome and bulbar involvement.
Oculopharyngeal muscular dystrophy	Tongue fasciculations do not occur
Spinobulbar muscular atrophy (Kennedy's syndrome)	X linked recessive disorder due to expanded trinucleotide (CAG) repeats in the androgen receptor gene. This presents as a lower motor neurone syndrome and bulbar involvement. Associated with tongue wasting, fasciculations, gynaecomastia, testicular atrophy, and diabetes.
Syphilitic amyotrophy	This is slowly progressive wasting of proximal upper limb muscles, fasciculations, and hyporeflexia whilst there is no sensory loss. There may be fasciculations on the tongue.
Old poliomyelitis	Some patients with old polio may develop a progressive wasting disease with prominent fasciculations.

What is the pathological basis for fasciculations?

Fasciculations result from spontaneous firing of large motor units formed by branching fibres of surviving axons that are striving to innervate denervated muscle fibres.

What other conditions cause fasciculations?

- After exercise in healthy adults
- Electrolyte disturbances (hypokalaemia and hypomagnesaemia)
- Thyrotoxic myopathy
- Cervical spondylosis
- Syringomyelia
- Hereditory Motor and Sensory Neuropathy (HMSN)

- Acute poliomyelitis (can also occur in cases of old polio)
- Neuralgic amyotrophy
- Syphilitic amyotrophy
- After tensilon test
- Benign giant fasciculations
- Spinal muscular atrophy
- Drugs (clofibrate, lithium, and salbutamol)

How would you investigate this patient?

There is no diagnostic test for MND. Investigations are aimed at excluding other diseases and should be tailored to the presenting symptoms.

What is the clinical course of motor neurone disease?

The mean age of onset is 60 years. The disease progresses segmentally, e.g. starting in one limb and involving other limbs sequentially. Mean survival is 3–5 years from onset. Progressive muscular atrophy and primary lateral sclerosis are associated with a better prognosis. Respiratory failure resulting from diaphragmatic weakness is the main cause of death.

What features would suggest a poorer prognosis?

- Older age at presentation
- Female sex
- Bulbar onset

How would you manage this patient?

Management should involve a multidisciplinary team and should be guided by the following principles:

- Respect for autonomy and choice
- Symptom control and quality of life
- Planning for the future and early involvement of palliative care

Symptoms requiring treatment include:

- Drooling—anticholinergic drugs, tricyclic anti-depressants, hyoscine patches, glycopyrrolate, radiotherapy to the parotids, and home suction devices
- Dysphagia—dietary advice and consider percutaneous endoscopic gastrostomy early
- Communication difficulties—speech and language therapist
- Pathological laughing or crying (emotional lability)—amitriptyline, lithium, and levodopa
- Fasciculations and muscle cramps—magnesium, vitamin E, diazepam, quinine, carbamazepine, and phenytoin
- Spasticity—physiotherapy and drugs e.g. baclofen, dantrolene, and tizanidine.
- Limb weakness—splints or neck supports and physiotherapy to aid posture.
- Respiratory symptoms—non-invasive respiratory support can be considered
- Depression—consider amitriptyline or selective serotonin re-uptake inhibitors (SSRIs)
- Pain—analgesia, physiotherapy, and occupational therapy

Do you know of any disease modifying treatments for this disease?

Riluzole is the only drug licensed in the UK for the treatment of MND, as a disease modifying therapy. It does not improve symptoms and does not prevent death. Evidence from placebo-controlled randomized controlled trials suggests a 3-month increased survival over an 18-month trial period.

Case 46 ◆ **Cerebellar Syndrome**

CASE PRESENTATION

*This patient is ataxic on the right. On examination of the upper limbs, there is **dysdiadochokinesis**,[1] impaired finger-nose testing with **dysmetria**[2] and an **intention tremor** (that worsens as the finger approaches the target)[3] on the right side. There is failure of the displaced right arm to find its original posture with the eyes closed (**rebound phenomenon**).[4] On examination of the lower limbs there is an **impaired heel–shin test**[5] on the right side. There is **hypotonia**[6] and **dyssynergia**[7] on the right side.*

*There is a **nystagmus**[8] with a fast component to the right. There is loss of smooth pursuit (**broken pursuit**).[9] The saccadic eye movements are abnormal with **hypermetric saccades**.[10]*

*The gait is **broad-based** and **ataxic** with a tendency to fall to the right.[11] Romberg's test is negative.[12] The **speech is slurred** and has an **explosive (staccato) character**.[13]*

The diagnosis is a right cerebellar syndrome.[14]

Clinical notes

Cerebellar syndrome is a common and straightforward neurological case in the MRCP (PACES) examination. There are many signs associated with this, and not all of them will be present. Remember, a cerebellar lesion will result in IPSILATERAL signs.

1. Dysdiadochokinesis is impairment of rapid alternating movements. Demonstrate this by asking the patient to tap the back of their hand with their other hand, with the tapping hand alternating between facing up and down. Sometimes, this may appear normal, and the dysdiadochokinesis will only become evident if you ask the patient to increase the amplitude of movements, i.e. the hand being tapped remains fixed, whilst the tapping hand starts approximately 30cm above it. A variant of this test is the thigh-tapping test, where the thigh is tapped as opposed to the opposite hand. Another test to demonstrate dysdiadochokinesis is to ask the patient to rapidly pronate and supinate the hand whilst keeping the elbow fixed. The movements will become irregular (dysdiadochokinesis) and movement will under and overshoot (dysmetria).

2. If done incorrectly, finger–nose testing, will not demonstrate ataxia, particularly in patients with subtle cerebellar signs. It is important for the target to be at a distance that is just below the patients arm reach length. Remember, it is at the extreme of the arm reach length where the intention tremor becomes marked and easily demonstratable. Dysmetria (past-pointing) is the incorrect velocity and amplitude of a planned movement and is often seen when patients reach beyond their intended target.

3. A cerebellar tremor is not present at rest and increases with voluntary movement, particularly when approaching a target. This is particularly seen in the finger–nose and heel–knee–shin tests.

4. The rebound phenomenon is an example of dysmetria.

5. There are many ways to do the heel–shin test. Often patients are asked to place the heel of one foot over the ankle of the other leg, and move the heel up and down the shin. The drawback of this technique is patients may rest the ankle on the shin, and use the contour of the shin to help guide movement. This may mask the ataxia. To overcome this problem, ask the patient to place the heel of one foot over the ankle of the other leg, and bring the heel up the shin to the knee. Then, rather than asking them to move the heel down the shin, ask them to make a semicircular arc in the air, over but not touching the shin, down to the ankle. This technique is more sensitive.

6. Cerebellar hypotonia occurs because under normal circumstances, the deep cerebellar nuclei send reinforcing signals to the motor cortex and the cerebellocortical tract, which increases the tone.

With cerebellar dysfunction, this is lost, and there is a slight decrease in tone. After some time, the hypotonia may disappear, as the motor cortex compensates by increasing its intrinsic activity.

7. Movements that involve more than one joint, i.e. finger–nose testing and heel–shin testing, appear to be broken up into parts. This is dyssynergia.

8. Cerebellar lesions produce coarse horizontal nystagmus. The fast component is *towards* the side of the lesion.

9. Demonstrate abnormalities of pursuit by asking the patient to follow the path of your finger as it slowly traces a large 'H' in front of them. In cerebellar disease, instead of smooth movements the movements will be jerky and broken up, termed 'broken pursuit'. Look for an internuclear ophthalmoplegia, where there is impaired adduction of the adducting eye and nystagmus of the abducting eye. This is highly suggestive of multiple sclerosis as an underlying cause.

10. Demonstrate abnormalities of saccades by asking the patient to keep their head steady and look alternatively between a hand and a finger held up in front of them shoulder width apart. You may observe hypo- or hypermetric saccades (saccades which under or overshoot the target respectively). This is another example of dysmetria.

11. The hallmark of cerebellar ataxia is the lack of coordination between different muscles. This is especially evident in the patient's gait. This will be broad-based, and the patient may lurch from side to side, with a tendency to fall to the side of the lesion. In patients with subtle cerebellar signs, the abnormal gait may manifest as difficulty walking heel-to-toe (tandem walking). This is the most sensitive clinical test for gait ataxia. In some cases where the gait appears normal, ask the patient to close the eyes and then walk—the patient will tend to walk towards the side of the lesion. Whilst the patient is seated and the trunk is supported, it will be difficult to look for truncal ataxia. Look carefully for this as the patient gets up. A lesion of the vermis will cause predominantly truncal ataxia, with relative sparing of the limbs. A lesion of the cerebellar hemisphere causes ipsilateral limb ataxia.

12. It is important to perform the Romberg's test when assessing a patient with cerebellar syndrome. A broad-based gait can also be seen in sensory ataxia (loss of proprioception). Patient's with cerebellar syndrome, given proprioception is intact, Romberg's test will be negative. In certain cases, i.e. alcoholic cerebellar degeneration and Friedreich's ataxia, there may be sensory impairment, and Romberg's test may be positive.

13. Cerebellar dysarthria is characterized by slurred speech. The words and syllables are broken up, and the speech has a scanning, yet explosive, character. There is a tendency to hesitate at the beginning of a word or syllable.

14. There are many causes of a cerebellar syndrome (for a more detailed list see the questions section), but certain causes may be easily looked for. Tell the examiner you would like to look for:

(a) **Demyelination (multiple sclerosis)**: internuclear ophthalmoplegia, optic atrophy

(b) **Alcoholic cerebellar degeneration**: stigmata of liver disease, peripheral neuropathy

(c) **Friedreich's ataxia**: pes cavus, pyramidal and dorsal columns signs in legs, depresses ankle jerks, extensor plantars

(d) **Posterior fossa space occupying lesions**: papilloedema, VI nerve palsy (false-localizing sign)—tumours in the posterior fossa frequently compress the 4th ventricle raising intracranial pressure

(e) **Paraneoplastic cerebellar degeneration**: *bilateral* cerebellar signs with features of malignancy, i.e. cachexia, clubbing, Horner's syndrome, lymphadenopathy, breast lumps (in females), prostate examination (in males) etc.

(f) **Hypothyroidism**: hypothyroid facies, dry skin, slowly relaxing reflexes, assess thyroid status

(g) **Drugs**: MedicAlert bracelet (especially phenytoin and lithium), ask to take a full drug history

Questions commonly asked by examiners

What are the common causes of cerebellar syndrome?

• Demyelination (multiple sclerosis)
• Alcoholic cerebellar degeneration

- Posterior fossa space occupying lesions
- Brainstem lesions
- Friedreich's ataxia
- Ataxia telangiectasia
- Hypothyroidism
- Vitamin E deficiency
- Abetalipoproteinaemia
- Paraneoplastic cerebellar degeneration
- Drugs (see below)
- Spinocerebellar degeneration
- von Hippel-Lindau syndrome
- Multiple systems atrophy (olivopontocerebellar atrophy)
- Arnold-Chiari malformation
- Dandy-Walker syndrome

Which drugs result in a cerebellar syndrome?

- Phenytoin
- Lithium
- Carbamazepine
- Phenobarbitone
- Chemotherapy agents

What primary tumours can affect the cerebellum?

Medulloblastoma and astrocytoma

Are there any signs that could help localize cerebellar lesions?

- Lesions of the vermis (midline cerebellar lesions) affect the trunk and axial muscles and cause truncal ataxia.
- Lesions of the neocerebellum (cerebellar hemispheres) cause ipsilateral limb ataxia.

What do you understand by the term 'pendular reflexes'?

This is best demonstrated with knee reflexes. With the knee crossed over and placed over the opposite leg, such that that the leg hangs freely, a tendon hammer is used to elicit the knee reflex. Under normal circumstances, the leg stops swinging after one or two excursions. In patients with cerebellar disease, the leg swings several times, to and fro, like a pendulum.

What do you know about paraneoplastic cerebellar degeneration?

This is a paraneoplastic manifestation seen with cancers of the ovary, uterus, breast, lung (small cell carcinoma), and Hodgkin's lymphoma. It is believed to be immune mediated, and high titres of autoantibodies can be found in the serum and CSF. These autoantibodies are a result of an immune response to the tumour and cross-react with cells of the nervous system. The onset of neurological symptoms often precede the diagnosis of the tumour, therefore recognition of this syndrome and detection of antibodies should prompt investigation for underlying malignancy. When the condition is associated with Hodgkin lymphoma, cerebellar disease often follows the diagnosis of lymphoma.

Symptoms often begin with acute onset of cerebellar dysfunction, usually over days to weeks, and rapidly progresses to involve both sides. Unilateral cerebellar dysfunction is against a diagnosis of paraneoplastic cerebellar degeneration.

Two main antibodies are recognized:

- **Anti-Yo** (anti-Purkinje cell antibodies): gynaecological and breast malignancies
- **Anti-Hu** (anti-neuronal nuclear antibodies): small cell carcinoma of the lung, carcinoma of the prostate, sarcomas, and neuroblastomas.

Case 47 ◆ Myotonic Dystrophy

Examiner's note

The most common instruction at this station is 'look at this patient, and examine as appropriate'. This instruction can often cause confusion and panic amongst candidates. Often from the clinical information provided, there may be a family history of respiratory complications following anaesthesia, which should lead one to suspect the diagnosis. Recognizing the myopathic facies, frontal balding, and ptosis should provide immediate clues to the diagnosis. It is important to pay particular attention to the grip, when shaking hands and introducing yourself to the patient. A slow-releasing grip is a useful pointer to the diagnosis.

CASE PRESENTATION

This patient has **myopathic facies**,[1] **frontotemporal balding**,[2] **ptosis**[3] (with a smooth forehead) and **cataracts**.[4] There is **wasting** of the **facial muscles, temporalis, masseter, sternomastoids**[5] and the **small muscles of the hands**.[6] There is **difficulty in opening the eyes after firm closure**.[7] On examination of the limbs there is **distal wasting and weakness** with impairment of fine movements of the hands and **foot drop**.[8] The **deep tendon reflexes are depressed**.[9] There is evidence of **myotonia**.[10] There is a **high steppage gait**.[11]

The diagnosis is **myotonic dystrophy**.[12]

Clinical notes

Before examining the patient, try to get as many clues as you can from just looking at and around the patient. The myopathic facies, frontal balding, and ptosis may be evident. Look for walking aids and look at the patient's shoes, especially noting ankle supports or orthoses, which would suggest a foot drop. Also look for scuffing at the front of the shoes, which results from foot drop.

1. Myopathic facies refers to a lifeless, lean, and expressionless face. Facial weakness produces a characteristic facial appearance with bilateral ptosis and flaccid muscles around the mouth and eyes. The face has a generally drooping appearance with the mouth often hanging open. With the presence of ptosis and daytime somnolence (common due to nocturnal hypoventilation), there may be an overall impression of a 'sleepy appearance'. It can be difficult to recognize myopathic facies, especially if mild. If you are not sure about the presence of myopathic facies, it is best to avoid this in your presentation.
2. Look carefully for balding. This may not be evident at first, as it may be camouflaged by hair covering the frontotemporal areas. Some patients may be wearing wigs, and it is important to note this.
3. Ptosis is often bilateral, but it can be unilateral.

4. Cataracts are usually posterior subcapsular. There may be evidence of previous cataract surgery.
5. There is wasting of the facial musculature that results in a long lean face. Demonstrate facial weakness by showing that you can easily overcome eye closure and show perioral weakness by asking the patient to whistle or blow as if they were blowing out a candle. Ask the patient to clench the teeth and palpate the temporalis and masseter muscles. Test the power of the sternocleidomastoid by asking the patient to turn the head to each side in turn, whilst palpating the contralateral sternocleidomastoid muscle). Place you hand over the forehead, and test neck flexion. In normal circumstances, the neck flexors are very strong and are not easily overcome.
6. Note the wasting of the small muscles of the hands with dorsal guttering and there may be hyperextension deformities at the MCP joints and flexion deformities at the interphalangeal joints.
7. Difficulty in opening the eyes after firm closure is a manifestation of myotonia.
8. Myotonic dystrophy is characterized by distal wasting and weakness, i.e. features of a distal myopathy.
9. The deep tendon reflexes may be depressed or lost.
10. Myotonia is defined as continued contraction of the muscle after voluntary contraction ceases, followed by impaired relaxation. The absence of a slow-releasing grip (grip myotonia) should not lead one to dismiss the diagnosis. Remember, that grip myotonia can be absent with advanced disease due to progressive wasting of the small muscles of the hands. Furthermore, there are pharmacotherapeutic measures that can relieve myotonia, which may make it difficult to elicit. Myotonia can be elicited at the hypothenar eminence by gentle percussion. This will produce a visible dent and which fills slowly due to delayed relaxation. You can also demonstrate myotonia by asking the patient to clench their fist and show they are unable to extend the fingers quickly after this. Similarly, it can also be demonstrated in the tongue, therefore one should inspect the tongue (tapping the tongue is usually not required for this).
11. Foot drop will manifest as a high-steppage gait.
12. Having recognized the facial features, demonstrated the characteristic wasting and features of myotonia, the diagnosis should be straightforward. Tell the examiner you would like to look for other associated features of this condition:
    (a) **Diabetes**: finger tip skin pricks (glucose testing), urinalysis, fundoscopy (diabetic retinopathy)
    (b) **Cardiomyopathy**: signs of heart failure
    (c) **Valvular heart disease**: mitral valve prolapse
    (d) **Arrhthymias**: irregular pulse of atrial fibrillation (AF) (25% of patients)
    (e) **Conduction defects**: look for permanent pacemakers
    (f) **Hypogonadism**: gynaecomastia, testicular atrophy
    (g) **Goitre**: nodular thyroid enlargement can occur (euthyroid), look for thyroidectomy scars

Questions commonly asked by examiners

What is the genetic basis of myotonic dystrophy?

It is an autosomal dominant disease caused by a trinucleotide repeat (CTG) expansion in the myotonin protein kinase gene on chromosome 19. The CTG trinucleotide is repeated 5–36 times in the normal population, but in patients with myotonic dystrophy it is expanded and repeated up to 2000 times. It demonstrates expansion (increased disease severity with successive generations) and anticipation (earlier onset with successive generations).

What other disorders involve trinucleotide repeat expansions?

* Fragile X syndrome
* Huntington's chorea
* Friedreich's ataxia
* Spinocerebellar ataxia
* Dentataorubropallidolysian atrophy

What are the cardiovascular complications of myotonic dystrophy?

- Resting ECG changes
  - Prolonged PR interval
  - Prolonged QTC interval
  - ST and T wave changes
  - Low voltage P waves
  - Dominant R wave in V_1
  - QRS widening
- Arrhythmias
  - Supraventricular tachycardia (most common)
  - Ventricular tachycardia
  - Atrial fibrillation and flutter (present in 25%)
- Conduction defects
  - First-degree heart block (present in 40% of cases)
  - Second-degree heart block
  - Third-degree (complete) heart block
- Mitral valve prolapse
- Cardiomyopathy
  - Left ventricular hypertrophy
  - Cardiac fibro-fatty changes
  - Myocardial myotonia

What are the endocrine complications of myotonic dystrophy?

- Diabetes mellitus (insulin resistance)
- Hypogonadism
- Nodular thyroid enlargement

What are the gastrointestinal complications of myotonic dystrophy?

- Dysphagia
- Reflux
- Delayed gastric emptying
- Hypomotility
- Malabsorption
- Bacterial overgrowth
- Megacolon

What are the respiratory complications of myotonic dystrophy?

- Weakness of respiratory muscles (hypoventilation)
- Respiratory failure following anaesthesia
- Pneumonia

What drugs can be used to help myotonia in these patients?

- Phenytoin
- Quinine*
- Procainamide*

[handwritten: Modafinil — CNS stimulant]

[handwritten: + NIV]

[handwritten: - orthotics / + physical activity. / - mobility Aids and Adaptive equipment]

---

* can worsen cardiac conduction

What do you know about myotonic dystrophy types 1 and 2?

Myotonic dystrophy type 1

This is the classical form of myotonic dystrophy (as described above)

Myotonic dystrophy type 2

This is similar to, but distinct from the classical myotonic dystrophy. Patients present with similar clinical features (balding, ptosis, cataracts, myotonia, hypogonadism), but there is proximal wasting and weakness. This is inherited as an autosomal dominant condition and is characterized by CCTG repeat expansions in the ZNF9 gene on chromosome 3. Because of clinical heterogeneity, the diagnosis of myotonic dystrophy type 2 should rely on DNA analysis alone.

What are the other causes of myotonia?

- Myotonia congenita (Thomsen's disease)—autosomal dominant; startle myotonia; a chloride ion channelopathy (CLC-1)
- Myotonia congenita (Becker's disease)—autosomal recessive; later onset; severe myotonia; a chloride ion channelopathy (CLC-1)
- Paramyotonia congenita—autosomal dominant; a sodium ion channelopathy (SCN4A); precipitants include exertion, stress, exposure to cold, sudden surprises, and potassium-rich foods
- Hyperkalaemic periodic paralysis—autosomal dominant; a sodium ion channelopathy (SN4A); precipitants include rest after exercise, stress, fasting, and potassium-rich foods
- Drugs, e.g. clofibrate   — low K+

What are other causes of distal wasting and weakness?

- Hereditary Motor Sensory Neuropathy
- Distal spinal muscular atrophy (a variant of spinal muscular atrophy)
- Inclusion body myositis
- Oculopharyngodistal myopathy
- Welander distal myopathy
- Finish distal myopathy
- Markesbury distal myopathy
- Miyoshi myopathy

Case 48 ♦ Peripheral Neuropathy

Examiner's note

This is the most common case encountered at the neurology station in the MRCP (PACES) examination. To make a diagnosis of peripheral neuropathy is relatively straightforward. However, many candidates fail to pick up extra marks that can easily be gained at this station, transforming a 'pass' into a 'clear pass', that can make all the difference between and overall pass and fail. Rather than diagnosing a peripheral neuropathy, try to be specific and get an impression of the pattern of loss, i.e. sensory, motor, or sensorimotor neuropathy. If it is sensory, is it large fibre (mostly joint position and vibration sense), or small fibre (mostly pain and temperature)? Try to look for potential causes, otherwise provide a list of differential diagnoses appropriate for type of neuropathy. The most common instruction in this case is to examine the lower limbs, but you may be instructed to examine the upper limbs. Peripheral neuropathy can present in many ways in the examination, and the following case presentations reflect this.

CASE PRESENTATION 1 (LOWER LIMBS)

On examination of the lower limbs,[1] the skin has a **shiny** and **dry** appearance with **loss of hair** up to the mid-calves. There are **ulcers** and **callosities** present on the soles of the feet.[2] The ankle joints are swollen and deformed, with abnormal range of movements (**Charcot joints**).[3] There is **distal wasting and weakness**.[4] The **reflexes are depressed** and the plantar responses are down-going.[5] There is **bilateral symmetrical sensory loss** in a **stocking distribution** with impairment of light touch, pinprick, joint position, and vibration sense.[6]

There is **ataxia** with a **wide-based** and **high-steppage gait**.[7] **Romberg's sign is positive**.[7]

The diagnosis is a **peripheral sensorimotor neuropathy**.[8]

CASE PRESENTATION 2 (UPPER LIMBS)

On examination of the upper limbs[1] there are no trophic changes with no evidence of ulcers and callosities.[2] There is **distal wasting and weakness**.[4] The **reflexes are depressed**.[5] Sensation is normal.[6]

The diagnosis is a **peripheral motor neuropathy**.[8]

CASE PRESENTATION 3 (LOWER LIMBS)

On examination of the lower limbs,[1] there is **loss of hair** up to the mid-calves, with **ulcers** and **callosities** present on the soles of the feet.[2] There is no wasting and weakness.[4] The reflexes are preserved.[5] There is **bilateral symmetrical sensory loss** in a **stocking distribution** with impairment of light touch, pinprick, joint position, and vibration sense.[6]

There is **ataxia** with a **wide-based gait**.[7] **Romberg's sign is positive**.[7]

The diagnosis is a **peripheral sensory neuropathy**.[8]

Clinical notes

1. Before examining for neurological signs, stand back and spend a little extra time to inspect carefully. A lot can be deduced even before you have physically examined a patient with peripheral neuropathy. Look around the patient. Look for walking aids and look at the patient's shoes, especially noting ankle supports or orthoses, which would suggest a foot drop. Also look for scuffing at the front of the shoes, which results from foot drop. Look for clues of reduced manual dexterity, suggesting a distal motor neuropathy, e.g. slip-on shoes (difficulty with laces) and absence of buttons on clothes. Look for deformities, such as pes cavus, which is suggestive of an inherited neuropathy.

2. Peripheral neuropathy can lead to a number of skin changes. The skin may be dry, thin, atrophic, and hypopigmented and there may be loss of hair. Look for callosities and ulcer formation. Repeated injuries and trauma may result in chronic infections, sometimes leading to osteomyelitis. Autonomic involvement may cause the limbs to appear warm, red, and swollen or they may be pale and cold due

to abnormal regulation of small blood vessels. Palpate the peripheral nerves to look for nerve thickening, especially the ulnar nerve at the elbow, the common peroneal nerve at the knee and the superficial peroneal nerve on the dorsum of the foot. Common causes of nerve thickening are: Hereditory Motor and Sensory Neuropathy (HMSN), amyloidosis, acromegaly, and leprosy.

3. Neuropathic joints (Charcot's joints) are swollen deformed joints with abnormal ranges of movement, and suggest loss of pain and proprioception. There may be marked crepitus. Any joint can be affected, but the ankle and elbow joints are more commonly affected in the upper and lower limbs respectively.

4. A motor neuropathy will manifest as a lower motor neurone pattern of weakness, with wasting, weakness, hyporeflexia, and down-doing plantars. In most cases, there is wasting and weakness in a distal-to-proximal gradient consistent with a length-dependent axonal degeneration. The longest motor fibres are affected first, and weakness begins in the toes and feet. As the polyneuropathy progresses, it ascends up the lower extremities. When the wasting and weakness reaches the levels of the knees, motor involvement of the hands will be seen, and the length-dependent process then begins in the upper limbs. Similar patterns of weakness may be seen with demyelinating polyneuropathies. Places to check for wasting are the first dorsal interossei (loss of bulk between thumb and first finger) and tibialis anterior. Look for wasting of the small muscles of the hands with dorsal guttering and for hyperextension deformities at the MCP joints and flexion deformities at the interphalangeal joints (long-standing cases).

5. Tendon reflexes are usually reduced or absent in a distal-to-proximal pattern of involvement, with the lower limbs affected more than the upper limbs. In small fibre neuropathy, large sensory afferents from muscle spindles are relatively preserved and the tendon reflexes may thus remain intact.

6. Sensory loss manifests in a 'stocking' distribution in the legs and a 'glove' distribution in the arms. In most generalized polyneuropathies, sensory symptoms begin in the most distal part of the longest sensory fibres, i.e. in the toes and feet. The pathological changes in most cases are those of a distal-to-proximal axonal degeneration. As the disease progresses, sensory loss ascends the lower extremities, typically in a symmetric fashion. When the sensory loss is at or above the level of the knee, the distal fingertips become involved, and the length-dependent process then begins in the upper limbs. Remember, not all modalities of sensation may be lost. If only pain and temperature sensation is lost, with preservation of light touch, vibration, and joint position sense, this suggests a small fibre neuropathy. If only joint position and vibration sense is lost with preservation of pain and temperature, this suggests a large fibre neuropathy.

7. A high steppage gait reflects loss of joint position sense at the ankles (sensory neuropathy) and/or foot drop (motor neuropathy). A sensory gait is wide-based, and the patients often watch the feet and ground carefully as they walk with visual input compensating for loss of joint position sense. As a result, if they stand with their feet together, and close their eyes, thereby removing visual input, they become unsteady. This is a positive Romberg's test. It is important to stand close to the patient, and be ready to support the patient should they become unsteady.

8. Having made a diagnosis of peripheral neuropathy, try to be more specific. This will gain extra marks.

   (a) **Is it a sensorimotor, sensory or motor neuropathy?** The above clinical features should make this straightforward

   (b) **If sensory, is it small fibre or large fibre neuropathy?** Often all modalities of sensation are affected, but it is important to be aware of the following differences:
   - Small fibre neuropathy: pain, temperature, and autonomic fibres affected
   - Large fibre neuropathy: vibration and proprioception affected

   (c) **Is there any autonomic involvement?** Often seen with small fibre neuropathy. Look for the skin appearances suggestive of autonomic dysfunction. Look for a resting tachycardia. Ask for a postural blood pressure.

It is important to be aware of the common causes of sensorimotor, sensory, and motor neuropathy (see below). If possible try to find a cause, as it may be obvious. Otherwise, conclude by providing a list of differential diagnoses. Tell the examiner, that you would like to take a complete drug history.

Questions commonly asked by examiners

What are the common causes of a sensorimotor polyneuropathy?
- Alcohol
- Diabetes
- Hypothyroidism
- Uraemia
- Sarcoidosis
- Vasculitis
- Paraneoplastic
- Chronic inflammatory demyelinating polyneuropathy/Guillain-Barré syndrome
- Hereditary motor and sensory neuropathies

What are the common causes of a motor neuropathy?
- Porphyria
- Lead
- Diphtheria
- Chronic inflammatory demyelinating polyneuropathy/Guillain-Barré syndrome
- Drugs (see below)

What are the common causes of a sensory neuropathy?
- Alcohol
- Diabetes
- Hypothyroidism
- Uraemia
- Sarcoidosis
- Vasculitis
- Paraneoplastic
- Vitamin B_{12} deficiency
- Amyloidosis
- Infections, e.g. leprosy, Lyme disease, and HIV
- Drugs (see below)

What are the causes of an autonomic neuropathy?
- Guillain-Barré syndrome
- Botulism
- Porphyria
- Paraneoplastic
- Diabetes
- Chagas disease
- HIV
- Amyloidosis

What do you understand by the term 'small fibre neuropathy'?
Small fibre neuropathies refer to a subtype of peripheral neuropathies characterized by impairment of small calibre sensory nerve fibres. This includes thinly myelinated A-delta fibres

(cold, pain, and autonomic) and unmyelinated C fibres (warmth). Vibration sense and proprioception (large calibre fibres) are relatively preserved. Causes include:

- Diabetes
- Alcohol
- Amyloidosis
- Leprosy
- Drugs, e.g. isoniazid, cisplatin, disulfiram, and metronidazole
- Heavy metals, e.g. gold, arsenic, and thallium
- Hypothyroidism
- Sjogren's syndrome
- Primary biliary cirrhosis
- HIV

What are the causes of demyelinating polyneuropathies?

- Chronic inflammatory demyelinating polyneuropathy
- Multiple myeloma
- Monoclonal gammopathy of undetermined significance (MGUS)
- Hereditory Motor and Sensory Neuropathy (HMSN) type 1 and 3
- Hereditary neuropathy with pressure palsy (HNPP)
- Refsum's disease
- POEMS syndrome
- Multifocal motor neuropathy
- HIV

What drugs can cause neuropathy?

Sensory	Motor	Sensorimotor
Isoniazid	Dapsone	Vincristine
Metronidazole		Vinblastine
Hydralazine		Paclitaxel
Disulfiram		Cisplatin
Chloroquine		Nitrofurantoin
Pyridoxine		Amiodarone
Colchicine		Gold
Flecainide		Allopurinol

What is the pathophysiology of peripheral neuropathies?

Peripheral nerves exhibit three main pathological reactions: wallerian degeneration, axonal degeneration, and segmental demyelination. The mechanisms by which specific disorders affect the peripheral nerves to produce these changes are largely unknown.

Wallerian degeneration

The axon degenerates distal to the site of the lesion, thus interrupting the continuity of the axon, e.g. focal neuropathies following trauma

Axonal degeneration ('dying-back phenomenon')

This is the most common form of pathological reaction in generalized polyneuropathies. Axonal degenerative polyneuropathies are symmetrical. Axonal degeneration occurs at the most distal end of the axon, and as the disorder progresses, the axons degenerate in a distal-to-proximal pattern.

Segmental demyelination

There is focal degeneration of the myelin sheath with sparing of the axon. This can be seen in focal mononeuropathies, but also in generalized sensorimotor or predominantly motor neuropathies. Segmental demyelination can also occur in some hereditary polyneuropathies.

What are the causes of mononeuritis multiplex?

- Diabetes
- Polyarteritis nodosa
- Churg-Strauss syndrome
- Wegner's granulomatosis
- Rheumatoid arthritis
- SLE
- Sjogren's syndrome
- Sarcoidosis
- Lymphoma
- Carcinoma
- Amyloidosis
- Lyme disease
- Leprosy

What conditions cause thickening of the peripheral nerves?

- Amyloidosis
- Hereditory Motor and Sensory Neuropathy (HMSN)
- Leprosy
- Acromegaly
- Neurofibromatosis

How would you investigate this patient?

- **Blood tests**
  - FBC
  - erythrocyte sedimentation rate (ESR)
  - U&E
  - LFT
  - Glucose
  - Thyroid function tests
  - Serum B_{12} and folate
  - Serum protein electrophoresis
  - Autoimmune profile
- **Urine tests**
  - Glucose
  - Bence-Jones proteins
- *Other tests (depending on initial findings):*
  - Nerve conduction studies
  - CSF analysis
  - Autonomic function tests
  - Nerve biopsy
  - Genetic testing

Case 49 ◆ Common Peroneal Nerve Palsy and L5 Root Lesion

CASE PRESENTATION

*This patient has **high steppage gait** with a right **foot drop**.[1] There is a scar over the neck of the right fibula.[2] There is **wasting of the anterolateral compartment** of the right calf[3] with **weakness of ankle dorsiflexion and eversion**. Ankle inversion is spared. There is **weakness of dorsiflexion of the first toe**.[4] The ankle jerk is preserved.[5] There is **loss of sensation over the lateral calf and dorsum of the foot**.[6]*

*The diagnosis is a right **common peroneal nerve palsy**.*

Clinical notes

1. A high steppage gait is characteristic of foot drop. The patient is unable to dorsiflex the foot at the ankle and so raises the foot high to allow the tips of the toes to clear the ground. Look for walking aids and look at the patient's shoes, especially noting ankle supports or orthoses, which would suggest a foot drop. Also look for scuffing at the front of the shoes, which results from foot drop.

2. Common peroneal nerve palsies are often associated with extrinsic compression at the level of the neck of the fibula. Shorts casts and braces can provide extrinsic compression. Other causes of common peroneal nerve palsy include knee surgery and fracture of the fibula. It is important to inspect for scars over the neck of the fibula.

3. Wasting of anterior tibial and peroneal group of muscles may be seen in long-standing cases.

4. The common peroneal nerve splits into 2 branches:
   (a) Superficial peroneal branch: foot everters and sensation to lateral calf and dorsum of foot.
   (b) Deep peroneal branch: foot and toe dorsiflexors and sensation to the web space between the 1st and 2nd toes.
      A common peroneal nerve lesion will cause weakness of ankle and toe dorsiflexion and ankle eversion. Ankle inversion will be spared. In mild cases, the weakness of foot eversion and dorsiflexion may only be evident by asking the patient to walk on the heels. In rare cases, if the deep peroneal branch is only affected, ankle eversion will be spared.

5. Deep tendon reflexes and plantar responses are not affected. The ankle jerk is not affected, and this is an important negative to mention in patients with a flaccid foot drop. The ankle jerk will be depressed with motor neuropathies, an important cause of foot drop.

6. With common peroneal nerve palsy, sensory loss is noted over the lateral calf and dorsum of the foot, but spares the 5th toe. If the deep peroneal branch only is affected, then the sensory loss will be limited to the dorsum of the web space between the 1st and 2nd toes.

CASE PRESENTATION

*This patient has **high steppage** gait with a right **foot drop**.[1] There are no scars.[2] The **straight leg raising test is positive**, and there is **weakness of hip abduction**. There is **weakness of ankle dorsiflexion, eversion, and inversion**. There is **weakness of dorsiflexion of the first toe**.[3] The ankle jerk is preserved.[4] There is **loss of sensation over the lateral calf and dorsum of the foot, extending up to the lateral thigh**.[5]*

*The diagnosis is a right **L5 nerve root lesion.***

Clinical notes

1. The most common cause of L5 nerve root lesion is L4–5 disc prolapse. When examining the gait, you would expect to find a high steppage gait, as with foot drop. It is often associated with back pain, and the patient may walk holding their back as they walk. There may be scoliosis.

2. Examine the back for scars, suggesting previous spinal surgery.

3. There is weakness of ankle and toe dorsiflexion and ankle eversion AND inversion. L4 and L5 also supply the tibialis posterior, which inverts the foot. Involvement of foot inverters differentiates L5 root lesion from common peroneal nerve palsy. Straight leg raising test (raising the straight leg to right angles at the hip) may be positive, as pain limits the movement. Another important difference between common peroneal nerve palsy and L5 root lesions is that in L5 root lesions, there will be weakness of hip abduction.

4. The deep tendon reflexes including plantar responses are not affected. L5 root lesions cause a depressed inner hamstring jerk.

5. The sensory involvement is similar to common peroneal nerve palsy, but may extend to the outer thigh up to the buttock.

Questions commonly asked by examiners

How would you differentiate clinically between a peroneal nerve and an L5 lesion?

	Common peroneal nerve palsy	L5 root lesion
Ankle inversion	Spared	Affected
Hip abduction	Spared	Affected
Straight leg raising test	Negative	Positive
Sensory loss	Lateral calf and dorsum of the foot	Lateral calf and dorsum of the foot further proximally up the lateral side of the leg
Inner hamstring jerk	Normal	Depressed
Pain	Usually painless	Often produce pain down the posterior-lateral aspect of the leg

Which investigations would help you differentiate between a peroneal nerve and an L5 lesion?

- Neurophysiology can confirm a common peroneal mononeuropathy and the site of injury. EMG should also be performed in an L4/5 muscle that is not innervated by the common peroneal nerve (e.g. tibialis posterior).
- MRI of the lumbar spine to exclude L5 lesion.

What is the course of the common peroneal nerve?

The common peroneal nerve arises as the smaller terminal branch of the sciatic nerve on the posterior aspect of the distal thigh. The sciatic nerve splits at or slightly above the popliteal fossa to form the tibial and common peroneal nerves. The common peroneal nerve winds around the neck of the fibula from posterior to lateral, where it is vulnerable to injury and divides into the superficial and deep peroneal nerves:

- **Superficial peroneal nerve** supplies peroneus longus and brevis (the everters) and sensation to the anterior lower leg and the medial and lateral dorsal foot.
- **Deep peroneal nerve** supplies tibialis anterior, extensor digitorum longus, extensor hallucis longus, and peroneus tertius (ankle and toe dorsiflexors) and sensation to the first dorsal web space.

What are the common causes of common peroneal nerve injury?

- **External compression***
  - ◆ Short braces
  - ◆ Plaster cast
  - ◆ Tourniquets
  - ◆ Leg crossing
  - ◆ Prolonged pressure due to positioning during surgery
  - ◆ Sudden weight loss**
  - ◆ Prolonged squatting (strawberry picker's palsy)***
  - ◆ Ganglion arising from the superior tibiofibular joint
  - ◆ Schwannoma
- **Trauma**
  - ◆ Direct trauma to the nerve
  - ◆ Fibular fractures
  - ◆ Following total knee arthroplasty or proximal tibial osteotomy
- **Causes of mononeuritis multiplex****

What are the causes of a flaccid foot drop?

Site of lesion	Example(s)
Muscle	Distal myopathies, e.g. myotonic dystrophy Spinal muscular atrophy Trauma, e.g. rupture of tibialis anterior tendon
Neuromuscular junction	Myasthenia gravis
Lower motor neurone	Motor neurone disease Causes of motor neuropathies
Lumbosacral plexus	Pelvic pathology
Cauda equina	Tumour (low cauda equina lesions)
L5 nerve root	L4/5 disc prolapse Neurofibroma Cauda equina tumours
Common peroneal nerve palsy	See above
Sciatic nerve palsy	Trauma Hip surgery Damage to sciatic nerve following intramuscular (IM) injection Neurofibroma

---

* The common peroneal nerve is particularly vulnerable as it winds around the head of the fibula, where it lies on the surface of the hard bone, covered only by skin.

** Lack of or loss of the fat pad over the fibular head due to sudden weight loss and/or thin body habitus predisposes to external compression.

*** The common peroneal nerve can be tethered as it dives into the peroneus longus muscle, making it susceptible to stretch injury at this level.

**** Leprosy is the commonest cause worldwide. Remember the other causes: diabetes, polyarteritis nodosa, Churg-Strauss syndrome, Wegner's granulomatosis, rheumatoid arthritis, SLE, Sjogren's syndrome, sarcoidosis, lymphoma, carcinoma, amyloidosis, and Lyme disease

What are the causes of a spastic foot drop?

Site of lesion	Example(s)
Internal capsule	Stroke
Parasagital cortex	Tumour
Cauda equina	Tumour (high cauda equina lesions)
Spinal cord	Causes of spastic paraparesis

Upper motor neurone weakness of the foot dorsiflexors can also produce a foot drop, which is often not so apparent. This is because the spasticity does not allow the leg to be lifted, nor the foot to flop.

What treatment would you offer this patient?
- Treat or remove the underlying cause (if possible)
- Physiotherapy
- Ankle foot orthoses

Case 50 ◆ Friedreich's Ataxia

CASE PRESENTATION

*This young patient has **pes cavus**,[1] **kyphoscoliosis**[2] and a **high-arched palate**.[3] The **speech is slurred** and has an **explosive (staccato) character**.[4] There is ataxia and the patient walks with a **broad-based gait** with a **tendency to fall to both sides**.[5] There is **bilateral gaze-evoked nystagmus**. There is loss of smooth pursuit (**broken pursuit**). The saccadic eye movements are abnormal with **hypermetric saccades** in all directions.[6] The pupillary reflexes are normal.[7]*

*There is **distal wasting and weakness** in the limbs in a **pyramidal distribution**.[8] The **lower limb reflexes are absent** with **extensor plantar responses**.[9] There is **bilateral limb ataxia** with **dysdiadochokinesis, impaired finger–nose test** with **dysmetria**, an **intention tremor** (that worsens as the finger approaches the target) and **impaired heel–shin test**.[10] There is **impaired vibration and proprioception** the in the feet.[11] **Romberg's test is positive**.[12]*

*This young patient demonstrates features of a cerebellar syndrome. The presence of pes cavus, pyramidal distribution of weakness, depressed reflexes with extensor plantar responses, and peripheral neuropathy would suggest a unifying diagnosis of **Friedreich's ataxia**.[13]*

Clinical notes

Candidates often miss the diagnosis of Friedreich's ataxia, and make a diagnosis of bilateral cerebellar syndrome. Look for clues that this is not a pure cerebellar syndrome. Look for hearing or visual aids, walking aids, or foot orthoses.

1. Pes cavus is an important clue here as it suggests longstanding peripheral neuropathy. This, combined with cerebellar ataxia is very suggestive of Friedreich's ataxia. Foot deformities such as pes cavus, foot inversion, and hammertoes may precede gait abnormalities.

2. Kyphoscoliosis is a frequent but non-specific finding. Severe scoliosis can result in cardiorespiratory morbidity—look for peripheral cyanosis.

3. Friedreich's ataxia is a cause of a high-arched palate. Other causes include Marfan's syndrome, Turner's syndrome, and tuberous sclerosis.

4. These are features of a cerebellar dysarthria.

5. The gait ataxia is a combination of both sensory and cerebellar type. This combination is often referred to as a 'tabetocerebellar gait'. Both cerebellar and sensory ataxia contribute to the wide-based gait. A high-steppage gait may also be seen.

6. A cerebellar nystagmus is a coarse horizontal nystagmus with the fast component *towards* the side of the lesion. In patients with bilateral cerebellar features (as in Friedreich's ataxia), this nystagmus will occur in both directions of lateral gaze. In 20% of patients, there may be a nystagmus in the primary position that increases on lateral gaze. Look for other eye signs, i.e. broken pursuit and hypo- or hypermetric saccades.

7. Pupillary reflexes are normal. This is an important negative finding. Although cerebellar signs are not present in tabes dorsalis, a similar pattern of weakness, depressed reflexes, extensor plantar responses, and posterior column signs may be seen. Tabes dorsalis will be associated with an Argyll Robertson pupil.

8. Wasting and weakness is often more marked in the lower limbs. Distal wasting of the upper limbs may be seen in 50% of cases. Pyramidal weakness is a characteristic pattern of upper motor neuron damage, where in the lower limbs, flexion is weaker than extension, and in the upper limbs, extension is weaker than flexion. Muscle tone is usually normal or reduced in Friedreich's ataxia. Patients with advanced disease have profound distal wasting and weakness of the legs and feet. Significant weakness of the arms is rare before the patient is wheelchair bound.

9. Tendon reflexes are depressed and often absent in most cases (due to degeneration of peripheral nerves). The knee and ankle jerks are most commonly affected. In 90% of patients, the plantar responses are extensor, whilst being absent in 10% of cases. It is a combination of pyramidal weakness and peripheral neuropathy that results in depressed deep tendon reflexes and extensor plantars.

10. Look for features of bilateral cerebellar ataxia. As the disease progresses, ataxia affects the trunk, arms, and legs. The arms may become grossly ataxic. Titubation of the trunk may appear.

11. In Friedreich's ataxia, there is gradual loss of vibration sense and proprioception from the disease onset, initially affecting the hands and feet. As the disease progresses, light touch, pain, and temperature sensation can become affected. When assessing proprioception, give the level at which the patient is able to detect small deflections up or down, for example, at the ankle joint.

12. A positive Romberg's test reflects loss of proprioception.

13. Patients are often young (onset <30 years). There are many features of Friedreich's ataxia, and thus it is worthwhile summarizing your clinical findings, and then presenting a unifying diagnosis. To demonstrate your knowledge of other associations, tell the examiner you would like to look for:

   (a) **Diabetes** (occurs in 10%): finger tip skin pricks, fundoscopy for evidence of retinopathy

   (b) **Optic atrophy** (occurs in 25%): fundoscopy to look for optic disc pallor

   (c) **Hypertrophic cardiomyopathy** (occurs in 50%): jerky carotid pulse, double apical impulse, systolic murmur

   (d) **Sensorineural deafness** (occurs in 10%): look for hearing aids

Questions commonly asked by examiners

What do you know about the molecular genetics of Friedreich's ataxia?

Friedreich's ataxia is an autosomal recessive condition, with the gene locus on chromosome 9q13. This is the most common autosomal recessive ataxia, and accounts for 50% of all hereditary ataxia. The mutation is a trinucleotide (GAA) repeat expansion in a gene encoding a protein called frataxin, which is involved in mitochondrial iron regulation and oxidative phosphorylation. Frataxin deficiency results in iron accumulation within the mitochondria of the affected cells.

Excess intracellular iron results in impairment of oxidative phosphorylation and free radical formation that results in cell death, particularly of the spinal cord neurones and peripheral nerves. In normal individuals, the GAA sequence is repeated up to 50 times. In Friedreich's ataxia, this sequence is repeated at least up to 200 times, and often more than 1000 times. Patients with larger number of trinucleotide repeats generally have an earlier age of onset and more severe manifestations.

What is the pathophysiology of Friedreich's ataxia?

This is a neurodegenerative disorder that primarily affects the spinal cord and spinal roots. The posterior columns, corticospinal, and spinocerebellar tracts show demyelination and depletion of large myelinated nerve fibres, resulting in fibrous gliosis. The spinal cord becomes thin and the dorsal root ganglia become atrophic. There is loss of large myelinated fibres in the sensory roots and peripheral nerves. Unmyelinated fibres in the sensory roots and peripheral nerves are relatively spared. The following pathophysiological mechanisms account for the clinical features observed in this condition:

Clinical feature	Pathophysiology
Loss of proprioception and vibration sense	Degeneration of the posterior columns
Hyporeflexia	Loss of large nerve fibres in the dorsal root ganglia
Cerebellar ataxia	Degeneration lateral and ventral spinocerebellar tracts, Clarke column, dentate nucleus, superior vermis, and dentatorubral pathways
Pyramidal weakness and extensor plantar responses	Degeneration of the corticospinal tracts (these tracts are relatively spared down to the cervicomeduallary junction, after which they are degenerated)

What is the differential diagnosis of depressed knee and ankle jerks with extensor plantar responses?

*   Combination of conditions (most common)
    *   Peripheral neuropathy and stroke
    *   Peripheral neuropathy and cervical myelopathy
    *   Cervical and lumbar spondylosis
*   Subacute combined degeneration of the cord (B_{12} deficiency)
*   Tabes dorsalis
*   Lesion of the conus medullaris
*   Friedreich's ataxia
*   Motor neurone disease

What is the age of onset of Friedreich's ataxia?

It typically presents in children aged 10–15 years, and almost always presents before 20 years of age.

What is the presenting symptom in these patients?

Gait ataxia is the most common presenting feature. Both lower limbs are usually affected equally. Some patients may present with unilateral ataxia (hemiataxia), but the ataxia soon becomes generalized.

What are the cardiac manifestations of this condition?

*   Inferolateral T-wave inversion on ECG (65% have ECG abnormalities)
*   Left ventricular hypertrophy

- Conduction defects
- Arrhythmias
- Chronic interstitial myocarditis
- Myocardial fibrosis
- Hypertrophic cardiomyopathy (seen in 50%)

How would you manage this patient?

There is no specific treatment for Friedreich's ataxia. Management should include regular review by a multi-disciplinary team that includes a neurologist, rehabilitation physician, genetic advisor, and therapists. The following should be considered:

- Physiotherapy to prevent deformities and exercises to maintain function of the limbs
- Ankle/foot orthoses
- Occupational therapy
- Orthopaedic correction of scoliosis and pes cavus
- Walking aids (most become wheelchair bound 15 years from onset)
- Hypoglycaemic drugs/insulin for diabetes
- Visual aids
- Hearing aids
- Symptomatic treatment of cardiomyopathy and arrhythmias

Are there attenuated variants of this condition?

Pes cavus or hammertoes occur in family members. Occasionally the ankle jerks may be absent.

What is the prognosis of this disease?

The disease progresses at a variable rate but most patients are unable to walk and become wheelchair bound after 15 years from onset. Death usually occurs in the fourth decade but increasing numbers are surviving beyond the fifth decade. Milder later onset variants have been diagnosed since genetic testing became available.

What other early onset recessive ataxias do you know about?

- Ataxia telangiectasia
- Abetalipoproteinaemia (Bassen-Kornzweig syndrome)
- Refsum's disease

Case 51 ◆ **Multiple Sclerosis**

Examiner's note

Multiple sclerosis is a demyelinating disorder of the central nervous system, characterized by lesions separated both in space and time, and patients may have a mixture of neurological signs. Such a mixture of signs can baffle candidates in clinical examinations, and it is important to be aware of the sites within the central nervous system, that are affected by demyelinating plaques. The multiple sclerosis patient in the MRCP (PACES) examination will often be young, and this may be an important clue to the diagnosis. The demyelinating plaques have predilection for the following sites:

- **Optic nerve**: optic atrophy, relative afferent pupillary defects
- **Brainstem**: internuclear ophthalmoplegia, facial sensory loss, facial weakness (UMN), rubral tremor, diplopia
- **Cerebellum**: ataxia, dysarthria
- **Spinal cord (corticospinal tracts)**: pyramidal weakness
- **Spinal cord (dorsal columns)**: loss of vibration and proprioception, Lhermitte's sign, pseudoathetosis.

Depending on the extent of involvement, the signs may be unilateral or bilateral, and not all of the above sites may be affected. In general, patients (young or middle-aged) with a mixture of eye, brainstem, cerebellar, pyramidal, and dorsal column signs should raise the suspicion of multiple sclerosis.

Candidates may be instructed to examine the eyes, upper limbs, or lower limbs. When examining, it is important to make general observations. A cerebellar dysarthria may be evident when introducing yourself to the patient. An intention tremor in the upper limbs may be noted when examining the lower limbs. This will provide useful indirect clues to cerebellar disease, and this in conjunction with pyramidal and/or dorsal column signs should help make the diagnosis. If instructed to examine the upper or lower limbs, it may be worthwhile to proceed directly to examining the eyes (nystagmus, internuclear ophthalmoplegia). If instructed to examine the eyes or lower limbs in a patient with slurred speech (suggestive of cerebellar dysarthria), which reveal pyramidal signs only, it may be worthwhile to proceed directly to examine the upper limbs for cerebellar signs. This will impress examiners!

Multiple sclerosis can present in many ways in the MRCP (PACES) examination. The following case presentations represent the typical presentations encountered in the examination. When presenting, it is best to use the term 'demyelinating disease'—a useful euphemism for multiple sclerosis.

CASE PRESENTATION 1 (INITIAL INSTRUCTION: 'EXAMINE THE EYES')

*This patient has dissociation of conjugate eye movements. Abduction is normal with impairment of adduction in both eyes. There is nystagmus in the abducting eye. When the abducting eye is covered, adduction of the opposite eye is normal (**internuclear ophthalmoplegia**).[1] The saccadic eye movements are abnormal with **hypermetric saccades** and there is **nystagmus** on looking to both sides.[2] The right optic disc is pale and has distinct margins (**optic atrophy**). The right pupil exhibits a loss of direct light reflex, whereas, the consensual light reflex is preserved (**afferent pupillary defect**). Visual field testing (using a red hat pin) reveals a **central scotoma** and **visual acuity is reduced** on the right.[3]*

Proceed as follows:[4]

*The **speech is slurred** with an **explosive (staccato) character**. There is bilateral ataxia in the bilateral upper limb with **dysdiadochokinesis, impaired finger–nose testing** and an **intention tremor**.[6] When the eyes are closed, there is unconscious writhing of the fingers (**pseudoathetosis**)[7] and there is failure of the displaced arms to find their original posture (**rebound phenomenon**).[6]*

*This patient has internuclear ophthalmoplegia (suggesting a lesion in the medial longitudinal fasciculus) and optic atrophy. There are cerebellar and dorsal column signs in the upper limbs. The most likely unifying diagnosis is **demyelinating disease**.*

Clinical notes

1. Internuclear ophthalmoplegia is due to a lesion in the medial longitudinal fasciculus. It results in weakness of adduction of the ipsilateral eye, with nystagmus on abduction of the contralateral eye. The key feature is weakness of ipsilateral adduction, and the nystagmus may or may not be present. This results in dissociation of conjugate eye movements. The adduction becomes normal when the contralateral (abducting) eye is covered. Multiple sclerosis is the most common cause, and often causes bilateral internuclear ophthalmoplegia (unilateral is less common).

2. Cerebellar eye signs include ocular dysmetria (hypo- or hypermetric saccades), broken pursuit and nystagmus towards the site of the cerebellar lesion. In patients with bilateral internuclear ophthalmoplegia AND cerebellar signs, the superimposition of dissociation of conjugate gaze movements and different forms of nystagmus associated with each can be confusing and present a diagnostic challenge to identify two separate components. In this situation, impairment of adduction is the key feature to look for in identifying internuclear ophthalmoplegia. With cerebellar disease, there may be nystagmus with a fast beat towards the side of lesion (may be in both directions with bilateral cerebellar signs). In this situation, it is best to look for cerebellar nystagmus when the abducting (contralateral) eye is covered. By covering the abducting eye, the adduction in the ipsilateral eye will normalize and it becomes much easier to appreciate a cerebellar nystagmus.

3. Optic atrophy results from optic neuritis. An afferent or relative afferent pupillary defect may be seen and the visual acuity may be reduced in the affected eye. There may be a central scotoma on visual field testing.

4. The presence of internuclear ophthalmoplegia, cerebellar eye signs, and/or optic atrophy should raise the suspicion of multiple sclerosis. Having introduced yourself to the patient, try to get an impression of the patient's speech. Is there a cerebellar dysarthria? Although, you have been instructed to examine the eyes, it would be reasonable to proceed to checking for cerebellar signs in the upper limb, rather than doing a complete examination of the upper limbs. It is best to start by asking the patient to put the arms out in front of them, and closing their eyes. Look for pseudoathetosis, and then examine for the rebound phenomenon. This initial manoeuvre will tell you if there are dorsal column signs in addition to cerebellar signs. Then proceed to examining for other cerebellar signs. Depending on the extent of involvement, cerebellar signs may be unilateral or bilateral.

CASE PRESENTATION 2 (INITIAL INSTRUCTION: 'EXAMINE THE UPPER LIMBS')

This patient displays **pyramidal weakness** *with* **hypertonia** *and* **hyperreflexia** *in the right upper limb.*[5] *There is ataxia on the right with* **dysdiadochokinesis, impaired finger-nose testing** *and an* **intention tremor**.[6] *When the eyes are closed, there is unconscious writhing of the fingers* **(pseudoathetosis)**[7] *and there is failure of the displaced arms to find their original posture* **(rebound phenomenon)**.[6] **Vibration sense and proprioception are impaired** *in the hands.*[7]

Proceed as follows:[8]

The **speech is slurred** *with an* **explosive (staccato) character.** *The saccadic eye movements are abnormal with* **hypermetric saccades** *and there is* **nystagmus** *on looking to the right.*[2] *The left optic disc is pale and has distinct margins* **(optic atrophy)**.[3]

This patient displays eye, cerebellar, pyramidal, and dorsal column signs. The most likely unifying diagnosis is **demyelinating disease**.

Clinical notes

5. Pyramidal weakness reflects involvement of the corticospinal tracts. This may be marked with gross weakness, hypertonia, and hyperreflexia. Wasting is not a feature of upper motor neurone lesions,

however, in long-standing cases, some wasting may be evident secondary to disuse atrophy. In other cases the weakness may be subtle and easily missed. A pyramidal pattern of weakness in the upper limbs results in weakness of extensors. Depending on the extent of involvement, pyramidal signs may be unilateral or bilateral.

6. In patients with marked pyramidal weakness, testing coordination and assessing for cerebellar signs may be difficult. Cerebellar signs in the upper limbs may be unilateral or bilateral and include dysdiadochokinesis, impaired finger–nose testing with dysmetria, dyssynergia, intention tremor, and the rebound phenomenon.

7. Dorsal column signs include loss of vibration sense and proprioception. The loss of sensory feedback with cervical cord lesions results in unconscious writhing movements of the fingers with the eyes closed (pseudoathetosis)—a sign of dorsal column involvement. Pain and temperature sensation can be affected, but this is uncommon (lateral spinothalamic tracts).

8. The presence of pyramidal, cerebellar, and/or dorsal column signs should be adequate to make the diagnosis of multiple sclerosis. Having introduced yourself to the patient, try to get an impression of the patient's speech. Is there a cerebellar dysarthria? Although, you have been instructed to examine the upper limbs, it would be reasonable to proceed to checking for eye signs. Look for internuclear ophthalmoplegia, cerebellar eye signs, and optic atrophy.

CASE PRESENTATION 3 (INITIAL INSTRUCTION: 'EXAMINE THE LOWER LIMBS')

This patient displays **pyramidal weakness** *with* **hypertonia, hyperreflexia** *with* **extensor plantar response** *in the left lower limb.*[9] *There is ataxia on the right, with* **dyssynergia** *and* **impaired heel–shin testing.**[10] **Vibration sense and proprioception are impaired** *in the feet.*[11,12]

Proceed as follows:[13]

The **speech is slurred** *with an* **explosive (staccato) character.** *The saccadic eye movements are abnormal with* **hypermetric saccades** *and there is* **nystagmus** *on looking to the right.*[2] *The left optic disc is pale and has distinct margins (***optic atrophy***).*[3]

This patient displays eye, cerebellar, pyramidal, and dorsal column signs. The most likely unifying diagnosis is **demyelinating disease**.

Clinical notes

9. Pyramidal weakness reflects involvement of the corticospinal tracts. This may be marked with gross weakness, hypertonia, and hyperreflexia. Wasting is not a feature of upper motor neurone lesions, however, in long-standing cases, some wasting may be evident secondary to disuse atrophy. In severe cases there may be contractures. Look for evidence of walking aids or a wheelchair, to get an idea of disability. In some cases the weakness may be subtle and easily missed. A pyramidal pattern of weakness in the lower limbs results in weakness of flexors. Depending on the extent of involvement, pyramidal signs may be unilateral or bilateral.

10. In patients with marked pyramidal weakness, testing coordination and assessing for cerebellar signs may be difficult. Cerebellar signs in the lower limbs may be unilateral or bilateral and include dyssynergia and impaired heel shin testing.

11. Look for the absence or presence of dorsal column signs (reduced vibration sense and proprioception). Pain and temperature sensation can be affected, but this is uncommon (lateral spinothalamic tracts).

12. If the patient is ambulant, examine the gait. Depending on the extent and pattern of involvement (cerebellar and pyramidal features), the findings on gait examination will be variable. A cerebellar gait is

wide-based and ataxic, with impaired heel-to-toe walking. With unilateral pyramidal weakness, there may a hemiplegic gait. With bilateral spastic weakness, there may be a 'scissor' gait. If there is dorsal column involvement, Romberg's test may be positive, and the patient may display a sensory gait. A sensory gait is wide-based and ataxic, and the patients often watch the feet and ground carefully as they walk with visual input compensating for loss of joint position sense. Ataxia in multiple sclerosis is usually mainly cerebellar.

13. The presence of pyramidal, cerebellar, and/or dorsal column signs should be adequate to make the diagnosis of multiple sclerosis. Having introduced yourself to the patient, try to get an impression of the patient's speech. Is there a cerebellar dysarthria? Although, you have been instructed to examine the lower limbs, it would be reasonable to proceed to checking for eye signs. Look for internuclear ophthalmoplegia, cerebellar eye signs, and optic atrophy.

CASE PRESENTATION 4 (INITIAL INSTRUCTION: 'EXAMINE THE LOWER LIMBS')

*This patient has **pyramidal weakness** in both lower limbs. There is bilateral **hypertonia, hyperreflexia**, with **extensor plantar responses**. Sensation is normal.[14]*

Proceed as follows:[15]

*The **speech is slurred** with an **explosive (staccato) character**. There is **nystagmus** to the right.[2] There is bilateral ataxia in the upper limbs with **dysdiadochokinesis, impaired finger–nose testing** with **dysmetria and** an **intention tremor**.[3]*

*This patient displays pyramidal signs (spastic paraparesis) in the lower limbs in addition to cerebellar signs. The most likely unifying diagnosis is **demyelinating disease**.*

Clinical notes

14. Multiple sclerosis can cause spastic paraparesis. Look for a sensory deficit. Although dorsal column involvement will result in impaired vibration sense and proprioception, this may be normal in some patients, obscuring the diagnosis. It is important to look for a sensory level (cord compression). Thus the finding of normal sensation is an important negative to mention.

15. In such cases with a patient with spastic paraparesis where there are no sensory signs in the legs, it is important to examine the upper limbs and/or the eyes to look for other features that would help make a diagnosis of multiple sclerosis. Having introduced yourself to the patient, try to get an impression of the patient's speech. Is there a cerebellar dysarthria? Is there a marked intention tremor? Is there an obvious nystagmus? Although, you have been instructed to examine the lower limbs, it would be reasonable to proceed to checking the eye for nystagmus and the upper limbs for cerebellar signs.

Questions commonly asked by examiners

What is the pathophysiology of multiple sclerosis?

Multiple sclerosis is an idiopathic demyelinating disorder of the central nervous system, characterized by demyelinating plaques both separated in space and time. It is regarded as an autoimmune disease, with candidate autoantigens including many myelin proteins, e.g. proteolipid protein, myelin oligodendrocyte glycoprotein, and myelin basic protein. What triggers the autoimmune process is not clear, but infections with human herpes virus 6 and Chlamydia pneumoniae have been implicated. Acute multiple sclerosis plaques develop when primed T-lymphocytes cross the blood brain barrier and activate macrophages. This inflammatory process results in demyelination, and the axons lose the ability for salutatory conduction, and inflammatory mediators further impede axonal conduction. Although there is relative sparing of axons, recent studies show that axonal damage does occur in acute attacks. Lesions characteristically involve the optic nerve, and the periventricular white matter of the cerebellum, brainstem, and spinal cord.

What are the different clinical categories of multiple sclerosis?

Relapsing-remitting (80–85%)
Short-lasting acute attacks followed by periods of remissions and a steady baseline state between relapses.

Secondary progressive (30–40%)
Gradual progressive deterioration that is seen in patients with the relapsing–remitting form of multiple sclerosis.

Primary progressive (10–15%)
Progressive deterioration from the onset of symptoms.

Progressive-relapsing (5–10%)
A variant of the primary progressive form of multiple sclerosis, where there is progressive deterioration, but with superimposed relapses.

What is Lhermitte's sign?

Neck flexion results in rapid tingling or electric shock-like feeling that passes down the spine and into the arms and legs. It indicates dorsal column involvement of the cervical spinal cord. Causes include:

- Multiple sclerosis
- Cervical myelopathy
- Cervical cord tumour
- Subacute combined degeneration of the cord

What is Uhtoff's phenomenon?

A raised body temperature, i.e. exercise, sauna, hot bath or shower, results in exacerbation of symptoms. The exact mechanism for this unclear, but it is believed to result from a heat-induced conduction block of partially demyelinated fibres.

What do you understand by internuclear ophthalmoplegia?

The medial longitudinal fasciculus starts below the posterior commissure and ends in the upper cervical spinal cord. In simplistic terms, it connects ipsilateral III nucleus (medial rectus-adduction) with the contralateral VI nucleus (lateral rectus-abduction) and is involved in the control of conjugate eye movement. A lesion in the medial longitudinal fasciculus primarily results in impairment of ipsilateral adduction. With normal abduction of the contralateral eye, there will be divergence, thus the abducting eye flicks back towards the nose to correct for this and continues abduction. This results in a few beats of nystagmus in the contralateral eye. The key feature of internuclear ophthalmoplegia is weakness of ipsilateral adduction, and nystagmus in the abducting eye may not be present. Causes include:

- Multiple sclerosis (most common)
- Brainstem lesions (infarction, tumours, and aneurysms)
- Wernicke's encephalopathy
- SLE
- Miller Fisher Syndrome
- Drug overdose (tricyclic antidepressants, phenytoin, and barbiturates)

What investigation is the most useful for confirming the diagnosis of multiple sclerosis?

An MRI scan is the most useful test for confirming the diagnosis of multiple sclerosis. Typical lesions appear as T2 hyperintense lesions in the periventricular white matter of the brain and spinal cord. Lesions that enhance with gadolinium reflect active disease, as enhancement corresponds to breakdown in the blood brain barrier. Often combinations of enhancing and non-enhancing lesions are seen reflecting the chronic nature of the multiple sclerosis. Hypointense T1 lesions may reflect axonal damage and chronic damage resulting in gliosis. Sometimes new lesions may appear as T1 hypointense lesions, reflecting marked oedema.

What is the role of CSF analysis in patients with multiple sclerosis?

CSF analysis is indicated if the diagnosis is uncertain and the neurological presentation and neuroimaging raises the suspicion of CNS infection. Up to 5% of patients with multiple sclerosis will have normal CSF findings. Typical findings include:

* Normal glucose
* Lymphocytosis
* Normal or slightly elevated protein
* Oligoclonal bands*

What are the causes of CSF oligoclonal bands?

* Multiple sclerosis
* Neurosarcoidosis
* Neurosyphilis
* CNS lymphoma
* Meninoencephalitis
* Neuromyelitis optica (Devic's disease)
* Acute disseminated encephalomyelitis
* SLE
* Subacute sclerosing panencephalitis
* Guillain-Barré syndrome
* Progressive multifocal leucoencepahalopathy
* Behcets disease
* Subarachnoid haemorrhage

What do you know about neuromyelitis optica (Devic's disease)?

This is an idiopathic inflammatory demyelination disease of the CNS that mainly affects the optic nerves and spinal cord. Most patients relapse, as they do with multiple sclerosis. However, patients with neuromyelitis optica have more severe attacks, with larger centrally located spinal cord lesions, and are seropositive for the neuromyelitis optica IgG (NMO-IgG). The immunological target of the NMO IgG is aquaporin-4, a water channel located at the foot processes of the astrocytes. In acute attacks, intravenous steroids are commonly used, and plasmapharesis can be used for steroid unresponsive patients. Immunosuppressive therapy is

---

* This demonstrates increased intrathecal IgG production, and if present only in the CSF and not in the serum, suggests CNS inflammation. It can be demonstrated in 95% of patients with multiple sclerosis, and the IgG index is elevated (>1.7). The IgG index = $[IgG_{CSF}/albumin_{CSF}]/[IgG_{serum}/albumin_{serum}]$; normal IgG index <0.77. There is no correlation between oligoclonal bands and the demyelination process, and oligoclonal bands can be present even in the presence of normal CSF igG levels. Once an oligoclonal response is established in the CSF, it can be maintained for the natural life of the patient.

indicated in patients with relapsing disease, and the most commonly used therapy is azathioprine alone or in combination with steroids.

What do you know about acute disseminated encephalomyelitis?

This is a monophasic demyelinating disorder of the CNS. It is a disease of the young, most commonly affecting children. Up to 75% of cases may be regarded as a post-infectious or post-immunization encephalomyelitis. Autoreactive T cells following an infection or immunization cross the blood brain barrier and target myelin antigens. Contrary to multiple sclerosis, where CNS lesions are heterogeneous in space, time, and composition, the lesions in acute disseminated encephalomyelitis are almost always of similar age and composition. MRI of the brain and spinal cord is the most widely used diagnostic tool. Lesions are often widespread, multifocal, or extensive (>50% of total white matter volume). To differentiate this from multiple sclerosis, it is important to look for dissemination in time of CNS demyelination, i.e. look for T1 hypointense lesions that would be a strong indicator of multiple sclerosis. Once the diagnosis is made and an acute infectious disorder excluded, the treatment is usually with high dose intravenous steroids, followed by prolonged oral steroid therapy. Other therapies including plasmapharesis, intravenous immunoglobulin (IVIG), and cyclophosphamide may be considered in steroid unresponsive patients.

What treatment options are available for multiple sclerosis?

General measures
- Patient education and counselling
- Physiotherapy
- Occupational therapy
- Walking aids and orthoses
- Visual aids

Management of acute attacks
- IV methylprednisolone*
- Plasma exchange (steroid unresponsive patients)

Prevention of relapses (disease-modifying therapies)

These therapies are used in relapsing-remitting form of multiple sclerosis:
- **Interferon-β**
  - Reduces the relapse rate by 33%
  - Associated with 50–80% reduction in inflammatory activity on MRI
  - Improve quality of life and cognitive function
  - Adverse effects include flu-like symptoms, myalgia, and fatigue (60% of patients)
  - Can result in neutralizing antibodies
- **Glatirimer acetate**
  - A synthetic polypeptide that competes with the auto-antigen, myelin basic protein
  - Reduces the relapse rate by 35%
  - Associated with 30–40% reduction in inflammatory activity on MRI
  - Usually well tolerated

---

* Steroids shorten the duration of acute relapses and hasten recovery, but do not affect the long-term course of the disease.

- **Mitoxantrone**
  - ◆ An anthracenedione chemotherapeutic agent
  - ◆ Reduces the relapse rate by 67%
  - ◆ Adverse effects include nausea and alopecia
  - ◆ Due to cumulative cardiotoxicity, can only be used for 2–3 years
- **Natalizumab**
  - ◆ A monoclonal antibody targeting α_4 integrin on leucocytes
  - ◆ Re-approved by FDA in June 2006 after initial concerns with links with progressive multifocal leucoencepahalopathy
  - ◆ Reduces the relapse rate by 67%
  - ◆ Associated with 80–90% reduction in inflammatory activity on MRI

Symptomatic treatment

- Spasticity: baclofen, tizanidine, gabapentin, and dantrolene
- Depression: SSRIs, tricyclic antidepressants
- Fatigue: amantidine, modafanil, SSRIs
- Pain: carbamazepine, tricyclic antidepressants
- Bladder dysfunction: self-intermittent catheterization, anti-cholinergic agents, α_1-antagonists
- Sexual dysfunction: counselling
- Erectile dysfunction: phosphodiesterase inhibitors (sildenafil)

What are the current recommendations for use of interferon-β therapy?

Interferon-β therapy is licensed for use only in patients with relapsing remitting form of multiple sclerosis, who have had at least 2 relapses in the previous 2 years and who are able to walk unaided.

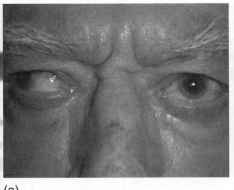
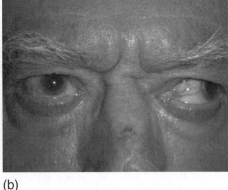

(a)   (b)

Figure 51.1 Bilateral internuclear opthalmoplegia. There is bilateral weakness of adduction with (a) right gaze and (b) left gaze.
Reproduced from Sundaram et al. Training in Ophthalmology. 2009, with permission from Oxford University Press.

Case 52 ◆ **Spastic Paraparesis**

CASE PRESENTATION

This patient has **wasting** *of the lower limbs with* **contractures**.[1] *There is bilateral* **pyramidal weakness**,[2] *with* **hypertonia**,[3] **hyperreflexia**,[4] **ankle clonus**[5] *and* **extensor plantar responses**.[6] *Sensation is impaired in the lower limbs, with a* **sensory level at the level of T9**[7,8]

There is no spinal deformity or tenderness. There is a **surgical scar over the thoracic spine**.[9]

This patient has **spastic paraparesis** *due to a lesion at the* **T9 level of the spinal cord**. *The presence of a surgical scar suggests previous surgery for trauma or spinal cord pathology, i.e. tumour. The presence of wasting and contractures suggests this has been longstanding.*[10]

Clinical notes

Before examining the patient, try to get as many clues as you can from just looking at and around the patient. Look for walking aids and look at the patient's shoes, especially noting ankle supports or orthoses, which would suggest a foot drop. Also look for scuffing at the front of the shoes, which results from foot drop. Spasticity can result in wearing of the lateral edges. Is there a wheelchair? This will provide an idea of patient disability. Look for an in-dwelling urinary catheter, which would suggest bladder involvement.

1. Wasting is often not a feature of upper motor neurone lesions. In long-standing cases, there is often global wasting due to disuse atrophy. Look for contractures in chronic immobilized patients. There may be scars over the tendons, representing previous corrective surgery for contractures and deformities.

2. In the lower limbs, pyramidal weakness is weakness of flexors: hip flexion, knee flexion, ankle dorsiflexion, and eversion.

3. Roll each knee from side to side looking for loss of the normal delay with which the foot follows the knee. Lift the knee from the couch and looking for the foot to 'jump up' off the couch. The patient needs to be warned first, and told to relax and keep the leg floppy.

4. In addition to looking for exaggerated contraction at the tested muscle (e.g. in quadriceps for knee jerk), look to see if there is 'spread' of contraction to other parts of the leg or the opposite leg, that would suggest a pyramidal lesion. For example, an ankle jerk test may also cause hamstring contraction on both sides. 'Crossed adductors' is also a useful sign of hyperreflexia: the adductor tendon is struck just above the medial aspect of the knee—it is normal if the same adductor contracts, but suggestive of a pyramidal lesion if the opposite adductor contracts as well (suggesting impaired descending inhibition).

5. To test for ankle clonus, hold the knee in the flexed position. Avoid testing for patellar clonus as this can cause pain.

6. The extensor response might be evident as big toe extension, fanning of all toes, or involuntary contraction of leg flexors (the latter of which may be confused with voluntary withdrawal, although this can sometimes be appreciated as occurring after a longer delay, and being more variable than a reflex withdrawal). In slight pyramidal disease, the extensor plantar response can be initially elicited on the dorsilateral part of the foot (Chaddock's manoeuvre). With increasing severity of pyramidal disease, the extensor plantar response may be elicited from the whole sole of the foot, and later beyond the foot. Oppenheim sign: extensor plantar response when the inner border of the tibia is pressed heavily. Gordon's sign: extensor plantar response when the Achilles tendon is pinched.

7. A sensory examination is important in a patient with spastic paraparesis. The presence of a sensory level will help localize spinal cord lesions. The presence of a sensory level in a patient presenting with

paraparesis should alert you to the possibility of spinal cord compression. Furthermore, certain patterns of sensory loss, will help determine the underlying cause (see below).

8. In patients with weak hip flexors or spasticity, heel–shin testing to test coordination may be imprecise and unreliable. However if the ataxia appears more than can be explained by weakness, especially if there is worsening of tremor as the target is approached (e.g. heel approaching knee or ankle), it would suggest that there is an additional ataxic component. A more reliable indicator of ataxia is demonstration of cerebellar signs in the upper limbs and/or eyes.

9. It is important that a brief examination of the spine is conducted at the end of the examination. Look for tenderness, scars, and deformities.

10. In patients who are ambulant, examine the gait. With bilateral spastic leg weakness, there will be a 'scissor' gait. There may be a 'high steppage' gait, indicating foot drop (upper motor neurone weakness of the foot dorsiflexors can also produce a foot drop, which is often not so apparent, because the spasticity does not allow the leg to be lifted, nor the foot to flop).

11. When presenting the findings, it is important to mention the absence and presence of a sensory level. If possible try to give a cause. This may be straightforward, as in the above case, otherwise present a differential diagnosis. In addition to sensory finding, in a patient with spastic paraparesis, the following feature can help identify the underlying cause:
    (a) Cerebellar signs (particularly in the upper limbs)
    (b) Fasciculations
    (c) Upper limb involvement
    (d) Wasting of the small muscles of the hands

Cause	Sensory signs	Other features to look for
Multiple sclerosis	Dorsal column signs	Cerebellar signs in the upper limbs; eye signs; pseudoathetosis
Cord compression, i.e. tumours	Sensory level	Absence of signs above the level of lesion
Trauma	Sensory level	Scars; deformity
Motor neurone disease	None	Fasciculations (limbs and tongue); bulbar involvement; wasting of small muscle of hands
Syringomyelia	Dissociated loss (preserved posterior columns and loss of spinothalamic)	Lower motor neurone weakness in upper limbs, wasting of small muscles of the hands, Horner's syndrome
Anterior spinal artery occlusion	Dissociated loss (preserved posterior columns and loss of spinothalamic)	Irregular pulse (AF)—a cause of embolic phenomena
Subacute combined degeneration	Dorsal column signs, peripheral neuropathy	Absent ankle jerks and extensor plantars; anaemia; jaundice; glossitis; splenomegaly
Taboparesis	Dorsal column signs	Absent ankle jerks and extensor plantars; Argyll Robertson pupils
Tropical spastic paraparesis	Dorsal column signs, peripheral neuropathy	Afro-Caribbean patient; proximal > distal weakness
Friedreich's ataxia	Dorsal column signs	Cerebellar signs; pes cavus; kyphoscoliosis
Cervical myelopathy	Dorsal column signs	Neck pain; Lhermitte's sign; inversion of bicep and suppinator reflexes; pseudoathetosis
Hereditary spastic paraparesis	None	Upper limbs normal
Parasagittal tumour	Cortical sensory loss	Papilloedema; history of headache

Questions commonly asked by examiners

What is the definition of spasticity?

This is defined as an increase in muscle tone due to hyperexcitability of the stretch reflexes, and velocity-dependent increase in tonic stretch reflexes.

What is the difference between spasticity and rigidity?

Rigidity represents a constant increased tone *throughout* the range of movement and is independent of velocity. Spasticity represents increased tone that is velocity-dependent, being more marked at the onset of the movement, and decreasing suddenly as passive movement is continued (clasp-knife phenomenon).

What is the pathophysiological basis for spasticity?

Spasticity results from enhanced stretch reflex activity. This may be manifested by increased muscle tone (tonic stretch reflexes) and exaggerated reflexes (phasic stretch reflexes). Normally, this reflex is activated whenever a muscle is rapidly stretched, causing the muscle to contract in order to resist the force that is stretching it. However, normal movement often requires this reflex to be switched off, and thus the brain sends inhibitory signals to the spinal cord. In upper motor neurone lesions, inhibitory inputs from the reticulospinal and other descending pathways to the motor and interneuronal circuits of the spinal cord are lost, resulting in α-motor neurone hyperexcitability. Denervation supersensitivity, shortening of motor neurone dendrites, and sprouting of dorsal root afferents may also play a role in α-motor neurone hyperexcitability.

What do you know about hereditary spastic paraparesis?

This is also known as familial spastic paraparesis and Stumpell-Lorrain syndrome. It is characterized by progressive, and often severe, spasticity in the lower limbs. Inheritance patterns can be X-linked, autosomal dominant, or recessive (autosomal dominant inheritance is the most common). It is caused by degeneration of the ends of the corticospinal tracts within the spinal cord. The ends of the longest corticospinal fibres are mostly affected, thus the legs are much more greatly affected than the arms. Although fibres supplying the arms may be affected, patients often don't have symptoms in the arms. Peripheral nerves are normal, however sensory impairment is seen in 10–65% of patients. It usually consists of diminished proprioception and vibration sense in the extremities, which reflects a central axonopathy, rather than a peripheral nerve involvement. Pes cavus can be seen, and reflects longstanding disease. Muscle wasting is uncommon, although mild muscle wasting can occur in patients who have had the disease for over 10 years, and this often affects distal muscles groups (small muscles of the feet and tibialis anterior).

What do you know about tropical spastic paraparesis?

This is also known as HTLV-1-associaited myelopathy and is characterized by a chronic progressive spastic paraparesis with sphincter disturbance and mild sensory involvement. It is common in regions of endemic HTLV-1 such as the Caribbean, Africa, Japan, and South America. The HTLV-1 virus is primarily transmitted through sexual contact, sharing of needles, blood products and by vertical transmission. Only 1–4% of affected individuals develop tropical spastic paraparesis. The incubation period from infection to onset of myelopathic symptoms ranges from months to years.

What do you understand by the term 'transverse myelitis'?

This is a broad term used to describe acute inflammation of cord. Inflammation tends to involve the cord diffusely at one or more levels, affecting all spinal cord function, with resultant bilateral motor, sensory, and sphincter deficit below the level of the lesion. It is, therefore, an important cause of paraparesis. Causes include:

- Bacterial infections (Lyme disease, mycoplasma, tuberculosis, and syphilis)
- Viral infections (HSV, VZV, CMV, EBV, HIV, HAV, influenza virus, and echovirus)

- Demyelination (multiple sclerosis and Devic's disease)
- Radiation myelopathy
- Anterior spinal artery occlusion
- Vasculitis

What treatment options are available to treat spasticity?

Physiotherapy
- Stretching exercises—help maintain full range of movement and prevent contractures
- Strengthening exercises
- Orthoses, casts, and braces to keep spastic limb in normal position
- Application of cold packs to spastic muscles can improve tone and function temporarily
- Electrical stimulation

Oral pharmacotherapy
- Benzodiazepines
- Baclofen
- Tizanidine
- Dantrolene
- Clonidine
- Gabapentin

Intrathecal pharmacotherapy
- Baclofen
- Phenol

Neurosurgery
- Selective dorsal rhizotomy (cutting selective nerve roots between L2 and S2)

Orthopaedic surgery
- Contracture release
- Tendon transfer
- Osteotomy

Other
- Botulinum toxin injections

Case 53 ♦ **Cervical Myelopathy**

Examiner's note

In cervical myelopathy, the key features that make the diagnosis are present in the upper limbs. If asked to examine the upper limbs, inversion of bicep and suppinator reflexes coupled with dorsal column signs should point to the diagnosis. In the lower limbs, the main findings are that of spastic paraparesis with dorsal column signs, and making the diagnosis of cervical myelopathy from only lower limb signs is difficult. In such cases, it is important to consider the differential diagnosis for such a presentation, and exclude other causes using other clinical signs (see below). In the MRCP (PACES) examination, the common instruction is to examine the upper limbs or, less frequently, the lower limbs. The following case presentations reflect this.

CASE PRESENTATION (UPPER LIMBS)

On examination of the upper limbs, there are **fasciculations** with **segmental wasting and weakness**, corresponding to **C5-C7 nerve roots**.[1] The **bicep and supinator jerks are absent** with **inversion of reflexes** and the **tricep jerk is brisk**.[2] There is **sensory loss (to all modalities of sensation) in the C5–C7 dermatomes**.[3] When the eyes are closed, and the hands outstretched and supinated, there is abduction of the little finger (**myelopathy hand sign**)[4] and there is unconscious writhing of the fingers (**pseudoathetosis**).[5]

The diagnosis is **cervical myelopathy**.[6]

Clinical notes

1. The main segments of the cervical cord that are affected are C5–C7, and there are lower motor neurone signs at this level with segmental wasting and weakness corresponding to these nerve roots. The muscle groups commonly affected include biceps (elbow flexion), brachioradialis (forearm suppination), and deltoids (shoulder abduction). As the small muscles of the hands are supplied by C8–T1, wasting of the small muscles of the hands is uncommon. In some cases, wasting of the small muscles of the hands may be seen, and this reflects vascular changes in the cord below the lesion. Fasciculations are seen in lower motor neurone lesions, and may be noted in the upper limbs.

2. The bicep and supinator jerks (C5–C6) will be absent. Inversion refers to absence of response at the tested locations (biceps or brachioradialis) with reflex contraction of myotomes innervated by lower segments of the cord than that being tested (usually finger flexors or triceps). This may lead to the paradoxical response of elbow extension following biceps testing! The lower motor neurones and pyramidal tracts are damaged at C5–C6, producing lower motor neurone signs at C5–C6 and upper motor neurone signs below. The combination of inverted bicep and suppinator jerks (C5–C6) and brisk tricep jerk (C7–C8) is termed the 'mid-cervical reflex pattern'.

3. The sensory loss will have a dermatomal pattern, and thus it is necessary to specifically test each dermatome in turn. Remember, the main segments that are affected are C5–C7, although C8–T1 segments may be affected in some cases. The thumb, middle, and index fingers are supplied by C6, C7, and C8, respectively. A C8 area of numbness extends more proximally in the forearm than the area of numbness expected from an ulnar neuropathy.

4. The **'myelopathy hand sign'** is a sensitive sign of pyramidal weakness in the upper limbs. This has also been termed the **'finger escape sign'**, and is defined as deficient adduction and/or extension of the ulnar 2 or 3 fingers. This can also be seen in ulnar nerve palsy and sensory testing should help differentiate this. Other signs in the hands include:

   (a) **Grip and release test**: normal individuals can open and close the fist up to 20 times in 10 seconds. Patients with cervical myelopathy have difficulty performing this manoeuvre and opening and closing fist is slow, difficult, and incomplete.

   (b) **Dynamic Hoffman sign**: the Hoffman sign is evidence for an upper motor neurone lesion and can be elicited by nipping the nail of the middle finger and observing a reflex contraction of the thumb and index finger. If Hoffman sign is negative in the resting position, it can be tested during active flexion and extension of the cervical spine as tolerated by the patient, and it may become positive during these manoeuvres. This is the dynamic Hoffman's sign and can be useful in diagnosing early cervical spondylitic myelopathy.

5. Dorsal column signs include loss of vibration sense and proprioception. The loss of sensory feedback with cervical cord lesions results in unconscious writhing movements of the fingers with the eyes closed (pseudoathetosis)—a sign of dorsal column involvement.

6. Although cervical myelopathy is the most commonly used term, it can also be referred to as cervical myeloradiculopathy.

CASE PRESENTATION (LOWER LIMBS)

On examination of the lower limbs, there is **pyramidal weakness** *with* **hypertonia, hyperreflexia, ankle clonus,** *and* **extensor plantar responses.**[7] *There is* **impaired proprioception and vibration sense** *in the lower limbs. There is a* **wide-based 'scissor' gait.**[8] **Romberg's test is positive.**[9]

This patient has **spastic paraparesis with dorsal column signs.**[1]. *The differential diagnosis includes:*

(a) **Cervical myelopathy**
(b) *Friedreich's ataxia*
(c) *Multiple sclerosis*
(d) *Taboparesis*
(e) *Subacute combined degeneration of the cord*

Clinical notes

7. In the lower limbs, the key findings are spastic paraparesis and dorsal column signs. It is important to remember, that in cervical myelopathy, signs exceed symptoms and spasticity often exceeds the level of weakness.

8. The gait disturbance is a combination of spastic paraparesis and a sensory ataxia. The patients often watch the feet and ground carefully as they walk with visual input compensating for loss of joint position sense.

9. Visual input compensates for loss of joint position sense. Ask the patient to stand with their feet together, and close their eyes, thereby removing visual input. If they become unsteady, this is a positive Romberg's test. It is important to stand close to the patient, and be ready to support the patient should they become unsteady.

10. Patients classically present with a combination of lower motor neurone signs (upper limbs) and upper motor neurone signs (lower limbs). This can be seen in cervical cord lesions, i.e. cervical myelopathy, and motor neurone disease. However, the presence of sensory signs excludes the latter. It is important to remember the differential diagnosis of spastic paraparesis and dorsal column signs, and be aware of the additional signs supportive of each diagnosis:

Causes of spastic paraparesis and dorsal column signs	Absent ankle jerks and extensor plantars	Additional features to look for
Cervical myelopathy	No	LMN signs in upper limbs, inversion of reflexes, neck collar*
Friedreich's ataxia	Yes	Pes cavus, kyphoscoliosis, cerebellar signs
Multiple sclerosis	No	Cerebellar signs, optic atrophy
Taboparesis	Yes	Argyll Robertson pupils
Subacute combined degeneration	Yes	Peripheral neuropathy (stocking distribution); anaemia; jaundice; glossitis; splenomegaly

* If the patient is wearing a neck collar, then this may suggest a diagnosis of cervical spondylosis and thus cervical myelopathy. Other indirect signs that may suggest degenerative disc disease are evidence of osteoarthritis, rheumatoid arthritis, and ankylosing spondylitis. It is therefore important to look at the patient and make a quick observation of hands, spine, and posture.

Questions commonly asked by examiners

What is the pathophysiology of cervical myelopathy?

The normal cervical spinal canal is 17–18mm in diameter (C3–C7). It accommodates the nerves, meninges, ligaments, and epidural fat. The most common aetiology of cervical myelopathy is canal stenosis. Congenitally narrow canals lower the threshold at which trivial trauma or degenerative changes encroach upon the spinal cord and resulting in cervical myelopathy. Causes of cervical myelopathy include:

- Cervical degenerative disc disease or spondylosis (most common)*
- Cervical cord tumours
- Ossification of the posterior longitudinal ligament
- Trauma

How would you investigate this patient?

Plain cervical X-rays (AP, lateral, and oblique)	Evaluate intervertebral disc spaces, facet joints, osteophyte formation and absolute sagittal diameter of the spinal canal.
Cervical myelography	Myelography with CT scanning is the best imaging test to assess spinal and foraminal stenosis. It is an invasive procedure involving intrathecal injection of a radio-opaque dye, and exposure to ionizing radiation. Therefore an MRI is preferred, and cervical myelography is used if there are contraindications to MRI.
MRI of the cervical cord	This is non-invasive and the preferred imaging modality to diagnose cervical spondylosis.

What is the treatment for cervical myelopathy?

Non-surgical treatment
- Simple analgesics
- Cervical intra-articular steroid injections
- Facet joint nerve blocks
- Physiotherapy: cervical neck collars, isometric cervical exercises
- Occupational therapy
- Psychosocial support

Surgical treatment
- Decompressive Discectomy and Foraminotomy
- Hemilaminectomy
- Laminoplasty

---

* This is the pathogenic factor in 55% of cervical myelopathy cases. Young adults may have few or no neck symptoms or signs (due to a so called 'soft' disc). Primary osteoarthritis is the commonest cause of this, but there also associations with conditions such as rheumatoid arthritis, ankylosing spondylitis, acromegaly, or achondroplasia. Degenerative cascades and narrowing of intervertebral disc space results in a decrease in height of the disc and a resultant increase in sagittal diameter with bulging of the disc into the canal. Reactive hyperostosis results in formation of osteophytes, and these can project posteriorly into the canal, thus reducing the space available for the cord and its blood supply.

Case 54 ◆ **Nystagmus**

1. Cerebellar nystagmus

CASE PRESENTATION

This patient has a **horizontal nystagmus** *with a* **fast component to the right**. *There is loss of smooth pursuit (broken pursuit). The saccadic eye movements are abnormal with hypermetric saccades.*

This is a *cerebellar nystagmus*, **with a** *right-sided cerebellar lesion.*

Clinical notes

1. A cerebellar nystagmus is a coarse horizontal nystagmus with the fast component towards the side of the lesion.
2. It is important to look for other cerebellar eye signs, i.e. broken pursuit and ocular dysmetria with hypo- or hypermetric saccades.
3. If other cerebellar eye signs cannot be demonstrated, then the differential diagnosis for the above findings would be:
    (a) Right-sided cerebellar lesion (fast component *towards* the side of the lesion)
    (b) Left-sided vestibular lesion (fast component *away* from the side of the lesion)
    Besides looking for the absence or presence of other cerebellar eye signs, there are other features one can look for to discriminate cerebellar and vestibular nystagmus (see below).

2. Vestibular nystagmus

CASE PRESENTATION 1

This patient has a **horizontal nystagmus** *with a* **fast component to the left**. *The nystagmus* **increases on left gaze**, *i.e.* **uni-directional**. *The nystagmus is* **suppressed by visual fixation** *and* **adapts to continued gaze**.

This is a **vestibular nystagmus**, *with a* **right-sided peripheral vestibular lesion**.

CASE PRESENTATION 2

This patient has **horizontal nystagmus** *with a* **fast component to the left on left gaze** *and a* **fast component to the right on right gaze**, *i.e.* **bi-directional**. *The nystagmus is* **not suppressed by visual fixation** *and* **persists on continued gaze**.

This is a **vestibular nystagmus**, *with a* **central vestibular lesion**.

Clinical notes

1. Vestibular nystagmus can be peripheral or central. Peripheral vestibular nystagmus can be mixed horizontal-rotatory or purely horizontal (never vertical). Central vestibular nystagmus can be horizontal, vertical, rotatory, or mixed.

2. Peripheral vestibular nystagmus is always unidirectional, and the fast component is away from the side of the lesion. Central vestibular nystagmus is often bi-directional, but can be uni-directional.

3. Alexander's law states that for:

   (a) **Peripheral vestibular nystagmus**: the nystagmus increases towards the direction of the fast component

   (b) **Central vestibular nystagmus**: the fast component changes with the direction of gaze, thus the nystagmus is left-beating on left gaze, right-beating on right gaze and up-beating on upward gaze

   Based on the above, the side of the vestibular lesion can easily be determined for peripheral vestibular nystagmus. As central vestibular nystagmus is bi-directional, the side of the lesion cannot easily be determined.

4. There are a number of important differences between *peripheral* and *central* vestibular nystagmus:

	Peripheral	Central
Oscillatory movements	Horizontal-rotatory Horizontal	Horizontal Vertical Rotatory Mixed
Direction	Always uni-directional	Bi-directional (can be unidirectional)
Fast component	Fixed; away from the side of lesion	Changes with direction of gaze
Visual fixation	Suppresses nystagmus	No effect
Continued gaze	Suppresses nystagmus (fatiguable)	No effect
Vertigo	Often present	Absent
Tinnitus and deafness	Often present	Absent
Tendency to fall	Uni-directional (towards the lesion)	Often multi-directional
Causes	Labyrinthitis Meniere's disease Acoustic neuroma Degenerative middle ear diseases Benign positional vertigo	Brainstem tumours Brainstem infarction Demyelination Syringobulbia Meningoencephalitis Alcohol

3. Ataxic nystagmus (internuclear ophthalmoplegia)

CASE PRESENTATION

This patient has dissociation of conjugate eye movements. Abduction is normal with **impairment of adduction** *in both eyes. There is* **nystagmus in the abducting eye**. *When the abducting eye is covered, adduction of the opposite eye is normal. There is* **diplopia** *in both directions of lateral gaze.*

This is **bilateral internuclear ophthalmoplegia**, *characterized by* **lesion in the medial longitudinal fasciculus**. *The most likely cause is demyelinating disease.*

Clinical notes

1. It results in weakness of adduction of the ipsilateral eye, with nystagmus on abduction of the contralateral eye. The key feature is weakness of ipsilateral adduction, and the nystagmus may or may not

be present. The impaired adduction on attempted horizontal gaze may be complete (the eye does not move past the mid-point), partial (the eye incompletely adducts, or adducts slower than normal speed). This results in dissociation of conjugate eye movements. The adduction becomes normal when the contralateral (abducting) eye is covered. This may be associated with diplopia.

2. Internuclear ophthalmoplegia is due to a lesion in the medial longitudinal fasciculus. Multiple sclerosis is the most common cause, and often causes bilateral internuclear ophthalmoplegia (unilateral is less common in multiple sclerosis). Myasthenia gravis can produce a pseudo- unilateral or bilateral internuclear ophthalmoplegia. Other causes include:

- Infarction
- Tumour
- Aneurysm
- Vasculitis
- Syphilis
- Trauma
- Wernicke's encephalopathy
- Arnold-Chiari malformation
- Drugs (tricyclic anti-depressants, phenytoin, barbiturates)

4. Pendular nystagmus

CASE PRESENTATION

*This patient has **horizontal, vertical, and rotatory nystagmus**, i.e. **multi-directional**. The **oscillations are of equal amplitude and velocity**, and there are **no fast and slow components**. The patient is **blind**.*

*This is a **pendular nystagmus (visual deprivation pendular nystagmus)**.*

Clinical notes

1. The most common form of pendular nystagmus is seen in patients who are blind. It is important to check for this. This is termed '**visual deprivation pendular nystagmus**'.

5. Downbeat nystagmus

CASE PRESENTATION

*This patient has **vertical nystagmus** that **beats downwards in the primary position**. The nystagmus **increases with downward and lateral gaze**.*

*This is a **downbeat nystagmus**, commonly associated with pathology at the level of the **foramen magnum**.*

Clinical notes

1. The fast component is in the downward direction.
2. With the eyes in this position, the nystagmus appears to be directed obliquely and downwards.

3. This has localizing value, and commonly indicates pathology at the level of the foramen magnum:
   - Arnold-Chiari malformation
   - Tumours
   - Syringobulbia
   - Platybasia
   - Spinocerebellar degeneration
   - Vertebrobasilar infarction
4. Other less common causes of downbeat nystagmus include:
   - Hypomagnesaemia
   - Wernicke's encephalopathy
   - Alcohol (acute or chronic)
   - Vitamin B12 deficiency
   - Lithium toxicity
   - Anticonvulsants (phenytoin, carbamazepine)

6. Upbeat nystagmus

CASE PRESENTATION

This patient has **vertical nystagmus** *that* **beats upwards in the primary position**. *The nystagmus* **increases on upward gaze**.

This is an **upbeat nystagmus**, *suggestive of a lesion in the* **anterior vermis of the cerebellum**.

Clinical notes

1. The fast component is in the upward direction. It is important to remember that convergence may enhance the nystagmus or convert to downbeat nystagmus.
2. Upbeat nystagmus can be classified as follows and has localizing value:
   (a) Increases on **UPWARD** gaze: **anterior vermis of the cerebellum**
   (b) Increases on **DOWNWARD** gaze: **medulla**
3. Other causes of upbeat nystagmus (where the location of the lesion is uncertain) include:
   - Organophosphate poisoning
   - Anticonvulsants (phenytoin and carbamazepine)
   - Wernicke's encephalopathy
   - Encephalitis
   - Meningitis

Questions commonly asked by examiners

What do you understand by the term 'jerk nystagmus'?

This is where the oscillations of the eyes are asymmetrical, i.e. the speed of oscillation to one side is slower than the speed of oscillation to the other side.

What do you understand by the term 'gaze-evoked nystagmus'?

This is a jerk nystagmus that occurs only when the eye are moved into eccentric gaze. This is the most common form of nystagmus encountered in clinical practice. Common types of gaze-evoked nystagmus include:

- Physiological nystagmus
- Cerebellar nystagmus
- Gaze-paretic nystagmus

What is physiological nystagmus?

This is also called 'end-point nystagmus' and occurs when a person looks beyond 40 degrees. It is a low amplitude horizontal nystagmus with the rapid component directed laterally. On looking laterally, the elastic pull of the stretched eye muscles and tendons pull the eyes centripetally towards the neutral position (slow phase). To overcome this, a gaze-holding network called the neural integrator generates a signal which results in a tonic contraction of the extraocular eye muscles and a rapid corrective movement back towards the direction of desired gaze (fast phase). Physiological nystagmus is an example of gaze-evoked nystagmus. Features differentiating a physiological from a pathological gaze-evoked nystagmus are:

Differentiating features	Physiological	Pathological
Amplitude	Smaller (<4 degrees)	Larger (>4 degrees)
Asymmetry in 2 directions of gaze	No	Yes
Other ocular abnormalities	Absent	Present

What is convergence-retraction nystagmus?

This is a manifestation of a dorsal midbrain syndrome (Parinaud syndrome). Convergence movements are saccadic, and therefore it is not a true nystagmus. Fast divergent eye movements are followed by slow convergent eye movements.

What is a seesaw nystagmus?

This is a pendular oscillation that consists of elevation and intorsion of one eye and depression and extorsion of the other eye that alternates every half cycle. This form of nystagmus is seen in patients with chiasmal lesions (loss of crossed visual inputs from the decussating fibres of the optic nerve at the level of the chiasm), and is therefore associated with bitemporal hemianopia.

What is a periodic alternating nystagmus?

This is a horizontal jerk nystagmus with the fast phase beating in one direction for 1–2 minutes, followed by an intervening neutral phase of 10–20 seconds and then the nystagmus beats in the opposite direction for 1–2 minutes and the cycle repeats itself. This is associated with disease in the midline cerebellum.

What is a gaze-paretic nystagmus?

This occurs secondary to weakness of the eye muscles to maintain an eccentric gaze position. This can be seen during the recovery phase of gaze palsies, myasthenia gravis, and Miller-Fisher syndrome. The recovery is sufficient to make conjugate eye movements, but not sufficient to maintain eye position. Following the initial saccadic eye movements, the eyes drift back towards the primary position, and rapid saccadic movements bring the eye back towards the direction of desired gaze.

Case 55 ◆ **Ophthalmoplegia**

Examiner's note

The most common instruction at this station is 'examine the cranial nerves'. It is important to remember, that ophthalmoplegia due to a specific nerve palsy may not be an isolated finding, and it may form part of multiple cranial neuropathies, or brainstem syndromes. It is not uncommon for candidates to miss other cranial nerve signs, after having made a diagnosis of a gaze palsy. The most common gaze palsies in the MRCP (PACES) examinations are VI and III nerve palsies. Although IV nerve palsy has been reported to occur, it is far less common. It is important to remember that myasthenia gravis can mimic specific gaze palsies, and it is important to look for this.

CASE PRESENTATION 1

This patient has a left **convergent strabismus** *at rest.[1] There is* **impaired abduction** *of the left eye.[2] There is* **diplopia**, *which is maximal on left* **lateral gaze**.[3] *Cover testing reveals that the outermost image comes from the left eye.[4]*

The diagnosis is a left **VI nerve palsy**.[5]

Clinical notes

1. Look at the eyes in the primary position. Note the position of each eye, in particular whether they are further apart than normal (divergent strabismus) or closer together than normal (convergent strabismus). The convergent strabismus of a sixth nerve palsy is due to unopposed action of the medial rectus muscle. In certain cases, the convergent strabismus may not be evident.
2. The VI nerve supplies the lateral rectus, leaving an isolated abduction deficit. This is easy to recognize.
3. Diplopia is worst on looking to the affected side.
4. In subtle cases, the eye movements may appear grossly intact. In such cases, the horizontal diplopia should alert one to suspect the diagnosis. If there is diplopia on left lateral gaze, then this could result from weakness of abduction of the left eye (lateral rectus) or weakness of adduction of the right eye (medial rectus). Cover testing is useful in this situation, as the outermost image comes from the affected eye.
5. Having made the diagnosis, provide a differential diagnosis:
   (a) Raised intracranial pressure
   (b) Inflammation: multiple sclerosis, sarcoidosis, giant cell arteritis
   (c) Infection: Lyme disease, syphilis
   (d) Neoplasm: pontine tumour
   (e) Vascular lesions: infarct, haemorrhage, basilar artery aneurysm
   (f) Cavernous sinus lesion: tumour, infection, thrombosis, and aneurysm
   (g) Subacute meningitis: carcinomatous, lymphomatous, fungal, tuberculous
   (h) Trauma
   (i) Mononeuritis multiplex*

---

* Diabetes, Polyarteritis nodosa, Churg-Strauss syndrome, Wegner's granulomatosis, Rheumatoid arthritis, SLE, Sjogren's syndrome, Sarcoidosis, Lymphoma, Carcinoma, Amyloidosis, Lyme disease, Leprosy

CASE PRESENTATION 2

This patient has **ptosis** *on the right.[1] There is a right* **divergent strabismus at rest***. The right eye movements are impaired and the* **eye is fixed in a down and out position.**[2] *The right* **pupil is fixed and dilated***.[3] There is diplopia, which is maximal on left superior gaze (***angulated diplopia***).[4]*

The diagnosis is a right **III nerve palsy***.[5]*

Clinical notes

The cell bodies for axons that travel in the occulomotor (III) nerve are located in the nucleus in the brainstem. The axons that are destined for each of the muscles originate from a specific subnucleus. The clinical signs in III nerve palsy are ipsilateral to the side of the lesion, as most axons of the muscles supplied are uncrossed from the nucleus to the eye. However, there are 2 exceptions:

- Levator palpebrae superioris is supplied from BOTH sides, i.e. crossed and uncrossed pathways from central caudal subnucleus.
- The superior rectus muscle is supplied from the superior rectus nucleus from the CON-TRALATERAL side.

Anatomically, the occulomotor nerve has a nuclear portion (contains cell bodies) that gives rise to the fascicular portion (contains axons). The fascicular portion can be further divided according to its anatomical course (intraparenchymal brainstem, subarachnoid, cavernous sinus, and orbital). Fascicular III nerve palsy is much more common than a nuclear III palsy. Fascicular III nerve palsy results in IPSILATERAL signs for all affected III nerve muscles, but in nuclear III nerve palsy, there is additional involvement of the superior rectus and levator palpebrae superioris on the contralateral side.

1. Involvement of the levator palpebrae superioris results in ptosis (often complete). The pupil is often covered as a result of this, and therefore when examining eye movements, it is important to lift the eyelid gently. In cases of a nuclear III nerve palsy, where the nucleus is affected, there may be partial ptosis on the contralateral side. This is because there is bilateral innervation and the axons for the levator palpebrae come from both sides of the central caudal subnucleus. In such cases, the ptosis is more complete ipsilateral to the side of the lesion.

2. The horizontal deviation is divergent due to weakness of the medial rectus. Vertical deviation occurs due to weakness of the superior rectus, inferior oblique (both elevators) and inferior rectus (depressor). The superior oblique is intact (IV nerve), and thus the eye is fixed in a down and out position. In cases of a nuclear III nerve palsy, there may be a weakness of elevation of the contralateral eye. This is because the superior rectus muscle is supplied from the superior rectus subnucleus on the contralateral side. The superior rectus nucleus output is totally contralateral with fascicles from the subnucleus on one side crossing through the subnucleus on the opposite side to the superior rectus muscle. A lesion of the superior rectus subnucleus results in bilateral superior rectus palsy. The eye contralateral to the side of the lesion is affected due to loss of cell bodies in the affected nucleus. The eye ipsilateral to the side of the lesion is affected due to involvement of the fascicles (that originate from the cell bodies of the subnucleus on the opposite side, but pass through diseased nucleus on the affected side). Thus a lesion of the superior rectus subnucleus causes bilateral elevation palsy.

3. If the pupil is affected, then this suggests involvement of the parasympathetic nerve fibres that originate from the Edinger-Westphal nucleus. This often results from extrinsic compressive lesions as these autonomic fibres are situated very superficially in the nerve trunk, and if the pupil is affected, it is termed a 'surgical III nerve palsy'. If the pupil is spared, it is termed a 'medical III nerve palsy'.

4. The diplopia is angulated, and maximal looking up and out.

5. Having made a diagnosis, provide a differential diagnosis:
   (a) Brainstem lesion: tumour, infarct, haemorrhage, and demyelination
   (b) Cavernous sinus lesion: tumour, infection, thrombosis, and aneurysm
   (c) Tentorial herniation
   (d) Posterior communicating artery aneurysm
   (e) Superior orbital fissure lesion: trauma, tumour, and granuloma
   (f) Subacute meningitis: carcinomatous, lymphomatous, fungal, and tuberculous
   (g) Mononeuritis multiplex

CASE PRESENTATION 3

The right eye is higher than the left eye in primary gaze.[1] With this, there is impairment of right eye movements, where the **adducted eye cannot look down***. There is* **vertical (angulated) diplopia***, which is* **maximal on looking down and away from the affected side***.[2] Cover testing reveals that the outermost image comes from the right eye.[3]*

The diagnosis is a right **IV nerve palsy***.[4]*

Clinical notes

1. The trochlear nerve supplies the superior oblique muscle, which causes the eye to look in and down. The affected eye appears higher in primary gaze due to weakness of the superior oblique muscle.
2. The diplopia is vertical or oblique. Patients may adopt a characteristic head tilt AWAY from the affected side to reduce the diplopia. Some patients may tilt their head towards the affected side, thus creating a wider separation between the images, and allows the patient to ignore one image! This is termed the 'paradoxical head tilt'.
3. In subtle cases, the eye movements may appear grossly intact. In such cases, the vertical diplopia should alert one to suspect the diagnosis, as IV nerve palsy is the most common cause for a vertical diplopia. Cover testing is useful in this situation, as the outermost image comes from the affected eye.
4. Having made the diagnosis, provide a differential diagnosis:
   (a) Trauma (most common)
   (b) Brainstem lesion: tumour, infarct, haemorrhage, and demyelination
   (c) Cavernous sinus lesion: tumour, infection, thrombosis, and aneurysm
   (d) Mononeuritis multiplex
   (e) Congenital

CASE PRESENTATION 4

This patient has **diplopia on looking to the right***. The eye movements appear to be grossly intact. The pupils are normal. Cover testing reveals that the outermost image comes from the left eye.*

This would suggest **impairment of the left medial rectus muscle***, and does not fit with a specific cranial neuropathy. The differential diagnosis would be:*

(a) Myopathies, e.g. Graves' ophthalmopathy
(b) Muscular dystrophies, e.g. occulopharyngeal dystrophy
(c) Myasthenia gravis

(d) *Miller-Fisher syndrome*
(e) *Myositis, e.g. orbital myositis*
(f) *Chronic progressive external ophthalmoplegia*
(g) *Trauma*

Clinical notes

This is a common problem encountered by candidates, where the occulomotor deficit and ophthalmoplegia does not fit with a specific gaze (cranial nerve) palsy. In such situations, it is important to remember that pathologies at the level of muscle or neuromuscular junction can present this way. The above case presentation lists a useful differential diagnosis.

In the above case presentation, there is a defect in adduction, and this raises the possibility of internuclear ophthalmoplegia. This would typically be associated with nystagmus in the abducting (opposite) eye, although this can be absent (remember, it is a failure of adduction that characterizes internuclear ophthalmoplegia). A useful way of differentiating internuclear ophthalmoplegia from other causes is to remember that in internuclear ophthalmoplegia, the adduction becomes normal when the contralateral (abducting) eye is covered.

Questions commonly asked by examiners

What are the main structures in the cavernous sinus?
- Cranial nerves: III, IV, VI, Va, and Vb
- Sympathetic carotid plexus
- Intracavernous carotid artery

What are the causes of a cavernous sinus syndrome?
- Thrombosis
- Aneurysms
  - Intracavernous carotid artery
  - Posterior communicating artery
- Carotico-cavernous fistula
- Tumours
  - Primary: meningioma, neurofibroma, nasopharyngeal carcinoma (direct extension)
  - Secondary: breast, lung, prostate
- Trauma
- Inflammation
  - Herpes zoster
  - Tuberculosis
  - Sinusitis
  - Sarcoidosis
  - Wegner's granulomatosis
  - Tolosa-Hunt syndrome

What clinical features are associated with cavernous sinus lesions?
- Unilateral III, IV, and VI nerve palsies
- Sensory loss in Va and Vb nerve distribution
- Loss of corneal reflex
- Painful ophthalmoplegia

- Proptosis (pulsating exophthalmos suggests a carotico-cavernous fistula)
- Conjunctival congestion
- Visual loss
- Papilloedema
- Retinal haemorrhages

What are the causes of upgaze palsy?

- Progressive supranuclear palsy
- Graves' ophthalmopathy
- Myasthenia gravis
- Miller-Fisher syndrome
- Muscular dystrophy
- Chronic progressive external ophthalmoplegia
- Parinaud syndrome

What do you know about Parinaud syndrome?

This is also known as 'dorsal midbrain syndrome' resulting from a lesion of the superior colliculus. Causes include pineal tumour, midbrain infarct or haemorrhage, hydrocephalus, and demyelination. Key features include:

- Upgaze palsy
- Loss of accommodation and light reflex
- Preserved convergence reflex
- Convergence retraction nystagmus
- Mydriasis

What do you know about aberrant regeneration following a complete III nerve palsy?

'Aberrant regeneration' also known as 'occulomotor misdirection' refers to abnormal and incomplete recovery that may follow a complete III nerve palsy, most commonly due to trauma or posterior communicating artery aneurysm. This classically results in:

- Adduction on attempted upgaze
- Lid retraction on attempted downgaze (pseudo-Graefe sign)
- Lid retraction on attempted adduction (horizontal gaze-eyelid synkinesis)
- Miosis on attempted adduction (pseudo-Argyll Robertson pupil)*

What do you know about primary progressive occulomotor misdirection?

This is where features of aberrant regeneration progressively occur, but without a history of complete III nerve palsy. This is characteristic of an intracavernous meningioma.

What is the mechanism of ophthalmoplegia in progressive supranuclear palsy?

Although voluntary eye movements cannot be elicited, if the patient is allowed to fixate on a point and the head is passively moved (Doll's head manoeuvre), the eyes display full range of movement within the orbit. This suggests that the occulomotor nuclei are intact, and that it is the descending supranuclear control of voluntary eye movements that is impaired.

What is chronic progressive external ophthalmoplegia?

This is characterized by slow progressive paralysis of extraocular muscles. Patients experience bilateral, symmetrical, and progressive ptosis followed by ophthalmoplegia (months to years later).

---

* This resembles the Argyll Robertson pupil, as the pupil is unreactive to light, but accommodation reflex is preserved. Miosis can occur with any direction of gaze, but it is seen most often with adduction.

The ciliary and iris muscles are not involved. Unilateral or asymmetric ptosis may develop. In some cases, ophthalmoplegia can occur without ptosis. It is the most frequent manifestation of mitochondrial myopathies, and may be associated with skeletal muscle weakness. Due to the symmetrical nature of this disorder, some patients may not complain of diplopia.

---

* Subtle hemiparesis may be observed by asking the patient to hold both arms outstretched with the palms facing upwards. Slight pronation and downward drift of the outstretched arm are sensitive indicators of even very mild hemiparesis.

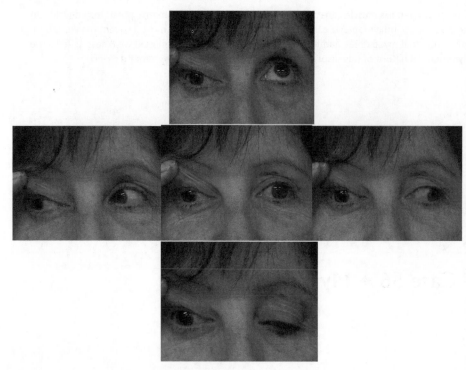

Figure 55.1 Right III nerve palsy as seen in different directions of gaze.
Reproduced from Sundaram et al. Training in Ophthalmology. 2009, with permission from Oxford University Press.

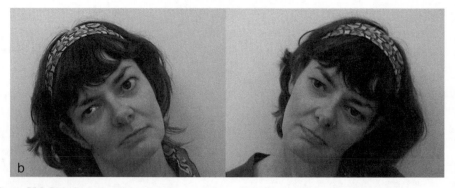

Figure 55.2 Right IV nerve palsy. In the primary position, the right eye is higher than the left eye (hypertropia), and there is vertical (angulated) diplopia. A head tilt to the left reduces the hypertropia with reduction in diplopia.
Reproduced from Sundaram et al. Training in Ophthalmology. 2009, with permission from Oxford University Press.

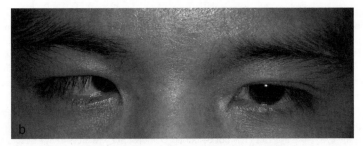

Figure 55.3 Right VI nerve palsy with the eyes in the primary position of gaze.
Reproduced from Sundaram et al. Training in Ophthalmology. 2009, with permission from Oxford University Press.

Case 56 ♦ **Myasthenia Gravis**

CASE PRESENTATION

This patient has **variable ptosis** *that is* **accentuated by sustained upgaze** *and* **improves following eye closure** *for a short period.*[1] *There is* **furrowing of the forehead** *to compensate for this weakness.*[2] *There is weakness of the occulomotor muscles with* **variable strabismus** *and* **diplopia.**[3]

There is **bilateral facial muscle weakness**, *with* **lack of facial expression**[4] *and a horizontal smile* **(myasthenic snarl).**[5] *There is* **jaw weakness** *and the jaw hangs open.*[6] *There is* **weakness of the neck muscles.**[7] *The patient sits with the hands under the chin to support the weak jaw and neck* **(jaw supporting sign).**[8] *The* **voice is weak** *with a* **nasal twang**, *and with prolonged vocalization, the speech becomes less distinct and more nasal.*[9]

On examination of the limbs, there is **proximal weakness** *with* **fatiguability.**[10] *There is no wasting. Deep tendon reflexes are normal. The sensation is normal.*[11]

The diagnosis is **myasthenia gravis.**[12]

Clinical notes

1. Ptosis is often unilateral but can be bilateral. If bilateral it is often asymmetrical. Muscle fatiguability can be demonstrated with ptosis: sustained upgaze increases eyelid weakness, whereas resting the eyelid by closure for a short period improves the weakness. After looking down for a short period (thus resting the eyelid muscles), the upper lid may overshoot and for an instant appear slightly retracted when the patient performs a saccade back to the primary position (because the eyelid weakness improves). This is the **'Cogan lid twitch sign'**.

2. Patients furrow the forehead, utilizing the frontalis muscle to compensate for the ptosis. This will be unilateral if the ptosis is unilateral.

3. Typically, the weakness of the extraocular muscles is asymmetrical, affects more than 1 extraocular muscle and is not limited to muscles innervated by a single cranial nerve. Weakness of both medial and lateral rectus muscles can result in a **'pseudo-internuclear ophthalmoplegia'** (weakness of adduction

of one eye with nystagmus in the abducting eye). An important feature in myasthenia gravis is that with sustained lateral gaze, the medial rectus of the adducting eye fatigues, and thus the nystagmus becomes coarser in the abducting eye. Remember, in true internuclear ophthalmoplegia, adduction becomes normal when the abducting eye is covered, and this will not be the case in myasthenia gravis. Fluttering of the ptotic eyelid may be seen during eye movements (**'lid hopping'**). Saccadic slowing may be seen due to fatiguability following repeated eye movements, and the saccades may have increased duration. This is termed **'intrasaccadic fatigue'**.

4. Bilateral weakness of the facial muscles is almost always present. This results in an expressionless face. It is important to demonstrate facial weakness by testing the facial muscle groups. Ask the patient to close the eyes—the eyelashes will not be buried. Demonstrate weakness of eye closure by asking the patient to close the eyes tight—this can be easily overcome using your finger and thumb. The **'peek sign'** has been described in myasthenia gravis—the eyes drift open to reveal the sclera during attempted eye closure. Ask the patient to seal the lips and inflate and keep the cheeks out—this may be easily overcome and air readily escapes through the lips when the cheeks are squeezed. In severe facial weakness, the lips cannot be easily opposed.

5. A 'myasthenic snarl' may be observed when the patient is asked to smile. This results because whilst there is contraction of the middle portion of the upper lip, the upper mouth corners fail to contract.

6. Demonstrate weakness of mouth opening by asking the patient to keep the mouth open—this can be easily overcome by applying gentle upward pressure on the chin. Jaw opening muscles often display normal strength, and jaw closure muscles are more frequently affected. This can be tested by exerting a sustained downward pressure on the chin while asking the patient to keep the jaw closed.

7. Weakness of neck muscles is common. The neck flexors are more severely affected than the extensors.

8. The jaw-supporting sign if present is pathognomic of myasthenia gravis. This may not be present at the beginning of the examination, but may become more evident later through the examination with fatiguability.

9. Weakness of the palatal muscles results in a weak and nasal quality speech. This may not be evident in the beginning. Ask the patient to count out loud—with progressive fatiguability the speech will become less distinct and more nasal.

10. Examination of the limbs will demonstrate proximal muscle weakness without wasting. Upper limb muscles are more likely to be affected than the lower limb muscles. Demonstrate fatiguability at the deltoid muscle by first testing shoulder abduction, and then asking the patient to repeatedly abduct and adduct the shoulder (usually 10–15 times). Then, re-test shoulder abduction, and in patients with fatiguable weakness, there will be marked increase in deltoid weakness. Alternatively, fatiguability can be demonstrated in a similar fashion for elbow extension. Avoid demonstrating fatiguability for elbow flexion, for 2 reasons: (a) in myasthenia gravis, the triceps are more likely to be affected than biceps, and (b) triceps are weaker than biceps, thus weakness is easier to demonstrate in the examination setting.

11. Sensory testing is normal in myasthenia gravis. It is important to be aware of other associated autoimmune diseases that may result in a neuropathy.

12. Tell the examiner that you would like to:
    (a) Look for evidence of **immunosuppressive therapy,** i.e. steroids (steroid purpura, cushingoid appearance)
    (b) Look for a **thymectomy scar**
    (c) Look for features of other associated **autoimmune diseases** (seen in 10% of patients):
        * **Hyperthyroidism**: tachycardia, tremor, goitre, features of Graves' disease (most common association)
        * **Hypothyroidism**: bradycardia, slow-relaxing ankle jerks, goitre
        * **Diabetes**: diabetic finger tip skin pricks (glucose testing), diabetic retinopathy, neuropathy
        * **SLE**: butterfly rash, arthropathy
        * **Rheumatoid arthritis**: symmetrical deforming arthropathy

- ◆ **Pernicious anaemia**: pallor, splenomegaly, neuropathy
- ◆ **Pemphigus**: flaccid blisters, oral lesions
(d) Take a detailed *drug history* (considering possibility of drug induced myasthenic syndrome)

Features of certain systemic diseases, e.g. rheumatoid arthritis may be clearly evident at inspection. In such cases, in the final presentation, a comment can be made about the presence of other autoimmune disease(s). This will impress examiners!

Questions commonly asked by examiners

What is the pathophysiology of myasthenia gravis?

This is an autoimmune disorder characterized by antibodies directed against the nicotinic acetylcholine receptors (nAChR) on the post-synaptic membranes of the neuromuscular junction. This results in impairment of neuromuscular transmission in the following ways:

- Complement-mediated destruction of the nAChRs
- Complement-mediated damage with resultant loss of normal folds of the post-synaptic membrane, thus decrease in area for insertion of newly synthesized nAChRs
- Functional blockade of nAChRs
- Accelerated endocytosis and breakdown of nAChRs
- Cross-linking 2 adjacent nAChRs by anti-AChR antibody

What the two broad clinical classifications for myasthenia gravis?

- Ocular myasthenia gravis (15%)—weakness is confined to the eyelids and extraocular muscles
- Generalized myasthenia gravis (85%)—generalized weakness

What proportion of patients have anti-nAChR antibodies?

The anti-AChR antibody is found in 80–90% of patients with myasthenia gravis (seropositive), whilst in the remaining population of patients such an antibody cannot be identified (seronegative). Seronegative patients often have ocular myasthenia gravis. More recently, it has been shown that most seronegative patients have antibodies against muscle-specific kinase (MuSK), which plays an important role in differentiation and clustering of nAChRs at the post-synaptic membrane. Patients with MuSK antibodies are usually female with prominent neck, bulbar, and respiratory weakness.

What drugs can exacerbate weakness in myasthenia gravis?

- Penicillamine
- Aminoglycosides
- Fluoroquinolones
- Macrolides
- β-blockers
- Calcium antagonists
- Quinine
- Quinidine
- Procainamide
- Lithium
- Phenytoin
- Lignocaine

If this patient has rheumatoid arthritis, what are the potential links?
- Association with autoimmune diseases (myasthenia gravis and rheumatoid arthritis)
- Penicillamine-induced myasthenia gravis (treatment of rheumatoid arthritis)

What other conditions may present in a similar fashion to myasthenia gravis?
- Botulism
- Lambert-Eaton myasthenic syndrome (LEMS)
- Mitochondrial myopathy (chronic progressive external ophthalmoplegia)
- Miller-Fisher syndrome
- Snake bites (cobra, kraits, and coral snakes)

What are the differences between LEMS and myasthenia gravis?

	Myasthenia gravis	Lambert-Eaton myasthenic syndrome
Antigenic target	Post-synaptic nAChR	Pre-synaptic V-gated Ca^{2+} channel
Diplopia	Common	Rare
Ptosis	Common	Rare
Tendon reflexes	Normal	Reduced ($\uparrow$ with exercise)
Weakness	Proximal weakness (upper LIMB (UL)>lower LIMB (LL))	Proximal weakness (LL>UL)
Autonomic dysfunction	No	Yes (cholinergic disturbance)
Associations	Autoimmune diseases	Small cell lung carcinoma (60% of cases) Autoimmune diseases
Female: male ratio	2:1	1:2
Single nerve stimulation	Normal	Decreased amplitude
Repetitive nerve stimulation	Decrement (3Hz stimulation)	Increment (20Hz stimulation)
Treatment	Acteycholinesterase inhibitors Immunotherapy	Treatment of tumour 3,4-diaminopyridine

What are the causes of a false positive tensilon test?
- Motor neurone disease
- Poliomyelitis
- Lambert-Eaton myasthenic syndrome
- Guillain Barré syndrome
- Myositis
- Botulism

What are the causes of false positive nAChR antibodies?
- First-degree relatives of patients with myasthenia gravis
- Motor neurone disease
- Lambert-Eaton myasthenic syndrome
- Thyroid ophthalmopathy
- Autoimmune hepatitis

- Primary biliary cirrhosis
- SLE
- Rheumatoid arthritis
- Penicillamine therapy

What do you know about the 'ice pack test'?

An ice pack is applied to the ptotic eyelid for 2–5 minutes, and improvement of ptosis is noted. This test has high sensitivity and specificity, but may be difficult for patients to tolerate.

What is Hering's law?

In patients with myasthenia gravis, when a ptotic eyelid is lifted manually, there is no longer a requirement for excessive eyelid innervation, and a result of reduction in eyelid innervation the other eyelid becomes ptotic.

What treatment options are available for myasthenia gravis?

Acteycholinesterase inhibitors

This is a symptomatic therapy and does not affect the disease process. Side-effects relate to increased muscarinic activity and include nausea, vomiting, abdominal cramps, diarrhoea, diaphoresis, increased lacrimation, salivation, and bronchial secretions.

Immunosuppressive therapy

Steroids are the most commonly used agents. Steroids may produce a transient increase in myasthenic weakness in up to 15% of patients, lasting up to 10 days, after which the strength improves. Steroid sparing agents include azathioprine, cyclosporin, and mycophenolate mofetil.

Plasma exchange

This produces a rapid improvement in symptoms and is effective in treating acute severe exacerbations or preparing patients for surgery. This improvement is temporary, lasting 6–8 weeks. The main complications are those relating to intravenous access.

Intravenous immunoglobulin

This produces a rapid improvement in symptoms and is effective in treating acute severe exacerbations or preparing patients for surgery. Often used in patients who are poor candidates for plasma exchange because of poor vascular access or septicaemia.

What is the role of thymectomy in patients with myasthenia gravis?

Myasthenia gravis (as well as other autoimmune disorders) results from loss of tolerance to auto-antigens. T lymphocyte tolerance to auto-antigens develops in the thymus. Thymic abnormalities are common in patients with myasthenia gravis (65% have thymic hyperplasia, and 15% have thymoma). Patients with thymoma have more severe and generalized weakness and higher titres of nAChR antibodies. Thymectomy in these patients can result in medication free remission. In the absence of thymoma, thymectomy is often considered as it increases the probability of remission or improvement. In the context of non-thymomatous myasthenia gravis, remission is more likely if there is thymus hyperplasia, high nAChR antibody titre and short duration of disease. At present thymectomy is routinely considered in all patients with thymoma, and in patients without a thymoma, who are aged <55 years and have generalized myasthenia. The remission rate increases with time, and the response to thymectomy may be delayed for several years.

Case 57 ◆ **Visual Field Defects**

Examiner's note

The most common instruction is to 'examine the cranial nerves'. You may be asked to examine the visual fields, and based on your findings, proceed to examine the remaining neurological symptoms appropriately. There many types of visual field defects, and the focus of the following case presentations is to reflect the most commonly encountered visual field defects, and being aware of associated features. It is important to remember, that in most circumstances, the visual field defect is one clinical manifestation of the neurological lesion, and having defined a particular defect, other associated clinical signs should be looked for.

Visual pathways

It is important to have a basic understanding of the visual pathways, and different patterns of visual field defects.

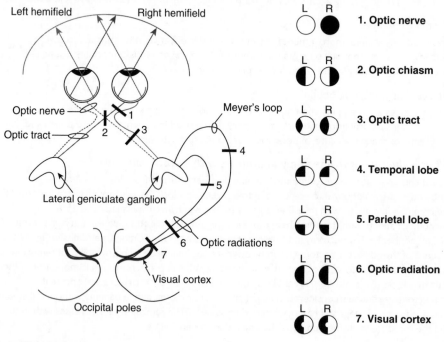

Figure 57.1 Visual pathways.

CASE PRESENTATION 1

*This patient has a right **congruous homonymous hemianopia**. This suggests a lesion behind the optic chiasm but more specifically behind lateral geniculate ganglion affecting the left optic radiation. The differential diagnosis includes:*

(a) *Cerebrovascular accident (infarct or haemorrhage)*
(b) *Intracranial tumour*
(c) *Trauma*

Clinical notes

1. A homonymous hemianopia indicates a lesion behind the optic chiasm. However, lesions of the optic tract produce incongruous defects, as fibres serving identical points in the homonymous fields from both eyes do not fully co-mingle in the anterior optic tract. Therefore lesions of the optic tract and lateral geniculate ganglion produce an incongruous and usually incomplete homonymous hemianopia. Lesions behind the lateral geniculate ganglion, affecting the optic radiation produce congruous visual field defects. Thus a right incongruous homonymous hemianopia would indicate a lesion of the left optic tract or lateral geniculate ganglion, whereas a right congruous homonymous hemianopia indicates a lesion in the posterior optic pathways, behind the lateral geniculate body, affecting the left optic radiation.

2. Having made the diagnosis of a right congruous homonymous hemianopia, look for the following:
   (a) Left craniotomy scars (previous trauma or surgery)
   (b) Right hemiparesis
   (c) Dysphasia (left [dominant] hemisphere involvement)

CASE PRESENTATION 2

*This patient has a **bitemporal hemianopia**. This suggests a lesion at the optic chiasm. The differential diagnosis includes:*

(a) *Pituitary tumour*
(b) *Craniopharyngioma*
(c) *Suprasellar meningioma*
(d) *Glioma*
(e) *Granuloma*
(f) *Metastasis*

Clinical notes

1. Bitemporal hemianopia is relatively straightforward to deduce from visual field testing. It is important to remember that pituitary tumours compress the optic chiasm from below, whilst craniopharyngiomas compress the optic chiasm from above. Chiasmal compression from below affects the lower nasal (upper temporal field) fibres first, then the upper nasal fibres. Chiasmal compression from above affects the upper nasal (lower temporal field) fibres first, then the lower nasal fibres. Thus pituitary tumours result in temporal hemianopia that progresses from upper to lower fields, and craniopharyngiomas result in temporal hemianopia from that progresses from lower to upper fields.

2. Having made the diagnosis of a bitemporal hemianopia, look for features of:
   (a) Pituitary tumour: acromegaly, Cushing's disease, hypopituitarism, and gynaecomastia
   (b) Granulomatous disease: sarcoidosis, tuberculosis
   (c) Metastasis: evidence of primary malignancy

CASE PRESENTATION 3

This patient has a right **homonymous upper quadrantonopia**. *This suggests a lesion in the left temporal cortex. The differential diagnosis includes:*

(a) Cerebrovascular accident (infarct or haemorrhage)
(b) Intracranial tumour
(c) Trauma
(d) Surgery

Clinical notes

1. Fibres from the upper quadrants leave the optic tracts to become the optic radiation that pass anteriorly to form Meyer's loops in the temporal lobe. These fibres loop back posteriorly to join the lower quadrant fibres in the parietal lobe. Temporal lobe lesions therefore result in a homonymous upper quadrantonopia.
2. Having made the diagnosis of a right homonymous quadrantonopia, look for the following:
   (a) Left craniotomy scars (previous trauma or surgery)
   (b) Right hemiparesis
   (c) Dysphasia (left [dominant] hemisphere involvement)

CASE PRESENTATION 4

This patient has a right **homonymous lower quadrantonopia**. *This suggests a lesion in the left (anterior) parietal cortex. The differential diagnosis includes:*

(a) Cerebrovascular accident (infarct or haemorrhage)
(b) Intracranial tumour
(c) Trauma

Clinical notes

1. The anterior parietal part of the optic radiation carries fibres from the lower quadrant. Thus lesions affecting the anterior parietal lobe result in a homonymous lower quadrantonopia. These fibres are quickly joined by upper fibres sweeping up from the temporal lobe, thus parietal lobe lesions often produce a complete homonymous hemianopia.
2. Having made the diagnosis of a right homonymous lower quadrantonopia, look for the following:
   (a) Left craniotomy scars (previous trauma or surgery)
   (b) Right hemiparesis

CASE PRESENTATION 5

*This patient has a right **nasal visual field defect**. The differential diagnosis includes:*

(a) *Chronic (open angle) glaucoma*
(b) *Retinal disease*
(c) *Lateral chiasmal compression*

Clinical notes

Demonstrating an isolated nasal visual field defect (nasal hemianopia) can often baffle candidates, but it can occur, and it is important to be aware of the principal causes. Having demonstrated such a defect, it is important to perform a fundoscopic examination with an ophthalmoscope. This will identify glaucoma or retinal disease.

1. Cupping of the optic disc (a hollowed-out appearance of the optic disc) is an important feature of chronic glaucoma. Generally, a cup: disc ratio >0.5 is a useful threshold for suspicion of glaucoma. As the disc cups posteriorly, the margins of the disc are steep and overhang the cupped portion of the disc. The retinal vessels as they climb up the sides of the cup appear hidden and this gives the appearance of vessels being broken off at the disc margin.

2. A nasal field defect can reflect disease in the temporal retina, and it is important to look for an area of chorioretinits, branch retinal artery occlusion or branch retinal vein occlusion.

3. Lateral chiasmal compression is rare but can occur due to dilatation of the intracavernous part of an atherosclerotic carotid artery and occurs in elderly female patients. This impinges on the lateral aspect of the chiasm. This unilateral defect can become bilateral if the chiasm is pushed against the carotid artery on the opposite side.

Questions commonly asked by examiners

Most questions that relate to visual field defect will relate to the underlying specific cause of the visual field defect.

What do you understand by the term 'homonymous' visual field defect?

The term 'homonymous' means an identical pattern of visual field defect in each eye, no matter how bizarre the visual defect may be.

What is the Foster-Kennedy syndrome?

This is ipsilateral optic atrophy, due to compression on the optic nerve, and contralateral papilloedema secondary to raised intracranial pressure. It is commonly caused by tumours on the inferior surface of the frontal lobe, e.g. olfactory grove meningioma or medial third sphenoid wing meningioma.

What is the cause of an ipsilateral blind eye and a contralateral upper quadrantonopia?

A lesion in the front of the optic chiasm affecting the ipsilateral optic nerve can also affect the crossing fibres that loop forwards before turning back into the optic tract. These fibres convey signals from the upper temporal field of the opposite eye. This will therefore result in ipsilateral blindness and contralateral upper quadrantonopia.

What is a scotoma?

This is small area of visual loss within the visual field. It can be classified as peripheral or central. Peripheral causes include chorioretinal lesions and central causes include macular and optic nerve disease.

What is a scintillating scotoma?

This is the most common visual aura that precedes a migraine attack. It often begins as a spot of flickering light in the centre of the visual fields. It then expands into shimmering arcs of white or coloured flashing light. These scotomas can obscure vision, and central vision eventually returns before the scotoma eventually disappears from the peripheral vision.

Case 58 ◆ Wasting of Small Muscles of the Hand

Examiner's note

Wasting of the small muscles of the hands is often seen in the context of other pathologies, but this may present as the focus of the neurology case in the MRCP (PACES) examination. The findings of distal wasting, weakness and possibly deformities (in long-standing cases) will be present in all cases. It is important to remember that generalized wasting of the small muscles of the hands suggests pathology affecting either the anterior horn cells, nerve roots or lower motor neurones that originate from C8–T1. This should be mentioned at the end of the presentation, to demonstrate your understanding of this basic, yet important, concept. Clues to a specific diagnosis will be based upon other motor and sensory findings.

CASE PRESENTATION 1

On examination of the upper limbs there is bilateral **distal wasting and weakness**. *There is* **wasting of the intrinsic muscles** *of the both hands (dorsal interossei, hypothenar and thenar eminences) with* **dorsal guttering**.[1] *There are* **hyperextension deformities at the metacarpophalangeal joints** *and* **flexion deformities at the interphalangeal joints**, *resulting in* **claw hands**.[2] *There is distal weakness, reflecting weakness of these muscle groups, and more specifically, there is* **weakness of finger and wrist extensors**.[3] *The deep tendon reflexes are depressed. Coordination and sensation are normal.*[4]

The **generalized wasting of the small muscles of the hands** *suggests pathology affecting either the anterior horn cells, nerve roots, or lower motor neurones that originate from C8–T1. There are* **lower motor neurone signs with no sensory signs**, *and the differential diagnosis for this would be:*

(a) **Peripheral motor neuropathy**

(b) **Motor neurone disease (progressive muscular atrophy)**[5]

CASE PRESENTATION 2

On examination of the upper limbs there is unilateral **distal wasting and weakness**. *There is* **wasting of the intrinsic muscles** *of the right hand (dorsal interossei, hypothenar, and thenar eminences) with* **dorsal guttering**.[1] *There are* **hyperextension deformities at the metacarpophalangeal joints** *and* **flexion deformities at the interphalangeal joints**, *resulting in a* **claw hand**.[2] *There is distal weakness,* *reflecting weakness of these muscle groups, and more specifically, there is **weakness of finger flexors** **and extensors and wrist extensors**.[3] Deep tendon reflexes are normal. There is **reduced sensation** **on the right in the C8–T1 dermatomes**. Coordination is normal.[4]*

*In addition, this patient has **finger clubbing** and **nicotine staining**. There is right partial ptosis, miosis, and anhidrosis, constituting a right **Horner's syndrome**.*

*The **generalized wasting of the small muscles of the hands** suggests pathology affecting either the* **anterior horn cells, nerve roots, or lower motor neurones that originate from C8–T1**. *The clinical signs suggest a **C8–T1 nerve root lesion**. In the presence of finger clubbing and a right Horner's syndrome, the most likely diagnosis is a **Pancoast syndrome** due to a right apical carcinoma of the lung.[5]*

Clinical notes

1. When inspecting wasted hands you must assess the pattern of wasting and ask 'does wasting preferentially affect median or ulnar-innervated muscles, or are they affected approximately in proportion?' If the former, then this suggests mononeuropathy is most likely. If the latter, then generalized wasting suggests anterior horn cells, nerve roots, or lower motor neurones that originate from C8–T1 are affected, i.e. motor neuron disease, C8–T1 radiculopathy, lower brachial plexus lesion, or motor neuropathy. Exceptions to this are combined median and ulnar nerve palsy (often unilateral, unlikely to have bilateral median and ulnar nerve palsy) and motor neurone disease (where the wasting is patchy-so-called 'split hand'). Carefully inspect for scars at the elbow, suggestive of ulnar nerve palsy.

2. In long-standing cases, a claw hand deformity may be seen. The features are:
   (a) Extension at the MCP joint
   (b) Flexion at the proximal and distal interphalangeal joints (PIP and DIP)
   This occurs due to weakness of the lumbricals and interossei, and unopposed action of the antagonist muscle groups:

	MCP	PIP	DIP
Flexion	Lumbricals, Interossei	Flexor digitorum sublimis	Flexor digitorum profundus
Extension	Extensor digitorum	Lumbricals, Interossei	Lumbricals, Interossei

   Not all conditions that result in wasting of the small muscles of the hands will produce a claw hand, as there MUST be differential muscle involvement with weakness of the lumbricals and interossei and preserved strength of extensors at the MCP and PIP joints. Only lower motor neurone lesions of C8–T1 nerves, C8–T1 nerve root lesions and brachial plexus lesions will produce such localized wasting of lumbricals and interossei that result in a claw hand deformity. A combined median and ulnar nerve palsy will produce a true claw hand.

3. Being able to elicit finger and/or wrist extensor weakness is an important sign—it suggests that there must be more than just median and/or ulnar neuropathies as a cause for wasting.

4. It is the presence of other motor and sensory signs that will point to a specific diagnosis. The following table lists the causes of wasting of the small muscles of the hands, and additional features which should be looked for:

   The specifics of each of the above have not been covered, and it is best to avoid the details of each of these rare distal myopathies, which will create unnecessary confusion. In the presence of lower motor neurone signs, distal myopathy should be considered. It is important to remember that clawing of hands is rarely seen in these cases. Although the lower motor neurones are intact, reflexes may appear to be depressed, and this purely reflects muscle weakness. Fasciculations do not occur, and if present should point specifically to a lower motor neurone pathology.

Site of lesion	Example	Pattern	Clawing	Motor signs	Sensory signs	Other features
Anterior horn cells at C8–T1	Motor neurone disease	Bilateral	Yes	Mixture of UMN and LMN signs; prominent fasciculations (may be seen in other LMN lesions); pure LMN signs can be seen in progressive muscular atrophy	None	Bulbar signs; tongue wasting and fasciculations
	Syringomyelia	Bilateral	Yes	LMN signs in upper limbs	Dissociated sensory loss; cape sensory deficit; painless scars on hands; Charcot joints	UMN signs in lower limbs (spastic paraparesis) Horner's syndrome; nystagmus (internuclear ophthalmoplegia)
	Heredirory Motor and Sensory Neuropathy	Bilateral	Yes	LMN signs	Sensory disturbance in a glove distribution	Pes cavus; essential tremor; inverted champagne bottle' appearance of legs
	Friedrich's ataxia	Bilateral	No	UMN signs; cerebellar signs	Dorsal column signs	Pes cavus; high-arched palate
	Cervical cord tumour (C8–T1)	Bilateral	No	Hand wasting only; reflexes not affected	C8 sensory level (C8–T1 sensory impairment)	UMN signs in lower limbs (spastic paraparesis); sphincter disturbance
	Meningovascular syphilis	Bilateral	Yes	LMN signs	Dorsal column signs	Absent ankle jerks and extensor plantars; Argyll-Robertson pupil
	Polyneuropathy (motor +/– sensory)	Bilateral	Yes	LMN signs	Sensory disturbance in a glove distribution (if sensory involvement)	Features associated with underlying cause
	Distal spinal muscular atrophy*	Bilateral	Yes	LMN signs	None	Pes cavus; distal wasting of the legs
	Old poliomyelitis	Unilateral	Yes	LMN signs	None	
C8–T1 nerve root	Pancoast syndrome	Unilateral	Yes	Hand wasting only; reflexes not affected	C8–T1 sensory loss	Horner's syndrome, clubbing, apical lung signs
	Neurofibroma	Unilateral	Yes	Hand wasting only; reflexes not affected	C8–T1 sensory loss	Neurofibromata; café-au-lait spots; axillary freckling

				Signs	Sensory	Additional features
Lower brachial plexus	Cervical myelopathy**	Bilateral	Yes	LMN signs in upper limbs; inverted reflexes	Dermatomal sensory loss (usually C5–7, but if hands are wasted, C8–T1 will also be affected); dorsal column signs	Cervical collar Pseudoathetosis; myelopathy hand sign; UMN signs in lower limbs (spastic paraparesis)
	Cervical rib (thoracic outlet syndrome)	Unilateral Bilateral	Yes	Hand wasting only; reflexes not affected	C8–T1 sensory loss	Supraclavicular bruit; absent brachial and radial pulses; pain in axilla and inner aspect of arm and hand; palpate cervical ribs
	Pancoast syndrome	As above				
Muscle disorder	Myotonic dystrophy	Bilateral	No	Hand-wasting; hyporeflexia; myotonia (may be absent)	None	Myopathic facies; ptosis; frontal balding; temporalis wasting
	Distal muscular dystrophies***	Bilateral	No	Hand wasting; hyporeflexia	None	Signs specific to individual muscular dystrophy
Other causes	Median and ulnar nerve palsy	Unilateral	Yes	Hand wasting; preserved finger and wrist extensors; reflexes not affected	Median and ulnar nerve distribution	
	Disuse atrophy	Bilateral (may be unilateral)	No	Hand wasting	None	Features of underlying disease, i.e. rheumatoid arthritis
	Cachexia	Bilateral	No	Generalized wasting	None	Feature of underlying cause of cachexia

* Distal spinal muscular atrophy is a variant of spinal muscular atrophy that is characterized by distal wasting and weakness. It may resemble Charcot-Marie-Tooth disease, but the key difference is the absence of sensory findings.

** The main segments of the cervical cord that are affected are C5–7, and there are lower motor neurone signs at this level corresponding to these nerve roots. As the small muscles of the hands are supplied by C8–T1, wasting of the small muscles of the hands is uncommon. In some cases, wasting of the small muscles of the hands may be seen, and this reflects vascular changes in the cord below the lesion. If C8–T1 is affected, then clawing of the hands may be seen in long-standing cases.

*** In general, muscular dystrophies result in proximal wasting and weakness. However, certain forms are characterized by distal wasting and weakness. These distal muscular dystrophies (or myopathies) include:

- Oculopharyngodistal myopathy
- Welander distal myopathy
- Finish distal myopathy
- Markesbury distal myopathy
- Miyoshi myopathy

5. Taking all the clinical signs into account (see table above), it should be clear which category of pathologies, accounts for the clinical picture:
   (a) Lesions affecting anterior horn cells (C8–T1)
   (b) Lesions affecting nerve root (C8–T1)
   (c) Lesions of the lower brachial plexus (innervated by C8–T1)
   (d) Muscle disorder
   (e) Mononeuropathies

   In the setting of the examination, the motor and sensory findings in the hands should direct you to look for other specific signs. However, in general terms, the following routine after examining the upper limbs may help you to remember, and broadly cover the causes of wasting of the small muscles of the hands encountered in the examination:

   ♦ **General:** Neurofibromatosis; rheumatoid arthritis (disuse atrophy); cervical collar (cervical myelopathy)
   ♦ **Face:** Tongue fasciculations (motor neurone disease); facies (myotonic dystrophy)
   ♦ **Eyes:** Horner's syndrome (Pancoast, syringomyelia); ptosis (myotonic dystrophy); internuclear ophthalmoplegia (syringomyelia)
   ♦ **Hands:** clubbing (Pancoast); myotonia (myotonic dystrophy)
   ♦ **Feet:** Pes cavus (Hereditary Motor and Sensory Neuropathy (HMSN), Friedreich's ataxia, old polio)
   ♦ **Legs:** 'Inverted champagne bottle' appearance (Hereditary Motor and Sensory Neuropathy (HMSN))
   ♦ **Gait:** Spastic paraparesis (syringomyelia, cervical myelopathy, motor neurone disease, C-cord tumour)

   The clinical signs may point to a specific diagnosis (see Case presentation 2). If this is not clear, then given that you have decided upon one of the above categories, it is best to provide a differential diagnosis for this (see Case presentation 1).

Questions commonly asked by examiners

The questions commonly asked at this station will reflect the underlying diagnosis. Please refer to questions covering each of the separate causes in other sections of the book.

What do you know about the innervation and action of hand muscles?

Muscle	Peripheral nerve	Nerve root	Action
Abductor pollicis brevis	Median nerve	C8 T1	Thumb abduction
Opponens policis	Median nerve	C8 T1	Thumb opposition
Dorsal interossei	Ulnar nerve	C8 T1	Finger abduction*
Palmar interossei	Ulnar nerve	C8 T1	Finger adduction*
Abductor digiti minimi	Ulnar nerve	C8 T1	Little finger abduction

* A useful pneumonic to remember for these is P-AD and (P̲almar-A̲D̲duct)
D-AB (D̲orsal-A̲B̲duct)

What do you know about the 'split hand syndrome'?

In some patients with motor neurone disease, the thenar muscles are more denervated than the hypothenar muscles. The first dorsal interosseous is even more denervated, and significantly involved before the thenar muscles. Thus the muscles on the lateral aspect of the hand are more greatly affected than the medial muscles. This has been termed the 'split hand' and has been reported to be specific for anterior horn cell disorders as opposed to C8 radiculopathies. It is not limited to motor neurone disease and can occur in spinal muscular atrophy and poliomyelitis.

Case 59 ◆ Syringomyelia

Examiner's note

Syringomyelia is a rare case, but does appear at the neurology station in the MRCP (PACES) examination. Many candidates often fear the diagnosis, but the clinical signs are straightforward to pick up, and if picked up, can be put together to make the diagnosis. Although signs can be present in the eyes, face, upper limbs, and lower limbs, it is examination of the upper limbs through demonstrating dissociated sensory loss that confidently makes the diagnosis. The most common instruction at this station is to 'examine the upper limbs'.

CASE PRESENTATION

This patient with **kyphoscoliosis**[1] *has* **surgical scars** *over the shoulders and a midline cervical scar.*[2] *On examination of the upper limbs there are* **fasciculations**,[3] *and the elbow joints are swollen and deformed, with abnormal range of movements (***Charcot joints***).*[4] *There are* **painless scars and ulcers over the fingertips**.[5] *There is* **distal wasting and weakness**, *with prominent* **wasting of the small muscles of the hands**.[6] *The* **deep tendon reflexes are absent**.[7] *There is* **dissociated sensory loss**[8,9] *(loss of pain and temperature sensation with preservation of joint sense and proprioception) in the upper limbs and upper chest.*[10] *The coordination is normal.*

The diagnosis is **syringomyelia**.[11]

Clinical notes

1. Kyphoscoliosis may occur due to involvement of median motor nuclei that supply paraspinal muscles. Left thoracic scoliosis is common

2. Surgical scars are common and should be carefully looked for in these patients. Shoulder replacements could be for osteoarthritis that is associated with cervical spondylosis (and therefore cervical radiculopathy), or Charcot's joints that may occur early in syringomyelia. A midline cervical scar suggests either laminectomies for cervical spondylosis, or syrinx decompression.

3. Classically, there are lower motor neurone signs in the upper limbs (corresponding to the length of the syrinx in the spinal cord, and lower motor neurone damage throughout its length) and upper motor neurone signs in the lower limbs. Prominent fasciculations may be seen in syringomyelia. Fasciculations are often limited to the actively wasting muscle.

4. Neuropathic joints (Charcot's joints) are swollen deformed joints with abnormal ranges of movement, and suggest loss of pain and proprioception. There may be marked crepitus. Any joint can be affected, but the elbow and shoulder joints are more commonly affected in the upper limbs.

5. Trophic and vasomotor changes are common in syringomyelia. Take extra time to examine the hands, and note the following:
    ◆   Painless scars and ulcers over the digits (loss of pain sensation)
    ◆   Callosities over the knuckles with thickened skin (loss of pain sensation)
    ◆   Oedema and excessive sweating (central autonomic dysfunction)
    ◆   Amputation of digits
    'La main succulente' is a term to describe the appearance of the hands due to the trophic and vasomotor disturbances: cold, oedematous, and cyanosed hands.

6. Syrinx extension into the anterior horns of the spinal cord damages the lower motor neurones and causes diffuse muscle atrophy. This begins in the hands and progresses proximally to include the forearms and shoulder girdle muscles. Weakness of shoulder girdle muscles may manifest as winging of the scapula. Wasting and weakness of the small muscles of the hand occurs early, and will always be present. Look for dorsal guttering. In long-standing cases, there may be hyperextension deformities at the MCP joints and flexion deformities at the interphalangeal joints, resulting in claw hands.

7. Areflexia occurs early in syringomyelia due to anterior horn cell compression and lower motor neurone damage. Wasting with hyperreflexia suggests motor neurone disease, whilst wasting with mixed hyperreflexia and areflexia and 'inverted reflexes' suggests cervical myelopathy (but this can occur with syringomyelia as well).

8. The anterior extension of the syrinx interrupts the anterior decussating spinothalamic fibres at the corresponding level in the spinal cord. The large sensory fibres of the posterior columns do not cross until in the medulla. Thus there is loss of pain and temperature sensations, whilst the posterior columns, i.e. joint position and vibration sense are preserved. This is termed 'dissociated sensory loss'. Sensory involvement occurs in a cape-like or suspended distribution across lower cervical and upper thoracic dermatomes—i.e. corresponding to the syrinx length and location. Although this classical sensory dissociation is associated with syringomyelia, it must be remembered that posterior columns may be affected if the syrinx expands posteriorly. In addition, there may be unilateral spinothalamic sensory loss due to the syrinx expanding towards the contralateral side.

9. A common error made by candidates in sensory testing is during testing pinprick sensation, i.e. pain. When using a pin to elicit a sharp stimulus, and then asking the patient whether he/she feels it by answering yes or no, the patient may feel the stimulus throughout the upper limbs and answering 'yes' throughout the examination, thus giving the candidate the false impression that pain sensation is intact. It is important to realize, that if pain sensation is impaired, *the patient may still feel the stimulus through light touch sensory pathways that are intact, but will not feel the sharp stimulus*. Therefore it is particularly important in this case (where detection of dissociated sensory loss is crucial in making the diagnosis) that the patient is asked specifically if each pinprick stimulus is sharp or dull.

   This simple error will make one miss the sensory findings, and given the lower motor neurone findings, make the incorrect diagnoses of motor neurone disease (progressive muscular atrophy) or motor neuropathy.

10. Sensory testing should be performed by testing each dermatome in the upper limb (C5–T1) and extend beyond this onto the trunk into the remaining thoracic dermatomes to demonstrate the location and extent of syrinx formation.

11. The presence of lower motor neurone signs and dissociated sensory loss in the upper limbs, points to a diagnosis of syringomyelia. Examination of the lower limbs will reveal upper motor neurone signs with spastic paraparesis. The syrinx most often develops in the cervical and thoracic segments of the spinal cord. To impress examiners, if time allows, one should specifically attempt to localize the syrinx. This can be done as follows:

    (a) **Testing sensation on the trunk** beyond T1 systematically to determine the lowest point of the syrinx.

    (b) **Look for Horner's syndrome.** This reflects damage to sympathetic neurones in the intermediolateral cell column, and suggests the syrinx extends superiorly to at least C8–T1.

    (c) **Test horizontal eye movements** and looking for internuclear ophthalmoplegia (impairment of adduction and nystagmus in the abducting eye). This reflects involvement of the medial longitudinal fasciculus, which extends down to C5. The presence of internuclear ophthalmoplegia suggests the syrinx extends superiorly to at least C5.

    (d) **Examine the lower cranial nerves (IX–XII).** Palatal weakness, wasted and fasciculating tongue, nasal speech, and weakness of sternomastoids and trapezius suggest bulbar palsy, and extension of the syrinx into the medulla (syringobulbia).

    (e) **Examine facial sensation.** The V nucleus is a long nucleus that extends from the brainstem down to C-cord. The upper portion of the nucleus receives sensory fibres from the inner face, and the lower portion of the nucleus receives sensory fibres from the outer face. Thus the lowest portion of the V nucleus may be affected before the syrinx reaches the medulla. This results in loss of sensation over the outer part of the face, whilst the sensation over the inner part of the face is intact. This pattern of dissociated facial sensory loss is also termed the 'balaclava helmet' distribution.

Questions commonly asked by examiners

What is syringomyelia?

This is the development of a fluid-filled tubular cavity (syrinx) in the central area of the spinal cord and originates in the spinal cord tissue. Hydromyelia is dilatation of the central canal of the spinal cord, and can be included in the definition of syringomyelia. The syrinx most often develops in the cervical and thoracic segments of the spinal cord.

What are the causes of syringomyelia?

CSF blockage

This is the most common type (50% of cases). The most common cause is Arnold-Chiari malformation. Other causes include basal arachnoiditis, basilar invagination, meningeal carcinomatosis, arachnoid cysts, or tumours (e.g. meningioma at the foramen magnum).

Spinal cord injury

This may occur in 1–3% of patients with spinal cord injury. The syrinx develops many years after the injury and occurs at the level of the original trauma. They are twice as likely to develop in the thoracic cord, than the cervical cord.

Intramedullary spinal tumours

Fluid accumulation can be caused by secretion from tumours themselves or haemorrhage. The most common tumours implicated are ependymoma or haemangioblastoma.

Idiopathic

What is the age of onset of symptoms?

This typically presents in the third or fourth decade. Rarely, it may present in childhood.

How can you explain the clinical signs seen in syringomyelia?

The syrinx extends through a segment of the spinal cord (often cervical and thoracic). The clinical signs can be subdivided as follows:

- At level of syrinx
  - The anterior horns of the spinal cord are affected thus damaging the lower motor neurones throughout its length. This results in lower motor neurone signs at the corresponding levels.
  - The decussating fibres of the spinothalamic tracts are affected throughout the length of the syrinx. The posterior columns are relatively spared. This results in a dissociated sensory loss.
- Below the syrinx
  - The corticospinal tracts are affected at the level of syrinx. This results in upper motor neurone signs below the level of the syrinx.

What fluid is contained within the syrinx?

The syrinx is filled with CSF, but has higher protein content. In cases where there is CSF blockage, the protein concentrations may be greater than 100mg/dL.

What are the other causes of dissociated sensory loss?

Anterior spinal artery occlusion

The anterior spinal cord is more vulnerable to ischaemia than the posterior spinal cord, especially in the watershed area of Adamkiewicz (T8–L2). The spinothalamic and corticospinal tracts are affected, and the posterior columns are spared.

Small fibre neuropathies

A subtype of peripheral neuropathies characterized by impairment of small calibre sensory nerve fibres. This includes thinly myelinated A-delta fibres (cold, pain, and autonomic) and unmyelinated C fibres (warmth). Vibration sense and proprioception (large calibre fibres) are relatively preserved. For a complete list of causes, see Case 48 Peripheral Neuropathy).

What medical treatments are available for syringomyelia?

There are no known medical treatments for this condition. It is important to establish the cause of syringomyelia. Surgical treatment is often necessary in these patients.

What surgical treatments are available for syringomyelia?

Cervical decompression

This comprises of suboccipital craniectomy, C1–3 laminectomy and duraplasty. This is used in patients with Arnold-Chiari malformation and decompresses the malformation at the foramen magnum.

Dorsolateral myelotomy

The syrinx is drained into the subarachnoid space through a longitudinal incision between the lateral and posterior columns at C2–3 (the dorsal root entry zone). This is usually done following decompression.

Shunt formation

A number of shunt procedures can be carried out. These include:

* Syringoperitoneal shunt
* Syringosubarachnoid shunt (through the dorsal root entry zone)
* Ventriculoperitoneal shunt (if ventriculomegaly and increased intracranial pressures are present)

Case 60 ◆ **Ulnar Nerve Palsy**

CASE PRESENTATION

This patient has **wasting and weakness of the small muscles** of the right hand in a pattern that **spares the thenar eminence**.[1] There are **extension deformities at the metacarpophalangeal joints** and **flexion deformities at the interphalangeal joints** of the 4th and 5th fingers. There is slight ulnar deviation of the 5th finger. This gives a clawed appearance to the hand (**main en griffe**).[2] There is **weakness of finger adduction and abduction**[3] and **weakness of adduction of the extended thumb**.[4] There is **weakness of flexion of the 4th and 5th fingers**.[5] Sensation is reduced over the 5th finger, the adjacent medial half of the 4th finger, and both the dorsal and palmar surfaces of the medial *portion of the hand (**sensory loss in the ulnar nerve distribution**).[6] The ulnar border of the forearm is spared,[7] and there is no weakness of wrist flexion (ulnar direction).[8]*

*The diagnosis is right **ulnar nerve palsy**. The most likely site of the lesion is distal to the elbow.[9]*

Clinical notes

1. Wasting of the small muscles of the hand is seen with dorsal guttering. Classically, there is **sparing of the thenar eminence**, which is supplied by the median nerve. This is important, and it is important to carefully inspect and examine the hypothenar and thenar eminences. The muscles of the hypothenar eminence are flexor digiti minimi, abductor digiti minimi and opponens digiti minimi.

2. This is the ulnar claw hand. It is important to remember the muscles responsible for extension and flexion at these joints, to be able to understand the mechanism of deformities:

	MCP	PIP	DIP
Flexion	Lumbricals, Interossei	Flexor digitorum sublimis	Flexor digitorum profundus
Extension	Extensor digitorum	Lumbricals, Interossei	Lumbricals, Interossei

    The 3rd and 4th lumbricals and interossei are supplied by the ulnar nerve, and serve as flexors at the MCP joints and extensors at the interphalangeal joints. The 4th and 5th fingers are extended at the MCP joints because the flexors at this joint are weak. The 4th and 5th fingers are flexed at the interphalangeal joints because the extensors at this joint are weak. The 5th finger may be deviated medially, as the extensor muscle (unopposed) inserts on the ulnar side of the MCP joint (**Wartenburg sign**). The ulnar claw hand is often seen with lesions at the wrist. Lesions at the elbow result in paralysis of the flexor digitorum profundus (ulnar half), the interossei and lumbricals. Thus both flexors and extensors are weak at the DIP joints of the 4th and 5th fingers and thus there are no flexion deformities.

3. The palmar interossei adduct the fingers (P-AD) and the dorsal interossei abduct the fingers (D-AB).

4. The adductor pollicis adducts the thumb, and the first dorsal interosseous adducts the index finger. These are important muscles that are responsible for the pincer grip, which is weak. The **Froment's sign** can be elicited to demonstrate this. Ask the patient to hold a piece of paper between the extended thumb and index finger. This grasp will be weak, and furthermore, the patient will flex the thumb at the interphalangeal joint to compensate for this weakness (flexor pollicis longus is innervated by the median nerve).

5. Gross weakness of finger flexion results from weakness of flexion at the 4th and 5th MCP joints. In lesions at the wrist, the flexor digitorum profundus is intact, thus flexion at the DIP joints is intact. In higher lesions, i.e. at the elbow, there will be weakness of flexion in the DIP joints. Holding the proximal portions of the fingers, and asking the patient to flex the fingertips can specifically tests for this.

6. The ulnar nerve supplies sensation to 5th finger, the adjacent medial half of the 4th finger, and both the dorsal and palmar surfaces of the medial portion of the hand. This is the classical pattern of sensory involvement in ulnar nerve palsy. Very occasionally, there may be exceptions to this rule, and this largely depends on the site of the lesion.

7. When examining sensation, it is important to note that sensation will be normal on the lateral aspect of the 4th finger. If this is abnormal, then this would suggest sensory loss in the C8 dermatome. If this is the case one should suspect a C8–T1 lesion (an important differential for wasting of the small muscles of the hands) and proceed to specifically check for sensory loss in the T1 dermatome.

8. Look for wasting at the ulnar border of the forearm. Lesions at the elbow, will result in weakness of the flexor digitorum profundus (ulnar portion) and flexor carpi ulnaris. These are important muscle groups to

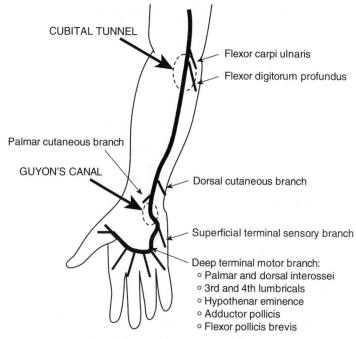

CUBITAL TUNNEL

Flexor carpi ulnaris

Flexor digitorum profundus

Palmar cutaneous branch

GUYON'S CANAL

Dorsal cutaneous branch

Superficial terminal sensory branch

Deep terminal motor branch:
  ○ Palmar and dorsal interossei
  ○ 3rd and 4th lumbricals
  ○ Hypothenar eminence
  ○ Adductor pollicis
  ○ Flexor pollicis brevis

Figure 60.1 The course of the ulnar nerve.

examine, and will be spared if the lesion is at the wrist. However, it must be remembered that in some cases where the lesion is at the elbow (especially in the lower elbow, i.e. around the cubital tunnel), these muscles groups may be spared. Testing the flexor digitorum profundus is mentioned above. By asking the patient to the flex the wrist in an ulnar direction, one can test the flexor carpi ulnaris. This will be weak, and the tendon of this muscle will not be palpable at the ulnar border of the wrist.

9. After having made the diagnosis of ulnar nerve palsy, it is important to comment on where the lesion would be. **The most common site for the lesion is at the elbow. It is important to examine the elbow, looking for evidence of scars, fractures, deformities, or arthritis.** This will provide useful clues. Before one can use the constellation of clinical signs to deduce the site of the lesion, it is important to understand the basic anatomy and course of the ulnar nerve.

The pattern of muscle involvement will greatly help in localization. Sensory testing will often reveal the classical ulnar sensory loss, with lesions at the elbow. However, lesions around the wrist may produce variable sensory findings. Candidates may become baffled when the sensory loss does not fit with the classical ulnar sensory pattern. It is therefore important to be aware of the sensory branches, and their cutaneous distributions. It is important to remember that there are 3 sensory branches of the ulnar nerve. The palmar and dorsal cutaneous branches do not pass through Guyon's canal. After the ulnar nerve passes through Guyon's canal it splits into the deep terminal motor and sensory branch. The cutaneous distributions are as shown in Figure 60.2.

Using the above patterns of motor and sensory signs, one can localize the site of the lesion. Remember the most common site of the lesion is at the elbow. For simplicity, it is best to describe the site as either 'at' or 'distal' to the elbow (as shown in Table 60.1). There are other less common sites for ulnar nerve compression at the wrist that will produce varying signs depending on which branches are affected which the candidate should be aware of (included below).

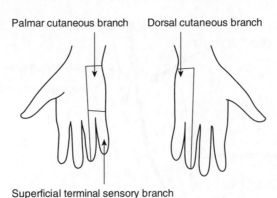

Palmar cutaneous branch   Dorsal cutaneous branch

Superficial terminal sensory branch

Figure 60.2 Cutaneous distributions of the ulnar nerve.

Table 60.1

Site of lesion	Wasting		Weakness				Sensory loss	Claw hand
	Hypothenar eminence and interossei	Ulnar border of forearm	Finger abduction and adduction	Flexion of 4th and 5th MCP joints	Flexion of 4th and 5th DIP joints	Ulnar flexion of wrist		
Elbow	Yes	Yes	Weak	Weak	Weak	Weak	Ulnar distribution	No
Distal to elbow	Yes	No	Weak	Weak	Preserved	Preserved	Ulnar distribution	Yes
Guyon's canal*	Yes	No	Weak	Weak	Preserved	Preserved	Palmar aspect of 5th and medial of 4th finger	Yes
Distal to Guyon's canal**	Yes	No	Weak	Weak	Preserved	Preserved	None	Yes

* A The deep terminal motor and superficial sensory branches are affected. The palmar and dorsal cutaneous branches are unaffected.
** The nerve is affected immediately after it comes out of the canal. The deep terminal motor branch is affected, but the superficial terminal sensory branch is unaffected.

Questions commonly asked by examiners

What are the causes of ulnar nerve palsy?

- **Lesions at the elbow**
  - ◆ Fracture
  - ◆ Arthritis
  - ◆ Compression during general anaesthesia
  - ◆ Compression by fibrous arch of flexor carpi ulnaris
- **Lesions at the wrist**
  - ◆ Ganglion
  - ◆ Tumour
  - ◆ Fracture
  - ◆ Aberrant artery
- **Mononeuritis multiplex**

What is 'tardy ulnar nerve palsy'?

This is slow and progressive development of ulnar nerve palsy. This often occurs in the setting of repeated trauma at the elbow of the progression of arthritis. Both the medial epicondylar region and the epicondylar groove are the classical sites for ulnar nerve involvement. Certain occupations can lead to this, i.e. leaning on elbows (secretaries using the telephone), or repeated flexion and extension at the elbow (decorators and carpenters).

Why are men more likely to develop peri-operative ulnar nerve palsies?

The tubercle of the ulnar coronoid process is larger in men, and women have greater fat content in the medial elbow overlying the tubercle of the ulnar coronoid process. Therefore, the ulnar nerve is more likely to be affected by compression at this site in men.

What is the 'benediction sign'?

This is another term used to describe the ulnar claw hand posture, as it resembles the hand posture a priest makes whilst giving a blessing.

What is the Guyon's canal?

This is a common anatomical area in the wrist, where entrapment of the ulnar nerve occurs. It is bounded proximally by the pisiform bone and distally by the hook of the hamate. The volar carpal ligament and the palmer brevis muscle cover the Guyon's canal.

What are the common sites for nerve entrapment at the wrist?

Site of entrapment	Notes
At the entrance of Guyon's canal	Affects all terminal branches (see above)
Just after the Guyon's canal	Affects the deep terminal motor branch. No sensory loss
At the site of the deep motor branch after the branch to hypothenar muscles have taken off	Weakness of interrosei only. Hypothenar eminence intact. No sensory loss
At the site of superficial terminal branch only	Sensory loss only (superficial terminal sensory branch only)

Case 61 ◆ **Radial Nerve Palsy**

CASE PRESENTATION

This patient has **wrist drop on the right***. There is weakness of extension at the wrist and at the metacarpophalangeal joints.[1] Extension at the interphalangeal joints is normal.[2]* **Finger abduction and adduction is normal** *(when the hand is held flat and the fingers are extended).[3]*

There is **weakness of forearm supination and elbow flexion** *(with the forearm held in between supination and pronation).[4]* **The tricep muscle as well as the tricep jerk is intact.[5]**

There is **sensory loss over the first dorsal interosseous***.[6]*

The diagnosis is **right radial nerve palsy***. The most likely site of the lesion is in the middle third of the humerus (spiral groove).[7]*

Clinical notes

1. Typically there is weakness of wrist and finger extension. Weakness of finger extension is due to weakness of extensors at the MCP joints.

2. Extension at the interphalangeal joints is preserved as the interossei and lumbricals are intact. This can be tested by passively extending the wrist, and asking the patient to straighten the fingers. The patient will be able to straighten them at the interphalangeal joints but not the MCP joints.

3. Finger abduction and adduction is served by the interossei muscles and these are supplied by the ulnar nerve. Finger abduction and adduction may appear weak in radial nerve palsy. However, if the hand is held flat on the table and the fingers are extended, abduction and adduction will be normal.

4. It is important to test the brachioradialis, as this will provide information on the site of the lesion. This will be affected if the lesion is at or above the middle third of the humerus (spiral groove).

5. It is important to test the tricep and tricep jerk, as this too provides information on the site of the lesion. These will be affected if the site of the lesion is at or above the upper third of the humerus (axilla).

6. Sensory loss is usually over the first dorsal interosseous space but can occur over the dorsum of thumb and index finger. If there is no sensory loss, then a lesion of the posterior interosseous branch (pure motor function) should be suspected. If the site of the lesion is high, i.e. above the upper third of the humerus (axilla), there will be additional sensory loss over the posterior surface of the forearm and over the tricep.

7. Depending on the site of the lesion, the clinical findings can be variable. It is important to be able to give the site of the lesion. The most common site for nerve involvement is at the spiral groove.

Questions commonly asked by examiners

What do you know about the anatomy of the radial nerve?

The radial nerve originates from the posterior cord of the brachial plexus, innervated by C5–T1 spinal roots. In the axilla, it gives off a branch to the tricep muscle and three sensory branches that supply the skin over the triceps and posterior forearm. It then wraps around the middle third of the humerus and travels down the spiral groove. After exiting the spinal groove, it supplies the brachioradialis and then divides into the posterior interosseous and sensory branches. The posterior interosseous nerve supplies the supinator muscle and dives into the supinator muscle through the fascia, under the arcade of Frohse, to supply the wrist and finger extensors. The sensory branch arises at the elbow and travels down the forearm to become superficial at the wrist.

Site of lesion	Wrist and finger extension	Forearm supination	Elbow extension	Sensory loss
Axilla	Weak	Weak	Weak	Posterior forearm and over the tricep First dorsal interosseous
Spiral groove	Weak	Weak	Spared	First dorsal interosseous
Proximal forearm*	Weak	Spared	Spared	None
Wrist**	Spared	Spared	Spared	First dorsal interosseous

* The posterior interosseous nerve is a branch of the radial nerve which has pure motor function. The posterior interosseous syndrome often occurs from compression of this branch as it penetrates the supinator muscle in the proximal forearm.
** The sensory branch of the radial nerve becomes superficial at the wrist.

What are the causes of radial nerve palsy?

- Axilla:
    - Trauma
    - Compression, i.e. improper use of crutches
- Spiral groove:
    - Trauma
    - Compression, i.e. Saturday night palsy
- Proximal forearm:
    - Trauma
    - Subluxation of the radius
    - Elbow synovitis
    - Large elbow bursa
    - Ganglion
    - Tumours, i.e. lipoma
    - Repetitive forearm supination (supinator muscle hypertrophy)
- Wrist:
    - Trauma
    - Compression, i.e. tight bracelet or handcuffs

Case 62 ◆ **Median Nerve Palsy**

CASE PRESENTATION

*This patient has **wasting of the thenar eminence**[1] with sparing of the hypothenar eminence.[2] There is an **'ape-hand appearance'** with the thumb externally rotated into the plane of the hand.[3] There is **weakness of thumb abduction, flexion, and opposition**.[4] There is **sensory loss over the palmar aspect of the first three and a half fingers**. Sensation over the thenar eminence is spared.[5]*

Distal thumb flexion, arm pronation, and wrist flexion is normal.[6] Tinel's and Phalen's sign are positive.[7]

The diagnosis is **median nerve palsy** *due to* **carpal tunnel syndrome.**[8]

Clinical notes

1. Thenar eminence wasting is a late sign in carpal tunnel syndrome and suggests long-standing, severe disease. In some cases only the outer half of the thenar eminence may be wasted (abductor pollicis brevis, opponens pollicis).

2. Hypothenar bulk is best tested by getting the patient to put their hands together in front of their face as if about to pray and comparing the thickness of two palms side-on. In the presence of thenar eminence wasting it is critical to ascertain whether ulnar and/or radial-innervated muscles are affected equally. If so, then one must consider other causes of weakness of the intrinsic muscles of the hand.

3. The thumb and index finger are permanently arrested in adduction and hyperextension position, due to weakness of flexion. There may also be a 'papal hand sign' which refers to selective extension of the index and middle fingers due to weakness of flexor digitorum superficialis and profundus (in which the latter is only weakened in 2nd and 3rd digits).

4. Remember the mnemonic of median-innervated muscles in the hand: **LOAF**—**L**umbricals 1+2, **O**pponens pollicis, **A**bductor Pollicis Brevis, **F**lexor Pollicis Brevis (superficial head). Isolating the muscle action of abductor pollicis brevis is difficult, since thumb abduction can also be served (rarely) by abductor pollicis longus (radial nerve). Similarly, the action of opponens pollicis can be difficult to isolate, as thumb opposition can also be served by flexor pollicis brevis (deep head) (ulnar nerve) and flexor pollicis longus (anterior interosseous nerve). In general **weakness of thumb abduction is a better indicator of thumb strength** than opposition and flexion that may involve muscles innervated by other nerves.

5. Numbness over the thenar eminence suggests involvement of the palmar cutaneous branch of the median nerve that arises proximally and courses OVER the transverse carpal ligament and hence SHOULD NOT be affected in a classical carpal tunnel syndrome.

6. These finding suggest a more proximal lesion of the median nerve, i.e. at the elbow. Weakness of distal thumb flexion (flexor pollicis longus), arm pronation (pronator teres) and wrist flexion (flexor carpi radialis) should be specifically looked for.

7. There are different provocative tests that can be used to aid diagnosis:

Tinel's sign	Tapping on the volar aspect of the wrist over the median nerve produces paraesthesia in the distribution of the median nerve
Phalen's sign	Flexion of the wrist at 90o for 60 seconds produces paraesthesia in the distribution of median nerve
Closed fist sign	Flexion of fingers into a closed fist for 60 seconds produces paraesthesia in the median nerve distribution
Compression test	Pressure by examiners thumb on the palmar aspect of patients wrist for 30 seconds produces paraesthesia in the median nerve distribution.

8. Having made the diagnosis of carpal tunnel syndrome, look for possible causes:
    (a) **Acromegaly**: prominent supraorbital ridges, enlarged nose, prognathism, macroglossia, bitemporal hemianopia
    (b) **Rheumatoid arthritis**: arthropathy, nodules, eye signs
    (c) **Trauma**: old radial fractures
    (d) **Hypothyroidism**: goitre (? previous thyroidectomy scar), features of hypothyroidism
    (e) **Amyloidosis**: macroglossia, thickened and palpable nerve
    (f) **Gout**: tophi (hands, feet, and ear)

(g) **Chronic renal failure/dialysis**: evidence of renal replacement therapy

(h) **Diabetes**: finger tip skin pricks (regular glucose testing), fundoscopy to look for retinopathy

(i) **Paget's disease**: enlargement of the skull, hearing aid, anterior bowing of the tibia

(j) **Idiopathic**: often middle-aged, obese females (ask for an occupational history)

Questions commonly asked by examiners

How common is carpal tunnel syndrome and what are its causes?

The prevalence is 9% in females and 0.6% in males.

What is the pathophysiology of carpal tunnel syndrome?

The aetiology of raised pressure in the carpal tunnel is multifactorial and both local and systemic factors play a role. The normal pressure in the carpal tunnel is approximately 2mmHg. Pressures as low as 20mmHg impede epineural blood flow in the median nerve, with the impairment of axonal nerve conduction at 30mmHg. Sensory and motor symptoms become evident at pressures of around 40mmHg. Increasing pressure eventually causes oedema in the epineurium and endoneurium. A pressure of 50mmHg for 2 hours will cause epineural oedema and if applied for 8 hours will increase endoneural fluid pressure 4-fold and block axonal transport. Pressures beyond this result in deterioration in neurological symptoms, and at 60–80mmHg, the intraneuronal blood flow is completely stopped. Increasing injury to the capillary endothelium results in protein leaking out into the surrounding tissues, which become more oedematous and a vicious cycle ensues. This is most marked in the endoneurium as more exudate and oedema accumulate here. The ability of the perineurium to resist pressure changes, its high tensile stress, and the difficulty of fluid to diffuse through it makes it analogous to a 'compartment syndrome' of the nerve. In the early stages, the neurological symptoms are intermittent and reversible, and this reflects impaired axonal conduction. Prolonged periods of elevated pressure results in segmental demyelination, and prolonged ischaemia results in secondary axonal loss and irreversible nerve dysfunction.

What would electro-diagnostic studies demonstrate?

Electro-diagnostic studies has 2 components, nerve conduction studies (NCS) and electromyography (EMG).

NCS

Median motor and sensory latencies and conduction velocities are measured across the wrist. A sensory latency greater than 3.5msec or motor latency greater than 4.5msec is considered abnormal. For a patient with unilateral involvement, a discrepancy between both hands greater than 1msec for motor latency and 0.5msec for sensory latency is also considered abnormal.

EMG

The abductor pollicis brevis is the key muscle to evaluate. This employs needle electrodes placed within the muscle to evaluate the activity of a single motor unit, which consists of nerve cells and the innervated muscle fibres. When the needle is inserted into the muscle, there is a short burst of electrical activity (insertional activity), but thereafter, normal muscle fibres are generally electrically silent, with occasional background impulses recorded by the needle. Patients may have increased insertional activity. Positive sharp waves and fibrillation potentials indicate recent muscle denervation, and can be found in patients with carpal tunnel syndrome.

What are the main sites of median nerve compression?

* Elbow (due to supracondylar ligament- ligament of Struthers)
* Pronator teres
* Anterior interosseous nerve
* Carpal tunnel

What is the pronator syndrome?

This is due to compression of the median nerve as it passes through the two heads of the pronator teres muscles just distal to elbow. It presents with pain on the volar surface of the forearm following sustained pronation of the forearm.

What do you know about anterior interosseous nerve palsy?

This can be caused by entrapment by the fibrous band between the deep head of the pronator and flexor digitorum superficialis, overuse of the forearm, and trauma. It presents as weakness of the index finger and the thumb and there are no sensory signs. The features are as follows:

- Weakness of flexor pollicis longus (thumb) and 1st flexor digitorum profundus (index finger)
- 'Pinch Sign': on forming a pinch between thumb and index finger, the DIP joint fails to flex
- 'Straight thumb sign': on grasping an object, the IP joint fails to flex

What treatments are there for carpal tunnel syndrome?

- Splint wrist in 30° extension (immediate but temporary relief)
- Local steroid injections
- Diuretics (temporary relief)
- Carpal tunnel decompression

Case 63 ◆ **Pupillary Abnormalities**

Examiner's note

Pupillary abnormalities may be the focus of a case at the Neurology station of the MRCP (PACES) examination. In this setting, the most common instruction is to 'examine the cranial nerves' or 'examine the eyes'. More often, they are present with other clinical signs that are associated with a specific underlying diagnosis. The following case presentations specifically focus on the most commonly encountered pupillary abnormalities.

CASE PRESENTATION 1

The direct and consensual reflexes are intact in both eyes.[1] During the **swinging torch test** *the* **right pupil dilates,** *whilst the* **left pupil demonstrates sustained constriction.**[2] *Visual acuity is reduced on the right.*[3]

This is a right **relative afferent pupillary defect**[4] *or* **Marcus-Gunn pupil** *that can result from optic nerve or retinal disease.*[5]

Clinical notes

1. The direct and consensual reflexes are intact when the eyes are tested separately.
2. The swinging torch test is a very reliable test for identifying a relative afferent pupillary defect. A steady light is shone into one eye, and then quickly switched to the other, and this is repeated back and forth.

Under normal conditions, as light on one pupil will cause both pupils to constrict, both pupils should remain constricted throughout this exercise. The principal behind the swinging torch test is that quickly switching from one to the other gives a relative indication of optic nerve function. In a relative afferent pupillary defect, the optic nerve functions adequately to provide a direct reflex on the affected side and a consensual reflex on the opposite side. During the swinging torch test, when the light is switched back to the affected side, the direct reflex (from the affected side) is weaker than the consensual reflex (from the opposite eye). The consensual reflex response from the opposite eye is that of pupillary dilatation, as the light source has been removed from the opposite eye. Thus the affected eye demonstrates abnormal pupillary dilatation when the light is shone onto the affected side.

3. Visual acuity is often reduced, but its presence does not correlate with the presence of a relative afferent pupillary defect. Certain conditions will result in marked reduction in visual acuity with a relative afferent pupillary defect, whilst other conditions spare the central vision.

4. It is important to remember that a relative afferent pupillary defect occurs with significant optic nerve or retinal disease *and* when there is a difference in the extent of disease between the two eyes. If each eye is affected equally, then there will not be a relative afferent pupillary defect. Bearing this in mind, it should be clear that bilateral relative afferent pupillary defect does not exist.

5. Tell the examiner that you would to perform fundoscopy to look for optic atrophy and evidence of retinal disease.

CASE PRESENTATION 2

Both pupils are **small** and **irregular**.[1] The **pupils react to accommodation but not to light**.[2] There is ptosis with wrinkling of the forehead.[3]

These are **Argyll Robertson pupils**, and the most likely aetiology is neurosyphilis.[4]

Clinical notes

1. Argyll Robertson pupils are usually small, and often the pupils demonstrate unequal sizes. A charcteristc feature of these pupils is that they are irregular, and this should be specifically looked for using an ophthalmoscope. Although the classical features may be more easily demonstratable in one eye, pupillary abnormalities are usually bilateral in the context of neurosyphilis, which is the most likely cause. In some cases of neurosyphilis, the pupils may be dilated.

2. The light reflex may be present, but this becomes very slow and eventually disappears. The accommodation reflex is preserved (a useful pneumonic is A-R-P: Accommodation Reflex Preserved). In cases where the light reflex may be present, it is important to remember that the accommodation reflex is always brisker than the light reflex.

3. Look for other eye signs of neurosyphilis, i.e. ptosis with wrinkling of the forehead. Wrinkling of the forehead results from compensatory overactivity of the frontalis muscle.

4. It is important to look for other features of syphilis (see Case 72 Neurosyphilis). Tell the examiner you would like to look for:
    ◆   Optic atrophy (syphilitic meningitis)
    ◆   Other cranial neuropathy affecting VIII, VII, and VI cranial nerves (syphilitic meningitis)
    ◆   Sensory ataxia (Positive Romberg's test)
    ◆   Loss of joint position and vibration sense
    ◆   Charcot joints and trophic ulcers
    ◆   Absent ankle jerks and absent plantar responses (tabes dorsalis)

- Absent ankle jerks and extensor plantar responses (taboparesis)
- Dementia (assess mental status)
- Aortic regurgitation (syphilitic aortitis)

CASE PRESENTATION 3

The **left pupil is dilated** and **reacts very slowly to light and accommodation**.[1] With a persisting light stimulus, the pupil eventually contracts, but excessively, to become smaller than the opposite pupil, and when the light stimulus is removed, the pupil gradually dilates to its normal size. There is delayed pupillary constriction with near vision, again excessively, to become smaller than the opposite pupil and delayed redilatation after near vision.[2]

This is a **myotonic pupil (Adie's tonic pupil)**. If this were associated with absent tendon reflexes, then this would be termed Holmes–Adie syndrome.[3]

Clinical notes

1. The myotonic pupil is a unilateral dilated pupil. Bilateral involvement can occur but is extremely rare. In chronic long-standing cases, the pupil may become chronically constricted. In some cases a myotonic pupil may be primarily miotic. In such cases, especially if there is bilateral involvement, differentiating this from an Argyll Robertson pupil can be difficult. The main differences between myotonic and Argyll Robertson pupils are:

	Argyll Robertson pupil	Myotonic pupil
Unilateral or bilateral	Usually bilateral	Usually unilateral
Pupil size	Usually small	Usually large
Light reflex	Absent	Slow and delayed response
Accommodation reflex	Preserved	Slow and delayed response
Reaction to mydriatics	Poor response	Normal response
Reaction to weak cholinergics	No response	Hyper-reactive
Other associated features	Other features of syphilis	Absent tendon reflexes

2. The myotonic pupil is characterized by slow (tonic) responses to light and accommodation. A delayed pupillary constrictor response to light and near vision occurs, but the constrictor response is often excessive. Similarly, there is also a delayed pupillary dilator response to dark and far vision.

3. Having demonstrated the features of a myotonic pupil, tell the examiner that you would like to check deep tendon reflexes (as this would constitute Holmes–-Adie syndrome), and look for evidence of autonomic dysfunction, i.e. postural hypotension (autonomic dysfunction can occur in Holmes–Adie syndrome).

Questions commonly asked by examiners

What nerve pathways are responsible for the light reflex?
- Afferent pathway: optic nerve → lateral geniculate body → pretectum (midbrain)
- Efferent pathway: Edinger-Westphal nucleus (midbrain) → occulomotor nerve

What are the causes of a relative afferent pupillary defect?
Optic nerve disorders
- Causes of optic neuritis (see Case 149 Optic Atrophy)

Retinal disorders

- Central (or severe branch) retinal vein occlusion
- Central (or severe branch) retinal artery occlusion
- Severe ischaemic diabetic retinopathy
- Retinal detachment (if macula is detached or >2 quadrants are detached)
- Severe macular degeneration (if unilateral and severe)
- Retinal infection (cytomegalovirus (CMV) and herpes simplex virus (HSV))
- Retinal and choroidal tumours (melanoma or retinoblastoma)

What is the site of lesion in Argyll Robertson pupil?

The exact site of the lesion is unknown, but damage to the pretectal region of the midbrain proximal to occulomotor nuclei is thought to be responsible for the Argyll Robertson pupil of neurosyphilis. This does not explain the small irregular pupils, and it is thought that separate local involvement of the iris is responsible for this.

What are the causes of Argyll Robertson pupils?

The most common cause is neurosyphilis. Other causes are rare and include:

- Diabetes
- Midbrain lesion
  - ◆ Tumour
  - ◆ Infarct
  - ◆ Haemorrhage
  - ◆ Demyelination
  - ◆ Syringobulbia
  - ◆ Sarcoidosis
- Lyme disease
- Wernickes encephalopathy
- Brainstem encephalitis

What is the site of the lesion in a myotonic pupil?

A myotonic pupil results from damage to the post-ganglionic parasympathetic fibres in the ciliary ganglion.

What do you know Holmes–Adie syndrome?

This is an idiopathic and benign disorder that is usually seen in middle-aged females. This is associated with absent deep tendon reflexes. The mechanism of areflexia is postulated to be a synaptic disorder of the spinal reflex pathways. There may be diffuse or localized autonomic disturbances including postural hypotension, hypohidrosis, and chronic diarrhoea.

What is Ross syndrome?

Ross syndrome is characterized by a triad of a myotonic pupil, hyopreflexia, and segmental hypohidrosis. There may be compensatory contralateral hyperhidrosis.

What is the effect of 0.1% pilocarpine on a myotonic pupil?

0.1% pilocarpine is a weak cholinergic agent and will have no effect on a normal pupil. In a myotonic pupil, the parasympathetic denervation results in acetylcholine supersensitivity, and thus a weak cholinergic agent results in pupilloconstrictor response.

What are the causes of mydriasis?

- III nerve palsy
- Myotonic pupil
- Mydriatic eye drops, i.e. tropicamide
- Parinaud syndrome
- Trauma
- Drugs: atropine, tricyclic antidepressants, anti-histamines, cocaine, amphetamine
- Carbon monoxide poisoning
- Deep coma or death

What are the causes of miosis?

- Infancy or advanced age
- Miotic eye drops, i.e. pilocarpine
- Argyll Robertson pupil
- Horner's syndrome
- Pontine haemorrhage or lesion
- Drugs: opiates, benzodiazepines, clonidine, phenothiazines
- Organophosphate poisoning
- Iritis

Why are pupils smaller in extremes of age?

Pupillary size is dependent on interaction between the sympathetic (pupillodilator) and parasympathetic (pupilloconstrictor) stimulation. The parasympathetic stimulation is mediated by the III nerve and is affected by the light reflex pathway. The sympathetic stimulation is inherent and not affected by external stimuli. The sympathetic tone is less in infancy and old age, and this results in a physiologically smaller pupil in extremes of age.

Which is the more potent stimulus for pupillary constriction, accommodation or light?

Accommodation is a much more potent stimulus for pupillary constriction as there are more nerve fibres mediating the accommodation reflex that the light reflex.

What is the 'reversed' Argyll Robertson pupil?

This is seen in encephalitis lethargica (epidemics of von Economo's encephalitis that resulted in progressive parkinsonism). The pupils react to light but not accommodation.

What do you know about a pseudo-Argyll Robertson pupil?

This is seen in aberrant regeneration following a complete III nerve palsy. This results in abnormal and incomplete recovery. A pseudo-Argyll Robertson pupil can occur in this situation. It resembles the Argyll Robertson pupil, as the pupil is unreactive to light, but accommodation reflex is preserved. In addition, miosis can occur with any direction of gaze, but it is seen most often with adduction.

Case 64 ◆ **Horner's Syndrome**

CASE PRESENTATION

This patient has **miosis,**[1] **partial ptosis**[2] *and (an apparent)* **enophthalmos**[3] *on the right. Pupillary light and accommodation reflexes are intact.*[1] *Eye movements are normal.*[4] *The* **ptosis can be overcome by voluntary upgaze.**[5] *There is also ipsilateral* **anhidrosis** *over the face, whilst the arm and the upper trunk are spared.*[6] *There is no evidence of heterochromia of the irides.*[7]

There is a **scar** *over the right side of the neck.*[8]

The diagnosis is a right **Horner's syndrome.** *The pattern of anhidrosis suggests a peripheral lesion proximal to the superior cervical ganglion, involving pre-ganglionic sympathetic fibres. The presence of a scar on the neck suggests this may be complication of neck surgery.*[9]

Clinical notes

1. Horner's syndrome is characterized by miosis, partial ptosis, enophthalmos, and anhidrosis (variable finding depending on the site of the lesion). Miosis results from impairment of the sympathetic pupillodilator fibres. The light and accommodation reflexes are intact in Horner's syndrome. However, as the sympathetic pupillodilator fibres are impaired, the pupil will not dilate (or dilates very slowly—a dilation lag) in response to dark (dim light) or far vision. The unilateral miosis can easily be missed if examining in a well-lit environment!

2. Look carefully at the patient's eyes in the neutral position especially noting the palpebral fissure in each eye (the distance between the upper and lower eyelids). The upper eyelid usually covers the upper edge of the iris but no part of the pupil. Ptosis is where all or part of the pupil is covered by the eyelid. Note if the ptosis is unilateral or bilateral. Complete ptosis does not occur in Horner's syndrome, as the upper eyelid is controlled by the levator palpebrae superioris (III nerve) and the Muller muscle (sympathetic fibres). The Muller muscles are affected in both the upper (causing partial ptosis) and lower eyelid (causing slight elevation of the lower eyelid). This results in narrowing of the palpebral fissure.

3. True enophthalmos does not occur, and the ptosis with narrowing of the palpebral fissures gives an impression of enophthalmos. It is best to describe this as 'apparent enophthalmos'.

4. It is important to note the absence of ophthalmoplegia excluding III nerve palsy or myasthenia gravis that remain important differential diagnoses. N.B. a III nerve palsy can either affect or spare the pupil, and if the pupil is affected it will be dilated.

5. A feature of partial ptosis in Horner's syndrome is that it can be overcome by voluntary upgaze.

6. The presence of anhidrosis is variable and depends on the site of the lesion. The pattern of anhidrosis has useful localizing value. The anhidrosis results in dry skin and this can be assessed crudely by gently stroking the skin with the side of a pen and comparing with the other side. Anhidrosis will cause the pen to glide over the surface of the skin more freely. It should be more formally assessed using sweating tests. It is important to particularly check for anhidrosis over each of the three areas: face, arm, and upper trunk. This will demonstrate to the examiner your understanding of the sympathetic pathways and the use of patterns of anhidrosis in localizing the site of the lesion.

Horner's syndrome results from interruption of the sympathetic pathway that starts at the hypothalamus and ends at the Muller muscles, pupil, and sweat glands. This comprises of three neurones:

FIRST ORDER NEURONE	Hypothalamus → brainstem → cervical cord → T1 root ganglion
SECOND ORDER NEURONE *(pre-ganglionic)*	T1 root ganglion → cervical sympathetic chain → superior cervical ganglion
THIRD ORDER NEURONE *(post-ganglionic)*	Superior cervical ganglion → Muller muscles, pupil and sweat glands

Lesions can be classified as central or peripheral. Central lesions affect first order neurones. Peripheral lesions affect second or third order neurones.

An understanding of the anatomy of the sympathetic pathway will help localize lesions according to the pattern of anhidrosis:

Site of lesion	Pattern of anhidrosis
CENTRAL	Face, arm and upper trunk
PERIPHERAL (pre-ganglionic)	Face only
PERIPHERAL (post-ganglionic)	Sweating unaffected

7. Look for heterochromia of irides, a feature of congenital Horner's syndrome. Iris pigmentation is under sympathetic control during development, which is complete by 2 years. Heterochromia does not occur in Horner's syndrome acquired later in life.

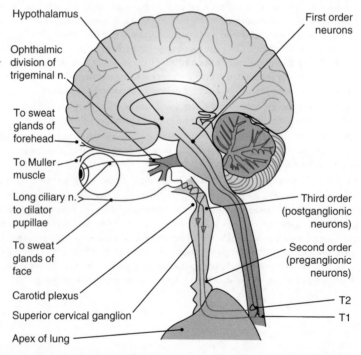

Figure 64.1 Interruption of sympathetic pathways in Horner's syndrome.

8. It is important to be aware of and look for the principal causes of Horner's syndrome. There are many causes of Horner's syndrome and a thorough general examination would be required for full assessment, and this will not be possible in a clinical examination setting. Once having made the diagnosis of Horner's syndrome, it would be appropriate to proceed and look for the following:

Neck	Scars (trauma, previous neck surgery, central venous catherization)
	Masses (tumour, lymphadenopathy, goitre)
	Aneurysms
Hands	Wasting, clubbing, nicotine staining and C8–T1 sensory loss (Pancoast syndrome)
	Wasting, fasciculations, and dissociated sensory loss (syringomyelia)
Chest	Apical lung signs (Pancoast syndrome)
	Sternotomy and thoracotomy scars (previous cardiothoracic surgery)
	Cervical rib

A diagnosis of Horner's syndrome is straightforward, but to gain extra marks is very easy (this could make the difference between an overall pass or fail)! To impress the examiner, the following points should be made:

(a) **Localization of lesion based on pattern of anhidrosis (see above).** Often in the examination setting, anhidrosis may be difficult to detect. If this is the case, DO NOT make up clinical signs, and tell the examiner that you are not able to do so, and that formal sweat testing would be indicated. It would be worthwhile pointing out to the examiner that this would be important, as the pattern of anhidrosis can help localize the lesion (this will demonstrate a better understanding of Horner's syndrome).

(b) **The underlying cause.** If the cause cannot be identified, you may provide a generalized differential diagnosis for Horner's syndrome, or can be more specific according to the type of neurone affected (first, second, or third order) if a clear pattern of anhidrosis can easily be demonstrated.

Questions commonly asked by examiners

What are the causes of unilateral ptosis?
- III nerve palsy
- Horner's syndrome
- Myasthenia gravis
- Congenital

What are the causes of bilateral ptosis?
- Myasthenia gravis
- Myotonic dystrophy
- Tabes dorsalis
- Bilateral Horner's syndrome, e.g. syringomyelia
- Chronic progressive external ophthalmoplegia
- Occulopharyngeal muscular dystrophy
- Nuclear III nerve palsy
- Miller Fisher syndrome
- Congenital

What are the causes of Horner's syndrome?

Site of lesion	Example
CENTRAL (first order neurone)	A – Demyelination B – Brainstem or spinal cord tumour C – Brainstem or spinal cord haemorrhage or infarction D – Syringomyelia E – Basal meningitis (syphilis, tuberculosis, carcinoma, lymphoma) F – Basal skull tumours G – Arnold-Chiari malformation H – Neck trauma
PERIPHERAL (second order neurone)	1 Pancoast tumour 2 Cervical rib 3 Neurofibromatosis 4 Neck surgery (thyroid or laryngeal) 5 Cardiothoracic surgery 6 Central venous catherization 7 Lymphadenopathy 8 Aneurysms or dissection (aorta, subclavian, or common carotid artery) 9 Birth trauma (lower brachial plexus)
PERIPHERAL (third order neurone)	A Internal carotid artery dissection B Carotico-cavernous fistula C Herpes zoster

What is the course of the sympathetic supply to the eye?

- The **first order neurones** originate from the posterolateral hypothalamus and pass via the brainstem to terminate in the intermediolateral cell column of the spinal cord at the level of C8–T1.
- The **second order neurones** (pre-ganglionic) exit the spinal cord at the level of T1, pass over the apex of the lung and enter the cervical sympathetic chain and synapse in the superior cervical ganglion (at the level of bifurcation of the common carotid artery)
- The **third order neurones** (post-ganglionic) exit the superior cervical ganglion and just after they exit the superior cervical ganglion, cervical ganglion vasomotor and sudomotor fibres branch off to travel along the external carotid artery to innervate the sweat glands and blood vessels in the face. The post-ganglionic fibres ascend along the internal carotid artery and enter the cavernous sinus and orbit. Fibres leave the carotid plexus via the long ciliary nerves to innervate the pupillodilator and Muller muscles.

How can you differentiate whether the lesion is post-ganglionic or not?

Pattern of anhidrosis

Post-ganglionic lesions do not affect sweating, as the main outflow to sweat glands and facial blood vessels is at or before the superior cervical ganglion.

Adrenaline 1:1000 eye drops

In post-ganglionic lesions, there is post-ganglionic denervation and thus a depletion of amine oxidase. This sensitizes the pupil to 1:1000 adrenaline. With pre-ganglionic and central lesions, amine oxidase is present which rapidly breaks down adrenaline. Thus in normal circumstances and in pre-ganglionic and central lesions adrenaline 1:1000 eye drops will have no effect, whereas in post-ganglionic lesions the pupil will dilate.

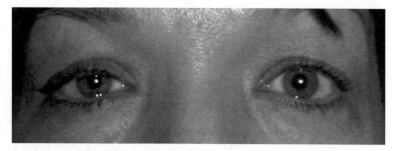

Figure 64.2 Right Horner's syndrome.
Reproduced from Sundaram et al. Training in Ophthalmology. 2009, with permission from Oxford University Press.

Hydroxyamphetamine 1% eye drops

Hydroxyamphetamine stimulates the release of noradrenaline from pre-synaptic (second order neurones) at the superior cervical ganglion. If the post-ganglionic fibres are intact, i.e. first or second order neurone lesions, the pupil will dilate to the same extent as the normal pupil. If the lesion affects the post-ganglionic neurone, the pupil will not dilate as well as the normal pupil.

Case 65 ◆ **Dysarthria**

Examiner's note

Dysarthria is often part of a more specific diagnosis, i.e. cerebellar disease, motor neurone disease (pseudobulbar or bulbar palsy), Parkinson's disease or syringomyelia (bulbar palsy). Rarely, it may be the sole focus of the Neurology case in the MRCP (PACES) examination. Candidates are often asked to assess the speech, which will lead on to demonstrating the features of the underlying diagnosis. Determining the pattern of dysarthria can sometimes be difficult, and this can only be acquired through experience and practice. Whilst examining the speech, try to make general observations and look for obvious signs of underlying disease, i.e. the resting tremor of Parkinson's disease that will provide useful pointers to the type of dysarthria you would expect to find.

Although there are many types of dysarthria, it is important to be able to pick up and describe the following four types of dysarthria. Often candidates can identify the type of dysarthria, but cannot describe the characteristic features, owing to a lack of descriptive terminology. The following case presentations cover the four most commonly encountered dysarthrias and different descriptive terminology that will help candidates to present their finding confidently and coherently.

CASE PRESENTATION 1

*This patient's speech is **indistinct** and **lacks modulation**. The speech is **slurred** with **imprecise consonants**, **omissions**, and **distortions** (particularly at word, phrase, and sentence endings). It is **irregular** and the patient speaks with **variable rates** and **intonation patterns**, being **jerky** and **explosive** whilst at other times a **slow** and **scanning** character. There are frequent inspiratory whoops between words and phrases.*

*This patient has an **ataxic dysarthria** suggesting cerebellar disease.*

Clinical notes

1. A lesion affecting the cerebellum or its outflow tracts results in a lack of coordination in the muscles of articulation, phonation, and respiration. This produces an ataxic dysarthria, as outlined above. The speech appears slurred, as a result of a lack of coordination between phonation and articulation especially at thr ends of words, phrases, and sentences. In principle this is analogous to ocular and limb dysmetria.
2. The lack of coordination between phonation, articulation, and respiration results in speech of variable lengths and tones, and therefore can appear jerky and explosive whilst at other times slow and scanning.
3. The lack of coordination between phonation and respiration results in abnormal respiration during words and sentences.
4. Having diagnosed an ataxic dysarthria, tell the examiner that you would like to demonstrate cerebellar signs in the eyes and limbs and examine the gait (see Case 46 Cerebellar Syndrome).

CASE PRESENTATION 2

*This patient's speech is **indistinct** and **lacks modulation**. The speech is **high-pitched** and **slow**. There is **imprecise articulation** and the **articulatory muscles are rigid**. There is a **harsh vocal quality** and the patient speaks with a **strained-strangled voice** and short phrases.*

*This patient has a **spastic dysarthria** suggesting pseudobulbar palsy (damage to bilateral corticobulbar tracts or bihemispheric disease).*

Clinical notes

1. A spastic dysarthria is outlined above and primarily reflects upper motor neurone weakness in the muscles of phonation and articulation.
2. It often results from *bilateral* pyramidal tract damage, and is unlikely to occur secondary to unilateral pyramidal tract damage. This is because most cranial nerve nuclei receive bilateral innervation from the corticobulbar tract, thus most pairs of cranial nerve motor nuclei receive upper motor neurone fibres from both hemispheres. This is an inherent safety mechanism, as following a unilateral pyramidal tract lesion both the ipsilateral and the contralateral cranial nerve nuclei will continue to receive cortical innervation, and paralysis will not occur. Thus the speech muscles will continue to function adequately, despite unilateral pyramidal tract damage. The exceptions to bilateral cortical innervation are cranial nerves VII and XII that only receive contralateral innervation from the pyramidal tract. Therefore a unilateral pyramidal tract lesion can result in unilateral (contralateral) weakness of the lower face and tongue protrusion, but this is unlikely to cause spastic dysarthria.
3. Having diagnosed a spastic dysarthria, tell the examiner that you would like to look for other features of pseudobulbar palsy (see Case 46 Cerebellar Syndrome).

CASE PRESENTATION 3

*This patient's speech is **indistinct** and **lacks modulation**. It has a **nasal quality**. The voice is **weak** with **low volume** and **unstable pitch**. There is **slurring of the labial and lingual consonants** and the patient speaks in short phrases.*

*This patient has a **flaccid dysarthria** suggesting bulbar palsy.*

Clinical notes

1. A flaccid dysarthria results from bilateral lower motor neurone weakness of the muscles of articulation. Palatal weakness results from bilateral IX nerve lesions. This gives a continuous nasal quality to the speech. X nerve involvement primarily affects phonation. Vowel prolongation (asking the patient to say 'aaaaah' or 'eeeeeeh') tests vocal cord function and integrity. The voice is weak with low volume, i.e. a whispering quality. The pitch is unsustained.

2. Bilateral V, VII, and XII nerve lesions primarily affect the articulatory muscles. This results in imprecise articulation slurred speech, and this can be particularly noted for the labial and lingual consonants (ask the patient to say 'ba-ba-ba-ba' and 'la-la-la-la').

3. Having diagnosed a flaccid dysarthria, tell the examiner that you would like to look for other features of bulbar palsy (see Case 46 Cerebellar Syndrome).

CASE PRESENTATION 4

*This patient's speech is **slow** and **monotonous** (lacking accents or emphasis). It is of **low volume** and **low pitch**. There is **variable articulatory precision** and the speech appears somewhat slurred. At times there are **silent intervals** or **inappropriate pauses followed by short bursts of rapid speech**.*

*This patient has a **hypokinetic dysarthria** suggesting unilateral or bilateral lesions of the substantia nigra or its projections (characteristic of Parkinson's disease).*

Clinical notes

1. A hypokinetic dysarthria is often used to describe the characteristic dysarthria seen in Parkinson's disease. This results from damage to the substantia nigra, a component of the extrapyramidal system. Loss of dopaminergic output results in the cardinal features of rigidity, bradykinesia, and tremor; this also affects muscles of articulation and phonation. Each of the cardinal features results in the pattern of dysarthria outlined above.
   - **Bradykinesia**: slow, monotonous and low volume
   - **Rigidity**: slow, low volume, and low pitch
   - **Tremor**: the speech may appear tremulous

2. A manifestation of bradykinesia is that movements are slow to start, but when they do they can become increasingly rapid and uncontrolled. This is particularly a feature of the characteristic 'festinant gait'. Such movements can also affect speech resulting in variable articulation, and speech that may appear slow to start, i.e. pauses of silent intervals, but which become rapid and uncontrolled.

3. Make general observations whilst examining the speech. Look for the expressionless face and the resting tremor. This will provide useful clues to the underlying diagnosis. Having diagnosed a hypokinetic dysarthria, tell the examiner that you would like to look for other features of Parkinsonism (see Case 43 Parkinson's Disease).

Questions commonly asked by examiners

The questions commonly asked for dysarthria will be specific and directed to reflect the underlying cause. Please refer to questions for cerebellar syndrome, Parkinson's disease, pseudobulbar, and bulbar palsy.

Case 66 ◆ **Dysphasia**

Examiner's note

Dysphasia is often part of a more specific diagnosis, i.e. a left hemisphere infarct. Rarely, it may be the sole focus of the Neurology case in the MRCP (PACES) examination. Candidates are often asked to assess the speech, which will lead on to demonstrating the features of hemiparesis or visual field defects. Determining the pattern of dysphasia can sometimes be difficult, and this can only be acquired through experience and practice. Assessing dysphasia often causes considerable panic and confusion amongst candidates, especially as different approaches to assessment are used and taught by different clinicians. The principles in assessment are simple, and there are 4 basic components of language function that should be tested and will lead one to diagnose the common patterns of dysphasia:

- **FLUENCY.** Can the patient complete phrases of normal length (5–10 words)? Ask the patient questions that require long answers, i.e. 'Can you tell me what you had for breakfast?'
- **COMPREHENSION.** Ask the patient to perform simple commands. This should be done without gesturing. Start with one-stage commands followed by two-stage then three-stage commands. Some patients with impaired comprehension may be able to perform simple one-stage commands, but unable to perform more complex two- or three-stage commands. Examples are as follows:
  - ◆ **One-stage:** 'Close your eyes'; 'Touch your nose'; 'Point to the chair'
  - ◆ **Two-stage:** 'Pick up this paper and fold it in half'; 'Close your eyes and then stick out your tongue'
  - ✦ **Three-stage:** 'Pick up this paper, fold it in half and then put it into your pocket'
- **REPITITON.** A commonly used phrase that the patient is asked to repeat is 'No ifs ands or buts'. However, it is best to use a sentence that contains both numbers and words, e.g. 'There are 7 trees and 4 seats in the garden'. This is because number and word repetitions can have different paraphasic distortions in conduction aphasia (see below).
- **NAMING.** Show the patient simple objects and ask them to name them, i.e. pen, key and watch.

The following case presentations reflect the most common types of dysphasia encountered in the MRCP (PACES) examination, and can easily be diagnosed using the above 4-component language assessment.

CASE PRESENTATION 1

*This patient's speech is **fluent**[1] but is **incomprehensible** with **paraphasia**[2] and **neologisms**.[3] **Comprehension is impaired**. **Repetition is impaired**.[4] The patient **lacks awareness** of the speech difficulty.[5] The articulation is normal.*

*This patient has **Wernicke's (sensory) dysphasia**. The causative lesion affects or disconnects Wernicke's area (dominant posterior peri-sylvian area: the posterior part of the dominant superior temporal gyrus).[6]*

Clinical notes

1. The speech is fluent, with long grammatically well-formed sentences, which contains almost no meaning. If the content of the speech is ignored, the form of the speech may sound normal.

2. Paraphasia describes new words, and this can be:

   (a) **Phonemic paraphasia**: similar sounding syllables with phonemic relationship to the original word, i.e. 'door' becomes 'floor'.

   (b) **Semantic paraphasia**: a different word but with semantic relationship to the original word, i.e. 'cup' becomes 'jug'.

3. Neologism is a new (non-existent) word that bears no semantic or phonemic relationship to the original word.

4. Repetition results in paraphasias and neologisms, which complicates (often lengthening) the original phrase. This is termed augmentation.

5. Patients often have a lack of awareness (anosognosia) of their speech difficulty or, at least, are not concerned about it. This lack of awareness and concern gives patients with Wernicke's dysphasia a worse prognosis than those with Broca's dysphasia (awareness is present). Some patients may develop awareness over time.

6. Tell the examiner you would like to examine the visual fields to look for a right homonymous upper quadrantonopia and the limbs for a right hemiparesis (left dominant hemisphere).

CASE PRESENTATION 2

This patient's speech is **not fluent**.[1] There is **difficulty in finding words**. The patient uses the wrong words and there are frequent grammatical errors.[2] **Comprehension is normal**.[3] **Repetition is impaired**.[4] The patient **has awareness** of the speech difficulty.[5] The articulation is normal.

This patient has **Broca's (expressive) dysphasia**. The causative lesion affects or disconnects Broca's area (dominant precentral area: the posterior part of the inferior frontal gyrus).[6]

Clinical notes

1. The patient's speech will appear slow and halting. In severe cases the patient may be unable to talk spontaneously.

2. Phrases may be short, telegraphic (omissions to reduce length of phrases, analogous to sending telegrams) and agrammatic. There is omission of function words (articles, pronouns, adverbs, prepositions, and conjunctions) and morpholoigical inflections (plurals, past tense). Noun, verbs, and adjectives may be retained, and the speech may be restricted to a noun–verb combination.

3. Although comprehension appears to be normal, especially if it is crudely assessed (as in clinical examinations), it is in fact *relatively spared*, and strictly is not completely normal. This is because Broca's area is also important for the ability to deal with grammar (especially the most complex parts). Comprehension of passive constructions may be abnormal, e.g. if you say 'the girl was attacked by the dog', the patient with Broca's dysphasia may interpret this as 'the dog attacked the girl'.

4. Repetition is abnormal often with omission of function words (articles, pronouns, adjectives, adverbs, prepositions, and conjunctions).

5. Patients with Broca's dysphasia are aware of their speech difficulty and errors in their speech. This often leaves them frustrated. Patients may have catastrophic reactions such as weeping.

6. Tell the examiner you would like to examine the limbs to look for a right hemiparesis (left dominant hemisphere).

CASE PRESENTATION 3

*This patient's speech is **not fluent**. It is **incomprehensible** with **paraphasia** and **neologisms**. There is **difficulty finding certain words**. The patient uses the wrong words and there are frequent grammatical errors. **Comprehension is impaired. Repetition is impaired**. The patient **has awareness** of the speech difficulty. The articulation is normal.*

*This patient has **global dysphasia** displaying features of both sensory and expressive elements. The causative lesion affects or disconnects both Wernicke's and Broca's areas and is commonly caused by a dominant middle cerebral artery territory infarct.[1]*

Clinical notes

1. Tell the examiner you would like to examine the visual fields to look for a right homonymous hemianopia and the limbs for a right hemiparesis (left dominant hemisphere).

CASE PRESENTATION 4

*This patient's speech is fluent. Comprehension is normal. Repetition is normal. The patient has **difficulty naming objects**.[1] The patient has awareness of the speech difficulty.*

*This patient has **nominal dysphasia**.[2] The causative lesion affects or disconnects the area around the dominant angular gyrus: the posterior part of the dominant superior temporal gyrus and adjacent inferior parietal lobe).[3]*

Clinical notes

1. The major feature of this dysphasia is the difficulty in naming objects, despite the patients being aware of what they are. This can be demonstrated in the following example: Hold out your pen and ask the patient to name the object. There will be no answer. If you proceed to ask 'Is it a key?', the patient will reply 'No'; 'Is it a book?', the patient will reply 'No'; 'Is it a pen?', the patient will reply 'Yes'. They will be able to answer 'yes' or 'no', but will not be able to name the object specifically.
2. This is also termed anomic dysphasia. All aspects of language appear normal except naming objects.
3. Tell the examiner you would like to examine the visual fields to look for a right homonymous hemianopia and the limbs for a right hemiparesis (left dominant hemisphere).

CASE PRESENTATION 5

*This patient's speech is fluent.[1] Comprehension is normal. **Repetition is impaired**.[2] The patient has **difficulty naming objects**.[3] The patient has awareness of the speech difficulty.*

*This patient has **conduction dysphasia**. The causative lesion affects the dominant arcuate fasciculus that connects Wernicke's and Broca's areas.*

Clinical notes

1. The speech is usually fluent, although in some cases this may be limited to brief runs of fluent speech. There may be paraphasias.

2. Poor repetition is the hallmark of this dysphasia, and patients will produce many paraphasias when trying to repeat. As the patients are aware of this, attempts will be made to correct the paraphasia and this is termed *condiut d'approche*. Patients may be able to repeat simple short words and phrases, but will not be able to repeat polysyllabic words and longer and more complex phrases. Number repetition often results in semantic paraphasia, whilst word repetition results in phonemic paraphasia. Therefore for testing repetition, it is best to ask patients to repeat sentences that contain both numbers and words (see examiner's note above).

3. The ability to name objects may or may not be impaired.

CASE PRESENTATION 6

This patient's speech is **fluent** but is **incomprehensible** with **paraphasia** and **neologisms**.[3] **Comprehension is impaired. Repetition is normal.**[1]

This patient has a **transcortical sensory aphasia**. The causative lesion affects or disconnects an area behind Wernicke's area at the temporo-occipito-parietal junction.[2]

Clinical notes

1. Transcortical sensory aphasia is *similar to Wernicke's dysphasia, except that repetition is normal.*

2. Tell the examiner you would like to examine the visual fields to look for a right homonymous hemianopia and the limbs for a right hemiparesis (left dominant hemisphere).

CASE PRESENTATION 7

This patient's speech is **not fluent**. There is **difficulty in finding words**. The patient uses wrong words and there are frequent grammatical errors. **Comprehension is normal. Repetition is normal.**[1]

This patient has a **transcortical motor aphasia**. The causative lesion affects the communication between Broca's area and pre-motor area (anterior cerebral artery territory infarct).[2]

Clinical notes

1. Transcortical motor aphasia is *similar to Broca's dysphasia, except that repetition is normal.*

2. Tell the examiner you would like to examine the limbs to look for a right hemiparesis (left dominant hemisphere).

Summary of common dysphasias

The diagram in Figure 66.1 shows the different locations of language areas in the brain:

Using this diagram, one can work out the characteristics of each dysphasia using the following three rules:

1. Lesions anterior to central sulcus affect fluency
2. Lesions below the sylvian fissure affect comprehension

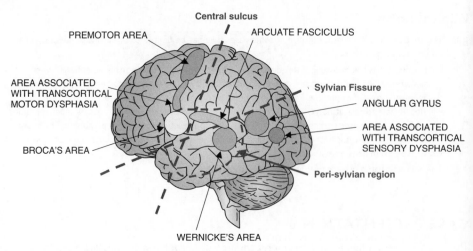

Figure 66.1 Location of language areas in the brain.

3. Lesions within the peri-sylvian area affect repetition

Dysphasia	Affected language components			
	Fluency	Comprehension	Repetition	Naming
Wernicke's	No	Yes	Yes	Yes
Broca's	Yes	Relatively spared	Yes	Yes
Global	Yes	Yes	Yes	Yes
Nominal	No	No	No	Yes
Conduction	No	No	Yes	Can be affected
Transcortical sensory	No	Yes	No	Yes
Transcortical motor	Yes	Relatively spared	No	Yes

Questions commonly asked by examiners

What is the difference between dysphasia and dysarthria?

Dysphasia is a disorder of language, whereas dysarthria is a disorder of speech.

What do you understand by the terms 'semantics' and 'syntax'?

Language is the process where thoughts become spoken. This process can be broken down into:

- Selection of words (semantics)
- Formulation of phrases and sentences (syntax)

Which cerebral hemisphere is responsible for language function?

Most language function resides in the dominant hemisphere. The left hemisphere is dominant in 97% of right-handed individuals, and 60% of left-handed individuals.

Where are locations for the different language areas in the brain?

Broca's area	Anterior pre-central area: posterior part of the inferior frontal gyrus
Wernicke's area	Posterior peri-sylvian area: posterior part of the superior temporal gyrus (first gyrus of the temporal lobe)
Angular gyrus	Temporo-occipital cortex: half way between the Wernicke's area and the visual cortex of the occipital lobe
Arcuate fasciculus	Connects the frontal and temporal cortex, i.e. Broca's and Wernicke's area, via the parietal lobe

What is the angular gyrus syndrome?

If the angular gyrus is affected, then in addition to the nominal dysphasia, alexia (inability to read) or dyslexia (difficulty with reading) and agraphia (inability to write) or dysgraphia (difficulty with reading) can also occur. This is a form of acquired illiteracy.

What do you know about transcortical dysphasias?

These dysphasias are not related to the primary lesions of the language cortex, but to areas connected to them. The primary feature is the preservation of repetition, but they may have lack of fluency, comprehension and difficulty naming objects. Transcortical dysphasias can be divided as follows:

Transcortical motor dysphasia	Lesion affects the communication between Broca's area and pre-motor area; resembles Broca's dysphasia, but repetition is spared
Transcortical sensory dysphasia	Lesion affects or disconnects an area behind Wernicke's area at the temporo-occipito-parietal junction; resembles Wernicke's dysphasia, but repetition is spared
Mixed transcortical dysphasia	Resembles global dysphasia, but repetition is spared

What language disorders can you see in patients with dementia?

Dysphasias can occur in dementia, and can resemble the fluent and non-fluent dysphasias described above. In general non-fluent dysphasias, i.e. Broca's type, usually occurs in non-Alzheimer's dementias, and fluent dysphasias, i.e. Wernicke's type, usually occur in Alzheimer's disease. Patients with advanced Alzheimer's disease typically display a transcortical sensory dysphasia.

Case 67 ◆ Cerebellopontine Angle Lesion

CASE PRESENTATION

*This patient has **impaired abduction of the left eye** with diplopia maximal on left lateral gaze. Cover testing reveals that the outermost image comes from the left eye.[1] There is **weakness of the upper and lower face** on the left.[2] Facial **sensation is reduced on the left** with sparing of the angle of the jaw.[3] There is **weakness of masticatory muscles** on the left.[4] There is **sensorineural hearing loss** on the left.[5] Movements of the palate, trapezius, and tongue are normal. There is no evidence of dysphonia.[6]*

The patient is **ataxic** on the left. There is a **nystagmus** with a fast component to the left. There is loss of smooth pursuit (**broken pursuit**). The saccadic eye movements are abnormal with **hypermetric saccades**. On examination of the upper limbs, there is **dysdiadochokinesis, impaired finger-nose testing**, with **dysmetria** and an **intention tremor**.[7]

This patient has multiple cranial neuropathies (V, VI, VIII, and VIII) and cerebellar signs. This suggests a **cerebellopontine angle lesion**.[8]

Clinical notes

1. This is a VI nerve palsy (see Case 55 Ophthalmoplegia). A VI nerve palsy may or may not be present. *If present*, the ophthalmoplegia may be very subtle with normal apparent eye movements, but with diplopia on lateral gaze. In these situations, cover testing will demonstrate weakness of the lateral rectus.

2. This is a lower motor neurone pattern of facial weakness, and is characterized by weakness of the upper *and* lower parts of the face (the frontalis and orbicularis occulis on the affected side are as weak proportionately as elevators of the angle of the mouth and orbicularis oris). Other features of VII nerve palsy include loss of taste on the anterior two-thirds of the tongue (you may test or ask about this), reduced ipsilateral tearing, hemifacial spasm, and hyperaesthesia of the posterior wall of the external auditory meatus (Hitselberg sign).

3. This is the sensory distribution of the V nerve. Often, the earliest sign of V nerve involvement in a cerebellopontine angle lesion is loss of the corneal reflex (and this may be the only sign present suggesting V nerve involvement). This will not require testing in the clinical examination setting, but it is important to tell the examiner that you would like to test for this.

4. This is the motor branch of the V nerve that supplies the muscles of mastication. Wasting and weakness on jaw closure, ipsilateral deviation of the jaw on keeping the mouth open or protruding the jaw demonstrate unilateral masticatory weakness. Ask the patient to move the jaw from side to side. There will be weakness on attempting to move the jaw to the side opposite the weakness (lateral pterygoid weakness).

5. Hearing can be crudely tested, and this will give an impression of perceptive deafness. To determine the pattern of hearing loss (sensorineural versus conductive), Rinne's and Weber's tests need to be performed. You may be expected to do this in the MRCP (PACES) examination.

   - **Rinne's test**: the 512Hz tuning fork is used to test air conduction (AC) and bone conduction (BC). AC is tested with the tuning fork in front of the ear and BC is tested with the base of the tuning fork against the mastoid process. Normally AC>BC, but in conductive hearing loss BC>AC. In sensorineural hearing loss, AC>BC, but both are reduced compared to the normal ear.

   - **Weber's test**: the base of the 512Hz tuning fork is placed on the centre of the forehead. Normally sound is heard in the middle. With conductive hearing loss, sound localizes to the affected side, whereas with sensorineural hearing loss, sound localizes to the normal side.

6. Having determined the pattern of cranial neuropathy described above, a cerebellopontine angle lesion should be considered. A large cerebellopontine angle lesion may extend and involve the lower cranial nuclei in order (IX X XI XII). Although these cranial nerves will be routinely tested in the cranial nerve examination, if normal, they are important negatives to mention in the case presentation:

   - IX: ipsilateral palatal weakness and deviation of the uvula to the normal side
   - X: hypophonia due to vocal cord paresis
   - XI: ipsilateral weakness of trapezius/sternocleidomastoid
   - XII: tongue deviation to the affected side

7. Having determined the pattern of cranial neuropathy described above, a cerebellopontine angle lesion should be considered, and it would be appropriate to proceed to examine for ipsilateral cerebellar signs (see Case 46 Cerebellar Syndrome).

8. Cerebellopontine angle lesions can present with variable clinical signs. Most often V, VII, and VIII nerves are affected. VI nerve involvement may or may not be present. The presence of cerebellar and lower cranial nerve (IX–XII) signs are late manifestations. It is important to remember that a combined VII and VIII nerve palsy can be caused by herpes zoster virus (Ramsay Hunt syndrome). This should be specifically looked for (vesicles or scars around the pinna, external auditory meatus, or eardrum). Tell the examiner that you would like to examine the ear with an otoscope.

Questions commonly asked by examiners

What is the cerebellopontine angle?

The cerebellopontine angle is a space filled with CSF outlined by the meninges of the cerebellopontine cistern. It is bound by the brainstem as its medial boundary; cerebellum as its roof; the petrous temporal bone as its lateral boundary; and the lower cranial nerves as its floor.

What are the causes of a cerebellopontine angle lesion?

- Acoustic neuroma
- Meningioma
- Cholesteatoma
- Haemangioblastoma
- Granuloma
- Medulloblastoma
- Nasopharyngeal carcinoma
- Basilar artery aneurysm
- Metastasis

What are the common causes of a cerebellopontine angle lesion?

Acoustic neuromas are the most common cause and meningiomas are the second most common cause. Together, acoustic neuromas and meningiomas account for 85% of cerebellopontine angle lesions.

What are the causes of sensorineural deafness?

Unilateral
- Cerebellopontine angle lesion

Bilateral
- Degenerative changes (presbycusis)
- Amphotericin
- Aminoglycosides
- Loop diuretics (high doses)
- Mumps
- Rubella

How would you investigate this patient?

An MRI of the brain is the best modality for imaging the cerebellopontine angle.

What treatment options are available for acoustic neuroma?

Surgical excision

This is the treatment of choice for eradication of the tumour.

Stereotactic radiotherapy

Multiple beams of radiation are directed to the tumour, resulting in arrest of tumour growth. It does not remove the tumour, thus is assocaited with high rates of recurrence.

Observation

This can be used in patients with small tumours, especially if asymptomatic or the hearing is good.

Case 68 ◆ Hemiparesis

Examiner's note

Hemiparesis is a very common case in the MRCP (PACES) clinical examination. Strokes are common, and often such patients are stable. Therefore these patients (often inpatients at the examination centre) may be used for clinical examination, especially at the last minute, when there may be an unexpected shortage of clinical cases. Compared to other more complicated cases at the Neurology station, for which the candidates thoroughly prepare, hemiparesis is regarded as a more simple and straightforward case, and it is common for candidates to under-prepare for this. This explains why many candidates may fail at this station. The instruction at this station is either to examine the upper or lower limbs. Therefore candidates may demonstrate unilateral weakness in one limb and fail to recognize that there is weakness in the other corresponding limb. The recognition of this will make the difference between diagnosis of a 'hemiparesis' or 'monoparesis', and potentially a 'pass' and a 'fail'. Although strictly instructed to examine either the upper or lower limbs, one can make general observations and often there are clinical clues to suggest weakness in the corresponding upper or lower limb that would lead to making the correct diagnosis of hemiparesis. The following cases presentations reflect such scenarios often faced by candidates.

CASE PRESENTATION 1 (UPPER LIMBS)

This patient has a **flexor posturing** *of the right upper limb[1] with* **dystonic posturing** *of the right hand.[2] There is a right* **pronator drift**.[3] *There is* **hypertonia**,[4] **hyperreflexia**[5] *(with* **spread**)[6] *and* **weakness in a pyramidal distribution**[7] *in the right upper limb. There is a* **positive Hoffman's sign**.[8] *There is* **reduced sensation** *(to pinprick and fine touch) in the right upper limb.[10]*

There is *extensor posturing of the right leg* **and there is a right** *circumducting gait* **(hemiplegic gait) and there is an** *expressive dysphasia.[12]*

The diagnosis is a **right hemiparesis**.[13]

CASE PRESENTATION 2 (LOWER LIMBS)

This patient has **extensor posturing** *of the left lower limb.[1] There is* **hypertonia**,[4] **hyperreflexia**[5] *(with* **spread**)[6] *and* **weakness in a pyramidal distribution** *in the left lower limb.[7] The left* **plantar response is extensor**.[9] *There is* **reduced sensation** *(to pinprick and fine touch) in the left lower limb.[10] There is a left* **circumducting gait**.[11]

There is a flexor posturing of the left upper limb **and** dystonic posturing of the left hand. **There is a** left pronator drift.[12]

The diagnosis is a **left hemiparesis**.[13]

Clinical notes

Before examining for neurological signs, stand back and spend a little extra time to inspect carefully. A lot can be deduced even before you have physically examined a patient with stroke. Look AROUND the patient. Look for walking aids and look at the patient's shoes, especially noting ankle supports or orthoses. Inspect the shoe tread for preferential wearing of the outer heel (weak ankle eversion and spared ankle inversion-pyramidal weakness). Also look for scuffing at the front of the shoes, which results from foot drop (can occur in hemiplegic patients).

1. Remember the characteristic posture of the hemiplegic patient: flexed upper limb and extended lower limb; often only one limb shows this posture. Remembering this posture will allow you to recall which sets of movements are weak, and which are spared when testing them at the bedside. In upper limbs: extensors are weak, while flexors are spared; whereas in the lower limbs: the flexors are weak and extensors are spared.

2. Look for dystonic posturing of the hemiplegic side. e.g. the shoulder is held adducted and internally rotated, whilst the wrist is flexed and the fingers held extended. This can sometimes be more obviously demonstrated by asking the patient to walk or to perform a mental arithmetic task. The sign suggests involvement of contralateral striatum and internal capsule.

3. Pronator drift is one of the most sensitive signs of unilateral upper motor neuron weakness and should always be tested for in neurological arm examination; fingers should be kept in adduction and forearms fully suppinated.

4. Spastic tone is differentiated from rigidity by noting that with spasticity the increase in tone is acceleration-dependent, i.e. it occurs most emphatically on suddenly moving a limb from rest. Hence the need to supinate the elbow rapidly is to feel a 'catch' just as the movement takes off in speed.

5. Test each reflex by comparison with the opposite side: e.g. right biceps with left biceps, then left supinator with right suppinator, etc. Avoid saying reflexes are 'brisk' as this can mean either normal or pathological. Decide after you've examined the whole system whether it would be consistent with everything else you've discovered, i.e. that the reflexes on one side are pathologically brisk, or the reflexes on the other side are pathologically reduced! It is more difficult if the reflexes are equally brisk on either side as this can be, and often is, normal.

6. Pathologically increased reflexes are suggested not only by an exaggerated response of the tested tendon, but by the presence of spread to other muscle groups. For example when testing biceps, look for finger flexion, or when testing ankles, look for thigh adduction. 'Crossed adductors' is also a useful sign of hyperreflexia: the adductor tendon is struck just above the medial aspect of the knee—it is normal if the same adductor contracts, but suggestive of a pyramidal lesion if the opposite adductor contracts as well (suggesting impaired descending inhibition).

7. The pyramidal pattern of weakness may be present, but severe hemiparesis will affect all muscles equally.

8. The equivalent of the Babinski sign in the upper limbs is the Hoffman's reflex. This can be elicited by flicking the middle finger (DIP joint) while inspecting the remaining digits, especially the thumb for flexion.

9. If extension of the big toe occurs with a delay, and is the same bilaterally, suspect a voluntary 'withdrawal response' (i.e. non-pathological). Flexion of the entire leg along with toe extension, or toe fanning, or other components of the pathological Babinski response.

10. Sensory testing for hemiplegia need not be too geographically detailed; it is important to know whether a hemisensory deficit is present or not. A lacunar stroke is classically only a motor or a only sensory hemideficit, whereas a large-vessel stroke will involve both. The proximal extent of the sensory deficit in hemisensory disturbance is highly variable and not specific for anatomical localization.

Also check sensation with light touch and ask 'does it feel the same on either side?' Central lesions may be associated with only a 'distortion' or even a heightening of perceived sensation (hyperaesthesia), rather than hypoaesthesia.

11. This is the classical hemiplegic gait. The affected leg will be stiff and extended. With each step, the patient will tilt the pelvis to the other side and the affected leg will 'circumduct', thus describing a semicircle. Foot drop can occur, and the toes may scrape the floor.

12. Given that you are formally instructed to examine either the upper or lower limbs, at the end of the examination you will have demonstrated weakness on one side (arm or leg). Now to make the correct diagnosis of 'hemiparesis' one needs to demonstrate weakness in the other corresponding limb. This can be formally demonstrated with a complete neurological examination, but in the MRCP (PACES) clinical examination, there will not be enough time, and furthermore you will be limited by your specific examination instructions! The following strategy can be used to help correctly diagnose a hemiparesis:

   (a) *'Examine the upper limbs'.* Having demonstrated arm weakness, observe for the abnormal extensor posture of the leg. Examine the gait—a hemiplegic gait will be extremely helpful. In patients with right hemiparesis, make some deductions about the patient's speech—an expressive dysphasia (left-dominant hemisphere) would be supportive of a left middle cerebral artery (MCA) territory infarction.

   (b) *'Examine the lower limbs'.* Having demonstrated leg weakness, observe for abnormal extensor posturing of the arm and dystonic posturing of the hand. Weakness of the upper limbs may be deduced from general inspection, introducing yourself (hand-shake) and examination of the gait. In patients with right hemiparesis, make some deductions about the patient's speech (see above).

13. Having presented your diagnosis, tell the examiner that you would like to:

   (a) Perform a complete neurological examination (upper and lower limbs; cranial nerves)
   (b) Assess visual field defects (homonymous hemianopia)
   (c) Assess patient's speech (particularly with right hemiparesis-left dominant hemisphere)
   (d) Fundoscopy for papilloedema (space occupying lesions)
   (e) Measure blood pressure
   (f) Assess pulse (AF)
   (g) Auscultate for carotid bruits
   (h) Check urinalysis (glycosuria)
   (i) Ask if the patient is right- or left-handed

Questions commonly asked by examiners

What are the common causes of hemiplegia?

- Cerebrovascular accident (ischaemic, haemmorhagic, or thrombosis)
- Tumour
- Demyelination
- Abscess
- Post-ictal (Todd's paresis)*
- Functional i.e. 'non-organic'

How can you differentiate between a cerebral and brainstem stroke?

Abnormalities of higher cerebral function e.g. aphasia, neglect, apraxia; homonymous hemianopia, and seizures suggest a cerebral stroke. Abnormalities of cerebellar function, or eye movements,

---

* Should not last for more than 1–2 days post-seizure (unless ongoing subclinical epileptic activity)

or Horner's syndrome; and presence of 'crossed signs' (e.g. right-sided III or VII cranial nerve palsy plus left-sided hemiplegia) suggest a brainstem stroke. Note that this distinction is not quite the same as that between anterior versus posterior circulation stroke, since a posterior circulation stroke may cause brainstem-cerebellar signs as well as a homonymous hemianopia and memory problems as the posterior circulation supplies the occipital cortex, hippocampus, and thalamus.

What is the relevance of knowing whether hemiplegia is due to a cerebral or brainstem cause?

In a cerebral stroke if the anterior circulation is affected, any identifiable carotid stenosis on the appropriate side may be causative. If a carotid stenosis is present and is ≥70% it is termed 'symptomatic' and requires an urgent carotid endarterectomy. Posterior circulation strokes should indicate either a vertebrobasilar stenosis or thrombosis, or cardioembolism.

What is the significance of unilateral arm weakness being significantly greater than unilateral leg weakness or vice versa?

This functional distinction may indicate whether the middle or anterior cerebral artery is preferentially affected: Middle cerebral artery lesions predominantly affect the arm and face, and anterior cerebral artery lesions predominantly affect the leg, the reason for this lying with the arterial supply of the motor homunculus. If both anterior and middle cerebral artery territories are affected on one side it points to carotid artery stenosis that may warrant an endarterectomy.

Why should you always test for both pain (or temperature) and joint-position sense (or vibration) in all patients with hemiplegia?

If there is a right-left dissociation between spinothalamic and dorsal-column sensory system deficits, with spinothalamic impairment on the opposite side to the hemiplegia, it suggests that the lesion is in the high-cervical cord and affects only half of the cord cross-section at this level, on the side of the hemiplegia. This would then constitute a Brown-Sequard syndrome (often due to a tumour or demyelination).

What are the clues to non-organic hemiparesis?

- Hoover's sign—on active hip extension the patient is unable to push the leg down into the bed, but on active hip flexion in the opposite (unaffected) leg it is noted the patient simultaneously extends the hip that had previously been found to be weak. This test relies on the normal pattern of agonist-antagonist pairs of movements that occur involuntarily with walking, and have been found to occur in the decorticate animal.
- Abductor sign—the examiner tells the patient to abduct each leg, and opposes this movement with his/her hands placed on the lateral surfaces of the patient's legs. The leg contralateral to the 'weak' abducted one (i.e. the sound leg) stays fixed in organic paresis, but moves in the hyper-adducting direction in non-organic paresis.
- Weak tongue protrusion to the side of the hemiparesis is the opposite to what would be expected with a straightforward pyramidal lesion e.g. stroke when the tongue deviates to the side of the hemiparesis and weakness occurs in protrusion to the opposite side.
- Variable or 'give-way' weakness.
- Observing the patient getting on and off the couch that may be incongruous with apparent weakness on the couch.
- Psychiatric co-morbidity.

Case 69 ◆ Involuntary movements

CASE PRESENTATION 1

This patient has **involuntary movements** that are **brief, irregular, non-repetitive, non-stereotyped** and appear **semi-purposeful**.[1] The movements are **randomly distributed** and move from one body part to the next.[2] The movements are **flowing** and have a **'dancing' quality**.[3] They are **present at rest** and **accentuated by activity**.[4] There is **abnormal posturing of the hands**, where the wrists are flexed and fingers hyperextended. The patient is unable to maintain a sustained posture, tongue protrusion, or eyelid closure (**motor impersistence**).[5] Attempting to make a handgrip, results in alternate squeezing and gripping (**milkmaid's grip**).[6]

The diagnosis is **chorea**.[7,8]

Clinical notes

1. The patient often tries to camouflage these movements by incorporating these choreic movements into subsequent purposeful acts, e.g. a jerk of the hand may be followed by scratching the forehead with the same hand.

2. The movements are irregular and random, and they flit from one body part to the next. The face and upper limbs are more affected than the lower limbs in Huntington's disease, tardive dyskinesia, and senile chorea. The lower limbs are more affected in Sydenham's chorea and neuroacanthocytosis.

3. Chorea can vary in severity from mild restlessness to intermittent exaggeration of gesture and expression and fidgeting movements of the hands to a continuous flow of disabling movement. In very mild forms, chorea can be difficult to distinguish from restlessness. The term chorea is derived from the Greek word khoreia—a choral dance. In the full blown syndrome, the movements appear to flow, and are often referred to as having a dancing quality.

4. Chorea can be accentuated by stress, anxiety, and activity. It disappears during sleep.

5. 'Motor impersistence' is an important feature of chorea. The tongue may appear to dart in and out of the mouth and has been termed a 'harlequin's tongue' or 'jack in the box tongue'.

6. The 'milkmaid's grip' is another example of motor impersistence, and can easily be assessed either with a simple handshake or asking the patient to squeeze your fingers. As a result of poor grip, patients often involuntarily drop objects.

7. It is important to differentiate chorea, athetosis, and choreoathetosis. Chorea refers to flowing rapid movements. Athetosis is a slow form of chorea with slow writhing movements that often affect the extremities. Choreoathetosis is a term used for chorea in the intermediate form, i.e. faster than writhing movements, but slower than flowing movements.

8. Having made the diagnosis of chorea, try to look for possible causes. There are many causes of chorea, but some causes can be easily looked for. Tell the examiner you would like to look for the following causes:
   - **Huntington's disease**: assess mental status (early dementia)
   - **Wilson's disease**: Kayser-Fleischer ring, stigmata of chronic liver disease, and akinetic-rigid syndrome
   - **Systemic lupus erythematosus**: butterfly skin rash, purpura, and arthropathy
   - **Polycythaemia rubra vera**: facial plethora and splenomegaly
   - **Thyrotoxicosis**: tremor, tachycardia, lid lag, and goitre (may be present)
   - **Drugs**: take a complete drug history

Chorea or other dyskinesias are manifestations of an extrapyramidal disorder, i.e. a disorder of the basal ganglia, and hence chorea often co-exists with Parkinsonism. If Parkinsonism is a prominent sign, especially if asymmetrical signs, it may be possible that the underlying diagnosis is Parkinson's disease and the chorea reflects levodopa therapy. It is important to remember, that patients with early-onset Huntington's disease (Westphal variant) may present with signs of Parkinsonism.

CASE PRESENTATION 2

This patient has **involuntary, stereotyped**, *and* **repetitive movements** *of the* **lips, tongue,** *and* **jaw** *of a* **choreiform nature**. *These include* **facial grimacing; tongue twisting and protrusions; lip smacking and puckering; jaw opening and closing;** *and chewing.*[1] *These movements are* **present at rest, diminish with activity**[2] *and are* **accentuated by distraction**.[3] *There are slow and writhing movements of the extremities (***athetosis***).*[4]

The diagnosis is **tardive dyskinesia**.[5]

Clinical notes

1. These movements are of variable amplitude and low frequency. Lip puckering, smacking, opening and closing may occur continuously. The patient may appear to be chewing constantly. The patient will be unable to maintain tongue protrusion (motor impersistence). Tardive dyskinesia may be seen in the upper face manifesting as excessive blinking and brow wrinkling.

2. Ask the patient to squeeze your fingers—the finger dyskinesias will diminish. Ask the patient to protrude the tongue—although tongue protrusion cannot be maintained for long, the tongue dyskinesias will diminish. Ask the patient to open the jaw—the orofacial dyskinesias will diminish.

3. Movements can be enhanced by distracting the patient's attention from the movements, e.g. ask the patient to pat the thighs with both hands using the palmar and dorsal surfaces of the hands alternately—this will accentuate the orofacial dyskinesia. This method of distraction may help in diagnosis in cases of mild tardive dyskinesia.

4. Tardive dyskinesia is often associated with athetosis. Ask the patient to remover his/her shoes and socks. This allows one to fully assess the movements of the hands and feet. Flexion and extension movements of fingers, wrists, toes, and ankles can be seen. Involuntary movements of the neck, trunk, and pelvis can also occur. Involuntary movements of the diaphragm and abdominal wall muscles can result in irregular respiration.

5. Tardive dyskinesia is commonly a result of long-term treatment with dopamine receptor antagonists. Tell the examiner that you would like to take a complete drug history.

Questions commonly asked by examiners

What is the difference between pyramidal and extrapyramidal systems?

	Pyramidal	Extra-pyramidal
Physiological movements	Voluntary	Involuntary
Pathological movements	Hypertonia, hyper-reflexia, paresis	Chorea, athetosis, ballism, myoclonus, dystonia, tremor, akathisia, rigidity
Anatomical pathways	Corticospinal tracts	Pathways involving the basal ganglia

What do you understand by the term 'dyskinesia'?

Dyskinesia is a term used to describe involuntary movement disorders and can be further subdivided into:

* Bradykinesia—e.g. rigidity (seen in Parkinsonism)
* Hyperkinesia—e.g. chorea, athetosis, ballism, myoclonus, dystonia, tremor, akathisia

What are the causes of chorea?

Inherited

* Huntington's disease
* Wilson's disease
* Benign familial chorea
* Paroxysmal choreoathetosis
* Neuroacanthocytosis
* Spinocerebellar ataxia

Acquired

* Sydenham's chorea
* SLE
* Polycythaemia rubra vera
* Thyrotoxicosis
* Hypoparathyroidism with hypocalcaemia
* Pregnancy (chorea gravidarum)
* Oral contraceptive pill
* Dopamine antagonists
* Cerebrovascular disease
* Senile chorea

What are the genetics of Huntington's disease?

This is an autosomal dominant disorder with 100% penetrance. It is characterized by CAG trinucleotide expansions in the gene that encodes the huntington protein on chromosome 4 (4p16). In normal individuals, the CAG trinucleotide sequence is repeated 9–34 times. Expansion of the CAG beyond the threshold of 36 repeats results in Huntington's disease. Like other trinucleotide repeat disorders, it demonstrates expansion (increased disease severity with successive generations) and anticipation (earlier onset with successive generations).

What are the clinical features of Huntington's disease?

* Rigidity (marked in the Westphal variant)
* Bradykinesia
* Chorea
* Myoclonus
* Dystonia
* Ataxia
* Slow saccadic eye movements*
* Cognitive impairment
* Psychiatric disturbance

---

* This classical eye movement abnormality occurs due to abnormalities of executive or frontal control. The patient has great difficulty making saccades without first trying to turn their head.

- Dysarthria
- Dysphagia

What do you about the pathophysiology of Wilson's disease?

This is an autosomal recessive disorder, caused by numerous mutations of the ATP 7B gene on chromosome 13 (13q14) that encodes for a copper-transporting ATPase (important for biliary copper excretion). Normally dietary copper is absorbed and transported to the liver, loosely bound to albumin where it becomes incorporated into an α_2-globulin to form caeruloplasmin, which is the main transport protein for copper and necessary for biliary copper excretion. In Wilson's disease, formation of caeruloplasmin is defective, thus there is failure of biliary copper excretion. Thus tissue and body levels of copper are high, serum caeruloplasmin is low and urinary copper is high (increased urinary excretion).

How do you diagnose Wilson's disease?

The diagnosis can be established by demonstrating a low serum caeruloplasmin (<300mg/L) and increased 24-hour urinary copper excretion (>100µg/day). The serum copper value has no diagnostic value. In doubtful cases, a liver biopsy (demonstrating a high copper content) may be required.

What are the clinical features of Wilson's disease?

- Neurological
  - Tremor ('wing-beating')
  - Bradykinesia
  - Rigidity
  - Chorea
  - Dystonia
  - Seizures
  - Dysarthria
  - Cerebellar signs
  - Psychiatric disturbances
- Hepatic
  - Hepatitis
  - Cirrhosis
  - Massive hepatic necrosis
- Metabolic
  - Hypoparathyroidism
  - Renal tubular acidosis (type 2)—Fanconi syndrome
- Other
  - Haemolysis
  - Arthropathy

What is the 'wing-beating' tremor in Wilson's disease?

In Wilson's disease, tremor is usually the initial symptom that occurs at rest, during action or is postural. The most characteristic pattern of tremor in Wilson's disease is a coarse, irregular, to-and-fro movement where the arms are held forward and flexed at the elbows ('wing-beating').

What are Kayser-Fleischer rings?

A Kayser-Fleischer ring is seen in almost all patients with neurological involvement. This is a green-brown discoloration usually in the upper pole of the cornea, and represents copper deposition in the Descemet's membrane.

What is the treatment for Wilson's disease?

- Low copper diets
- Zinc supplementation
- Penicillamine therapy
- Liver transplantation

What do you know about neuroacanthocytosis?

This is a rare, multisystem degenerative disorder that is characterized by acanthocytes (deformed erythrocytes with spicules) and abnormal movements. It has a variable pattern of inheritance—autosomal dominant, recessive, or X-linked inheritance. Choreic and dystonic movements of the face, tongue, and lip biting are virtually diagnostic. Other features include chorea (predominantly of the lower limbs), axonal neuropathy (50% of cases), areflexia, seizures, and psychiatric disturbance. Compared to Huntington's disease, cognitive impairment is minimal. A raised plasma creatine kinase level is seen. The diagnosis is made by the family history, acanthocytes on peripheral blood film, and raised creatine kinase level. The mean age of onset is 30 years, and the disease progresses with death occurring within 15 years. There is no cure, and the treatment is largely supportive.

What do you know about Sydenham's chorea?

This is a delayed complication of group A β-haemolytic streptococcal infections. It is considered to be an immune autoantibody mediated disorder, cross reactivity between streptococcal antigens and caudate and subthalamic nuclei. The age of onset is 5–15 years, and is commonly seen in females. This results in chorea, muscular weakness, and psychiatric disturbance (irritability and obsessive-compulsive disorder). The chorea is symmetrical and consists of more finer and rapid movements than those in Huntington's disease. It has a self-limiting course (5–15 weeks), but can recur in 20% of patients. Treatment is often not necessary, as it has a good prognosis for recovery. In patients with severe generalized chorea, treatment with tetrabenazine or valproate can be considered.

Which drugs can cause tardive dyskinesia?

Long-term treatment with dopamine (D_2 receptor) antagonists can cause tardive dyskinesia. Traditionally, neuroleptics that inhibit dopamine receptors are associated with tardive dyskinesias. Drugs that are commonly implicated include:

- Phenothiazines
- Butyrophenones
- Metoclopramide

What is pathophysiology of tardive dyskinesia?

Long-term therapy with dopamine antagonists leads to upregulation and supersensitivity of D_2 receptors in the basal ganglia. When dopamine antagonists are stopped, or even reduced slightly, there is an exaggerated response of the post-synaptic D_2 receptor to low concentrations of dopamine.

What is the temporal relationship between drug therapy and tardive dyskinesia?

Tardive dyskinesia is often the result of long-term neuroleptic drug therapy, and requires exposure for at least 3 months. Tardive dyskinesia begins during drug therapy or within 4 weeks of discontinuation of therapy.

What is the treatment for tardive dyskinesia?

The mainstay of therapy is cessation of offending medication. Generally pharmacotherapy including anticholinergics or benzodiazepines is ineffective.

What are other examples of involuntary movement disorders?

(a) Dystonia

Involuntary sustained muscle contractions that result in abnormal movements and posture, e.g. occulogyric crisis, torticollis, trismus, blepharospasm, writer's cramp.

(b) Myoclonus

Involuntary, brief, shock-like movements or jerks; physiological examples include hiccups and hypnic jerks whilst falling asleep; pathological examples include myoclonic epilepsy, metabolic encephalopathy, Creutzfeldt-Jakob disease, anoxic brain injury, Whipple's disease.

(c) Akathisia

Uncontrollable restlessness and an inner feeling of unease.

(d) Ballism

Involuntary large amplitude proximal limb movements; often occur on one side (hemiballism); commonly caused by a cerebrovascular accident in the contralateral subthalamic nucleus.

Case 70 ◆ **Bulbar and Pseudobulbar Palsy**

CASE PRESENTATION 1

This patient's speech is **indistinct** *and* **lacks modulation***. It has a* **nasal quality***. The voice is* **weak** *with* **low volume** *and* **unstable pitch***. There is* **slurring of the labial and lingual consonants** *and the patient speaks in short phrases.[1] There is* **bilateral palatal weakness***.[2] The* **tongue is wasted, flaccid, and fasciculating***. The* **jaw jerk is absent***.*

The diagnosis is **bulbar palsy***.[6]*

CASE PRESENTATION 2

This patient's speech is **indistinct** *and* **lacks modulation***. The speech is* **high-pitched** *and* **slow***. There is* **imprecise articulation** *and the* **articulatory muscles are rigid***. There is a* **harsh vocal quality** *and the patient speaks with a* **strained-strangled voice** *and short phrases.[1] There is* **bilateral palatal weakness***.[2] The* **tongue is small, immobile, and spastic***.[3] The* **jaw jerk is brisk***.[4] There is* **emotional lability***.[5]*

The diagnosis is **pseudobulbar palsy***.[6]*

Clinical notes

1. Bulbar palsy is associated with a flaccid dysarthria, whilst pseudobulbar palsy is assocaited with a spastic dysarthria (see Case 65 Dysarthria).

2. There is weakness of the soft palate. Ask the patient to say 'aah' and carefully inspect the soft palate for movement. In both bulbar and pseudobulbar palsy, there is palatal weakness. Bulbar palsy has a LMN pattern of palatal weakness (reduced or absent gag reflex), whilst pseudobulbar palsy has an UMN pattern of palatal weakness (brisk gag reflex). Testing the gag reflex is often not required in the setting of MRCP (PACES) examination, as it can cause discomfort, but it is important you tell the examiner, that you would like to do so.

3. Ask the patient to open the mouth and inspect the tongue for wasting and fasciculations *inside* the mouth. Fasciculations may be clearly visible, and are often present on the sides of the tongue. Both are a sign of LMN lesions, i.e. bulbar palsy. Although the tongue may appear shrunken in pseudobulbar palsy, wasting is not a feature. Next ask the patient to protrude the tongue and check lateral movements, by asking the patient to move it side to side. In bulbar palsy, there will be reduced movements and the tongue will be flaccid. In pseudobulbar palsy, the tongue appears shrunken, immobile, and stiff—there will be difficulty in protruding the tongue from the mouth.

4. Testing the jaw jerk is often not required in the setting of MRCP (PACES) examination, but it is important you tell the examiner that you would like to do so. If required to do so, show the patient what you intend to do to them on yourself first, emphasizing that you will strike the chin gently. A pathologically brisk response will occur to a slight stimulus.

5. Emotional lability (spontaneous laughter or crying is a feature of pseudobulbar palsy).

6. There are many causes of bulbar and pseudobulbar palsy. Tell the examiner that you would like to examine further to look for underlying causes. A detailed list of causes is provided below, but the following conditions can be easily looked for:

   (a) **BULBAR PALSY**:
      - **Motor neurone disease**: fasciculations in limbs; mixed upper and lower motor neurone signs in limbs
      - **Syringobulbia**: dissociated sensory loss; painless ulcers on hands; wasting of small muscles of the hands; Horner's syndrome; internuclear ophthalmoplegia; UMN signs in upper and lower limbs; spastic gait
      - **Poliomyelitis**: asymmetric limb wasting and weakness; limb deformities
      - **Myasthenia gravis**: ptosis; diplopia; myopathic facies; muscle fatiguability

   (b) **PSEUDOBULBAR PALSY**:
      - **Motor neurone disease**: see above
      - **Bihemispheric vascular disease**: UMN signs in limbs
      - **Multiple sclerosis**: cerebellar signs; internuclear ophthalmoplegia; optic atrophy

It is important to remember, that motor neurone disease can produce mixed upper and lower motor neurone signs, and thus both features of bulbar and pseudobulbar palsy may be present, i.e. tongue fasciculations, spastic dysarthria, and brisk jaw jerk.

Questions commonly asked by examiners

What are the causes of bulbar palsy?

A true bulbar palsy is one that is caused by LMN disease. Bulbar palsy can also be caused neuromuscular junction and muscle disorders. In patients with muscle disease, the pharynx is only mildly affected, thus the clinical features may be subtle. Patients with acute myasthenia or generalized myasthenia can mimic the presentation of an acute ischaemic bulbar palsy.

Disorders of lower motor neurones (true bulbar palsy)
- Motor neurone disease
- Brainstem vascular disease (basilar ischaemia)
- Syringobulbia
- Brainstem tumour
- Poliomyelitis
- Guillain-Barre syndrome
- Neurosyphilis
- Subacute meningitis

Disorders of neuromuscular junction (myasthenic bulbar palsy)
- Botulism
- Myasthenia gravis

Disorders of muscle (myopathic bulbar palsy)
- Muscular dystrophies (facio-scapulo-humeral and occulopharyngeal dystrophy)
- Polymyositis

What are the causes of pseudobulbar palsy?
- Motor neurone disease
- Bihemispheric vascular disease
- Brainstem tumour
- Multiple sclerosis
- Trauma

Why is pseudobulbar palsy only seen with bilateral lesions?

Most cranial nerve nuclei receive bilateral innervation from the corticobulbar tract, thus most pairs of cranial nerve motor nuclei receive UMN fibres from both hemispheres. This is an inherent safety mechanism, as following a unilateral pyramidal tract lesion, both the ipsilateral and contralateral cranial nerve nuclei will continue to receive cortical innervation, and paralysis will not occur. The exceptions to bilateral cortical innervation are cranial nerves VII and XII that only receive contralateral innervation from the pyramidal tract.

Case 71 ◆ **Old Poliomyelitis**

CASE PRESENTATION

This patient's right leg[1] is **hypoplastic[2]** *with proximal and distal* **wasting and weakness, hypotonia, hyporeflexia (areflexia),** *and* **absent plantar responses.[3] Sensation is normal.** *There is* **pes cavus[5]** *on the affected side, with* **surgical scars** *over the ankle and foot.[4]*

The diagnosis is **old poliomyelitis** *(affecting the right leg).[6]*

Clinical notes

Before examining the patient, try to get as many clues as you can from just looking at and around the patient. Look for walking aids, arm and hand splints, and look at the patient's shoes, especially noting ankle supports or orthoses, which would suggest a foot drop. Also look for scuffing at the front of the shoes, which results from foot drop.

1. In poliomyelitis, the findings are often unilateral, although bilateral involvement can be seen. The lower limbs are more commonly affected than the upper limbs.

2. When one limb is shorter than the other, it suggests growth impairment since childhood. Poliomyelitis will not result in shortening of a limb if it occurs in adulthood.

3. There is an LMN pattern of weakness. Patients may have contractures with fixed flexion deformities (long-standing immobility) or previous joint fixation surgery that may limit the motor examination. Fasciculations occur during the acute infection and are usually not seen in the setting of old poliomyelitis. However, some patients may develop a late progressive wasting disease with prominent fasciculations (post-polio syndrome).

4. Poliomyelitis is an important cause of pes cavus.

5. Look carefully for scars especially over the foot and ankle. Patients may have had tendon transposition surgery (for foot drop) and joint fixation surgery (arthrodesis). In the setting of arthrodesis, the joint will be fixed and movement will not be possible. In patients with long-standing immobility, corrective surgery may be necessary for releasing contractures and restoring limb function. As a result of long standing asymmetric weight bearing, patients may develop arthritis, spinal degenerative disorders and scoliosis. Look for deformities, and evidence of joint replacement surgery (especially hips and knees).

6. The presence of LMN signs (often unilateral) with the absence of sensory signs in a patient with hypoplastic limbs would suggest old poliomyelitis. If the findings are bilateral, then the differential diagnosis would be causes of motor neuropathies and motor neurone disease (progressive muscular atrophy). In patients with bilateral weakness and pes cavus, it may be confused with Hereditory Motor and Sensory Neuropathy (HMSN). It is important to remember that in poliomyelitis there are NO sensory signs.

Questions commonly asked by examiners

What do you know about the poliovirus?

The polioviruses are Enteroviruses in the Picornaviridae family. There is a single strand of ribonucleic acid (RNA) surrounded by a protein capsid without a lipid envelope. This makes the poliovirus resistant to lipid solvents and stable at low pH. There are 3 different strains of this virus (type 1–3), with type 1 accounting for 80% of the paralytic illness.

What is the pathophysiology of poliomyelitis?

The poliovirus is transmitted through the faeco-oral route or ingestion of contaminated water. The virus replicates in the oropharyngeal and the gastrointestinal mucosa during the incubation period (1–3 weeks). The virus then drains into cervical and mesenteric lymph nodes and subsequently enters the blood stream. The poliovirus enters the nervous system by crossing the blood brain barrier and axonal transportation from a peripheral nerve. Only 5% of patients have nervous system involvement. There are 5 different clinical syndromes caused by poliovirus:

1. Abortive poliomyelitis
- This is seen in 95% of cases
- Patients are either asymptomatic or have mild symptoms reflecting a pharyngitis or gastroenteritis

2. Non-paralytic (pre-paralytic) poliomyelitis
- Headache, fever, sore throat, and gastrointestinal symptoms
- Irritability, neck and back stiffness may occur (meningism)

- Symptoms usually last 1–2 weeks
- Some patients may progress to paralytic poliomyelitis

3. **Paralytic poliomyelitis**
   - Flaccid limb paresis followed by atrophy (usually after 3 weeks)
   - Patients may complain of paraesthesias in the affected limb, although sensation is intact
   - The recovery may complete, partial, or absent

4. **Paralytic poliomyelitis with bulbar involvement**
   - Pure bulbar involvement without limb involvement can be seen in children (especially if tonsils and adenoids have been removed)
   - Bulbar with spinal involvement is often seen in adults
   - Bulbar involvement results in dysphagia, dysphonia, and facial weakness
   - If the brainstem reticular formation is affected, respiratory failure and vasomotor disturbance (cardiovascular instability) can occur

5. **Encephalitis**
   - This is very rare and is assocaited with a high mortality
   - Results in agitation, confusion, stupor, and coma

What is the post-polio syndrome?

This is the development of progressive wasting and weakness several years (as long as 30 years) after acute poliomyelitis. The exact pathogenesis is not known, although ongoing viral replication or reactivation has been suggested.

What is the differential diagnosis of acute flaccid paralysis?

- **Infection**
  - ◆ Viral
    - – Poliomyelitis
    - – Enterovirus 71
    - – Coxsackie A7
    - – Japanese encephalitis
    - – West Nile virus
    - – Tick paralysis
    - – Paralytic rabies
  - ◆ Bacterial
    - – Botulism
    - – Diphtheria
    - – Lyme disease
- **Neuropathy**
  - ◆ Guillain-Barré syndrome
  - ◆ Acute intermittent porphyria
  - ◆ Lead poisoning
  - ◆ Buckthorn poisoning
- **Spinal disease**
  - ◆ Acute transverse myelitis
  - ◆ Spinal cord compression
  - ◆ Spinal cord infarction

What vaccines are available for prevention of poliomyelitis?

Inactivated polio virus (IPV)—Sabin vaccine

- Consists of all three strains of the virus that have been inactivated or destroyed
- Given by injection
- Stimulates serum IgM, IgG, and IgA (not secretory IgA) production

Oral live attenuated polio virus (OPV)—Salk vaccine

- Consists of all three strains of the virus that have are live but attenuated
- Oral administration at 2, 4, and 6–18 months followed by a booster at 4–6 years of age
- Results in an attenuated infection of the oropharynx and the gut
- Stimulates serum IgM, IgG, and IgA (and secretory IgA) production
- Results in excretion of live virus, thus a small incidence of vaccine assocaited paralytic poliomyelitis in unimmunized contacts, especially if immunocompromised

Case 72 ◆ Neurosyphilis

Examiner's note

This is uncommon in the current era, but given that tabes dorsalis and taboparesis are late manifestations of syphilis, there are patients with clinical signs following infection many years previously, which appear in the MRCP (PACES) examination. These cases can cause confusion amongst candidates, but a basic understanding of the pathophysiology will greatly help discern the clinical signs one encounters. In simple terms, in tabes dorsalis there are slow degenerative changes in the posterior roots and dorsal columns of the spinal cords. Thus one would expect to find LMN signs and dorsal column signs. In taboparesis, there is additional cortical degeneration that results in additional pyramidal signs.

In neurosyphilis, the lower limbs are more commonly affected than the upper limbs, and the most common instruction is to 'examine the lower limbs'. The following case presentations reflect this.

CASE PRESENTATION 1 (LOWER LIMBS)

*On examination of the lower limbs, the ankle joints are swollen and deformed, with abnormal range of movements (**Charcot joints**).[1] There are **ulcers** and **callosities** present on the soles of the feet.[2] There is proximal and distal **wasting and weakness, hypotonia, hyporeflexia** and **absent plantar responses**.[3] There is **loss of joint position and vibration sense**. There is **ataxia** with a **wide-based gait** and **Romberg's sign is positive**.[4]*

*In addition, there are **Argyll Robertson pupils** with **ptosis** and **wrinkling of the forehead**.[5]*

*The diagnosis is **tabes dorsalis**.[6]*

CASE PRESENTATION 2 (LOWER LIMBS)

*On examination of the lower limbs, the ankle joints are swollen and deformed, with abnormal range of movements (**Charcot joints**).[1] There are **ulcers and callosities** present on the soles of the feet.[2] There is proximal and distal **wasting and weakness, hypertonia, brisk knee jerks, absent ankle jerks**, and **extensor plantar responses**.[3] There is **loss of joint position and vibration sense**. There is **ataxia** with a **wide-based 'scissor' gait** and **Romberg's sign is positive**.[4]*

*In addition, there are **Argyll Robertson pupils** with **ptosis** and **wrinkling of the forehead**.[5]*

*The diagnosis is **taboparesis**.[6]*

Clinical notes

1. Dorsal column signs include loss of joint position and vibration sense and can result in neuropathic joints. Neuropathic joints (Charcot's joints) are swollen deformed joints with abnormal ranges of movement, and suggest loss of pain and proprioception. There may be marked crepitus. Any joint can be affected, but the ankle joint is more commonly affected in the lower limbs.

2. Loss of joint position and vibration sense may lead to alteration of weight bearing characteristics, and thus it is important to note ulcers and callosities on the feet.

3. In tabes dorsalis, there are degenerative changes in the posterior roots of the spinal cord, and this results in an LMN pattern of weakness. The deep tendon reflexes and plantar responses may be absent. In general paresis of the insane, there is a progressive frontotemporal meningoencephalitis with cortical atrophy. The spastic paraparesis is cortical in origin. Taboparesis is a combination of tabes dorsalis and general paresis of the insane, thus there may be a mixture of UMN and LMN signs. The key differentiating feature is the presence of extensor plantar responses that will suggest taboparesis as the underlying diagnosis. Other UMN signs may or may not be present. The differential diagnosis for absent ankle jerks and extensor plantars includes:

    - Combination of conditions (most common)
        - Peripheral neuropathy and stroke*
        - Peripheral neuropathy and cervical myelopathy*
        - Cervical and lumbar spondylosis
    - Subacute combined degeneration of the cord (B_{12} deficiency)*
    - Taboparesis*
    - Lesion of the conus medullaris
    - Friedreich's ataxia*
    - Motor neurone disease

4. A sensory gait is wide-based, and patients often watch the feet and ground carefully as they walk with visual input compensating for loss of joint position sense. As a result, if they stand with their feet together, and close their eyes, thereby removing visual input, they become unsteady. This is a positive Romberg's test. It is important to stand close to the patient, and be ready to support the patient should they become unsteady.

5. The clinical signs above suggest a motor and sensory neuropathy. It is the presence of Argyll Robertson pupils that point to syphilis as the underlying cause, and thus a diagnosis of tabes dorsalis or taboparesis. Argyll Robertson pupils are bilateral small irregular pupils that are usually small, and often the pupils demonstrate unequal sizes. A characteristic feature of these pupils is that they are irregular and react to accommodation but not to light. In cases where the light reflex may be present, it is important to remember that the accommodation reflex is always brisker than the light reflex. Wrinkling of the forehead results from compensatory overactivity of the frontalis muscle.

---

* Denotes causes of absent ankle jerks, extensor plantars, and dorsal column signs.

6. Having made the diagnosis of tabes dorsalis or taboparesis, tell the examiner you would like to look for other manifestations of syphilis:
   - Optic atrophy (syphilitic meningitis)
   - Other cranial neuropathy affecting VIII, VII, and VI cranial nerves (syphilitic meningitis)
   - Dementia (general paresis of the insane)—assess mental status
   - Aortic regurgitation (syphilitic aortitis)

Questions commonly asked by examiners

What is the pathophysiology of syphilis?

Syphilis is a sexually transmitted disease caused by Treponema pallidum, with humans being the only hosts. These spiral organisms enter the body through abrasions of the skin and mucous membranes and attach to host cells through the action of muccopolysaccharidases. The characteristic syphilitic lesion (gumma) results from necrosis and obliterative endarteritis of the terminal arterioles with fibroblastic proliferation and lymphocyte infiltration, and can be found throughout the body. There are three phases of disease:

(A) PRIMARY

- Painless ulcer (chancre) with regional lymphadenopathy

(B) SECONDARY

Organ system	Clinical features
GENERAL	Acute febrile illness, generalized lymphadenopathy
SKIN/MUCOUS MEMBRANES	Scaly maculopapular rash (palms and soles); condylomata lata (coalescing fleshy papular lesions in warm moist areas); alopecia; mouth ulcers (snail track ulcers); pharyngitis
EYES	Uveitis; iritis; choroidoretinitis; optic atrophy
NERVOUS SYSTEM	Cranial neuropathies; sensorineural deafness
OTHER	Hepatosplenomegaly; arthritis

(C) TERTIARY

- Cardiovascular manifestations: aortitis and its sequelae (aortic regurgitation and aortic aneurysm)
- Neurological manifestations: see below

What are the different clinical patterns of neurosyphilis?

Clinical pattern	Features
Meningovascular syphilis	This occurs 3–4 years after the primary infection and is characterized by endarteritis with perivascular inflammation with fibroblastic intimal proliferation. This predisposes to cerebrovascular thrombosis and infarction. It can present as cranial neuropathy (VIII, VII, VI, and II), cerebral or spinal stroke.
Tabes dorsalis of the insane	This occurs 10–30 years after the primary infection and is characterized by slow progressive degeneration of the dorsal columns and posterior roots of the spinal cord. Bladder incontinence and sexual dysfunction is common. 'Lightening pains'—sudden electric shock-like sensation spreading rapidly throughout the limbs and trunk often occurs early—resulting in severe pain crises in 90% of patients.

General paresis	This is also known as 'dementia paralytica' and occurs 20–30 years after the primary infection, and represents a progressive frontotemporal meningoencephalitis that results in cortical atrophy. It is characterized by a perivascular and meningeal inflammatory reaction with degeneration of the cortical parenchyma with resultant fibrosis and gliosis. There is insidious onset of psychiatric symptoms and all patients have dementia within 5 years. The accompanying spastic paraparesis is cortical in origin.

What is the definition of neurosyphilis?

Invasion of the CNS occurs early in untreated syphilis, and neurosyphilis is defined as a CSF white blood cell (WBC) > 20 cells/μL or a positive CSF VDRL test.

What is the treatment for acute syphilis?

Penicillin (tetracycline if penicillin allergy).

How can you diagnose syphilis?

- Dark field microscopy
- Direct visualization of the spirochete organism from exudates collected from skin lesions
- Venereal disease research laboratory (VDRL) test*
- Treponema pallidum haemagglutination assay (TPHA) test**

What are the causes of a false-positive VDRL test?

- Rheumatoid arthritis
- SLE
- Autoimmune hepatitis
- Pregnancy
- Infection mononucleosis
- Malaria
- Infection with non-venereal treponemal infections (yaws and pinta)

What are the causes of a false-positive TPHA test?

This test is usually specific for syphilis, but infection with B. burgdorferi (Lyme disease) can cause a false positive result (VDRL test will be negative in such cases).

Case 73 ◆ Facial Nerve Palsy

CASE PRESENTATION

This patient has **right-sided facial weakness** affecting the **upper and lower parts of the face** (equally in frontalis and orbicularis oculi, as for orbicularis oris and elevators of the mouth angle).[1] There is no

---

* Syphilitic infection produces a non-specific IgE anti-cardiolipin antibody. Cardiolipin is used as the antigen to test for this.

** Syphilitic infection produces a specific anti-treponemal antibody.

hearing deficit.[2] There is no ophthalmoplegia.[3] The facial sensation is normal.[4] There are no cerebellar signs.[5] The parotid gland is not enlarged and is normal to palpation.[6] There is no tenderness over the parotid gland and the preauricular area.[7]

The diagnosis is **right lower motor neurone facial nerve palsy (Bell's palsy)**.

Clinical notes

1. In general, LMN lesions affect both upper and lower parts of the face, but due to bilateral innervation in UMN lesions, there is frontalis sparing. However, this general rule regarding distinction of upper versus lower motor neuron lesions is not absolute. Some weakness of frontalis and orbicularis oculis may be apparent with a dense stroke, mimicking a 'Bell's palsy'; conversely, an LMN Bell's palsy may involve lower facial fibres predominantly.

2. Hyperacusis can be tested by noting that a tuning fork sounds louder on the affected side with the prongs held close to the ear. If this is present then a lesion proximal to the stapedius nerve root is suggested, e.g. within the middle ear. Deafness, or tinnitus, might signify a lesion within the internal auditory canal, e.g. acoustic neuroma, or a large brainstem lesion.

3. Look carefully for ophthalmoplegia. An ipsilateral VI nerve palsy, or ipsilateral gaze palsy would suggest a hemi-brainstem cause of the facial palsy. If so, test also for ipsilateral facial sensation impairment or a contralateral hemiparesis, which may also be associated. The VI nerve may be involved in cerebellopontine angle lesions.

4. A simple Bell's palsy may be associated with subjective reports of tingling or numbness on the same side, but not should show objective numbness. If there is ipsilateral facial numbness (V nerve involvement), then consider a cerebellopontine angle lesion.

5. The presence of ipsilateral cerebellar signs would suggest a cerebellopontine angle lesion.

6. Parotid tumours or surgery can cause peripheral facial nerve palsy.

7. Tenderness may reflect an acute/subacute viral or 'idiopathic' Bell's palsy.

8. Tell the examiner you would like to:

    (a) Inspect the ear and examine the ear with an otoscope (vesicles of Ramsay-Hunt syndrome)

    (b) Formally test the taste function

    (c) Enquire about asymmetric tear production*

Questions commonly asked by examiners

What are the causes of Bell's (LMN) palsy?

*   **Idiopathic** (accounts for >95% of cases)**
*   **Structural lesion**
    *   **Brainstem**: demyelination, stroke, tumour
    *   **Cerebellopontine angle**: acoustic neuroma
    *   **Middle ear**: infection
    *   **Parotid gland**: infection, tumour, surgery
*   **Mononeuritis multiplex***

---

* The significance of hypolacrimation on the affected side is that it indicates a lesion proximal to the geniculate ganglion (as most cases of 'idiopathic' Bell's palsy are). Conversely, hyperlacrimation with movements of the mouth ('crocodile tears') indicates aberrant reinnervation that may occur after many months with a Bell's palsy.

** These are most likely viral in origin, especially herpes simplex virus infections.

*** These include diabetes, polyarteritis nodosa, Churg-Strauss syndrome, Wegner's granulomatosis, rheumatoid arthritis, SLE, Sjogren's syndrome, sarcoidosis, lymphoma, carcinoma, amyloidosis, Lyme disease, leprosy.

What tests would you do?

In typical acute Bell's palsy developing over 1–2 days, no tests are required other than possibly a random glucose (due to association with diabetes mellitus). However, if other cranial nerve signs are present, including a bilateral Bell's palsy, or if the history is slowly progressive, or with prominent pain, then an MRI brain should be requested. In idiopathic Bell's palsy the facial nerve usually shows T2 hyper-intensity in its proximal (suprageniculate) course. Other tests to be considered include:

- **Blood tests**: C-reactive protein (CRP), ESR, serum ACE, Lyme serology, HIV serology, autoantibodies (including anti-ganglioside antibodies).
- **Nerve conduction studies** (if Guillain-Barré syndrome is a possibility)
- **Lumbar puncture** (if multiple cranial nerve, or peripheral nerve lesions occur, suggesting a mononeuritis multiplex, polyradiculopathy, or meningeal infiltration)

What treatment would you recommend?

- High-dose oral prednisolone e.g. 60–80mg OD for 5 days provided started within first week.
- Oral acyclovir is also sometimes given in first week although the evidence for this is less strong. Intravenous acyclovir may be used for Ramsay-Hunt syndrome.
- Corneal protection—eye lubricant and tape to close eye should be given in cases where eye cannot be voluntarily closed.

What are the complications of a Bell's palsy?

- Persistent facial weakness
- Corneal abrasions
- Pain and/or sensory disturbance in the distribution of the facial nerve
- Aberrant reinnervation causing crocodile tears (tearing while talking or eating), or jaw-eyelid synkinesia
- Hemifacial spasm

Case 74 ◆ **Muscular Dystrophy**

1. Facio-scapulo-humeral dystrophy

CASE PRESENTATION

*This patient has **myopathic facies**.[1] There is generalized **wasting and weakness of the facial muscles**.[2] There is no ptosis.[3] There is no evidence of frontotemporal balding.[4] Eye movements are normal.[5] There is **wasting and weakness of the upper limb girdle muscles**[6] and the **upper arms**.[7] The superior margins of the scapulae are visible from the front above the clavicles[8] and there is **winging of the scapulae**.[9] There is **abdominal muscle weakness** and the **lower abdominal muscles are weaker than the upper abdominal muscles** (**Beevor's sign**).[10] There is bilateral **weakness of foot dorsiflexion** (anterior tibialis muscle) with foot drop.[11] The lower limb girdle muscles are intact.[12]*

*The diagnosis is **facio-scapulo-humeral dystrophy**.[13]*

Clinical notes

Before examining the patient, try to get as many clues as you can from just looking at and around the patient. Look for walking aids and look at the patient's shoes, especially noting ankle supports or orthoses, which would suggest a foot drop. Also look for scuffing at the front of the shoes, which results from foot drop. One fifth of patients become wheelchair bound. If a wheelchair is present, don't miss it!

1. Myopathic facies refers to a lifeless, lean, and expressionless face. This is also seen in myotonic dystrophy.

2. Weakness is initially seen in the facial muscles, starting in the orbicularis oculi, orbicularis oris, and zygomaticus. The weakness may be asymmetrical. Patients have difficulty with eye closure, smiling, whistling, and pursing their lips.

3. The eyelid muscles are not affected and ptosis is not present. This is an important negative, as myotonic dystrophy produces similar myopathic facies but with ptosis. Myasthenia gravis can also present with facial weakness and ptosis.

4. Frontotemporal balding would indicate myotonic dystrophy.

5. The extraocular muscles are spared, and there is no ophthalmoplegia. This is an important negative to mention, as ophthalmoplegia in the context of facial weakness would suggest myasthenia gravis.

6. Shoulder weakness is the presenting symptom in greater than 80% of cases. There is weakness of scapular fixation that accounts for this. Although the deltoid muscle is usually spared, weakness of shoulder abduction is predominantly due to weak scapula fixation. If the scapula is stabilized manually against the chest wall, there will be a reduction in weakness. Remember, asymmetrical weakness can occur.

7. The bicep and tricep muscles are selectively involved with sparing of the forearm muscles.

8. The scapula is placed more laterally than normal and the superior margins may be visible from the front reflecting wasting of the upper limb girdle muscles.

9. Ask the patient to place the arms out in front of them. Weakness of the lower trapezius muscle results in characteristic upward movement of the scapula (winging of the scapula). Remember asymmetric weakness can occur and one scapula may appear to be more greatly affected.

10. Weakness of abdominal muscles can result in lumbar lordosis and a protuberant abdomen. The lower abdominal muscles are selectively involved whilst the upper abdominal muscles are spared. This results in the Beevor's sign—a very specific sign for facio-scapulo-humeral dystrophy. Whilst the patient is supine, ask the patient to flex the neck or raise the head form the couch. This will result in contraction of the abdominal muscles. In normal circumstances, the upper and lower portions of the abdominal muscles will contract equally, and the umbilicus will remain in a central position. If the upper abdominal muscles are stronger than the lower abdominal muscles, then the umbilicus will be displaced upwards (a positive Beevor's sign).

11. Weakness of foot dorsiflexion follows shoulder weakness. Tibialis anterior muscle weakness is highly characteristic.

12. The lower limb girdle muscles are not affected in 50% of patients. When affected it often occurs late.

13. The winging of the scapula with myopathic facies (with or without foot drop) should point to the diagnosis. Tell the examiner you would like to proceed as follows:

    (a) Look for hearing aids and assess hearing (sensorineural deafness occurs in 75% of patients)

    (b) Perform fundoscopy (retinal telangiectasia occur in 60% of patients)

2. Duchenne's and Becker's Muscular dystrophy

CASE PRESENTATION 1

*This **young**[1] patient is **wheelchair-bound**.[2] There is generalized **wasting and weakness** predominantly affecting the **neck** and **proximal muscles of the upper and lower limb**. The **neck flexors are*** *more affected than the neck extensors. The **wrist extensors are more affected than wrist flexors**. The **tibialis anterior is more affected than the gastrocnemii and solei muscles**.[4] There are **contractures**[5] in the lower limbs and there is **pseudohypertropthy of the calf muscles**.[6] The **deep tendon reflexes are reduced**.[7] There is **kyphoscoliosis**[8] and there is an **inability to generate a forceful cough**.[9] There is sparing of the facial musculature.[10]*

*The diagnosis is **Duchenne's muscular dystrophy**.[11]*

CASE PRESENTATION 2

*This **young**[1] patient is **ambulant** and has a **waddling gait**.[2,3] There is **wasting and weakness** predominantly affecting the **proximal muscles of the upper and lower limb**. There is preserved power of the neck muscles.[4] There is **pseudohypertropthy of the calf muscles**.[6] The **deep tendon reflexes are reduced**.[7] There is sparing of the facial musculature.[10]*

*The diagnosis is **Becker's muscular dystrophy**.[11]*

Clinical notes

Duchenne's muscular dystrophy (DMD) and Becker's muscular dystrophy (BMD) have similar clinical features, but patients with DMD have more severe and earlier onset of weakness. Patient's with DMD develop severe cardiorespiratory failure and usually die in their early 20s. Patients with BMD have a greater life expectancy (usually into their 40s, but some can survive longer) and are more likely to occur in the MRCP (PACES) examination. However, patients with DMD have appeared in the MRCP (PACES) examination, and it is important to be aware of the differences, and the features pointing to either DMD or BMD. Remember, these are X-linked recessive conditions, and the patient is most likely to be male.

1. It is important to note the patient's age. Patients with DMD have more severe and earlier onset of weakness. The usual life expectancy with DMD is 20–25 years. Patients with BMD have a greater life expectancy, usually 40–50 years, but there is greater phenotypic variability and they may survive to 60–70 years.

2. It is important to note if the patient is ambulant, as ambulatory status may help differentiate DMD from BMD. DMD clinically manifests at 3–6 years with a waddling gait and most patients are wheelchair bound by 12 years. If a child is ambulant after the age of 13 years, the diagnosis of DMD should be questioned, and these patients will usually have BMD. The age at which BMD patients become non-ambulatory is 30 years, but many patients with BMD may ambulate independently into the fourth decade of life. A waddling gait can be observed in the ambulant patient, i.e. BMD: a wide-based gait with the trunk moving side to side, and the pelvis drops on each side as the foot leaves the ground. The hip extensor weakness results in a forward tilt of the pelvis, resulting in hyperlordosis of the spine to maintain posture. Other causes of waddling gait include polymyositis and osteomalacia/rickets.

3. In ambulant patients, i.e. BMD, one can look for the Gower sign. The Gower sign points to proximal weakness in the hip extensors, and the patient pushes on the knees in order to stand. Strictly speaking, the Gower sign is used to describe patients moving from lying supine to standing, by climbing up their own body. This is not recommended for the examination as it is not very dignified for the patient and is unlikely to add any extra information.

4. In muscular dystrophies, the general pattern of weakness is in a proximal-to-distal direction. There are rare distal myopathies that predominantly result in distal weakness (see Case 47 Myotonic Dystrophy). In both DMD and BMD, the pattern of weakness is similar, but the onset is earlier and the weakness is severe in DMD. There is progressive generalized weakness predominantly affecting the neck and proximal musculature. This often starts in the legs, later affecting the neck and arms. Eventually there is

distal weakness—the tibialis anterior (often early) and wrist extensor muscles are involved. The neck flexor, wrist extensor, and tibialis anterior strength is preserved early in BMD, but these muscles become compromised with disease progression.

5. Contractures of the limbs occur early in patients with DMD usually at the Achilles tendon and hip and knee flexors. The contractures are initially supple and are often treated with different surgical procedures. Look carefully for scars around the Achilles tendon that may reflect previous tendon surgery.

6. Calf pseudohypertrophy occurs due to fibro-fatty infiltration of the necrotic calf muscles and compensatory hypertrophy of the calf muscles secondary to weakness of the anterior tibial muscles.

7. Loss of deep tendon reflexes reflects muscle fibre loss. Initially they are reduced, but eventually they disappear. However, the ankle jerk may remain intact even in the later stages of the disease.

8. Asymmetric weakness of the paraspinal muscles results in kyphoscoliosis, that contributes to respiratory failure.

9. Ask the patient to cough. A poor cough reflects weakness in the thoracic musculature. Look for evidence of ambulatory oxygen, indicating severe respiratory failure.

10. The facial musculature is usually spared.

11. It should be relatively straightforward to differentiate between DMD and BMD based on age, severity of weakness, and ambulatory status. The following table summarizes the difference in clinical findings.

	DMD	BMD
Age of onset	3–6 years	5–25 years
Age at which non-ambulatory	12 years	30–50 years
Weakness	Severe	Less severe
Pattern of weakness	Proximal limb muscles	Proximal limb muscles
	Neck (flexors>extensors)	Neck (flexors>extensors)
	Tibialis anterior (early involvement)	Tibialis anterior (early involvement)
	Wrist extensors	Wrist extensors
Contractures	Early	Late
Kyphoscoliosis	Early	Late
Calf pseudohypertrophy	Prominent	Mild

After having given the diagnosis, tell the examiner that you would like to look for other associated features:

(a) **Dilated cardiomyopathy**: displaced apex beat, murmurs (functional mitral regurgitation)
(b) **Pulmonary hypertension**: right ventricular heave, loud P_2
(c) **Respiratory failure**: bedside spirometry

Questions commonly asked by examiners

What is muscular dystrophy?
Muscular dystrophies encompass a group of disorders of progressive weakness caused by the progressive degeneration of skeletal muscles.

What is the common pattern of weakness seen in muscular dystrophies?
The classical pattern of weakness observed is proximal-to distal weakness.

Which muscular dystrophies are characterized by distal as opposed to proximal muscle weakness?
- Oculopharyngodistal myopathy
- Welander distal myopathy

- Finish distal myopathy
- Markesbury distal myopathy
- Miyoshi myopathy
- Hereditary inclusion body myopathy
- Distal nebulin myopathy
- Myopathy with ringed muscle fibres
- Limb-Girdle muscular dystrophy type 2B

What are the genetics of facio-scapulo-humeral dystrophy?

This is an autosomal dominant condition in 80% of affected individuals and occurs sporadically in the rest. The gene(s) that are affected have not been identified, but have been localized to chromosome 4 (4q35).

What is the genetic basis of Duchenne and Becker's muscular dystrophy?

Both DMD and BMD are X-linked recessive disorders caused by a mutation in the dystrophin gene (Xp21). All males carrying the gene are affected and females are not affected but are carriers. This means that 50% of their sons will be affected and 50% of their daughters will be carriers.

What is the molecular basis of Duchenne and Becker muscular dystrophy?

Dystrophin is the largest gene described to date and occupies 2% of the X-chromosome. It is expressed in the skeletal, smooth and cardiac muscle as well as the brain. Dystrophin is important in maintaining the structural integrity of the muscle fibres. Loss of dystrophin results in sarcolemmal breakdown, calcium influx into muscles cells, oxidative stress and injury, and ultimately muscle cell death. In DMD, the levels of dystrophin are less than 5%. However, in BMD, the levels are 30–70% of normal, thus resulting in milder clinical features.

Do you know of any other muscular dystrophies?

Emery-Dreifuss muscular dystrophy

There are two forms, type 1 and type 2, and both are due to mutations of genes encoding nuclear envelope proteins. Type 1 is an X-linked recessive condition and caused by a mutation in the EMD gene (Xq28) that codes emerin. Type 2 is an autosomal dominant condition caused by a mutation in the LMNA gene that codes laminin A and C. These are characterized by scaupulo-humero-peroneal wasting (with winging of the scapula) and weakness, early contractures of the elbow, ankle, and neck, and cardiac conduction defects. Contractures often occur before weakness, and contribute significantly to the disability. In general type 1 and type 2 variants are clinically indistinguishable, but type 2 is associated with (a) weakness before contractures; (b) prominent winging of the scapulae; and (c) more severe cardiac conduction defects.

Oculopharyngeal muscular dystrophy

This is an autosomal dominant disorder characterized by slowly progressive ptosis, dysphagia, and dysarthria. Onset is in the fifth or sixth decade. Ptosis is often accompanied by frontalis overactivity and extension of the neck to enable the patient to see.

Limb girdle muscular dystrophies

These are a group of heterogeneous disorders that are inherited in an autosomal recessive (more common) and autosomal dominant pattern. In general, patients with an autosomal dominant form have a later onset and slower course compared to autosomal recessive forms. There are many different forms, and they are characterized by progressive weakness of the shoulder and pelvic girdle muscles, although there is phenotypic variability amongst the different forms. They may be mild or severe. The face and hands are usually spared. Calf pseudohypertrophy and cardiomyopathy may occur.

Case 75 ◆ **Brainstem Syndrome**

Examiner's Note

There are multiple variations of brainstem syndromes. It is not necessary to know them all. It is important to be aware of the specific pointers that indicate brainstem dysfunction. Often brainstem syndrome causes considerable panic and confusion, and candidates try to complicate matters by trying to identify a specific brainstem syndrome. The key is to confidently and competently identify the abnormal neurological signs and be aware of signs that indicate brainstem dysfunction. Furthermore, there are several important conditions that mimic brainstem dysfunction—especially of peripheral nervous system origin—and the candidate would be expected to include these within the differential diagnosis. The clinical pointers of brainstem dysfunction are:

(a) Ophthalmoplegia, especially if involving more than one eye movement
(b) Conjugate gaze palsy—when both eyes are affected equally in their movement in one direction
(c) Pupil involvement—either as a third nerve (including nuclear) lesion, or as a central Horner's syndrome
(d) Nystagmus, especially if vertical
(e) Crossed signs, i.e. sensory and/or motor dysfunction affecting the limbs on one side and the face/bulbar muscles on the other side.
(f) Ataxia in combination with any of the above signs
(g) Bilateral pyramidal signs, e.g. extensor plantars or quadriparesis
(h) Respiratory or autonomic involvement

CASE PRESENTATION 1 (INITIAL INSTRUCTION: 'EXAMINE THE CRANIAL NERVES')

This patient has a **complex ophthalmoplegia**[1] *with* **impaired adduction** *of the right eye, and impaired abduction of the left eye* **(VI nerve palsy)**.[2] *There is a* **bilateral ptosis**[3] *but pupils are unaffected.*[4] *There is* **up-beating nystagmus**[5] *but no internuclear ophthalmoplegia. There is left sided* **lower motor neurone facial weakness (VII nerve palsy)**.[6] *The remainder of the cranial nerves are normal.*

The patient has evidence of a **brainstem syndrome** *that is multifocal, affecting both sides of midbrain and pons. The likeliest causes are vascular, neoplastic, or inflammatory. Toxins such as alcohol in Wernicke's encephalopathy, or anticonvulsants can also cause complex disorders of eye-movements and should be considered.*

I would like to examine the limbs specifically for pyramidal and cerebellar signs, and perform fundoscopy to look for optic atrophy as demyelination may be an underlying cause. I would like to take an alcohol and drug history.[7]

Clinical notes

1. This term can be reasonably applied to any eye movement disorder where there are more than two abnormalities. It focuses the discussion by effectively saying that the underlying disorder is multifocal or diffuse.

2. It is better to describe the ocular movement deficit, rather than committing oneself to a cause, e.g. partial 3rd nerve palsy, since impaired adduction, for example, could equally be due to a supranuclear gaze palsy, lesion in the medial longitudinal fasciculus/paramedian pontine reticular formation, or a muscular/neuromuscular lesion, e.g. thyroid eye disease and myasthenia.

3. Bilateral ptosis in the presence of a 3rd nerve palsy suggests a lesion of the oculomotor nucleus, although myopathy or myasthenia may mimic.

4. Pupils are typically constricted with pontine lesions; dilated with midbrain lesions.

5. Vertical nystagmus always indicates a brainstem or vermis lesion. Down-beating localizes the lesion to the cervicomedullary junction (e.g. Arnold-Chiari malformation) or anterior vermis, whereas up-beating may occur with lesions anywhere in the brainstem.

6. A VII nerve palsy on the same side as an VI nerve palsy suggests a lesion in the lower pons.

7. This case presentation demonstrates multiple cranial nerve signs that can easily confuse the candidate. The key is to identify and present the clinical signs confidently and conclude that this is likely due to brainstem dysfunction, but you would like to conduct a complete neurological examination. Complete the presentation by providing a broad differential diagnosis.

CASE PRESENTATION 2 (INITIAL INSTRUCTION: 'EXAMINE THE CRANIAL NERVES AND PROCEED AS APPROPRIATE')

On examination of the cranial nerves, this patient has a right-sided **Horner's syndrome**,[1] *a* **horizontal nystagmus** *with a fast component to the right*,[2] *right-sided* **facial numbness**[3] *(impairment of pain and temperature sensation), right-sided* **palatal paralysis**[4] *with a* **diminished gag reflex**.[5] *There is* **weakness of the sternocleidomastoid muscle**[6] *on the right. The tongue does not deviate on protrusion*.[7] *This patient has* **dysarthria**.[8]

Proceed as follows:

On examination of the limbs, there are **right-sided cerebellar signs** *and there is* **left-sided impairment of pain and temperature sensation**.[9] *There are no pyramidal signs*.[10]

This patient has a **lateral medullary syndrome**.[11]

Clinical notes

1. Always look for a Horner's syndrome if there are other brainstem signs as it is often subtle (it might only be manifest as a slight ptosis without pupillary difference). However, remember that the presence of lower cranial nerve signs and a Horner's syndrome on the same side can also be caused by a peripheral sympathetic chain disturbance, e.g. carotid aneurysm or dissection, or a skull base mass lesion. The latter however, would not cause pyramidal or cerebellar signs.

2. This is a cerebellar nystagmus.

3. Facial sensation should be tested by pinprick, first in each of the three trigeminal dermatomes (forehead, cheek bone, and chin) on each side and, secondly, along centrifugal lines from the centre of the nose outwards (e.g. to the angle of the jaw and neck, and another towards the vertex). The former method tests separate peripheral divisions of the trigeminal nerve; the latter method tests for a brainstem pattern of trigeminal spinothalamic sensory dysfunction. The spinal nucleus of the V nerve extends caudally to the upper cervical spinal cord. The upper part of the nucleus supplies the central face and the lower part supplies the outer face. Hence as brainstem lesions are located progressively more caudal from the midpons, the uppermost part of the spinal nucleus is spared and this results in a sensory disturbance where the outer parts of the face are affected whilst sparing more central areas,

i.e. nose and mouth. This is called an 'onion-ring pattern' of 'balaclava helmet distribution' sensory disturbance.

4. Palatal weakness on one side is indicated by the uvula being dragged to the normal side. This is a test of the X nerve (vagus nerve).

5. A diminished gag reflex indicates IX nerve dysfunction (glossopharyngeal nerve). The IX nerve can only be assessed by testing sensation of the pharynx, or the afferent limb of the gag reflex. You will not need to perform this in the exam! The efferent component of this reflex is mediated by the X nerve.

6. This indicates XI nerve dysfunction (accessory nerve). Remember that each sternocleidomastoid is tested by turning the head to *opposite* side. Inspection for atrophy, during isometric contraction, may be more sensitive of a unilateral deficit than testing power.

7. It is important to look for XII nerve involvement. The XII nerve nucleus is located in the medial medulla and is not affected in the lateral medullary syndrome. Look for unilateral wasting, ipsilateral deviation with tongue protruded directly forward, and weakness of lateral pointing away from lesion side (tested by patient pushing tongue against inside of cheek against examiner's thumb pushed from outside).

8. Dysarthria might reflect either bulbar weakness, facial weakness, or cerebellar dysfunction. There may be hoarseness due to vocal cord paralysis.

9. The lateral medullary syndrome is characterized by
    (a) Ipsilateral Horner's syndrome
    (b) Ipsilateral cerebellar signs
    (c) Ipsilateral V (spinothalamic), IX, X, and XI nerve signs
    (d) Contralateral spinothalamic signs (below the lesion)
    'Crossing' of weakness or sensory disturbance is highly suggestive for a unilateral brainstem syndrome owing to crossing of corticospinal tract and spinothalamic sensory fibres caudal to the mid-brainstem.

10. If the lateral medullary syndrome is caused by occlusion of the posterior inferior cerebellar artery, there are no pyramidal signs. However, there may also be occlusion of the vertebral artery and thus the pyramidal tracts will be affected resulting in contralateral hemiplegia. It is therefore important to note the absence or presence of pyramidal signs.

11. This is one of the commonest unilateral brainstem stroke syndromes and consists of a combination of: dysphonia with palatal weakness (patient may also be nil by mouth and have a gastrostomy); ipsilateral facial numbness (and possibly contralateral trunk and limb numbness); Horner's syndrome; and nystagmus/ataxia. It is typically caused by a PICA infarct, i.e. posterior inferior cerebellar artery occlusion, that itself may be secondary to a vertebral artery stenosis or dissection.

Questions commonly asked by examiners

What investigations should be performed for a brainstem syndrome?
Imaging:

*   **CT head**: may show a large brainstem tumour or stroke, especially haemorrhage. Will also indicate whether obstructive hydrocephalus is present as a result of a compressive brainstem lesion. In the latter circumstance, an urgent neurosurgical opinion is required as an extraventricular drain, or ventriculo-peritoneal shunt, may be indicated.

*   **MRI head**: a more sensitive test in showing stroke, tumour, demyelination, abscess.

*   **MRI head with Gadolinium enhancement**: this may be useful to reveal meningeal disease, e.g. basilar meningitis, sarcoid, neoplastic meningitis.

*   **MRA head and neck**: this is an important follow-up investigation if an acute brainstem infarct is revealed on regular MRI, as vertebral dissection may be the underlying cause and would possibly prompt the use of anticoagulation.

*   **CXR**, e.g. for tuberculosis, sarcoidosis, and lung malignancy.

Laboratory:

- **Blood tests** such as liver function tests (LFTs), red cell transketolase levels, ESR, autoanti-bodies, anti-neuronal, and Purkinje-cell antibodies and anticonvulsant levels if epileptic.
- **Lumbar puncture**: only to be done if there is no mass lesion, and the diagnosis is unclear. Hence a lesion that respects an arterial territory in a patient whose clinical deficit appeared abruptly, suggesting a straightforward ischaemic stroke, does not need a lumbar puncture. If demyelination is a possibility, but multiple sclerosis is not a certainty (given the appearance of the rest of the brain and spinal cord), a lumbar puncture specifically for unpaired oligoclonal bands is useful.

Other:

- Brainstem and somatosensory evoked potentials if multiple sclerosis is being considered.

If an MRI brain is normal in a brainstem syndrome, what should you consider?

- Toxic or metabolic brainstem dysfunction, e.g. Wernicke's syndrome or anticonvulsant use
- Basilar meningitis or viral rhomboencephalitis, e.g. enterovirus
- Peripheral lesion that masquerades as a brainstem syndrome, e.g. myasthenia gravis, botulism or Miller-Fisher syndrome

What are the causes of a unilateral brainstem syndrome?

The arterial supply of the brainstem respects the mid-sagittal plane and so arterial infarcts are often unilateral, e.g. PICA or AICA (anterior inferior cerebellar artery infarction). However, a vertebrobasilar thrombosis or dissection may cause multiple bilateral brainstem infarcts as right and left pontine branches exit a common basilar artery stem. Furthermore, multiple sclerosis lesions tend to be centred around specific arterial branches and so it is not uncommon for a multiple sclerosis plaque to cause unilateral brainstem signs.

What is the significance of unilateral deafness in the presence of other brainstem signs?

One would consider a cerebellopontine angle tumour (ipsilateral facial and corneal numbness and facial palsy); anterior inferior cerebellar artery infarct, especially due to cardioembolism or vasculitis, or a basilar meningitis.

What are the associations of brainstem dysfunction in an alcoholic?

- Meningitis, especially pneumococcus
- Wernicke's encephalopathy
- Central pontine demyelination

What are the causes of Wernicke's encephalopathy; how would you confirm it, and how do you treat it?

Wernicke's encephalopathy is caused by thiamine (vitamin B1) deficiency due to malnutrition in the setting of chronic alcoholism or repetitive vomiting, e.g. hyperemesis gravidarum, gastric outlet obstruction. It is classically triggered by a high carbohydrate feed, e.g. dextrose hydration in a patient with low thiamine stores.

It can be confirmed by raised red cell transketolase levels, or MRI brain showing petechial hemorrhages of mamillary bodies. Treated with daily intravenous vitamin B1 until neurological signs improve, e.g. for 1–2 weeks, when oral therapy can be substituted. Alcoholic rehabilitation may also be required.

Where is the lesion in lateral medullary syndrome?

This syndrome results from a wedge-shaped infarct in the lateral medulla and inferior surface of the cerebellum.

What are the causes of lateral medullary syndrome?

Occlusion of one of the five arteries may result in this syndrome:

1. Posterior inferior cerebellar artery (most common)
2. Vertebral artery
3. Superior lateral medullary artery
4. Middle lateral medullary artery
5. Inferior lateral medullary artery

What is the medial medullary syndrome?

This is caused by occlusion of the lower basilar artery or the medial branches of the vertebral artery. This results in:

- Ipsilateral XII weakness
- Contralateral hemiplegia (sparing the face)
- Contralateral loss of joint position and vibration sense

Do you know of other eponymous brainstem syndromes?

Eponymous syndrome	Clinical features	
	Ipsilateral signs	Contralateral signs
Weber's	III nerve palsy	Hemiplegia
Millard-Gubler	VI and VII nerve palsy	Hemiplegia
Foville's	VI and VII nerve palsy; lateral conjugate palsy	Hemiplegia
Benedikt's	III nerve palsy	Cerebellar signs

Station 5 ◆ **Brief Clinical Consultations**

General Approach

Supplementary Cases

A. Endocrine

D. Eyes

Brief Clinical Consultations

General approach to brief clinical consultations

Structure of the station

The new Station 5, Integrative Clinical Assessment involves two 10-minute encounters, each known as a 'Brief Clinical Consultation'. Following an introductory referral, the candidate has 8 minutes to undertake a focused history and examination to solve a clinical problem, answer any questions the patient may have and explain their investigation and/or treatment plan to the patient. The remaining 2 minutes are spent with the examiners, to relate the relevant physical findings and differential diagnosis. Remember, you are *not* expected to take a complete history or conduct a complete and thorough examination, as you would in the other stations.

Scenarios for this station

Candidates should be prepared to encounter scenarios relating to:
1. Old Station 5 cases, i.e. skin, eye, locomotor, and endocrine systems.
2. Other stations of the examination (stations 1 and 3).
3. Medical problems encountered in everyday practice, i.e. chest pain, hypotension, jaundice, and deterioration in renal function.

In principle, this station can include any possible inpatient and outpatient medical scenario, and therefore providing a comprehensive selection of cases will never be feasible. Some patients may not display a wealth of clinical signs, and this often occurs in everyday practice.

The candidate should understand the key principles, and develop the art of integrative clinical assessment. This will ensure success in any clinical scenario provided. This integrated approach is a test of higher clinical reasoning and professionalism, rather than a simple test of clinical skills—this should be kept in mind when preparing for this station. The compilation of 20 cases in this section is designed to achieve this, and encourages the candidate to adopt a uniform style, and a thoughtful approach and strategy in tackling this station.

General approach to the station

(a) Candidate information *(5 minutes)*

- Explanatory referrals are provided in the 5 minute interval before the station.
- Read these carefully, and identify the clinical problem(s).
- Develop a differential diagnosis based on the limited information available, even before seeing the patient.
- A preliminary differential diagnosis will initially help guide the focused history.

(b) Focused history and examination *(7 minutes)*

- The history and examination should not be seen as separate components, where the history is followed by the examination.
- Instead, both history and examination should be integrated. It is acceptable to take a history, then examine, and then to re-focus on the history.
- The examination of the patient should begin as soon as you set your eyes on the patient.
- Look for any obvious signs that may prompt a diagnosis.
- Begin with open questions, centred on the patient's symptoms.
- Try to refine the differential diagnosis at every stage of the consultation.
- Conclude the history with closed specific questions to further refine the differential diagnosis.
- It is important to establish the *patient's agenda*, using the techniques illustrated in the communication skills section of this book (Volume 2).
- For inpatient scenarios, don't forget to look at the observation chart, drug chart, glucose chart, etc.
- If the diagnosis is clear, the examination should be conducted to demonstrate the associated clinical features and answer the current clinical problem.
- If the diagnosis is unclear, the examination should reflect the working differential diagnosis.
- With an integrated approach to assessment, a lot of information can be deduced in the limited time provided with the patient.

(c) Feedback to the patient *(1 minute)*

- This is an important part of any clinical encounter, and you will be marked on this.
- Explain the diagnosis or differential diagnoses, using the techniques of *checking* and *repetition*, and avoiding the use of *jargon*.
- Relate these to the patient's symptoms to help patient understanding.
- Explain your initial plans for further investigation and management, again avoiding jargon.
- Address the patient's concerns.
- Conclude with a final check of patient understanding, and ask if there are any other questions.

(d) Feedback to the examiner *(2 minutes)*

- Summarize the key history and examination findings.
- Provide a diagnosis or differential diagnoses, giving supporting evidence.
- Outline an investigation and management plan (in greater detail than that given to the patient).

Case 76 ◆ **Neck Lump**

A. Candidate information

Role: *On-call medical registrar*

This lady has been admitted for elective carpal tunnel decompression for carpal tunnel syndrome. She is scheduled for discharge today. She has no other significant medical history. She has raised concerns about a neck swelling she has noticed over the last 8 months. The surgical doctor has requested a review by the medical registrar.

Task: *Assess for likely cause of neck swelling and explain to the patient if further investigations are necessary.*

B. Patient information

Age: 45 years

Problem: Neck swelling

Over the last 18 months you have been troubled by carpal tunnel syndrome, which has not responded to conservative measures. You have been admitted for a left carpal tunnel decompression procedure. Over the last 10 months you have noticed a neck lump. This has become more noticeable more recently, and your family members have commented about it. There is no associated swallowing or breathing difficulty. You have noticed a 10kg weight loss over the recent 5 months despite having an increased appetite. With this you have noticed increased stool frequency.

You have no other previous medical history. Besides using simple analgesic medications for carpal tunnel syndrome you have not been taking any regular medications.

You have a family history of thyroid problems, and both your mother and sister have previously had thyroid surgery. Unfortunately, your mother was diagnosed with stomach cancer 3 years ago after endoscopy, where she initially presented with a lump in the neck and weight loss.

With your neck lump, you have been particularly concerned that this too may be cancer. As a result of your heightened anxiety you have not been able to sleep very well. Your friends and family have commented about a change in your eyes, and describe your eyes as having a 'fixed staring look'. You feel that this is due to a lack of sleep.

You will ask the doctor:

(a) *Is this cancer, because my mother was diagnosed with stomach cancer when she was found to have a lump in her neck?*
(b) *Do I need further investigations?*
(c) *Can I go home today?*

C. Examiners' information

A good candidate will be able to:

- *Establish symptoms of thyrotoxicosis*
- *Enquire about other gastrointestinal symptoms to explore the possibility of gastrointestinal malignancy*
- *Establish thyroid status*
- *Examine the neck swelling and demonstrate this to be a goitre*
- *Confirm exophthalmos*
- *Examine for other features of Graves' disease (eye signs, thyroid acropachy, and pretibial myxoedema)*
- *Re-assure the patient that her symptoms are due to an overactive thyroid gland as opposed to malignancy, and explain the finding of a goitre*
- *Conclude that this is Graves' disease*
- *Explain the need for further investigations*

D. Focused history

History of presenting complaint

- How long has the neck swelling been present?
- Does it move with swallowing?
- Has it increased in size?
- Are there any swallowing or breathing difficulties?
- Is there any associated pain or tenderness?
- Has there been a change in voice?
- Are there any symptoms of thyroid disease?
    - Hyperthyroidism: weight loss, increased appetite, heat intolerance, palpitations, sweating, insomnia, diarrhoea, and anxiety.
    - Hypothyroidism: weight gain, decreased appetite, cold intolerance, lethargy, constipation, and depression.
- Are there any features to suggest Graves' disease:
    - Visual disturbance?
    - Double vision?
    - Skin rashes?
- Are there any other gastrointestinal symptoms, i.e. abdominal pain, haematemesis, and melena? (screening questions for gastrointestinal malignancy).

Previous medical history

- Is there a history of thyroid problems?
- Has the patient previously had a thyroid function test? If so, what was the result?

Family history

- Is there a family history of thyroid disease?
- If so, what was the diagnosis, and what treatments were undertaken?

Drug history

- Review patient's drug chart

Patients concerns
- What concerns does the patient have?
- Does the patient have any thoughts as to what this could be?

E. Focused examination

Examine thyroid state
- Hyperthyroidism: tachycardia, restlessness, palmar erythema, tremor, lid lag, and retraction
- Hypothyroidism: bradycardia, slowness of movement, slow relaxing deep tendon reflexes

Examine goitre
- Establish thyroid swelling (moves with swallowing)
- Determine characteristics of thyroid swelling
- Symmetry
- Tenderness
- Retrosternal extension
- Bruit
- Lymphadenopathy

Examine for features of Graves' disease
- Thyroid eye signs (exophthalmos and ophthalmoplegia)*
- Thyroid acropachy
- Pretibial myxoedema

F. Diagnosis
- Graves' disease
- Hyperthyroidism

This patient has symptoms of hyperthyroidism. The weight loss and gastrointestinal symptoms may suggest gastrointestinal malignancy, especially with a family history. However, the clinical findings of thyrotoxicosis, goitre, and exophthalmos, indicate Graves' disease as the underlying cause. Furthermore, there is strong family history of thyroid disease.

This patient has carpal tunnel syndrome, which can be associated with hypothyroidism. This may confuse candidates, but the signs of thyrotoxicosis and Graves' disease are clearly present and should not prevent making the correct diagnosis. There are many other causes of carpal tunnel syndrome, and this may be coincidental!

G. Feedback to the patient

Explain diagnosis
- *'There is a swelling of the thyroid gland, which appears to be overactive.'*
- *'The overactive thyroid gland secretes excess thyroxine hormone, and this accounts for the symptoms of weight loss, diarrhoea, anxiety and insomnia.'*
- *'One particular form of thyroid disease can affect other tissues in the body, particularly the muscles of the eyes. This is known as Graves' disease. The examination findings suggest that the eye muscles are involved to some extent, and suggests this diagnosis. The eye involvement often improves with treatment.'*

---

* If there are signs of thyroid eye disease, then check visual acuity

Address patient concerns

- 'The examination findings suggest that your symptoms are due to an overactive thyroid gland and not due to an underlying cancer. Although your mother presented with a neck lump when she was diagnosed with stomach cancer, that neck lump would likely have been a swollen lymph gland. However, your examination findings suggest a thyroid swelling and not a lymph gland swelling.'
- 'Further investigations are necessary: blood tests to check thyroid function, and ultrasound scan of the neck.'
- 'Although the investigations can be conducted as an outpatient, since you have symptoms of an overactive thyroid gland, it may best to await the results of thyroid function tests and be reviewed by the endocrinologist whilst an inpatient.'
- 'If there were evidence of an overactive thyroid gland, it would be best to initiate anti-thyroid therapy prior to discharge.'

H. Feedback to the examiner

Further investigations

- Blood tests (including thyroid function tests and thyroid antibodies*)
- Ultrasound scan of the neck
- Isotope scan (^{99m}Tc)

Further management

- Await results of thyroid function tests to confirm thyrotoxicosis
- If confirmed, anti-thyroid therapy, i.e. carbimazole (first-line) or propylthiouracil
- Non-selective beta-blocker (symptom control)
- Protective measures for exophthalmos:
  - Eyedrops and lubrication
  - Sleep upright (with the eyes taped closed)—reduces lid oedema
  - Lateral tarsorrhaphy to protect the cornea
  - Smoking cessation—smoking increase the risk of oedema and congestion
  - Prism glasses can help with diplopia

I. Additional reading

Volume 1

Supplementary Endocrine Case 97 Goitre

Supplementary Endocrine Case 98 Assessment of Thyroid State

Volume 2

Station 2 Case 20 Neck Lump

---

* Thyroid-stimulating hormone (TSH) receptor antibody (TSH rAb) or thyroid stimulating immunoglobulin (TSI) [Graves' disease], and antithyroid peroxidase enzymes antibody (anti-TPO) [Hashimoto's thyroiditis]

Case 77 ◆ **Leg Swelling**

A. Candidate information

Role: On-call medical registrar

This lady is currently an inpatient on the general medical ward. She has been admitted 10 days ago with breathlessness and oedema. She has been treated for congestive cardiac failure and had responded well to intravenous diuretics. She had been switched to oral diuretic therapy yesterday and was scheduled for discharge if her weight had remained stable. Her previous medical history includes hypertension, type 2 diabetes, ischaemic heart disease, and rheumatoid arthritis. Since this morning, she has complained of painful leg swelling. The sister on the ward has requested an urgent medical opinion, as this lady was potentially scheduled for discharge today.

Task: Assess for likely cause of leg swelling and explain to the patient if further investigations are necessary.

B. Patient information

Age: 72 years

Problem: Right calf swelling

You have been troubled by breathlessness on exertion, and have had three admissions with fluid overload. This is your fourth admission with congestive cardiac failure. You have responded well to intravenous diuretics and have now started on oral diuretics. You have been mobilizing on the ward and your daily weights have remained stable.

This morning you have noticed a gradual onset of pain in the right calf. Two days ago, you had a mechanical fall on the ward where you tripped over some bags by the side of your bed. You fell to the floor and sustained a trivial injury to your right calf against the side of a chair. You were able to get up, and there was no subsequent calf pain. Last night everything appeared to be fine, but this morning the right calf appears painful and swollen. Although you are able to weight-bear and mobilize, it is uncomfortable. There is no chest pain or breathlessness.

You have a previous history of hypertension, diabetes, previous myocardial infarction, and rheumatoid arthritis. Following the myocardial infarction 3 years ago, you had coronary angioplasty with 3 coronary stents. The rheumatoid arthritis has been well controlled. You have never had deep vein thrombosis (DVT) or pulmonary embolism (PE).

You feel that this is a muscular injury and wish to be prescribed painkillers so that you can go home. You are very keen to go home. However, the ward sister is concerned about the leg swelling and has asked the on-call doctor to review.

You will ask the doctor:

(a) This is a muscular injury. Why is the ward sister concerned?
(b) Will I need further investigations?
(c) Can I go home today?

C. Examiners' information

A good candidate will be able to:

- Establish the history of acute unilateral calf swelling and tenderness
- Relate the timing of events, particularly the recent leg trauma
- Enquire about thrombotic risk factors
- Review the drug chart particularly noting for anticoagulant therapy and/or DVT prophylaxis
- Examine the lower limb appropriately reflecting the appropriate differential diagnoses
- Enquire about symptoms of possible pulmonary embolism
- Explain to the patient the possible diagnosis of DVT and the need for further investigation and management
- Address the patient's concerns

D. Focused history

History of presenting complaint

- Establish the specifics of current admission.
- Enquire about the efficacy of diuretic therapy.
- When did the patient note the swelling?
- Establish the relationship of onset of the swelling with trauma.
- Is it unilateral or bilateral?
- How extensive is the swelling?
- Is there any evidence of bruising or injury?
- Is there associated
  - ◆ pain?
  - ◆ numbness?
  - ◆ paraesthesia?
  - ◆ change in skin colour?
- How has it affected the patient? Can the patient weight bear and walk?
- Is there any chest pain or breathlessness?

Previous medical history

- Previous history of DVT/PE
- Thrombophilia
- Establish any contra-indications to anticoagulation (treatment for DVT)

Family history

- Thrombophilia

Drug history

- Review patient's drug chart
- Specifically note the use of anticoagulant therapy. In the context of limb trauma, anti-platelet or anticoagulation can increase bleeding risk and risk of compartment syndrome. If patient is on oral anticoagulation therapy, check the international normalized ratio (INR) (often written on the chart). Furthermore, if a patient is therapeutically anticoagulated, it reduces the likelihood of DVT (although DVT can occur in patients with therapeutic anticoagulation!).
- Has DVT prophylaxis (low molecular weight heparin and/or thrombo-embolus deterrent (TED) stockings) been prescribed?

Patients concerns
- What concerns does the patient have?
- Does the patient have any thoughts as to what this could be?

E. Focused examination

Review the observation chart
- Temperature (fever suggests possible infection, i.e. cellulitis)
- Heart rate (tachycardia can be seen in PE)
- Oxygen saturations (hypoxia is seen in PE)

Examine lower limbs
- Establish asymmetrical leg swelling
- Assess the extent of leg swelling
- Note any trophic changes (erythema, blue-brown discoloration secondary to venous hypertension)
- Look for presence of pitting oedema to assess the efficacy of diuretic therapy
- Is the swelling soft or tense?*
- Assess peripheral pulses*
- Assess sensation*

Examine the chest
- Assess jugular venous pressure (JVP). An elevated JVP suggests fluid overload or pulmonary hypertension (secondary to pulmonary embolism). This patient has had an admission for congestive cardiac failure. A euvolaemic state has been achieved following diuresis, and in this context, an elevated JVP would suggest pulmonary embolism.
- Signs of pulmonary hypertension (parasternal heave and loud P_2)
- Assess for pulmonary congestion (bibasal crepitations)
- Assess for signs of pulmonary embolism (consolidation, pleural rub)

F. Diagnosis

- *Possible DVT*

In the above case, the differential diagnosis of unilateral leg swelling is

(a) DVT
(b) Ruptured Baker's cyst (given history of rheumatoid arthritis)
(c) Compartment syndrome (given history of trauma).

When taking a focused history, one needs to have a clear differential diagnosis in mind. This patient was originally admitted with bilateral lower limb oedema, which responded to diuretic therapy. It will be important to determine the effect of diuretic therapy, prior to the onset of unilateral leg swelling.

---

* The presence of tense leg swelling with neurovascular deficit following trauma should raise the suspicion of compartment syndrome.

G. Feedback to the patient

Explain diagnosis
- 'The examination findings suggest that a clot may have developed in veins of the leg (DVT).'
- 'The current admission has been for heart failure and has resulted in a period of relative immobility. Immobility is a recognized risk factor for DVT.'

Address patient concerns
- 'Although a muscular injury remains a possibility, we need to exclude a DVT—the most likely diagnosis. This is easy to diagnose and treat. If a DVT is untreated, the clot can extend and cause further complications by breaking off and impacting in the blood vessels in the lung (pulmonary embolism). This can potentially be life-threatening.'
- 'The treatment for DVT is medication to thin the blood. Given that the suspicion of DVT is high, you will commence this treatment immediately (low molecular weight heparin injection), and I will arrange a doppler ultrasound scan of the leg.'
- 'If the diagnosis is confirmed on doppler ultrasound scan, then you will need to take warfarin tablets, instead of injections for 3-6 months.'

H. Feedback to the examiner

Further investigations
- Blood tests (including full blood count (FBC), C-reactive protein (CRP), D-dimer, creatinine kinase (CK) and coagulation profile)
- electrocardiogram (ECG) (tachycardia and/or features of right ventricular strain)
- Chest X-ray (CXR) (if chest signs are present)
- Doppler ultrasound scan of the leg

Further management
- Anticoagulation (initially with low molecular weight heparin and then formally with warfarin if DVT confirmed)
- Analgesia
- Await results of doppler ultrasound scan of the leg

I. Additional reading

Volume 2
Station 2 Case 12 Ankle Swelling

Case 78 ◆ **Palpitations**

A. Candidate information

Role: *On-call medical registrar*

This gentleman has been admitted with a community-acquired pneumonia and is currently an inpatient receiving intravenous antibiotics. He is currently on the third day of antibiotic therapy and is making good progress. Earlier this morning, he noticed palpitations. They were rapid and irregular. The ward sister has taken routine observations and noted a pulse rate of 125 and blood pressure of 118/70. She has requested an urgent medical registrar review.

Task: Assess the patient and assess for possible arrhythmia. Advise on further investigation and treatment.

B. Patient information

Age: 32 years

Problem: Palpitations

You have been admitted to the medical ward for the last 3 days with pneumonia. You have been receiving intravenous antibiotic therapy and are making a progressive recovery. You are still experiencing breathlessness and require supplementary oxygen.

This morning, upon waking you noticed that your heart rate was rapid. It felt irregular. There was no chest pain. There has been no deterioration in breathlessness. Initially you thought it was anxiety, as previously panic attacks have resulted in similar palpitations. However, this is different as the palpitations have been persistent and the pulse rate is much faster. The ward sister has taken routine observation and the pulse rate was 125 beats per minute. You had not felt particularly anxious earlier, but now having learnt of a fast pulse rate you are extremely concerned and anxious.

You have a previous history of infrequent panic and anxiety attacks. You have no other significant medical history. There is no significant family history of medical problems.

You are smoker and have minimal alcohol intake

You will ask the doctor:

(a) Is this anxiety? If not, why is my pulse rate so fast?
(b) Will I require treatment with anxiolytics drugs?
(c) Does a fast heart rate reflect worsening of the pneumonia?

C. Examiners' information

A good candidate will be able to:

- *Obtain a history of palpitations*
- *Establish previous cardio-respiratory history and other potential precipitants of arrhythmia*
- *Establish an irregular pulse without haemodynamic compromise*
- *Conclude the most likely diagnosis is atrial fibrillation secondary to infection*
- *Assess pulse and blood pressure with an appropriate cardiovascular examination*
- *Explain to patient the likely diagnosis of atrial fibrillation and need for further investigation (ECG, blood tests, and echocardiogram) and management (rate-control and anticoagulation)*
- *Address the patient's concerns*

D. Focused history

History of presenting complaint

- Establish the specifics of the current admission and response to treatment.
- When did the patient notice the palpitations?
- Are they persistent or intermittent?
- Are they fast or slow?
- Do they feel regular or irregular? [Ask the patient to tap them out to establish pattern].
- Is there associated
  - chest pain?
  - breathlessness?
  - dizziness?
- Is there calf swelling and tenderness? (DVT with subsequent PE should be suspected in immobile patients as a possible cause of atrial fibrillation).

Previous medical history

- Previous history of palpitations
- Cardiorespiratory disease
- Hyperthyroidism

Drug history

- Review patient's drug chart
- Nebulizer therapy can cause tachycardia

Patients concerns

- What concerns does the patient have?
- Does the patient have any thoughts as to what this could be?

E. Focused examination

Review the observation chart

- Temperature (persisting fever indicates poor response to antibiotic therapy)
- Heart rate (assess the trend in heart rate—a sudden marked increase in baseline heart rate without an obvious cause suggests this is not a physiological response and is most likely to represent an underlying arrhythmia).
- Blood pressure (assess the trend in blood pressure—a hypotensive state requires emergency treatment of arrhythmia)
- Oxygen saturation

Examine cardiovascular system

- Assess pulse
- Assess JVP—an elevated JVP suggests fluid overload or pulmonary hypertension (secondary to PE). In a euvolaemic state, an elevated JVP would suggest PE.
- Listen for murmurs (particularly mitral valve disease)
- Assess for signs of congestive cardiac failure, i.e. S_3, S_4 (will not be present in atrial fibrillation), pulmonary congestion, and peripheral oedema

Examine the respiratory system

- Establish signs of pneumonia (lung consolidation)
- Assess for congested lung fields

F. Diagnosis

- Atrial fibrillation secondary to pneumonia

There are many causes of an irregular pulse. Although an irregular pulse is suggestive, it is not diagnostic of atrial fibrillation. This will need to be confirmed with an ECG. A confounding factor in the history is panic attacks and anxiety. However, the history and examination reveals a persistently elevated and irregular pulse rate—this is more likely to represent an arrhythmia as opposed to anxiety. As with all patients with atrial fibrillation, it will be important to exclude thyroid disease, as hyperthyroidism may potentially explain this patient's previous history of anxiety.

G. Feedback to patient

Explain diagnosis

- 'A persistently rapid and irregular pulse is most likely to be a rhythm disturbance of the heart known as atrial fibrillation. This is the most common rhythm disturbance encountered in patients.'
- 'Infection is a common precipitant, and it is likely the pneumonia has triggered this.'

Address patient concerns

- 'A persistently elevated and irregular pulse is unlikely to be related to anxiety and is most likely a rhythm disturbance of the heart. We need to confirm this by performing an ECG.'
- 'This has been triggered by infection, and does not necessarily suggest a worsening of infection, especially as there has been an improvement since admission.'
- 'If atrial fibrillation is confirmed on ECG, it will require treatment with drugs to slow the heart rate. This is often temporary, and once the infection has cleared, the heart rhythm often normalizes.'
- 'Blood tests will be necessary (to check the electrolytes and thyroid function).'
- 'We will also need to do an echocardiogram to look for structural heart problems.'
- 'Atrial fibrillation is associated with increased risk of clot formation in the heart, so patients often take medications to thin the blood. Although the risk is small in young patients without structural heart disease, this is recommended in the first instance, although it may be temporary if the heart rhythm normalizes.'

H. Feedback to the examiner

Further investigations

- Blood tests (including FBC, urea and electrolytes (U&E), CRP)
- ECG
- CXR (signs of pulmonary congestion)
- Echocardiogram (structural heart disease)

Further management

- Correction of electrolytes
- Rate-control therapy with β-blockers or non-dihydropyridine calcium channel blockers (verapamil and diltiazem). Digoxin can be added if further rate control is required.

- Anticoagulation (low molecular weight heparin and then warfarin if atrial fibrillation persists).*

I. Additional reading

Volume 2

Station 2 Case 11 Palpitations

---

* In patients with acute atrial fibrillation secondary to infection, restoring sinus rhythm is not advised, unless there is haemodynamic compromise. It is important to treat the underlying infection and adopt a rate-control strategy in the first instance. Often, when the infection is treated, the rhythm will revert back to sinus rhythm. Occasionally, atrial fibrillation may persist after treatment of infection. In such cases, it is important to exclude the presence of underlying structural heart disease. If atrial fibrillation persists after adequate treatment of infection, then sinus rhythm can be restored with electrical DC cardioversion after 4 weeks of therapeutic anticoagulation with warfarin (INR: 2–3). It would be appropriate to initiate anticoagulation therapy with low molecular weight heparin and if sinus rhythm is spontaneously restored following treatment of infection, then this may be discontinued. If atrial fibrillation persists, then warfarin may be initiated with a view to DC cardioversion after 4 weeks of therapeutic anticoagulation.

Case 79 ◆ Transient Visual Disturbance

A. Candidate information

Role: On-call medical registrar

This lady has been admitted to the medical ward with cellulitis of the right leg. She has been receiving antibiotic therapy for the last 5 days, and has now been switched to oral therapy. She is scheduled for discharge tomorrow provided her clinical status and inflammatory markers remain stable. This afternoon, she experienced 2 episodes of transient loss of vision with full recovery. She feels well in herself and is keen to go home. She has mentioned the visual disturbances to the ward nurse, who has been concerned and therefore requested a review by the on-call doctor. Her previous medical history includes hypertension, type 2 diabetes, and atrial fibrillation (diagnosed many years ago). Her medications include aspirin, metformin, bisoprolol, ramipril, and simvastatin.

Task: Assess the patient; ascertain the cause for visual disturbance; and address patient's concerns.

B. Patient information

Age: 82 years

Problem: Visual disturbance

You have been admitted to the medical ward for the last 5 days with a cellulitis. You have been receiving intravenous antibiotic therapy and have been switched to oral therapy today. Following the ward round earlier today, you may potentially be discharged tomorrow, provided your blood tests improve and you do not spike a fever.

This afternoon, just before lunch you noticed sudden loss of vision affecting the left eye. When asked to describe the visual disturbance, it was like a 'curtain coming down over your field of vision'. This lasted for half an hour, after which your vision normalized. After approximately 3 hours, it recurred, again affecting the left eye. You are short-sighted and use your spectacles only when really necessary, but have never experienced this before. There was no associated weakness of the limbs. Infrequently in the past you have had blurring of the vision in both eyes, but this has been associated with hypoglycaemia, which resolves rapidly on intake of sugary foods. The ward nurse checked your glucose and it was normal at 6.8mmol/L.

Your previous medical history includes hypertension, type 2 diabetes, and atrial fibrillation. The atrial fibrillation was diagnosed 5 years ago where you saw a cardiologist who recommended warfarin. You were not keen on warfarin, as you did not want to be inconvenienced by regular blood tests and were therefore asked to continue with aspirin. You have been diagnosed with diabetes for 10 years and have annual eye checks. You have been told there are minor eye changes in the eyes which will be kept under annual review.

You have been frightened by this episode, and are concerned this may happen again. You are the main carer for your husband who suffers from Alzheimer's dementia, and wish to be in the optimum state of health.

You will ask the doctor:

(a) What is the cause of this visual disturbance?
(b) Will this happen again?
(c) Can this be prevented?
(d) Will this preclude my discharge tomorrow?

C. Examiners' information

A good candidate will be able to:

- Obtain a history of visual disturbance
- Establish previous history of diabetic eye disease
- Enquire about hypoglycaemic symptoms
- Enquire about previous reluctance to warfarin therapy
- Examine the pulse, the carotids (for bruits), and precordium (murmurs)
- Examine the eyes (visual acuity, visual fields, eye movements, and fundoscopy)
- Conclude that this a transient ischaemic attack, most likely a complication of atrial fibrillation
- Explain the need for further investigations (echocardiogram, carotid dopplers, computerized axial tomography (CT), or magnetic resonance imaging (MRI) Head)
- Explain the need for warfarin therapy
- Address the patient's concerns

D. Focused history

History of presenting complaint

- When did you notice the visual disturbance?
- Can you describe the onset of visual disturbance? Was it sudden or gradual?
- Can you describe the visual disturbance? Was it partial or complete?

- Did it affect one or both eyes?
- Is it intermittent or persistent?
- How long did it last?
- Did you get complete recovery? Did it recur?
- Enquire about symptoms associated with stroke:
    - Facial or limb weakness?
    - Facial or limb sensory disturbance?
    - Double vision?
    - Headache?
    - Speech disturbance?
- Enquire about symptoms associated with polymyalgia rheumatica/temporal arteritis:
    - Headache?
    - Scalp tenderness?
    - Jaw claudication?
    - Joint aches and pains?
- Did you measure the blood glucose? If so, what was it?

Previous medical history
- Previous history of visual disturbance
- Enquire about cardiovascular risk factors
- In patients with diabetes, it is important to establish:
    - Previous diabetic control
    - Microvascular and microvascular complications
    - History of diabetic eye disease (diagnosis and previous treatments)
    - Hypoglycaemic attacks (frequency and characteristics of such attacks)
- Atrial fibrillation
- Migraines
- Polymyalgia rheumatic/temporal arteritis

Drug history
- Review patient's drug chart
- If there is a history of atrial fibrillation, what is the current anti-thrombotic therapy?
- Has warfarin even been mentioned or recommended?
- If patient has previously declined warfarin, why?
- Are there any contraindications to warfarin therapy?

Patients concerns
- What concerns does the patient have?
- Does the patient have any thoughts as to what this could be?

E. Focused examination

Review the observation chart
- Heart rate (establish irregular pulse and check adequacy of rate-control)
- Blood pressure (check adequacy of blood pressure control; contributes to ABCD criteria, see below)
- Look at the glucose chart (are there hypoglycaemic periods?)

Examine cardiovascular system
- Assess pulse (rate and rhythm)
- Listen for carotid bruits
- Listen for murmurs (particularly mitral valve disease)

Examine the eyes
- Test visual acuity. Test each eye separately.
- Assess visual fields
- Assess eye movements
- Perform fundoscopy
- Palpate temporal arteries (temporal arteritis is common in the elderly)

Examine the nervous system
- This may not be possible given the time constraints, and in such cases it is acceptable to tell the examiner that you would like to conduct a complete neurological examination assessing the cranial nerves and limbs.
- If time allows, a truncated neurological examination may be conducted by assessing for facial weakness and limb power and reflexes.

F. Diagnosis

- Amaurosis fugax or transient ischaemic attack (TIA) as a complication of atrial fibrillation.

The differential diagnosis of *monocular* visual disturbance in this patient is:

(a) TIA (atrial fibrillation, diabetes, hypertension)
(b) Diabetic maculopathy (diabetes)
(c) Retinal or vitreous haemorrhage (diabetes, hypertension)
(d) Central retinal vein or branch occlusion (diabetes, hypertension)
(e) Temporal arteritis (age)

Given the patient's previous medical history, the above differential diagnosis should be borne in mind. The focused history and examination should be specifically tailored to look for these.

This patient has had two episodes of transient monocular visual disturbance in the characteristic pattern of amaurosis fugax that is highly suggestive of TIA. She has a history of atrial fibrillation and is not anticoagulated with warfarin, which would otherwise be strongly indicated in this patient with increased thromboembolic risk. As most TIAs last minutes rather than hours, the initial diagnosis is usually made on the patient's history. Focal neurological signs have usually resolved by the time the patient presents. The ABCD score can be used to identify which patients require admission and urgent assessment. Although TIAs affecting the eyes have better prognosis than hemispheric TIAs, two separate TIAs constitute a diagnosis of crescendo TIAs, thus an increased risk of stroke. This warrants urgent inpatient assessment.

G. Feedback to the patient

Explain diagnosis
- *'Your visual disturbance has been caused by what is known as a transient ischaemic attack (mini-stroke).'*
- *'Atrial fibrillation is associated with increased risk of clot formation in the heart. It is likely a small clot has formed in the heart and entered the circulation to block small arteries in the brain and the eyes.'*

Address patient concerns

- 'Warfarin therapy in atrial fibrillation prevents complications such as stroke. Although aspirin reduces this risk (risk reduction of 22%), warfarin is associated with a greater reduction in risk (risk reduction of 66%).'
- 'This transient visual disturbance has occurred twice and can occur again. Other forms of stroke with facial/limb weakness and/or speech disturbance can also occur. Warfarin will reduce this risk, and is strongly recommended.'
- 'Further investigation will be necessary: echocardiogram, carotid dopplers, and CT/MRI head.'
- 'TIA is a medical emergency and indicates unstable blood flow to the brain with an increased risk of subsequent stroke. This requires immediate assessment by a stroke physician. Given that there have been two episodes, the risk of stroke is higher, and these investigations should be arranged as an inpatient, and initiation of warfarin is recommended prior to discharge.'

H. Feedback to the examiner

Further investigations

- Blood tests (including lipid profiles, HbA_{1C} and erythrocyte sedimentation rate (ESR)*)
- Echocardiogram (valvular heart disease, left atrial size and presence of cardiac thrombus)
- Carotid dopplers (carotid stenoses)
- CT/MRI head

Further management

- Initiation of warfarin (provided there are no contraindications)
- Optimization of cardiovascular risk factors
- Up-titrate lipid lowering therapy (aim total cholesterol <4.0mmol/L and low density lipoprotein (LDL) <2.0mmol/L)
- Improve blood pressure control
- Improve glycaemic control (pending HbA_{1C})
- Up-titrate rate-control therapy if necessary

I. Questions commonly asked by examiners

Why is TIA considered a medical emergency?

A TIA is the only warning that a stroke may be imminent and precedes ischaemic stroke in 15–26% of patients. The risk of stroke in the first 48 hours is 5% and in the first 7 days after a TIA is approximately 8%. Thus following a TIA, there is an opportunity to intervene, and to help prevent a more damaging ischaemic stroke. This window of opportunity is small and requires patients to have rapid specialist stroke specialist assessment.

What do you know about the ABCD² criteria for TIAs?

The 7 day risk of stroke after a TIA can be predicted using the ABCD² score, based on Age, Blood pressure, Clinical features, and Duration of symptoms. Those with an ABCD² score of 6 have the highest risk of stroke, with approximately 33% of such patients suffering a stroke at 7 days post-TIA. Patients with ABCD² score >4 are considered at high risk for stroke and should be admitted and undergo intracranial imaging with 24 hours of onset of symptoms [NICE guidelines (2008)]

---

* If suspecting temporal arteritis.

	Criteria	Sub-criteria	Score
A	Age	Age >60 years	1
B	Blood pressure	Systolic >140mmHg and/or	
		Diastolic >90 mmHg	1
C	Clinical features	Unilateral weakness	2
		Speech disturbance	1
		Other	0
D	Duration of symptoms	>60 minutes	2
		10–59 minutes	1
		<10 minutes	0
	Presence of Diabetes mellitus		1

What is the definition of crescendo TIAs?

This is defined as two or more TIAs within 1 week. This warrants urgent admission for investigation and management.

Which patients with TIA require admission and urgent assessment?

- All patients with a suspected TIA require urgent specialist assessment and investigation.
- Patients with crescendo TIAs, those with an ABCD score ≥4, and those on warfarin should be admitted immediately to the stroke unit for urgent assessment, investigation, and management.
- Patients on warfarin therapy need urgent imaging to exclude intracranial haemorrhage.
- All patients with an ABCD score <4 should be referred to a Neurovascular Clinic or TIA clinic. They should be seen and have intracranial imaging within 7 days of the event.

What is the role of carotid endartarectomy in TIA and stroke?

According to the NICE guidelines (2008),[1] all patients with TIA and non-disabling stroke should have:

- Carotid imaging within 1 week of onset of symptoms
- Those with carotid stenosis >70% should be referred for carotid endartarectomy within 1 week, and have carotid endartarectomy within 2 weeks of onset of symptoms.

J. Additional reading

Volume 1

Station 3 Central Nervous System Case 68 Hemiparesis

Volume 2

Station 2 Case 11 Palpitations

Station 2 Case 28 Visual Disturbance

---

[1] National Institute for Clinical Excellence Stroke: diagnosis and initial management of acute stroke and transient ischaemic attack (TIA). London: NICE, 2008.

Case 80 ◆ Tall Stature

A. Candidate information

Role: *Medical registrar (endocrinology outpatient clinic)*

This young gentleman has tall stature. Most of his paternal family appear to have tall stature. This has never really been investigated, as it has been attributed as a family trait. He has no significant medical history. Following a routine check, he was noted to have mild gynaecomastia. I wonder if there is an endocrine basis for the tall stature. Thank you for your assessment.

Task: *Assess for the likely cause of tall stature and consider further investigations if necessary.*

B. Patient information

Age: 23 years

Problem: Tall stature

You have strong family history of tall stature, with your father, brother, and paternal uncles all being very tall. Ever since you can remember, you have always been taller than your peers. You have never really taken notice of it, and have considered it a family trait.

Recently, you visited the GP with a flu-like illness. The GP noted mild swelling of tissue below the nipples, and felt that there may be a hormonal problem that may account for the tall stature. You have always had this soft tissue swelling below the nipples, and have never really been bothered by it.

You have no previous medical history.

You have no significant family history. You do not smoke and do not consume alcohol. You are a student at university.

You have been particularly concerned by your GP's comments, and fear that you may have a hormone problem.

You will ask the doctor:

(a) Is this a hormone problem?
(b) Do I need further investigations?

C. Examiners' information

A good candidate will be able to:

- *Recognize a marfanoid habitus from the outset of the consultation.*
- *Establish the family history of tall stature*
- *Enquire about possible associations and complications of Marfan's syndrome.*
- *Examine for gynaecomastia, and appreciate that there is no significant gynaemcomastia.*
- *Examine systematically for features of Marfan's syndrome.*
- *Appreciate that a marfanoid habitus can be seen with other conditions, and look for these*

- *Address patient's concerns.*
- *Explain the need for further tests to confirm the diagnosis of Marfan's syndrome.*

D. Focused history

History of presenting complaint

- Enquire about tall stature.
  - Has the patient always been tall?
- Enquire about gynaecomastia.
  - When did the patient first notice it?
  - Is it progressive or intermittent?
  - Is it getting worse?
  - Is it tender?
- Enquire about symptoms indicative of endocrine disease (as a cause of tall stature).
  - Hyperthyroidism: weight loss; increased appetite; heat intolerance; palpitations; sweating; insomnia; diarrhoea; and anxiety?
  - Acromegaly: headaches; visual disturbance; change in appearance; change in hat glove or shoe size; increased sweating?
  - Klinefelter's syndrome (primary hypogonadism): decreased facial, pubic, and body hair; infertility?
- Enquire about features of Marfan's syndrome.
  - Joint aches and pains (joint hypermobility)
  - Back pain (kyphoscoliosis and dural ectasia)
  - Stretch marks
  - Vision (myopia)

Previous medical history

- Complications of Marfan's syndrome, e.g. pneumothorax, visual disturbance (lens dislocation), herniae, kyphoscoliosis (+/− corrective surgery)

Family history

- Is there a family history of tall stature? If so, has this been investigated?
- A family history of pneumothoraces and aortic dissection may suggest Marfan's syndrome.
- A family history of thyroid disease and thyroidectomy may suggest MEN2b (which can also have a marfanoid habitus)

Drug history

- Enquire about medications that can potentially cause gynaemcomastia.

Patients concerns

- What concerns does the patient have?

E. Focused examination

The key is to recognize a marfanoid habitus early in the consultation. Given the initial referral was centred on 'possible' gynaecomastia, it is important to start by looking for this. In this case, this patient does not have gynaecomastia, and the remainder of the examination should be directed at identifying features associated with a marfanoid habitus and Marfan's syndrome.

Examine for gynaecomastia

- Differentiate gynaecomastia form 'pseudogynaecomastia' due to adiposity.*

Examine musculoskeletal system

- Tall stature (arm span > height; pubis–sole > pubis–vertex)
- Kyphoscoliosis (look for scars of previous corrective surgery)
- Arachnodactyly (thumb and wrist signs)
- Hyperextensible joints
- Pes planus

Examine the face and eyes

- High-arched palate
- Heterochromia of the irides
- Iridodonesis
- Blue sclera

Examine the chest

- Pectus excavatum
- Pectus carinatum
- Scars (previous pneumothoraces)

Examine cardiovascular system

- Aortic regurgitation
- Mitral regurgitation

Examine for features of other syndromes associated with marfanoid habitus

- MEN2b: mucosal neuromas (lips and tongue), hypertension (phaechromocytoma)
- Homocystinuria: livedo reticularis, mental retardation

F. Diagnosis

- Marfan's syndrome

This patient does not have true gynaecomastia. A marfanoid habitus and a strong family history of tall stature, suggests Marfan's syndrome is the most likely diagnosis. This will need to be confirmed.

There are many causes for gynaecomastia, but the differential diagnosis for gynaecomastia and tall stature include:

(a) Klinefelter's syndrome (most common)
(b) Thyrotoxicosis**
(c) Acromegaly**

It is important to remember that a marfanoid habitus does not constitute a diagnosis of Marfan's syndrome. The differential diagnosis of a marfanoid habitus is:

(a) Marfan's syndrome
(b) Homocystinuria
(c) MEN2b

---

* Pseudogynaecomastia is due to adiposity and palpation of glandular tissue should help differentiate this. Place your thumb and forefinger on opposite sides of the areola, and feel for the presence of a firm disc of mobile glandular tissue.

** These conditions can cause tall stature in adolescence before fusion of growth plates

It is important to look for features associated with these conditions. In the above case, a strong family history of tall stature supports Marfan's syndrome (autosomal dominant), but MEN2b also has autosomal dominant inheritance. However, the absence of an associated family history of thyroid disease would not support a diagnosis of MEN2b.

F. Feedback to patient

Explain diagnosis

- 'Your examination findings suggest a diagnosis of Marfan's syndrome.'
- 'This syndrome can be inherited and is associated with tall stature. It would explain the strong family history of tall stature.'

Address patient concerns

- Explain that there is no evidence of glandular tissue swelling below the nipples, and the tall stature is unlikely to reflect a hormonal problem.
- The examination findings support a diagnosis of Marfan's syndrome, and this is the most likely cause of tall stature.
- This syndrome can affect the heart valves, the large blood vessel that originates from the heart (aorta), the eyes, and the spine.
- You would like to arrange tests to look for these features and help confirm the diagnosis.
- Confirming this diagnosis is important, as individuals with Marfan's syndrome should be followed up regularly to look for associated complications. This is important, as if appropriately detected and treated, this can be life saving.

H. Feedback to the examiner

Further investigations

- Echocardiogram
- Slit-lamp eye examination
- X-ray of pelvis for protrusio acetbulae
- X-ray of spine for scoliosis of >20° or spondylolisthesis
- MRI spine (ductal ectasia)
- Genetic testing (fibrillin gene mutation)

Further management

- Annual ophthalmological evaluation
- Serial echocardiographic surveillance (frequency depends on severity of involvement)
- Family screening of first-degree relatives (echocardiogram ± ophthalmological examination).

I. Additional reading

Volume 1

Supplementary Endocrine Case 104 Gynaecomastia
Supplementary Locomotor Case 113 Marfan's Syndrome

Case 81 ◆ **Cold Hands**

A. Candidate information

Role: *On-call medical registrar*

This lady has been admitted with fast atrial fibrillation following a viral illness. She has been initiated on digoxin and β-blocker for rate-control. An echocardiogram has demonstrated a structurally normal heart. She has been commenced on warfarin anticoagulation, and is scheduled for discharge once adequate rate control has been achieved with a view to outpatient DC cardioversion. Whilst on the wards she has complained of painful cold hands, and has been reviewed by the on-call surgical registrar who has noted good peripheral pulses and feels this is not due to peripheral vascular disease. He has requested a medical review.

Task: *Establish the underlying cause and advise on further investigation and treatment*

B. Patient information

Age: 35 years

Problem: Cold hands

You have been admitted with palpitations following flu-like symptoms over the preceding week. The doctors have diagnosed atrial fibrillation. A scan of your heart has been normal. The current plan is to control the heart rate with medications, initiate warfarin therapy, and to arrange an electrical shock treatment as an outpatient to restore the normal rhythm. Since starting the medications, the heart rate has settled remarkably, but is still irregular. However, you have noticed that both your hands have become persistently cold and painful.

You have noticed poor circulation in both your hands for the last two years. It is often intermittent and usually occurs outdoors in cold weather. This has been reduced to some extent by wearing gloves outdoors. Recently, this has now started to occur indoors, and you find that wearing gloves indoors on most days helps prevent this. On exposure to the cold, the hands become immediately white and then blue. On warming the hands, they become intensely red and painful. You have not seen your doctor about this. There is no history of joints aches, muscle pains, or swallowing problems. You have no previous medical history.

You are a smoker and are taking the oral contraceptive pill. You work as a teacher at your local primary school, and with the increasing problem of poor circulation in your hands, you are finding it difficult to engage in outdoor activities for the children.

You are extremely concerned about the persistent nature of the symptoms since your admission to hospital, and are surprised by the opinion of the surgical doctor who has told you that the blood supply to the hands is normal.

You will ask the doctor:

(a) What is the cause of the cold and painful hands?
(b) Are the medications making it worse?
(c) What can I do to prevent this?

C. Examiners' information

A good candidate will be able to:

- *Recognize this patient has Raynaud's*
- *Try to differentiate Raynaud's phenomenon from Raynaud's disease*
- *Look for possible underlying associated disease (Raynaud's phenomenon)*
- *Establish potentiating factors: smoking, contraceptive pill, and β-blocker*
- *Examine the hands and look for underlying systemic disease*
- *Establish that this is most likely Raynaud's disease, but systemic diseases must be excluded*
- *Explain diagnosis to patient and need for further investigation and treatment*
- *Advise on adjustment of life-style measures*
- *Suggest to stop the β-blocker and replace this with non-dihydropyridine calcium antagonist for continuing rate-control.*

D. Focused history

History of presenting complaint

- Establish the specifics of the current admission.
- When did the symptoms start? Establish the temporal pattern of events since admission, i.e. after starting rate-control medications.
- Is it intermittent or persistent?
- Has this happened before?
- What happens when the hands are exposed to the cold? Establish triphasic response with characteristic colour changes of Raynaud's.
- Are there any exacerbating or relieving factors?
- Is there symmetrical involvement?
- Enquire about other sites that may be involved, i.e. tip of the nose, earlobes, and toes
- Are there any symptoms to suggest underlying rheumatolgical or systemic disease? Enquire about:
  - Joint aches and pains
  - Muscle aches and pains
  - Swallowing difficulty
  - Rashes

Previous medical history

- Rheumatological disease
- Hypothyroidism
- Cardiovascular risk factors (atherosclerosis)

Drug history

- Review patient's drug chart
- Enquire about drugs that can potentiate Raynaud's: Ergot alkaloids, bromocriptine, β-blockers, oral contraceptive pill, ciclosporin, clonidine, chemotherapeutic agents (bleomycin, cisplatin), and interferon-α

Social and occupational history

- Smoking history
- Occupational risk factors (vibration injury)

Patients concerns
- What concerns does the patient have?
- Does the patient have any thoughts as to what this could be?

E. Focused examination

When conducting your examination, remember the difference between Raynaud's disease and Raynaud's phenomenon:

	Raynaud's disease	Raynaud's phenomenon
Age	Usually <40 years	Usually >40 years
Associated conditions	None	Many systemic diseases (see below)
Symmetrical involvement	Yes	No (can involve one hand)
Nail fold capillaries	Normal	Abnormal
Tissue necrosis or gangrene	Never occurs	Can occur
ESR	Normal	Elevated
Serological findings (antinuclear autoantibody (ANA))	Negative	Positive

Examine the hands
- Symmetrical/asymmetrical involvement
- Nail-fold capillaries
- Tissue gangrene necrosis
- Assess upper limb pulses

Look for other areas of involvement
- Tip of the nose
- Earlobes
- Toes

Look for associated conditions

There are many systemic associations with Raynaud's phenomenon. Given the time constraints in the examination, the following conditions can be easily diagnosed:

- **Systemic sclerosis**: tight sclerotic facial skin, telangiectases, sclerodactyly, and calcinosis
- **Systemic lupus erythematosus (SLE)**: butterfly skin rash and arthropathy
- **Rheumatoid arthritis**: arthropathy, subcutaneous nodules, episcleritis, and scleritis
- **Dermatomyositis**: heliotrope rash, Gottron papules, proximal weakness, and tenderness
- **Polymyositis**: proximal weakness and tenderness
- **Cervical rib**: supraclavicular bruits, reduced upper limb pulses

Review observation chart
- Check adequacy of rate-control

F. Diagnosis

- Raynaud's disease (potentiated by β-blocker therapy)

This patient gives a classical history of Raynaud's. Her symptoms have worsened since admission, when rate-control therapy with digoxin and β-blocker was initiated. The most likely culprit is the β-blocker.

It is important to differentiate between Raynaud's disease and phenomenon (see table above). The history and examination should focus specifically on establishing this, and to determine any underlying rheumatological disease.

G. Feedback to the patient

Explain diagnosis

- 'The history and examination findings suggest that you may have Raynaud's disease.'
- 'This condition causes an abnormal constricting response of the small blood vessels that supply blood to the hands. This exaggerated constricting response can be triggered by exposure to cold.'
- 'The beta-blockers initiated on this admission can make the constricting response and the symptoms worse.'

Address patient concerns

- Beta-blockers can worsen the symptoms of Raynaud's disease, and will be discontinued. An alternative rate-control drug will be initiated.
- Other contributing factors in Raynaud's disease include smoking and the use of the oral contraceptive pill.
- Although specific treatments for Raynaud's are available, conservative measures help reduce the symptoms considerably. Smoking cessation and discontinuation of the oral contraceptive pill is recommended. Avoid exposure to cold weather and keep the hands warm, i.e. use gloves.
- Certain conditions can be associated with Raynaud's and you will request some investigations.

H. Feedback to the examiner

Further investigations

- The following tests can be requested to look thoroughly for associated systemic disease in Raynaud's phenomenon:

Investigations	Rationale
FBC	Haematological and autoimmune disorders
U&Es	Renal impairment and/or dehydration
LFT	Chronic liver disease (hepatitis B and C)
CK	Polymyositis, dermatomyositis
Clotting	Antiphospholipid syndrome (elevated APTT)
Glucose (fasting glucose)	Diabetes
Thyroid function tests	Hypothyroidism
ESR	Auto-immune disease
Full autoimmune profile	Auto-immune disease
Rheumatoid factor	Rheumatoid arthritis
C3 and C4 complement	Auto-immune disease, cryoglobinaemia
Cryoglobulins	Cryoglobinaemia
Cold agglutinins	Cold agglutinin diseases, i.e. Mycoplasma
Serum protein electrophoresis	Paraproteinaemia
CXR	Cervical rib

Further management

- Stop β-blocker
- Stop oral contraceptive pill (consider alternative contraception)

- Initiate alternative rate-control therapy, i.e. non-dihydropyridine calcium antagonist*
- Smoking cessation
- Avoid exposure to cold
- Recommend hand-warmers, e.g. gloves

I. Additional reading

Volume 1

Supplementary Skin Case 119 Scleroderma

Supplementary Skin Case 127 Raynaud's Phenomenon

Case 82 ◆ Chest Pain and Swallowing Difficulty

A. Candidate information

Role: *On-call medical registrar*

This lady has been admitted to the medical ward with retrosternal chest pain. Her cardiovascular risk factors include a family history, hypertension, and hypercholesterolemia. Her ECG and CXR have been normal. Her cardiac enzymes have been negative. This morning she complained of similar retrosternal chest pain. This was relieved by drinking a glass of milk. Her symptoms have now recurred. The ward nurse has performed an ECG. This has been reviewed by the on-call ward doctor who has not found any abnormality. He has requested a review by the medical registrar.

Task: *Establish the underlying cause and advise on further investigation and treatment*

B. Patient information

Age: 48 years

Problem: Chest pain and swallowing difficulty

You have been admitted to the medical ward with recurrent episodes of chest pain. These have been occurring over the last two years. You have been told that you have not had a heart attack, but need further investigations to exclude coronary artery disease. The chest pains are often worse first thing in the morning and during the night. The pains occur in the centre of the chest and radiate to the neck and throat. They are not related to exertion. There is no associated nausea or breathlessness. Your exercise capacity is excellent. You find that having milk-based breakfast helps with your symptoms. Prolonged periods of hunger potentiate your symptoms. You remember when dieting earlier in the year, you were noticeably troubled by these symptoms. Occasionally you would notice an acid taste in the mouth.

---

* These include verapamil and diltiazem. Calcium antagonists may be of further benefit in Raynaud's due to their vasodilating effects.

Since taking gaviscon which you acquired over the counter, your symptoms had much settled. Last week your GP started simvastatin for high cholesterol. Given your cardiovascular risk factors, he initiated aspirin for cardiovascular protection. Your symptoms have now worsened considerably despite using gaviscon more frequently. This morning you had similar symptoms relieved by drinking a glass of milk. The symptoms returned by lunch time. You were hungry and tried to relieve the symptoms by having an early lunch. Unfortunately, you had trouble swallowing the sandwich. It felt as if it were getting 'stuck in the lower part of the chest'. Eventually you were able to swallow it with a drink. You have never had swallowing difficulties before.

Your previous medical history includes hypertension and hypercholesterolaemia. Your medications include aspirin, bendrofluamethiazide, and simvastatin.

You have a strong family history of ischaemic heart disease. Your father died at the age of 40 years with a heart attack. Both your brothers aged 35 and 38 years have had coronary artery bypass surgery. Your sister aged 51 years has had an angioplasty 2 years ago after a heart attack. You are extremely concerned about the persistent nature of the symptoms as they bear resemblance to your sisters symptom's prior to her attack.

You will ask the doctor:

(a) Am I having a heart attack?
(a) Why am I having swallowing difficulties?

C. Examiners' information

A good candidate will be able to:

- Recognize that the cause of chest pain is gastro-oesophageal reflux
- Recognize the cutaneous manifestations of scleroderma
- Look for other associated clinical features of scleroderma
- Enquire about Raynaud's phenomenon
- Conclude that the dysphagia is likely to reflect an oesophageal stricture or oesophageal dysmotility in the context of scleroderma
- Explain the diagnosis to patient and address the patient's concerns
- Suggest stopping the aspirin and initiate proton pump inhibitor
- Explain the need for further investigations—blood tests including autoimmune screen and the need for endoscopy.

D. Focused history

History of presenting complaint
- How long have the symptoms been present?
- What are the characteristics of the chest pain:
  - Onset? (Gradual or sudden)
  - Nature? (dull, sharp, or burning)
  - Location?
  - Radiation?
- Exacerbating and relieving factors:
  - Exertion?
  - Deep breathing? (pleuritic)

- ♦ Hunger?
- ♦ Eating?
- ♦ Posture, i.e. lying down or sitting up? (lying down can increase discomfort in gastro-oesophageal reflux and pericarditis)
- Are there any associated symptoms?
  - ♦ Breathlessness?
  - ♦ Palpitations?
  - ♦ Nausea and sweating?
  - ♦ Abdominal pain?
  - ♦ Acid taste in mouth?
- Enquire about dysphagia.
  - ♦ Have you experienced this before?
  - ♦ Is it particularly with solid, liquids, or both?
  - ♦ Can you point where 'the food gets stuck'?
  - ♦ Is there a history of weight loss?
  - ♦ Has there been haematemesis or melena?
  - ♦ Has there been a change in bowel habit?
  - ♦ Is there any difficulty in speech or regurgitation through the nose? (neuromuscular dysphagia)

Previous medical history

- Scleroderma
  - ♦ Ask about tight skin of face and hands
  - ♦ Enquire about arthritic symptoms
- Raynaud's phenomenon
  - ♦ Ask about cold hands and characteristic triphasic colour change in response to cold.
- Previous gastric history
  - ♦ Peptic ulcer disease
  - ♦ Gastro-oesophageal reflux

Drug history

- Review patient's drug chart
- Are there any drugs that may potentiate gastro-oesophageal reflux symptoms, i.e. aspirin, nonsteroidal anti-inflammatory drugs (NSAIDs) and steroids

Patients concerns

- What concerns does the patient have?
- Does the patient have any thoughts as to what this could be?

E. Focused examination

The key is to recognize scleroderma early in the consultation (the main focus of this station). The examination should focus on demonstrating the features and associations of scleroderma.

Examine for cutaneous features of scleroderma

(a) Face

- Sclerotic skin over the face (smooth, shiny, and tight)
- Loss of facial wrinkles

- Perioral puckering with restrictive mouth opening
- Pinched nose
- Telangiectasia

(b) Hands
- Sclerotic skin over the fingers (smooth, shiny, and tight)
- Sclerodactyly with flexion deformities
- Dilated nail-fold capillaries
- Dystrophic nails
- Atrophy of soft tissue
- Digital ulceration and gangrene
- Calcinosis
- Raynaud's phenomenon

Look for systemic involvement in scleroderma
- Auscultate heart: pericardial rub (pericarditis, a cause of chest pain), loud P_2 (pulmonary hypertension)
- Auscultate lungs: bibasal crepitations (interstitial lung disease)

Review observation chart
- Blood pressure (renovascular disease in scleroderma)
- Oxygen saturations (interstitial lung disease)

Inspect oral cavity
- Evidence of tooth decay (acid reflux)

F. Diagnosis

- Scleroderma
- Gastro-oesophageal reflux
- Dysphagia secondary to oesophageal stricture or oesophageal dysmotility

This patient gives a history of chest pain and dysphagia. Although she a strong cardiovascular risk profile, it should be clear from the history that the chest discomfort does not sound like cardiac ischaemia. Previously her symptoms have been due to gastro-oesophageal reflux, and have been aggravated by aspirin therapy. The dysphagia that she has developed on this admission is new. This could be secondary to oesophageal stricture from long-standing gastro-oesophageal reflux or oesophageal dysmotility in the context of scleroderma.

The signs of scleroderma should be evident from the outset of the consultation. This should guide the focused history and examination. The differential diagnosis of chest pain in scleroderma is:

(a) Gastro-oesophageal reflux
(b) Oesophageal stricture
(c) Pericarditis
(d) Pleuritis (pleurisy)

G. Feedback to the patient

Explain diagnosis
- *'The examination findings suggest that you may have scleroderma—a condition which causes thickening of the skin and can also affect other organs. The foodpipe and stomach can be affected in this condition.'*
- *'The symptoms prior to admission were due to heartburn, with reflux of acidic contents of the stomach into the oesophagus (foodpipe). The aspirin therapy may have worsened these symptoms.'*

* 'Long-standing heartburn can result in a narrowing or stricture of the foodpipe. Also, scleroderma can affect the muscle of the foodpipe, making it less able to propel the food forward into the stomach. Both these conditions may account for the swallowing difficulties noted on this admission.'

Address patient concerns

* Although there are strong cardiovascular risk factors, the symptoms do not reflect a heart attack.
* The chest discomfort is due to a combination of heartburn and stricture of the food pipe. Furthermore, swallowing difficulties with food getting stuck in the foodpipe may cause chest discomfort.
* The examination findings suggest a diagnosis of scleroderma. Further tests are necessary to confirm this, and you will request a specialist review by the rheumatologist.
* It would be best to stop aspirin and that you will initiate medications to suppress the acid production in the stomach.
* An endoscopy is warranted to further investigate the foodpipe and ascertain the cause of swallowing difficulty.

H. Feedback to the examiner

Further investigations

* Full blood count
* Autoimmune profile
  * Anti-centromere
  * Anti-ScL 70 (topoisomerase 1)
  * Anti RNA polymerase I, II, and III
  * Anti-nuclear antibody
  * Rheumatoid factor
* ECG
* Barium swallow
* Endoscopy

Management plan

* Stop aspirin*
* Proton pump inhibitors for reflux symptoms
* Prokinetic drugs for dysmotility
* Review with results of above investigations
* A specialist rheumatology review
* An exercise treadmill test (can be arranged as an outpatient)**

G. Additional reading

Volume 1

Supplementary Skin Case 119 Scleroderma

---

* Although aspirin therapy would be indicated for cardiovasculttar protection, there is no absolute indication for aspirin therapy. If aspirin is not tolerated, then it should be discontinued. Alternatively, an enteric-coated aspirin preparation with proton-pump inhibitor therapy may be appropriate.

** Although the chest pain does not appear to have a cardiac basis, if there are any concerns, especially in the context of a strong cardiovascular risk profile, then an exercise treadmill test may be considered as a non-invasive test.

Supplementary Skin Case 127 Raynaud's Phenomenon

Volume 2

Case 83 ◆ Tremor

A. Candidate information

Role: *On-call medical registrar*

This gentleman has been admitted with breathlessness and lower limb oedema. He has been treated for an infective exacerbation of asthma and has responded well to nebulizers, steroids, and antibiotics. He was initiated on intravenous diuretics for the lower limb oedema with good effect. An echocardiogram this morning has demonstrated good cardiac function. During the admission he has noticed a tremor of his arms and hands, and has become increasingly concerned and anxious. His previous medical history includes anxiety and panic attacks, bipolar disorder, asthma, and hypertension. He has no previous cardiac history. His medications on admission included amlodipine, lithium, salbuatmol, and becotide inhalers. Oral frusemide has now been added.

Task: *Assess for likely cause of tremor and arrange further investigations if necessary.*

B. Patient information

Age: 49 years

Problem: Tremor

You have been admitted with a productive cough (yellow sputum), worsening breathlessness and wheeze for the last 5 days. You have been treated for a chest infection and asthma with nebulizers, steroids, and antibiotics and your breathing has improved. You have a long-standing history of asthma, which is usually well controlled and you have never been admitted into hospital for treatment of asthma. Your best peak-flow measurement is 540L/min. On admission this was reduced to 200L/min, but this has improved. You are a non-smoker and there are no known aggravating factors for your asthma. On admission, the doctor noted mild swelling of the ankles, and the doctor initiated intravenous diuretics. This swelling has been present for the last 6 months, and you have never taken any notice of it. The swelling has disappeared and you are inconvenienced by the need to pass urine frequently. The admitting doctor was concerned that the ankle swelling may be attributed to poor heart function and you have had an echocardiogram, which in fact has demonstrated good heart function.

Since admission, you have noticed a worsening tremor of both arms and hands. You have noticed increasing difficulty with coordinating hand movements as a result of this and you find it difficult to write and eat. You are very anxious about this. This morning when going to use the toilet, you felt unsteady. The nurse helped you back to your bed, and gave you a nebulizer. You have previously suffered with episodic tremors, and your GP had told you this was likely to be secondary to anxiety. You admit you have been very anxious, but the tremor has never been this bad to intrude with your activities.

You have a previous history of asthma, anxiety and panic attacks, bipolar disorder, and hypertension. Your medications include salbutamol and becotide inhalers, lithium and amlodipine, and frusemide (started on this admission). Previously, your blood pressure has been well-controlled. There is no family history of tremor. You do not drink alcohol.

You will ask the doctor:

(a) What is the cause of this troublesome tremor? Is this anxiety related?
(b) Can I be prescribed medication to relieve this?
(c) Can I stop the diuretics? I've had trouble with getting up at night to pass water.

C. Examiners' information

A good candidate will be able to:

* Establish the specifics of the current admission.
* Take an appropriate and concise history of the tremor.
* Establish a differential diagnosis of the tremor: (a) salbutamol, (b) lithium toxicity, and (c) anxiety
* Focus the history and examination around the differential diagnoses
* Establish that this is an intention tremor, and reflects cerebellar dysfunction
* Demonstrate cerebellar signs
* Conclude that this is most likely lithium toxicity potentiated by diuretic therapy
* Conclude that the ankle swelling is secondary to amlodipine therapy, and that there is no need for diuretics, especially with a normal echocardiogram.
* Address patient's concerns
* Explain the need for further investigations (electrolytes, thyroid function, and lithium level)

D. Focused history

History of presenting complaint

* When did you notice the tremor?
* Is intermittent or constant? Is it progressive?
* Which parts of the body are affected?
* Is it present at rest?
* Are there any exacerbating or relieving factors?
  * Voluntary movements?
  * Rest?
  * Anxiety or emotional stress?
* Are there any symptoms of cerebellar dysfunction?
  * Incoordination?
  * Unsteadiness and difficulty in walking?
* Are there any symptoms of lithium toxicity?
  * Nausea and vomiting?
  * Abdominal cramps?
  * Diarrhoea?

- ◆ Confusion?
- ◆ Seizures?
- Enquire about symptoms of thyroid disease.
  - ◆ Hyperthyroidism: weight loss, increased appetite, heat intolerance, palpitations, sweating, insomnia, diarrhoea, and anxiety
  - ◆ Hypothyroidism: weight gain, decreased appetite, cold intolerance, lethargy, constipation, and depression *(hypothyroidism is a complication of chronic lithium use)*
- How does the tremor interfere with daily activities?

Previous medical history
- Thyroid disease
- Anxiety
- Essential tremor
- 8Akinetic rigid syndromes (Parkinson's disease)

Family history
- Essential tremor

Drug history
- Review patient's drug chart
- Look for medications that can cause tremor: anticonvulsants, bronchodilators, cyclosporin, and lithium. Has there been a change in dose of medications?
- Look for medications that potentiate lithium toxicity: diuretics, ACE inhibitors, and NSAIDs.

Social history
- Enquire about alcohol consumption*

Patients concerns
- What concerns does the patient have?
- Does the patient have any thoughts as to what this could be?

E. Focused examination

There are many causes of tremor, and one cannot look for all the causes in the limited time provided. When assessing a patient with tremor, it is important to determine the characteristics of the tremor, before looking for specific causes.

Assess the tremor
- Physiological tremor (anxiety, sympathomimetics, thyroid disease)
- Resting tremor (akinetic-rigid syndromes)
- Intention tremor (cerebellar disease)

Then proceed to examine for specific causes:

Examine for cerebellar signs
- Dysarthria (can be assessed during history taking)
- Dysdiadochokinesis

---

* Chronic alcohol abuse can cause cerebellar disease as a cause of tremor. Furthermore, it is important to establish alcohol intake for inpatients, as patients who drink excess alcohol may develop withdrawal symptoms, manifesting as tremor!

- Impaired finger–nose testing with dysmetria
- Nystagmus
- Wide based and ataxic
- Truncal ataxia

Examine thyroid state

- Hyperthyroidism: tachycardia, restlessness, palmar erythema, tremor, lid lag, and retraction
- Hypothyroidism: bradycardia, slowness of movement, slow relaxing deep tendon reflexes

Examine for akinetic-rigid syndromes

- Resting tremor
- Bradykinesia
- Rigidity (cogwheel and lead-pipe rigidity)

This patient displays cerebellar signs, and with a history of lithium use, it is important to determine the key factors that potentiate lithium toxicity.

Examine fluid status

- Dehydration and hypovolaemia potentiates lithium toxicity
  - ◆ Check heart rate and blood pressure (review observation chart)
  - ◆ Assess mucous membranes, skin turgor, and JVP

F. Diagnosis

- Lithium toxicity (potentiated by diuretic therapy)

The differential diagnosis for tremor in this patient is:

(a) Salbutamol therapy
(b) Lithium
(c) Anxiety

This patient displays cerebellar signs shortly after initiation of intravenous diuretic therapy. Given that he is previously on lithium therapy, lithium toxicity should be strongly considered.

The diuretic therapy was initiated for ankle swelling, presumably for congestive cardiac failure. However the echocardiogram demonstrates good cardiac function, and in the absence of symptoms and signs of cardiac failure, the most likely cause of ankle oedema is amlodipine therapy.

G. Feedback to the patient

Explain diagnosis

- *'From the examination, it seems as if the lithium you are taking is the most likely cause for the tremor.'*
- *'Lithium can interact with many medications that affect its clearance from the blood. Diuretics, the 'water tablets,' can result in increased lithium levels in the blood.'*

Address patient concerns

- Although anxiety and salbutamol can cause tremor, on examination, the pattern of tremor suggests lithium is the cause. The levels are likely to have increased following diuretic therapy. A blood test will be necessary to check the lithium levels and salts in the blood.
- The diuretics are not necessary as the echocardiogram demonstrates good heart function, and the most likely cause of ankle swelling was the use of amlodipine.

- Given this, the diuretics will be discontinued. One can consider changing the blood pressure medication (if the mild ankle swelling is intrusive).
- Explain that at this stage you would not recommend prescribing a drug to alleviate the tremor, and it would be best to await the results of the blood tests. The cessation of diuretics will hopefully optimize the salt levels in the blood and help reduce the symptoms.

H. Feedback to the examiner

Further investigations

- U&Es
- Thyroid function tests*
- Serum lithium levels**
- ECG***

Further management

- Stop diuretics
- Intravenous fluids to correct hypovolaemia
- Optimize electrolytes, i.e. K^+ and Mg^{2+}
- Await the results of blood tests
- Further management depends on the results of the lithium levels****
- Consider changing amlodipine to an alternative antihypertensive (if ankle oedema is intrusive)

I. Additional reading

Volume 1

Station 3 Central Nervouse System Case 46 Cerebellar syndrome

Supplementary Endocrine Case 98 Assessment of Thyroid State

Volume 2

Station 2 Case 32 Tremor

---

* Hyperthyroidism can result in a physiological tremor. Furthermore, chronic lithium therapy can predispose to hypothyroidism, which can potentiate lithium toxicity.

** A repeat level should be checked several hours later after intravenous hydration to disclose any trend. Serial levels may be warranted in cases of sustained-release tablets.

*** Chronic lithium toxicity is frequently associated with non-specific and diffuse ST segment depression and T-wave inversion. Lithium toxicity may result in arrhythmias and heart block.

**** The mainstay of treatment is fluid therapy. The goal of saline administration is to restore glomerular filtration rate, normalize urine output, and enhance lithium clearance. Haemodialysis is indicated for patients who have renal failure (unable to eliminate lithium) and patients with congestive heart failure or liver disease (cannot tolerate hydration). Haemodialysis should be considered in patients who develop severe signs of neurotoxicity such as profound altered mental status and seizures. In patients with symptoms, an absolute level ≥4 mEq/L (acute toxicity) and a level ≥2.5 mEq/L (chronic toxicity) should also be considered for haemodialysis.

Case 84 ◆ **Diarrhoea**

A. Candidate information

Role: On-call medical registrar

This gentleman has been an inpatient on the respiratory ward for four days. He was admitted with severe community acquired pneumonia and has responded well to antibiotic therapy with amoxicillin and clarithromycin and supplemental oxygen therapy. He has developed diarrhoea over the last three days. Initially this was mild and settled, but has returned today. He has had four severe episodes since this morning. He complains of diffuse abdominal pains and cramps. The ward nurse has taken routine observations and noted a pulse rate of 98 beats per minute and a blood pressure of 98/50. She is concerned that he is dehydrated and has requested a medical review.

Task: Assess the patient and advise on further therapy.

B. Patient information

Age: 55 years

Problem: Diarrhoea

You have been admitted to the respiratory ward with pneumonia and have responded well to intravenous antibiotic therapy. You have been an inpatient for four days. On the second day of your admission you developed loose stool, but this settled. However, since this morning you have had four large episodes of watery diarrhoea. There is generalized abdominal pain with severe cramps. There is no blood or mucous in the diarrhoea. You feel thirsty.

There is no history of recent travel. You have not been in contact with individuals with diarrhoea.

Previously you have noticed the development of loose stools following courses of oral antibiotic therapy, but this has been mild and self-limiting. You have suffered from constipation for the last two years and attribute this to a poor diet–primarily due to a poor appetite. You have noticed an unintentional weight loss of 1 stone over the last year. You take regular senna and lactulose to maintain a healthy bowel habit.

There is a family history of bowel cancer, and your father and uncle were diagnosed aged 72 and 74 years respectively. Your father died due to advanced cancer with metastases, and your uncle underwent curative surgery.

You do not smoke and consume minimal alcohol.

You feel it is the antibiotics that have precipitated the diarrhoea.

You will ask the doctor:

(a) What is the cause of the diarrhoea?
(b) As you have improved considerably, can you stop the antibiotics?

C. Examiners' information

A good candidate will be able to:

- Establish the specifics of the current admission.
- Take an appropriate and concise history of the diarrhoea.
- Enquire about tolerability of previous antibiotic therapy.
- Enquire about previous history of gastro-intestinal disease.
- Assess fluid status and examine the abdomen.
- Consider the differential diagnosis of antibiotic-associated diarrhoea or possible manifestation of atypical pneumonias.
- Request appropriate investigations electrolytes, stool tests (microscopy, cultur,e and C. difficile toxins), atypical pneumonia screen and abdominal X-ray.
- Advise rehydration, stop laxatives, continue current antibiotic therapy, and initiate oral metronidazole therapy.
- Appreciate that previous altered bowel habit, weight loss, and loss of appetite need further investigation, especially given a strong family history of bowel cancer.

D. Focused history

History of presenting complaint
- Establish specifics of current admission
- Establish the specifics of the diarrhoea:
  - Onset?
  - Frequency (day and night)?
  - Consistency?
  - Exacerbating or relieving factors?
  - Is there associated blood or mucous?
- Are there any associated symptoms?
  - Fever?
- Abdominal pains and cramps?
- Abdominal distension?
- Weight loss?
- Nausea and vomiting?
- Establish usual bowel habit.
- Enquire about risk factors for legionella: inhalation of aerosolized mist from water sources, e.g. whirlpools, showers, cooling towers, and air-conditioning systems
- Enquire about recent travel.
- Enquire about contact with individuals with gastrointestinal symptoms.

Previous medical history
- Chronic respiratory disease (risk factor for Legionella)
- Gastrointestinal disease
- Inflammatory bowel disease
- Malignancy
- Hyperthyroidism

Family history
- Gastro-intestinal malignancy

Drug history
- Review patient's drug chart
- Is the patient on laxatives?
- Have any prophylactic measures to prevent antibiotic-associated diarrhoea been taken? (probiotic preparations)

Smoking history
- Smoking is a risk factor for Legionella pneumonia

Patients concerns
- What concerns does the patient have?
- Does the patient have any thoughts as to what this could be?

E. Focused examination

Review observation chart
- Check heart rate and blood pressure (review observation chart)
- Check for spikes in temperature since admission

Examine fluid status
- Assess mucous membranes, skin turgor, and JVP
- Ask for postural blood pressure measurements

Assess nutritional status
- Cachexia
- Temporal wasting
- Reduced triceps fold thickness

Examine the abdomen
- Clubbing (inflammatory bowel disease and gastro-intestinal malignancy)
- Abdominal distension
- Abdominal tenderness
- Examine for masses
- Bowel sounds

F. Diagnosis
- Antibiotic-associated diarrhoea
- Diarrhoea secondary to atypical pneumonia (Legionella and mycoplasma)

This patient has diarrhoea following antibiotic therapy, which is the most likely cause. Of course, one cannot exclude the possibility of diarrhoea associated with atypical pneumonias. Another important feature in the history is previous history of altered bowel habit (constipation), weight loss, loss of appetite, and a family history of bowel malignancy. This will require investigation in due course.

G. Feedback to the patient

Explain diagnosis
- 'The diarrhoea is most likely caused by antibiotics, although sometimes diarrhoea can be associated with certain types of pneumonias.'

Address patient concerns

- As the current admission has been for a severe pneumonia, it is important to continue with the antibiotics, since there has been a clinical improvement.
- The regular use of laxatives will be contributory, and this will have to be discontinued temporarily.
- The diarrhoea has resulted in dehydration, and rehydration with intravenous fluids is necessary.
- Oral antibiotics are necessary to cover antibiotic-associated diarrhoea.
- Further investigations will be necessary: blood tests, stool tests, and abdominal X-ray.

H. Feedback to the examiner

Further investigations

- U&Es
- Thyroid function tests*
- Inflammatory markers *(has there been a rise inflammatory markers?)*
- Tests for atypical pneumonia:
  - Mycoplasma: complement fixation tests, IgM antibodies
  - Legionella: urinary Legionella antigen, direct immunoflorescence, or PCR (polymerase chain reaction) of respiratory specimens
- Abdominal x-ray (ileus or toxic megacolon)

Further management

- Intravenous fluids (with potassium replacement if necessary)
- Continue current antibiotic therapy (consider changing antibiotics)
- Oral metronidazole (first line) or oral vancomycin (second line)
- Withhold laxatives temporarily
- Recommend outpatient investigations, i.e. colonoscopy, given a history of altered bowel habit, weight loss, and loss of appetite with a strong family history of bowel cancer

I. Questions commonly asked by examiners

What is the definition of antibiotic-associated diarrhoea?

This is defined as unexplained diarrhoea that occurs in association with antibiotic treatment.

When does diarrhoea develop in antibiotic-associated diarrhoea?

This can develop between 2 hours and up to 2 months after antibiotic use.

How common is antibiotic-associated diarrhoea?

The incidence ranges between 5–25% depending on the type of antibiotic.

What organisms are implicated in antibiotic-associated diarrhoea?

- Clostridium difficile (most common—accounts for 25% of cases)
- Clostridium perfringens
- Staphylococcus aureus
- Klebsiella oxytoca
- Candida spp.
- Salmenella spp.

---

* Hyperthyroidism is a cause for diarrhoea. Furthermore, this lady has had a long-standing history of constipation, and it is important to exclude hypothyroidism as a potential cause.

How can antibiotic-associated diarrhoea be prevented?

- Limit antibiotic use
- Probiotics (Saccharomyces boulardii and lactobacillus)

How is C.difficile diagnosed?

- Detection of stool cytotoxins A and B
    - ELISA based tests (false negative rate=10% – these tests increase negative predictive value)
    - RT-PCR has high sensitivity and specificity for toxin B.
- Stool culture is not commonly used, since 30% of hospitalized patients are colonized without disease, and anaerobic culture takes 3 days.

What is the management of diarrhoea associated with C.difficile?

- Stop causative antibiotic (this may not be possible if it is necessary to treat original infection; consider changing antibiotics to those less implicated in antibiotic-associated diarrhoea—aminoglycosides, sulfonamides, macrolides, vancomycin, and tetracycline)
- Treat dehydration and correct electrolyte disturbance
- Avoid the use of anti-peristaltic drugs (loperamide or opiates)
- Oral antibiotic therapy: metronidazole (first line) and oral vancomycin (second line)
- Observe infection-control hospital guidelines

When should oral vancomycin be used?

- Intolerant to metronidazole
- Poor response to metronidazole
- Pregnancy

Can metronidazole or vancomycin therapy be given intravenously?

Ideally, the treatment should be oral since C. Difficile is restricted to the lumen of the colon. Only metronidazole (not vancomycin) can be given intravenously as this can result in adequate colonic concentrations.

What are the complications of C.difficile infection?

- Pseudomembranous colitis
- Toxic Megacolon
- Ileus
- Perforation
- Shock

J. Additional reading

Volume 1

Volume 2

Case 85 ◆ Deterioration in Renal Function

A. Candidate information

Role: *On-call medical registrar*

This lady has been admitted to the medical ward with cellulitis of the left leg. She has been on intravenous antibiotics (flucloxacillin and benzylpenicillin) for four days and has responded well to therapy. Her previous history includes type 2 diabetes and hypertension. Her glycaemic control was initially managed with an insulin infusion, but this has been switched back to her usual diabetic medication, which consists of metformin and insulin. Her renal function on admission was normal. Today, her blood tests have been phoned through urgently to the ward with Na 132mmol/L, K 6.8mmol/L, Ur 34.1, Cr 651. The patient feels well in herself and has not voiced any complaints. The ward sister, who took the urgent phone call, has asked for an urgent medical review.

Task: Assess the patient, establish cause of renal dysfunction and advise further investigation and treatment.

B. Patient information

Age: 58 years

Problem: Deterioration in renal function

You have been admitted to the ward with severe cellulitis of the left leg. You have been treated with intravenous antibiotics for four days with good improvement. Following the ward round earlier today, the consultant was keen to switch to oral antibiotic therapy from tomorrow. You have repeat blood tests today, which show that your kidney function has deteriorated. However, you feel well in yourself.

When asked specifically, you have noticed that over the last two days, you have passed very little urine. Today at 6am, you passed very little urine and have not passed any since. You admit that you haven't been drinking much fluid recently as you have felt unwell with the cellulitis. There is no abdominal pain and your bowel habit is normal. There is no chest pain but you feel a little more breathless than usual. There are generalized aches and pains and you feel lethargic.

You have a previous medical history of diabetes and hypertension. Your regular medications include aspirin, simvastatin, ramipril, frusemide, metformin, and insulin. You have regular diabetic checks and you have been told you have background diabetic retinopathy. Your kidney function previously has been normal, but at your last check you were told there was a slight increase in protein in the urine.

Last year, your mother was admitted with pneumonia and her kidney function deteriorated significantly. The doctors said she had renal failure. She had to be admitted to the intensive care unit for dialysis. You are becoming increasingly worried that you may also have renal failure.

You will ask the doctor:

(a) What is the cause of the deterioration in kidney function?
(b) Do I have renal failure?
(c) Will I need to have dialysis?

C. Examiners' information

A good candidate will be able to:

- Establish the specifics of the current admission
- Enquire about urinary symptoms
- Enquire about previous history of renal disease and microvascular complications of diabetes
- Assess the fluid status and look for signs of fluid overload
- Conclude the hypovolaemic status of the patient
- Consider the broad differential diagnosis of acute renal failure
- Arrange appropriate investigations (blood tests, acid-base status, screening tests for renal failure, CXR, ECG, and renal ultrasound scan)
- Initiate appropriate treatment (intravenous fluids, correction of hyperkalaemia, cessation of nephrotoxic medications, and accurate monitoring of fluid balance)
- Address the patient's concerns

D. Focused history

History of presenting complaint

- Has there been a reduction in urine output?
- Enquire about urinary symptoms:
    - Haematuria?
    - Dysuria?
    - Urinary frequency?
- Are there any symptoms of uraemia?
    - Restlessness?
    - Pruritis?
    - Fatigue?
    - Confusion? (metabolic encephalopathy)
    - Chest pain? (uraemic pericarditis)
- Enquire about symptoms of fluid overload:
    - Breathlessness?
    - Orthopnoea?
    - Paroxysmal nocturnal dyspnoea?
    - Oedema?
- Enquire about symptoms suggesting hypovolaemia:
    - Fluid intake?
    - Diarrhoea?
    - Thirst?
    - Postural dizziness?
- Enquire about any recent investigations with contrast (contrast nephropathy)

Previous medical history

- Is there a history of renal disease?
    - Previous known renal function tests
    - Renal calculi
- Hypertension (enquire about control)
- Polycystic kidney disease

- Diabetes
  - Enquire about glycaemic control
  - Enquire about microvascular complications (proteinuria or microalbuminuria)
- Rheumatological disease
- Prostatic disease (in males)

Drug history
- Review patient's drug chart
- Nephrotoxic medications

Patients concerns
- What concerns does the patient have?

E. Focused examination

Review observation chart
- Heart rate, blood pressure, and oxygen saturations
- Fluid balance charts
- Urine output (if documented)
- Glucose readings (renal failure results in reduced insulin metabolism thus predisposes to hypoglycaemia)

Examine fluid status
- Hypervolaemia
  - Raised JVP
  - Third or fourth heart sound
  - Bibasal lung crepitations
  - Oedema
- Hypovolaemia
  - Reduced JVP
  - Dry mucous membranes
  - Reduced skin turgor

Examine for uraemia
- Restlessness and confusion
- Pruritis
- Flapping tremor of outstretched hands (metabolic encephalopathy)
- Pericardial rub (uraemic pericarditis)

Examine abdomen
- Palpable kidneys (polycystic kidney disease)
- Palpable bladder (urinary retention)

F. Diagnosis

- Acute renal failure (pre-renal)

Remember, the broad differential diagnosis for acute renal failure. The history and examination should focus on determining the aetiology. The differential diagnosis for acute renal failure can be sub-divided into

(a) Pre-renal: hypovolaemia

(b) Renal: glomerulonephritis, tubulointerstitial nephritis, acute tubular necrosis
(c) Post-renal: urinary obstruction

In this patient, the most likely cause is pre-renal due to hypovolaemia (poor fluid intake with concurrent diuretic therapy). Another possibility is tubulointerstitial nephritis secondary to penicillins.

G. Feedback to the patient

Explain diagnosis

- 'The blood tests show that your kidneys are not working properly. This is sometimes called 'kidney failure' but may be reversible. The most likely cause is dehydration.'

Address patient concerns

- As a result of poor kidney function, the potassium level in the blood is high and this needs treatment.
- Although the most likely cause is dehydration, other causes of renal failure need to be excluded.
- Further tests will be necessary, including blood tests, ECG, urine tests, and renal ultrasound scan.
- It is important to initiate intravenous fluids, and closely monitor the urine output carefully and this will require insertion of a urinary catheter.
- At this stage, it is difficult to tell whether dialysis will be needed, but this will largely be determined by the response to adequate rehydration. A repeat blood test will be requested following rehydration and correction of the potassium level.

H. Feedback to the examiner

Further investigations

- ECG (to look for features of hyperkalaemia)
- CXR (if suspecting fluid overload with pulmonary congestion)
- Blood tests
    - Establish acid-base status
    - Repeat U&E after intravenous fluids and correction of hyperkalaemia
    - Autoimmune profile
    - ESR
    - Calcium and phosphate
    - CK
    - Serum protein electrophoresis
    - Serum bicarbonate
- Urine tests
    - Urinalysis
    - Urine microscopy for cells, crystals and casts
    - Urine for Bence-Jones protein
    - Urine osmolality
    - Urine: Plasma osmolality ratio
    - Urine: Plasma creatinine ratio
    - Urinary sodium
- Ultrasound scan of the renal tract

Further management
* Stop nephrotoxic medications
* Adjust antibiotic doses for renal dysfunction*
* Correct hyperkalaemia (calcium gluconate and insulin/dextrose infusion)
* Intravenous fluids to optimize volume status (this may require monitoring of central venous pressure)
* Urinary catheter to monitor hourly urine output
* Stop metformin. Insulin infusion to optimize glycaemic control. Monitor glucose closely**
* Accurate fluid-balance charts
* If persistent oliguria or anuria, despite optimization of fluid status, then consider haemofiltration

I. Questions commonly asked by examiners

What are the indications for haemofiltration in acute renal failure?
* Refractory acidosis
* Refractory hyperkalaemia (despite adequate treatment)
* Pulmonary oedema
* Uraemic encephalopathy

How can you differentiate between pre-renal renal failure and renal failure due to intrinsic (renal) disease?
In renal failure due to intrinsic disease, the kidneys lose the ability to concentrate urine and sodium excretion is inappropriately increased. In pre-renal renal failure, the ability to concentrate urine is preserved.

	Pre-renal	Renal
Urine osmolality	>500	<350
Urine: Plasma osmolality	>1.5:1	<1.1:1
Urine: Plasma creatinine	>20:1	<20:1
Urinary sodium	<20mmol/L	>50mmol/L

What do you know about the different types of urinary casts?
* **Tubular casts**: acute tubular necrosis or interstitial nephritis
* **Hyaline casts**: Tamm-Horsfall glycoprotein
* **Granular casts**: non-specific
* **Red cell casts**: glomerulonephritis
* **White cell casts**: acute tubular necrosis or pyelonephritis

---

* If the cause of renal failure is penicillin therapy, then one would consider stopping penicillin, and replacing with alternative antibiotics if clinically indicated. However, the most likely cause is pre-renal (dehydration) and given that strong clinical indication for antibiotic therapy (severe cellulitis), then it is appropriate to continue penicillin in the first instance, but to make dose adjustments for renal dysfunction.

** Insulin is metabolized by the kidneys. In acute renal failure, the insulin requirement therefore decreases. This must be remembered when correcting hyperkalaemia with insulin/dextrose infusions and using insulin infusions for glycaemic control. It is important to monitor glucose carefully in this setting, and beware of hypoglycaemia.

J. Additional reading

Volume 1

Case 86 ◆ **Skin Rash**

A. Candidate information

Role: *On-call medical registrar*

This gentleman has been admitted with severe urinary tract infection. He is currently being treated with intravenous augmentin and gentamicin. Shortly after the admission, he has developed a troublesome rash affecting his truck and upper limbs. Two days ago he was seen by the on-call doctor who prescribed anti-histamines, which initially helped the symptoms. However, the rash has since deteriorated and the patient is extremely distressed. It is intensely pruritic and the patient has difficulty sleeping at night. He has a history of hypertension, diabetes, and ischaemic heart disease (coronary angioplasty 4 months ago). His regular medications include aspirin, clopidogrel, gliclazide, ramipril, simvastatin, and bisoprolol. The ward sister is extremely concerned as the rash is spreading.

Task: *Assess the patient and establish the cause(s) for the rash. Advise on further treatment.*

B. Patient information

Age: 82 years

Problem: Widespread rash

You have been admitted to the hospital with fever and pain on passing urine. You have been diagnosed with a severe urinary tract infection and have been initiated on intravenous antibiotic therapy. The admitting doctor found an enlarged prostate on examination and has requested a specialist urology opinion. On admission, you complained of persistently swollen ankles that worsen towards the end of the day. The doctor told you that this was likely a side-effect of your blood pressure tablets (amlodipine) and prescribed an alternative drug (ramipril). You were told that this would be better for you given that you have ischaemic heart disease and diabetes.

Shortly after the admission you developed a rash composed of red wheals on the lower part of the trunk. This has now progressed to involve most of your trunk including your back and upper arms. It is intensely itchy, and you are finding it increasingly difficult to sleep at night. Two days ago, an on-call doctor prescribed anti-histamines, which provided temporary relief from itching. However, they are now not controlling the symptoms, and the rash has since worsened. There is no swelling of the neck or throat. You do not complain of difficulty in breathing.

Your previous medical history includes hypertension, diabetes, and ischaemic heart disease. You underwent successful coronary angioplasty 4 months ago, and have been instructed to continue aspirin and clopidogrel for 1 year, after which you must continue with aspirin therapy life-long. You have no drug allergies. Previously your doctor has prescribed you penicillins on a number of occasions, and you have not experienced any problems.

Your wife was recently admitted with an increasing red rash on arm (after an infected cannula site). She was diagnosed with cellulitis and required prolonged treatment with antibiotics. You are concerned that this is cellulitis, and feel the antibiotics for the urinary tract infection may not cover the cellulitis.

You will ask the doctor:

(a) *Is this cellulitis?*
(b) *Do I need different antibiotics?*

C. Examiners' information

A good candidate will be able to:

- Acquire a history of the rash, and correlate this with recently prescribed drugs.
- Enquire about previous rashes, allergies, and tolerance to penicillins
- Examine the rash.
- Inspect oral cavity for upper airway and tongue swelling
- Examine for features of respiratory compromise
- Establish that this is an urticarial rash and there are no features of angio-oedema
- Conclude that this is drug-induced urticaria (likely secondary to ACE inhibitor)
- Advise discontinuation of the offending drug
- Initiate steroids and anti-histamines
- Recommend alternative anti-hypertensive therapy

D. Focused history

History of presenting complaint
- Enquire about characteristics of the rash:
  - Onset?
  - Distribution?
  - Intermittent or persistent?
  - Colour?
  - Colour blanching on pressure?
  - Flat (papular) or raised (macular)?
  - Exacerbating factors? (cold, heat, trauma, stress, sun rays, allergens, or contact with substances)
  - Relieving factors?
  - Associated pain or itching?
  - Oozing or discharge?
- Does the rash appear at sites of trauma? (Koebner phenomenon)
- Is there a history of bee or wasp stings?
- Is there involvement of the face, lips, mouth, and tongue?
- Are there any symptoms of respiratory compromise, i.e. breathlessness, stridor, and wheeze?
- Are there any potential precipitants, i.e. new perfume, clothing, jewellery, washing power, soap?
- Are there any gastro-intestinal symptoms, i.e. abdominal pain, vomiting, and diarrhoea?

Previous medical history

- History of atopy (allergic rhinitis, eczema, and asthma)
- Angio-oedema
- Urticaria pigmentosa
- Other conditions that can present with urticaria:
  - Hyperthyroidism
  - SLE
  - Lymphoma
  - Viral or febrile illness

Family history

Angio-oedema

Drug history

- Review patient's drug chart
- Are there any new medications?
- Are there any food or drug allergies?

Patients concerns

- What concerns does the patient have?
- Does the patient have any thoughts as to what this could be?

E. Focused examination

Review observation chart

- Check heart rate and blood pressure (review observation chart)
- Check for spikes in temperature since admission (fever suggests infection)
- Respiratory rate and oxygen saturations (assess for respiratory compromise)

Examine rash

- Distribution?
- Macular or papular?
- Colour? Does it blanch with pressure?
- Vesicles?
- Oozing?
- Scaling?
- Excoriation marks?
- Inspect sites of trauma (Koebner phenomenon)

Assess for evidence of respiratory compromise

- Inspect face, lips, mouth, and tongue for swelling
- Stridor
- Wheeze

F. Diagnosis

Explain diagnosis

- Drug-induced urticaria (allergic drug rash)

New drugs that have been initiated on this admission include penicillin and ramipril. Given that penicillin has previously never caused problems, the most likely culprit is ramipril.

G. Feedback to the patient

Explain diagnosis

- 'The pattern of the rash resembles that of an allergic rash.'

Address patient concerns

- 'This is most likely an allergic rash and is not cellulitis.'
- 'Given that previously penicillin has been tolerated and has not caused problems, this is unlikely to be related to the antibiotics. The most likely culprit is ramipril, and this will be stopped.'
- 'As this is not cellulitis, there is no need to change antibiotic therapy, and you should continue the current antibiotics for the urinary infection.'
- 'Reassuringly, there are no signs of a severe allergic reaction, i.e. airway involvement.'
- 'The cessation of the offending drug and initiation of steroids and anti-histamines will reduce the rash and help symptoms.'

H. Feedback to the examiner

Further investigations

- FBC (eosinophilia)
- CRP (a rise in inflammatory markers indicates worsening infection or cellulitis)
- U&Es (following initiation of ACE inhibitor therapy)

Further management

- Stop offending drug, i.e. ramipril
- Short course of oral steroids
- Anti-histamines
- Consider alternative anti-hypertensive therapy

I. Questions commonly asked by examiners

What are the common causes of drug-induced urticaria?

- Penicillin
- Cephalosporins
- NSAIDs
- Opiates
- ACE inhibitors
- Hydralazine

What do you know about hereditary angio-oedema?

This is an autosomal dominant condition characterized by C1-esterase inhibitor deficiency. This results in increased C1-esterase levels, with a resultant decrease in C2 and C4 levels. Patients present with angio-oedema (not urticaria) and often there is a painful macular rash. Laryngeal involvement results in stridor, breathlessness, and respiratory compromise. Gastrointestinal involvement results in abdominal pain and vomiting. Precipitating factors include infection, trauma, and stress. Treatment is with C1-esterase inhibitor concentrate or fresh frozen plasma with steroids.

What do you know about urticaria pigmentosa?

This condition is characterized by the development of reddish-brown macules and papules with urticarial wheals following trauma to the skin (friction, rubbing, and itching). Precipitants include alcohol, NSAIDs, codeine, and morphine. Treatment is generally to avoid drugs and precipitating factors and the use of anti-histamines.

J. Additional reading

Volume 1
Supplementary Skin Case 125 Purpura

Case 87 ♦ **Chest Pain**

A. Candidate information

Role: On-call medical registrar

This gentleman has been admitted to the ward with fever and breathlessness. He has a history of HIV diagnosed 3 years ago and has not previously been on retroviral therapy. He has been treated for pneumocystis jiroveci pneumonia (PCP) with high dose co-trimoxazole. He had improved considerably and his supplementary oxygen requirements had reduced considerably, with oxygen saturations of 96% on room air. This morning whilst mobilizing from his bed to the toilet, he developed sudden onset of left-sided chest pain and breathlessness. He is a smoker and has a strong family history of ischaemic heart disease. Routine observations taken by the ward sister demonstrate a heart rate of 102 beats per minute, blood pressure of 138/78 mmHg and oxygen saturations of 90% on room air. She has requested an urgent medical registrar review.

Task: Assess the patient and advise on further investigations and treatment.

B. Patient information

Age: 55 years

Problem: Chest pain

You have been diagnosed with HIV 3 years ago following health insurance screening tests. You have been admitted with fever and breathlessness, and have been diagnosed with a specific pneumonia, which the doctors term as PCP. You have now been on intravenous antibiotic therapy for 1 week, and have improved considerably. You are no longer requiring supplementary oxygen. This afternoon, whilst getting up from the bed to go the toilet, you develop severe left-sided chest pain with associated breathlessness. It is sharp in nature and increased by movement and deep inspiration. There is no radiation. There is no associated nausea, sweating, cough, sputum, or haemoptysis. There is no calf pain, swelling, or tenderness.

Besides HIV, you have no other significant medical history. You do not take regular medications and there are no allergies.

You are a smoker and smoke up to 20 cigarettes per day. You drink minimal alcohol

You have a strong family history of coronary artery disease with both your brothers suffering heart attacks aged 55 and 51 years. Your current symptoms resemble that of your brothers' symptoms when they had heart attacks. Given this and the strong family history, you are concerned that you may be having a heart attack.

You will ask the doctor:

(a) Am I having a heart attack?
(b) If not, what is it?
(c) Will I need more tests?

C. Examiners' information

A good candidate will be able to:

- Establish the specifics of the current admission.
- Acquire a concise and appropriate history of chest pain, and establish this is pleuritic chest pain.
- Enquire about thrombotic risk factors.
- Formulate an appropriate differential diagnosis of pleuritic chest pain AND hypoxia (pneumothorax and pulmonary embolism).
- Examine the chest to look for signs of pneumothorax or pulmonary embolism.
- Examine calves for clinical evidence of deep vein thrombosis.
- Request appropriate initial investigations: ECG and CXR. Subsequent investigations depend on the results of these.
- Initiate appropriate management: oxygen, analgesia, and review with results of the investigations. If pneumothorax is excluded, then anticoagulation and CT pulmonary angiogram to exclude pulmonary embolism.

D. Focused history

History of presenting complaint

- How long have the symptoms been present for?
- What are the characteristics of the chest pain:
  - Onset? (Gradual or sudden)
  - Nature? (dull, sharp or burning)
  - Location?
  - Radiation?
- Exacerbating and relieving factors:
  - Exertion?
  - Deep breathing? (pleuritic)
  - Hunger?
  - Eating?
  - Posture, i.e. lying down or sitting up? (lying down can increase discomfort in gastro-oesophageal reflux and pericarditis)
- Are there any associated symptoms?
  - Breathlessness?
  - Palpitations?
  - Nausea and sweating?
  - Abdominal pain?
  - Acid taste in mouth?
  - Cough, sputum, or haemoptysis?

Previous medical history
- Ischaemic heart disease.
  - Enquire about cardiovascular risk factors
  - A recent myocardial infarction can result in pericarditis (Dressler's syndrome)—this is associated with pleuritic chest pain
- Chronic respiratory disease
- Pneumothorax
- Thromboembolic disease
- Thrombophilia

Family history
- Ischaemic heart disease
- Thrombophilia

Drug history
- Review patient's drug chart
- Has the patient been prescribed DVT prophylaxis?
- Is the patient on retroviral therapy?
- Is the patient on pentamidine prophylaxis?*

Smoking history
- Smoking increases the risk of pneumothorax

Patients concerns
- What concerns does the patient have?
- Does the patient have any thoughts as to what this could be?

E. Focused examination

Review observation chart
- Check heart rate and blood pressure
- Respiratory rate and oxygen saturations (assess for respiratory compromise)

Examine chest
- Musculoskeletal chest pain: palpate for chest wall tenderness, look for evidence of chest trauma
- Pneumothorax: tracheal deviation to the opposite side, ipsilateral reduction in chest expansion, hyper-resonance, and reduction in breath sounds
- PE: often no signs, but a pleural rub or features of consolidation may be present.

Examine heart
- Features of pulmonary hypertension: raised JVP, parasternal heave, and loud P_2
- Pericardial rub (pericarditis is a cause of pleuritic chest pain, but will not explain the hypoxia)

Examine legs
- Calf swelling and tenderness (clinical evidence of deep vein thrombosis)

---

* Pentamidine prophylaxis increases the risk of PCP-associated pneumothorax.

F. Diagnosis

- The differential diagnosis for pleuritic chest pain AND hypoxia. is:

(a) PE

(b) Pneumothorax (complication of PCP)

This patient has a strong cardiovascular risk profile, and is concerned he is having a myocardial infarction. It is crucial to be able to discriminate between cardiac and non-cardiac chest pain. The history of pleuritic chest pain is clear, and this is against a diagnosis of cardiac ischaemia. Therefore, the patient can be reassured.

In the absence of clinical signs of pneumothorax, the most likely diagnosis is a PE. PE should be considered in hospitalized patients who may be relatively immobile. PCP-associated pneumothorax is seen in approximately 5% of patients with PCP, and thus pneumothorax must be considered in the differential diagnosis for this patient. A pneumothorax must be excluded prior to commencing anticoagulation for PE, as this may warrant aspiration +/– intercostal drain insertion.

G. Feedback to the patient

Explain diagnosis

- 'The cause of chest pain is not clear.'
- 'A clot in the lung (pulmonary embolism) can occur in patients who are hospitalized, as immobility is a risk factor.'
- 'Some patients with PCP pneumonia can have small cysts on the lung that can rupture, resulting in the accumulation of air around the lung (pneumothorax). Smoking increases this risk of this.'

Address patient concerns

- The characteristics of the chest pain do not suggest a heart attack. However, an ECG will be requested.
- Initially, it is important to exclude a pneumothorax and you will arrange a chest X-ray to look for this.
- If the chest X-ray does not show a pneumothorax, then one must consider the possibility of pulmonary embolism. This can be diagnosed using a CT pulmonary angiogram.'
- The oxygen levels in the blood are low, and this warrants supplementary oxygen. Analgesia can be given to control the pain.
- The specific treatment depends on what these investigations will show and the exact cause.

H. Feedback to the examiner

Further investigations

- Arterial blood gas
- ECG
- CXR
  - Request a pulmonary artery (PA) film to look for pneumothorax
  - If the clinical suspicion of a pneumothorax is high, but the PA chest radiograph is normal, a lateral chest or lateral decubitus film should be requested.
  - A CXR can also demonstrate other causes of pleuritic chest pain, i.e. consolidation or collapse
- CT pulmonary angiogram (if clinical suspicion of PE)
- Doppler ultrasound of leg (if clinical suspicion of DVT)

Further management
- Oxygen
- Analgesia
- If CXR confirms pneumothorax, then aspiration +/– intercostal drain
- If CXR does not show a pneumothorax, then anticoagulate with low molecular weight heparin and request CT pulmonary angiogram to look for PE
- If CT pulmonary angiogram does not show a PE, then consider other causes of pleuritic chest pain:
  - (a) Pleurisy
  - (b) Pericarditis
  - (c) Musculoskeletal chest pain

The hypoxia in the above case is against these diagnoses. However, the hypoxia may be a manifestation of PCP. It is important to remember that in extreme cases, severe pleuritic chest pain can result in voluntary splinting of the chest and hypoventilation, which can lead to hypoxia. In such cases, adequate analgesia is helpful—both therapeutically and diagnostically.

Other issues to address:
- Check CD4 count and initiate anti-retroviral therapy (highly active anti-retroviral therapy— HAART)
- PCP prophylaxis (pentamidine)

I. Questions commonly asked by examiners

What is the differential diagnosis of pleuritic chest pain?
- Pulmonary embolism
- Pneumonia
- Malignancy
- Pleurisy
- Pneumothorax
- Musculoskeletal chest pain
- Pericarditis

What ECG changes are seen in pericarditis?
- Global saddle shaped ST segment elevation
- PR (per rectum) segment depression

What are the causes of pericarditis?
- Viral infections (coxsackie, adenovirus, echovirus)
- Bacterial infections (mycoplasma, haemophilus, tuberculosis)
- Connective tissue disease (rheumatoid arthritis, SLE)
- Drugs (hydralazine, procainamide)
- Dressler's syndrome (post myocardial infarction or cardiac surgery)
- Uraemia

What are the risk factors for PCP-associated pneumothorax?[1]
- Smoking

---

[1] Metersky ML, Colt HG, Olson LK, Shanks TG. AIDS-related spontaneous pneumothorax: risk factors and treatment. Chest. 1995;108:946–51.

- History of pentamidine chemoprophylaxis
- Pneumatoceles identified on CXR*

J. Additional reading

Volume 1

Station 1 Respiratory Case 19: Pneumothorax

Volume 2

Station 2 Case 9 Chest Pain

Station 2 Case 18 HIV Treatment

Case 88 ◆ Swollen Knee

A. Candidate information

Role: On-call medical registrar

This lady has been admitted for severe community acquired pneumonia. She has responded well to intravenous antibiotics and has been converted to oral antibiotic therapy (amoxicillin and clarithromycin). Over the last two days she has noticed a swollen right knee. It is increasingly painful and warm to touch. She is finding it increasing difficult to weight bear. Her previous medical history includes atrial fibrillation, hypothyroidism, hypertension, and chronic back pain. Her medications on admission include warfarin, thyroxine, bendroflumethiazide, atenolol, and paracetamol. She is scheduled for discharge tomorrow, and the ward sister is concerned that this may not be possible given her painful swollen knee. She has requested a medical review.

Task: Assess for likely cause of swollen knee and advise further investigations and treatment.

B. Patient information

Age: 78 years

Problem: Swollen and painful right knee

You have been admitted to the medical ward with pneumonia. You have responded very well to intravenous antibiotics and have been switched to oral antibiotic therapy. This morning on the ward round, your doctors were happy with your progress and have scheduled discharge tomorrow with a course of oral antibiotic therapy.

Two days ago, whilst on the ward you tripped over the chair by the side of the bed. You fell to the floor and sustained a trivial injury to your right knee. You were able to get back into bed. The following morning, the right knee appeared slightly swollen, but it was not painful. Given that it felt to be a trivial injury, you

---

* Pneumothorax is thought to develop primarily in the setting of a rupture of cystic lesions that may be present in active disease or from previous infection.

did not take much notice of it. Since then, the swelling has been gradually increasing, but there had been no associated pain. This morning on the ward round, you did not mention it to the doctors, as you did not want to potentially delay discharge, as you are very keen to go home. However, throughout the day, the swelling has become noticeably larger and it is now becoming increasingly painful. You find it difficult to weight bear. You have alerted the ward sister to this.

You have a history of atrial fibrillation, hypertension, hypothyroidism, and long-standing back pain. Your medications include warfarin, thyroxine, bendroflumethiazide, atenolol, and paracetamol. You have no allergies. Besides back pain, you have never suffered from joint swelling, aches, or pains. However, you do notice that the joints in the hands are stiff in the morning, but this gets better throughout the day. You attribute this to old age. You are limited by your back pain, and you mobilize with a stick.

You have been particularly concerned that the knee swelling will delay discharge.

You will ask the doctor:

(a) Will I be able to go home tomorrow?
(b) Will I need further tests? If so, can they be done as an outpatient?

C. Examiners' information

A good candidate will be able to:

- Establish specifics of current admission
- Obtain history of joint swelling, with an appropriate differential diagnosis in mind.
- Enquire about previous history of rheumatological disease, and suspect the possibility of rheumatoid arthritis (morning stiffness)
- Examine the swollen knee for effusion and ruptured Baker's cyst.
- Examine the calves to explore the possibility of DVT.
- Conduct a general examination to look for rheumatological disease
- Recognize the warfarin–macrolide interaction and the potential for increased INR and bleeding tendency.
- Establish the link between trauma and knee swelling, and given the interaction between macrolide and warfarin, conclude that this is most likely to be a traumatic effusion (haemarthrosis).
- Address patient's concerns
- Explain the need for further investigations: blood tests, X-ray of right knee, and joint aspiration

D. Focused history

History of presenting complaint
- How long has the joint swelling been present?
- Which joints are affected?
- Is there swelling of the adjacent tissues? (ask about calf swelling, pain, and tenderness—could this be DVT?)
- Is it getting worse?
- Are there any precipitating factors? (trauma)
- Are there any exacerbating or relieving factors?
- Is there is a history of fever, rigors, or chills?
- Is there associated pain? Is the pain present at rest? Is the pain only on movement of the joint?

- Are you able to weight bear?
- Is there any discoloration of the overlying skin and tissues?
- Are there associated:
  - Genitourinary symptoms? (reactive or gonococcal arthritis)
  - Gastrointestinal symptoms? (seronegative arthritis with inflammatory bowel disease)
- Do you suffer from joint stiffness, aches, and pains?

Previous medical history
- Previous joint replacements
- Rheumatoid arthritis
- Osteoarthritis
- Gout
- Pseudogout (enquire about related conditions*)
- Bleeding disorders i.e. haemophilia (haemarthrosis)

Drug history
- Is the patient on anticoagulation? Note drug interactions with warfarin that may potentially increase bleeding risk. Check for anticoagulation chart and INR values if available.
- Are there any medications that may increase the risk of gout? (diuretics, low-dose aspirin, cyclosporin, tacrolimus)
- Review the analgesic medications.
- Is the patient on DVT prophylaxis? (unlikely if patient is therapeutically anticoagulated with warfarin)

Social history
- Is there a history of recent travel? Lyme disease can cause a monoarthritis. Areas endemic for Lyme disease (New Forest, Northeastern United States)

Patients concerns
- What concerns does the patient have?
- Does the patient have any thoughts as to what this could be?

E. Focused examination

Review observation chart
- Check heart rate and blood pressure
- Respiratory rate and oxygen saturations (PE as a complication of DVT)
- Fever (septic arthritis)

Examine the joint
- Establish swelling of knee joint (compare with contralateral joint)
- Inspect overlying skin. Erythema suggests active inflammation or infection
- Is the joint warm to touch? Warmth suggests active inflammation

---

* Haemochromatosis, hypothyroidism, hyperparathyroidism, acromegaly, diabetes.

- Check patellar tap sign*
- Always check if swelling extends into the popliteal fossa and upper third of the calf (Baker's cyst)
- Check passive and active movements of the joint (ensure this is not painful for the patient!)
- If there is no joint swelling, then examine the calves. Could this be a DVT?

Examine for rheumatological disease
- Inspect hands, arms, face, and feet. Look for the following:
  - Rheumatoid arthritis
  - Scleroderma
  - SLE
  - Osteoarthritis
  - Psoriasis and/or psoriatic arthropathy
  - Chronic tophaceous gout
  - Ankylosing spondylitis

Look for evidence of coagulopathy
- Purpura and echymoses
- Evidence of prolonged bleeding (recent venepuncture sites)

F. Diagnosis
- Traumatic joint effusion (haemarthrosis).

In this patient, the differential diagnosis of an acutely swollen joint is:

(a) Haemarthrosis (trauma and potential for increased bleeding tendency)
(b) Rheumatoid arthritis (history of morning joint stiffness)
(c) Gout (chronic diuretic therapy)
(d) Pseudogout (hypothyroidism)
(e) Osteoarthritis
(f) Septic arthritis (this should always be considered in an acute swollen joint)

Although joint effusion may occur in the setting of trauma or overuse, super-imposed on underlying joint pathology, i.e. rheumatoid arthritis or osteoarthritis, a rapidly increasing joint effusion after trauma, should raise the suspicion of haemarthrosis. This is further suggested by an increased bleeding tendency that can result from the warfarin–macrolide interaction. The history is suggestive of a number of underlying rheumatological diagnoses, and the clinical examination should focus specifically on identifying these.

G. Feedback to the patient

Explain diagnosis
- 'The most likely cause of a swollen knee following injury is possible bleeding into the joint.'
- 'The use of warfarin increases bleeding risk, even following trivial injury. The antibiotics can interact with the warfarin levels, increasing the overall rise of bleeding.'

---

* With one hand above the knee joint, apply pressure to drive the fluid from the suprapatellar pouch into the knee joint. With the index finger of the other hand, press the patella from above with a jerky movement. If the patella rebounds, then this suggests fluid in the knee joint. If there is too little or too much fluid, then the patellar tap sign will be negative.

Address patient concerns
- Further investigations are necessary: blood tests, X-rays and joint aspiration. If there has been bleeding into the joint, then the joint aspiration will be therapeutic as well as diagnostic. If the joint aspirate yields no blood, then the joint fluid can be sent for further tests to identify the cause.
- The discharge will be delayed, as this needs further investigation and treatment. These investigations cannot be organized as an outpatient.
- Joint aspiration cannot be performed if the blood is too thin (high INR) as this may increase bleeding. It is important to withhold the warfarin and request an up-to-date blood test and depending on the result, the effect of warfarin may require reversal, before it is safe to aspirate the joint with a needle.
- In the meantime bed rest is advised and analgesic medications will be prescribed.

H. Feedback to the examiner
Further investigations
- Blood tests
  - FBC
  - CRP
  - Clotting
  - Blood cultures (if suspecting septic arthritis)
  - Serum uric acid
  - Rheumatoid factor and autoimmune profile (if suspecting rheumatological disease)
- X-ray of the joint(s)
- Joint aspirate
  - Gram stain and culture
  - Crystals (negative birefringence—gout, positive birefringence—pseudogout)

Further management
- Analgesia
- Bed-rest (movement and weight bearing can increase bleeding in haemarthrosis)
- Await results of clotting and correct INR if necessary (fresh frozen plasma +/– vitamin K)
- Aspirate joint

I. Additional reading
Volume 1
Supplementary Locomotor Case 108 Rheumatoid arthritis
Supplementary Locomotor Case 111 Gout
Supplementary Locomotor Case 112 Osteoarthritis

Volume 2
Station 2 Case 12 Ankle Swelling
Station 2 Case 23 Joint Pains

Case 89 ◆ **Loss of Vision**

A. Candidate information

Role: On-call medical registrar

This lady has been admitted for an infected leg ulcer and is currently receiving intravenous antibiotics. This afternoon she has developed sudden loss of vision. She has a previous history of type 2 diabetes, hypertension, and ischaemic heart disease. The ward sister has checked her glucose and it is 7.1mmol/L. Her routine observations are stable. The ward sister has requested an urgent medical review.

Task: Assess the patient and determine the causes of visual disturbance. Advise on further investigation and treatment

B. Patient information

Age: 78 years

Problem: Sudden loss of vision

You have been admitted to the medical ward with infected leg ulcers. You are currently receiving intravenous antibiotics and are making a slow but progressive recovery. This afternoon after lunch, you developed sudden painless loss of vision in the right eye. You were not able to read the newspaper and not able to recognize faces. However, you could differentiate between dark and light. There was no associated headache or limb weakness. You tested each eye in turn and found only the right eye to be affected. The left eye was not affected. However, the vision has improved now, but is not normal.

Your previous medical history includes type 2 diabetes, hypertension, and ischaemic heart disease (coronary artery bypass graft surgery 5 years ago). You have never complained of chest pain after your heart operation. The diabetes was diagnosed 15 years ago and you have since been under regular follow-up in the diabetes clinic. You have regular eye checks, and at the last visit you were told you had minor eye changes. You have never required laser treatment for your eyes. Your kidney function is normal, except that your doctor has told you that you have small amount of protein in the urine, and this can occur in diabetes. You complain of numbness and pins and needles in your feet. Over the last 2 years you have developed ulcers on your feet and have required two previous hospital admissions for intravenous antibiotics. You do not usually wear glasses for vision.

Your medications include aspirin, ramipril, simvastatin, insulin, and metformin. You are allergic to penicillin, which results in widespread and rash and facial swelling.

Very infrequently you have experienced hypoglycaemic attacks, and this results in feeling faint and blurring of your vision in both your eyes. These symptoms resolve rapidly with intake of sugary foods. The visual disturbance today is different to previous hypoglycaemic attacks, and furthermore the glucose levels when checked by the ward sister were satisfactory. Your sister suffered with transient visual disturbance, and she was diagnosed with a mini-stroke. You are concerned you have had a stroke.

You will ask the doctor:

(a) Have I had a stroke?
(b) Will my vision improve?

C. Examiners' information

A good candidate will be able to:

- *Obtain a history of visual disturbance*
- *Establish previous history of diabetic eye disease*
- *Enquire about hypoglycaemic symptoms*
- *Examine the pulse, the carotids (for bruits), and precordium (murmurs)*
- *Examine the eyes (visual acuity, visual fields, eye movements, and fundoscopy)*
- *Conclude that the cause of visual disturbance is diabetic maculopathy*
- *Address patient's concerns*
- *Request investigations: ECG, carotid dopplers, and echocardiogram*
- *Request ophthalmology review*

D. Focused history

History of presenting complaint

- When did you notice the visual disturbance?
- Can you describe the onset of visual disturbance? Was it sudden or gradual?
- Can you describe the visual disturbance? Was it partial or complete?
- Did it affect one or both eyes?
- Is it intermittent or persistent?
- How long did it last?
- Did you get complete recovery?
- Enquire about associated symptoms:
  - Facial or limb weakness?
  - Facial or limb sensory disturbance?
  - Double vision?
  - Headache?
  - Speech disturbance?
- Did you measure the blood glucose? If so, what was it?

Previous medical history

- Previous history of visual disturbance
- Enquire about cardiovascular risk factors
- In patients with diabetes, it is important to establish:
  - Previous diabetic control
  - Microvascular and microvascular complications
  - History of diabetic eye disease (diagnosis and previous treatments)
  - Hypoglycaemic attacks (frequency and characteristics of such attacks)
- Atrial fibrillation

rug history

Review patient's drug chart

If there is a history of atrial fibrillation, what is the current anti-thrombotic therapy?

atients concerns

What concerns does the patient have?

Does the patient have any thoughts as to what this could be?

. Focused examination

eview the observation chart

Heart rate (check adequacy of rate-control)

Blood pressure (check adequacy of blood pressure control)

Look at the glucose chart (are there hypoglycaemic periods?)

xamine the eyes

Test visual acuity. Test each eye separately.

Assess visual fields

Assess eye movements

Perform fundoscopy (diabetic retinopathy)

xamine cardiovascular system

Assess pulse (rate and rhythm)

Listen for carotid bruits

Listen for murmurs (particularly mitral valve disease)

. Diagnosis

Diabetic maculopathy

uring the history and examination, it is important to remember the principal causes of onocular visual disturbance in a diabetic patient:

) Transient ischaemic attack (diabetes, hypertension)

) Diabetic maculopathy (diabetes)

) Retinal or vitreous haemorrhage (diabetes, hypertension)

) Central retinal vein or branch occlusion (diabetes, hypertension)

his patient has *persisting* monocular visual loss. Fundoscopy demonstrates diabetic maculopathy, d is the focus of this case. Diabetic maculopathy is the main cause of visual loss in patients with n-proliferative diabetic retinopathy. This warrants urgent ophthalmology referral.

the patient had *transient* visual loss in the absence of fundoscopic signs of significant diabetic e disease (maculopathy, haemorrhages, retinal detachment) then one should consider naurosis fugax as the cause.

. Feedback to the patient

xplain diagnosis

'From the examination, I can see important diabetic changes in the eyes, which explain why you have lost your vision in that eye.'

Address patient concerns
- The examination findings do not support stroke as a cause of visual disturbance.
- Diabetes can affect the eyes in many ways, but sometimes certain changes are more important, especially if they compromise vision. In such cases, urgent ophthalmology opinion should be sought, as if untreated there is a risk of permanent visual loss.
- Laser therapy reduces the risk of visual loss by 50% and increases the chance of visual improvement.

H. Feedback to the examiner

*Further investigations**
- Blood tests
  - FBC
  - Glucose
  - HbA_{1C}
  - U&Es
  - Lipids
- Urine tests
  - Urinalysis
  - 24 hour urine collection for proteinuria

Further management
- Urgent ophthalmology review for focal laser photocoagulation therapy.

I. Additional reading

Volume 1

Supplementary Eyes Case 146 Diabetic retinopathy

Volume 2

Station 2 Case 28 Visual disturbance

Station 2 Case 19 Diabetes

---

* Investigations should not delay urgent ophthalmology referral. These investigations can be requested to assess diabetic control, risk factors for worsening diabetic retinopathy, and looking for other microvascular complications of diabetes. These can be subsequently addressed. Risk factors for worsening diabetes include poor glycaemic control, hypertension, anaemia, diabetic nephropathy (proteinuria), hyperlipidaemia (increased risk of leakage and hard exudates), and pregnancy.

Case 90 ♦ Drooping Eyelid

A. Candidate information

Role: On-call medical registrar

This gentleman was admitted with acute aortic dissection and underwent emergency aortic surgery and aortic valve replacement. He is 10 days post-op, and is making a slow and progressive recovery. He is currently on the rehabilitation ward. His only previous medical history is hypertension, and he has been on amlodipine tablets for many years. Over the last few days, the physiotherapist has been noticing drooping of the right eyelid. She has told the surgical doctor on the ward who has requested a medical review.

Task: Assess the patient and advise on further investigation and treatment.

B. Patient information

Age: 51 years

Problem: Drooping right eyelid

You were admitted to hospital 10 days ago with severe chest pain. A tear in the aorta (aortic dissection) was diagnosed on CT scan. You did not notice any drooping of the eyelid at this stage. The aortic dissection required emergency major surgery, and this has been successful. The aorta was replaced and you have also received a tissue aortic valve because the aortic valve was also leaky. You were initially in the intensive care unit before being transferred to the cardiothoracic ward. Post-operatively you have been treated for a chest infection. Besides this, there have been no complications. You have made a slow but progressive recovery and are currently on the rehabilitation ward. Over the last 3 days, your physiotherapist has noticed drooping of the right eyelid. You have also noticed it now, although this could have been present from before, but it certainly wasn't present before the surgery. You initially thought that this was due to tiredness and lack of sleep. However, this has persisted and the physiotherapist has mentioned this to the ward doctor. You do not re-call this problem prior to having surgery. There are no other associated symptoms, i.e. headache, double vision, visual disturbance, or limb weakness. There has been no change in your voice.

You have a history of hypertension and you are taking a tablet for that. You cannot remember your medication list. You have no allergies.

You are a smoker (5 cigarettes per day) and consume 6–8 units of alcohol per week.

You are concerned about the persisting nature of the drooping eyelid and are concerned that this will be permanent.

You will ask the doctor:

(a) What has caused this? Is it a stroke?
(b) Is this permanent?
(c) Will it get better?

C. Examiners' information

A good candidate will be able to:

- *Obtain an appropriate history for ptosis with a broad differential diagnosis in mind*
- *Establish the onset of ptosis in relation to surgery, and conclude this developed post-operatively*
- *Enquire about the type of valve used, as this will affect if the patient can have MRI*
- *Recognize the association between thoracic surgery and Horner's syndrome*
- *Look for features of Horner's syndrome*
- *Examine for other potential causes and associations of ptosis, i.e. ophthalmoplegia and fatiguability*
- *Address patient's concerns*
- *Explain the need for further investigations: bloods, CXR, CT chest, and CT/MRI brain*

D. Focused history

History of presenting complaint

- Establish the specifics of the current admission.
- Was type of valve was used? Tissue versus metallic. *(Metallic valves will preclude the use of MRI)*
- How long has the ptosis been present? Was it present before surgery?
- Establish the onset of ptosis in relation to the surgery
- Did you notice it, or did someone else notice it?
- Is it complete or incomplete?
- Is it unilateral or bilateral?
- Is there anything that makes the ptosis worse?
- Is the ptosis worse at the end of the day?
- Have you noticed any double vision?
- Have you noticed any change in pupil size?
- Does the eyeball appear sunken?
- Have you noticed any change in sweating affecting the face, arms, and chest?
- Enquire about other associated symptoms:
  - Headache?
  - Facial or limb weakness?
  - Fatiguability?
  - Weight loss, productive cough, and haemoptysis? *(Prior to operation, as screening symptoms for lung malignancy)*

Previous medical history

- Remember the causes of Horner's syndrome:
  - PERIPHERAL
    - Pancoast tumour (ask about weight loss, cough, haemoptysis)
    - Neck surgery (thyroid or laryngeal disease)
    - Cardiothoracic surgery
    - Central venous catheterization
    - Lymphadenopathy
  - CENTRAL
    - Syringomyelia
    - Demyelination
    - Neck trauma

- Myasthenia gravis
- Myotonic dystrophy

Drug history

- Drug-induced myasthenia can be caused by aminoglycosides, penicillamine, phenytoin, lignocaine, procainamide, macrolides, fluoroquinolones, and lithium

Social history

- Is there a history of smoking? (risk factor for Pancoast tumour)

Patients concerns

- What concerns does the patient have?
- Does the patient have any thoughts as to what this could be?

E. Focused examination

Examine the eyes

- Is the ptosis unilateral or bilateral?
- Assess eye movements (ophthalmoplegia in III nerve palsy and myasthenia gravis)
- Check for heterochromia of the irides (congenital Horner's syndrome)
- Is ptosis accentuated on upward gaze? (myasthenia gravis)
- Check for pupillary reflexes (miosis-Horner's syndrome, mydriasis-III nerve palsy)
- If relative afferent pupillary defect noted, fundoscopy to look for optic atrophy (demyelination as a cause for Horner's syndrome)

Following examination of the eyes, the presence of partial ptosis, miosis, and the absence of ophthalmoplegia should indicate Horner's syndrome as the diagnosis. Proceed as follows:

Look for other features of Horner's syndrome

- Enophthalmos
- Anhidrosis (assess the pattern and extent of anhidrosis)

Examine to look for causes of Horner's syndrome

- Horner's syndrome has many causes, and to look for clinical signs relating to each takes time. A reasonable strategy is to examine the neck, hands, and chest:

Neck

- Scars (trauma, previous neck surgery, central venous catherization)
- Masses (tumour, lymphadenopathy, goitre)
- Aneurysms

Hands

- Wasting, clubbing, nicotine staining, and C8–T1 sensory loss (Pancoast syndrome)
- Wasting, fasciculations, and dissociated sensory loss (syringomyelia)

Chest

- Apical lung signs (Pancoast syndrome, apical collections)—*percuss for apical dullness*
- Cervical rib (supraclavicular bruit)

If the examination of the eyes does not indicate Horner's syndrome or III nerve palsy, then look for other causes of ptosis.

Look for other causes of unilateral ptosis

- Myasthenia gravis (fatiguability)
- Myotonic dystrophy (myopathic facies frontotemporal balding, temporalis wasting, myotonia)

F. Diagnosis

*   Horner's syndrome (as a complication of cardiothoracic surgery)

The differential diagnosis for unilateral ptosis is:

(a) III nerve palsy
(b) Horner's syndrome
(c) Myasthenia gravis (including drug-induced myasthenia gravis)
(d) Myotonic dystrophy (often bilateral, but can be unilateral)
(e) Congenital

The above conditions can be differentiated by history and examination. Horner's syndrome is characterized by a miosis, partial ptosis, enophthalmos, and anhidrosis. It may be a complication of aortic dissection, and it is important to establish the onset of ptosis in relation to (a) symptoms of aortic dissection at the time of presentation, and (b) time of surgery. Given that this patient has developed ptosis post-operatively, a post-operative complication of cardiothoracic surgery is the most likely cause. However, it is important to focus the examination on looking for the other principal causes of Horner's syndrome.

G. Feedback to patient

Explain diagnosis

*   'The cause of the drooping eyelid is a condition called Horner's syndrome. This is caused by compression of the nerves supplying the eyelid.'
*   'Although there are many causes, it can occur following cardiothoracic surgery, and this is the most likely cause. During the operation there is stretching of the blood vessels and nerves in the neck, and following the operation, there can be small collections of fluid and blood in the tissues, resulting in localized swelling, and compression of the nerves.'

Address patient concerns

*   'A stroke cannot be excluded, but it is rare for a stroke to cause such an isolated defect.'
*   'As a complication of surgery, this resolves with time as nerve function often improves. However, in some cases it may be permanent, but it is difficult to tell at this stage.'
*   'Although the cause is most likely a post-operative complication of surgery, you will arrange tests to exclude other causes. Importantly, it will be important to exclude a stroke with CT or MRI scan.'

H. Feedback to patient

Further investigations

*   Chest radiograph
    *   Cervical rib
    *   Apical ling lesions, e.g. Pancoast tumour
*   CT chest
    *   Apical lung lesions
    *   Post-operative intra-thoracic collections, i.e. apical lung haematoma
*   CT/MRI head and brainstem*

---

* Following valve surgery, it is important to determine the type of prosthesis and compatibility with MRI. MRI is the investigation of choice as it can identify other pathologies (e.g. demyelination) and is superior for imaging the brainstem.

Further management
- Await the results of the above investigations and manage accordingly

I. Questions commonly asked by examiners

How common is Horner's syndrome following cardiothoracic surgery?

Horner's syndrome has been reported in 1.3% of patients following thoracic surgery or thoracic trauma.[1]

What are the mechanisms of Horner's syndrome in a patient following thoracic surgery?
- Direct injury of cervical sympathetic chain
- Pressure of chest drain tube on the sympathetic chain at the lung apex
- Post-operative collection or haematoma at the lung apex

J. Additional reading

Volume 1

Case 91 ◆ Headaches and Visual Disturbance

A. Candidate information

Role: *Medical registrar (outpatient clinic)*

This gentleman has a history of hypertension, hypercholesterolaemia, and impaired glucose tolerance. More recently he complains of headaches and visual disturbance. The blood pressure has been difficult to control and the reading today in clinic is 164/80. His current medications include ramipril, atenolol, and simvastatin. He has a busy and stressful office job and his work primarily involves working with computers. His social factors may be contributory, but his poor blood pressure control is the likely factor. Thank you for your assessment.

Task: *Assess the patient and determine the causes of headaches and visual disturbance. Advise on further investigation and treatment.*

---

[1] Kaya et al. Horner's syndrome as a complication in thoracic surgical practice. Eur J Cardiothorac Surg. 2003; 24:1025–8.

B. Patient information

Age: 52 years

Problem: Headaches and visual disturbance

You have been referred by your GP who is concerned about your persisting headaches and occasional visual disturbance. Over the last year you are noticing an increasing frequency of headaches. There is no known precipitant and these can occur intermittently. They often respond to simple analgesics, i.e. paracetamol. Over the last 2 months you have noticed some visual disturbance. You do not wear glasses for your vision, and a recent eye check performed by your optician was satisfactory. Although your vision is clear, you find that at times you are not completely aware of your surroundings and often bump into people and objects unintentionally.

If asked by the candidate, you have noticed a change in facial appearance over the last 2 years, but have taken little notice of it. You have noticed that your hands have become larger, as evidenced by an increase in glove size. You enjoy DIY and gardening, and feel that your enlarging hands may be secondary to skin thickening as a result of this manual work. You find that you sweat more profusely, but attribute this to a busy life-style.

Your previous history includes hypertension and hypercholesterolemia. Following a recent check you were told you had 'impaired glucose tolerance' indicating possible early diabetes. You work in a busy office environment and have recently been promoted. This has placed increased stress on you and you find that you are working long days in front of a computer screen.

You regularly check your blood pressure at home, but it is often elevated at the GP surgery. Your GP feels that the headaches and visual disturbance may be due to inadequate blood pressure control. You feel that your symptoms are related to stress and your working environment. However, you are concerned about the headaches and visual disturbance, as they persist even when not working, e.g. whilst on holidays.

You will ask the doctor:

(a) Are my symptoms related to stress?
(b) Can poor blood pressure control account for my symptoms?
(c) Will I need further tests?

C. Examiners' information

A good candidate will be able to:

- *Obtain a history of headaches and visual disturbance.*
- *Conclude from this history that the central vision is intact, but it is the peripheral vision that is affected.*
- *Recognize a link between hypertension, impaired glucose tolerance, headache,s and visual disturbance—acromegaly, and direct specific questions in relation to this.*
- *Enquire about blood pressure control.*
- *Conduct a general examination to look for features of acromegaly.*
- *Address patient's concerns.*
- *Explain possible diagnosis to patient and the need for further investigations: glucose, HbA1C, oral glucose tolerance test, serum IGF-1, pituitary function tests, and MRI head (pituitary gland)*

D. Focused history

History of presenting complaint

- Headaches:
  - How long have the headaches been present for?
  - Enquire about the nature of the headaches, i.e. location, character, radiation.
  - What the precipitating and relieving factors?
  - Are they intermittent or persistent?
  - Are there any associated symptoms:
    - Facial or limb weakness?
    - Facial or limb sensory disturbance?
- Visual disturbance:
  - How long have you had the visual disturbance?
  - Can you describe the onset of visual disturbance? Is it sudden or gradual?
  - Can you describe the visual disturbance? Is it partial or complete?
  - Does it affect one or both eyes?
  - Is it intermittent or persistent?
  - Is there a relationship between headaches and visual disturbance?
- Acromegaly (screening questions):
  - Have you noticed a change in your appearance?
  - Have you noticed a change in your hat, glove, or shoe size?
  - Do you have increased sweating?

Previous medical history

Enquire about other systemic manifestations of acromegaly:

- Hypertension
- Diabetes/impaired glucose tolerance
- Arthritis
- Carpal tunnel syndrome
- Goitre

Drug history

- Enquire about medications, side-effects, and compliance

Patients concerns

- What concerns does the patient have?
- Does the patient have any thoughts as to what this could be?

E. Focused examination

The main focus of the examination should be to look for features of acromegaly. Given that this case was centred on a referral for inadequate blood pressure control as a possible cause for symptoms, it is important to start by requesting a blood pressure reading.

Examine eyes

- Visual fields (bitemporal hemianopia)

Examine the face
- Prominent supraorbital ridges
- Enlarged nose and lips
- Prognathism
- Interdental separation
- Macroglossia

Examine the hands
- Large sweaty hands (broad palms and spatulate fingers)
- Thickened skin on dorsum of hands
- Features of carpal tunnel syndrome (look for previous carpal tunnel release scars)

Examine the skin
- Hypertrichosis
- Gynaecomastia
- Skin tags (axillae)
- Acanthosis nigricans

Examine for other features of acromegaly
- Goitre
- Arthropathy

F. Diagnosis

- Acromegaly

The focus of this case is acromegaly. A history of headaches, visual disturbance, hypertension, and impaired glucose tolerance is highly suggestive of acromegaly. The examination findings of acromegalic facies and bitemporal hemianopia should not cause diagnostic difficulties.

The key in this station is to recognize acromegaly early in the consultation. The history should begin with open questions centred on the symptoms, and conclude with specific closed questions focusing on acromegaly.

G. Feedback to the patient

Explain diagnosis
- 'From the exmination, it seems as if your symptoms are caused by acromegaly (a condition which results in increased levels of growth hormone in the body).'
- 'This is caused by an increase in size of the pituitary gland, which lies along the bottom surface of the brain. This is why you have been getting headaches and altered vision. The increased growth hormone levels explain the changes in your appearance and the increased sweating.'

Address patient concerns
- Although social stressors and busy working life may account for symptoms of headache and visual disturbance, possibly through poor blood pressure control, the examination findings support a diagnosis of acromegaly.
- To confirm this, blood tests and an MRI scan of the head (to look specifically at the pituitary gland) will be arranged.

H. Feedback to the examiner

Further investigations

- Blood tests
  - ◆ FBC
  - ◆ Prolactin
  - ◆ Serum IGF-1
  - ◆ Oral glucose tolerance test (suppresses growth hormone in normal individuals)
- MRI head—pituitary adenoma

Further management

- Transsphenoidal hypophysectomy
- Pharmacological treatment is used as an adjunct, or where surgery is contraindicated or declined.
  - ◆ Somatostatin analogues (octreotide, lanreotide)
  - ◆ Dopamine agonists (cabergoline, bromocriptine)
- Radiotherapy

I. Additional reading

Volume 1

Volume 2

Case 92 ◆ **Back Pain and Breathlessness**

A. Candidate information

Role: *Medical registrar (outpatient clinic)*

This gentleman has been complaining of severe back pain over the last 3 years following a road traffic accident. This has progressively got worse, now requiring higher doses of simple analgesics. His back pain is worse in the mornings and improves with analgesics by the afternoon. He uses paracetamol and ibuprofen regularly. Over the last 3 months he has noticed increasing breathlessness on exertion, with a noticeable reduction in exercise tolerance. He has no other significant medical history. Thank you for your assessment.

Task: *Assess the patient and determine the causes for symptoms. Advise on further investigation and treatment.*

B. Patient information

Age: 38 years

Problem: Back pain and breathlessness

You have been referred by your GP. For the last 3 years you have been complaining of lower back pain. This initially developed after a road traffic accident. You did not sustain any fractures and have not had any spinal surgery. You remember being seen in the Accident and Emergency department where you were told that the X-rays were normal. Since then you have been using paracetamol and ibuprofen as and when you need. However, over the last 5 months, you have noticed that the back pain is increasing in severity. It is particularly worse in the mornings and you have trouble getting out of bed. This improves considerably by the mid-morning after analgesic medications, which you have now started taking regularly. You do not complain of any other join aches or pains.

Over the last 3 months you have also noticed increasing breathlessness on exertion. Previously your exercise tolerance had been unrestricted, but you find yourself breathless on rapidly going up 2 flights of stairs. There is no chest pain. There is no dizziness.

You have no other previous medical history. You do not smoke and consume occasional alcohol. Your mother suffers with severe rheumatoid arthritis, diagnosed in her 40s, who you recall as originally presenting in the same fashion. She was told her rheumatoid condition affects her lungs. Your father died aged 78 years of a heart attack and subsequent heart failure 5 years ago. The back pain affects your daily activities, especially in the mornings, but is fortunate that you are self-employed and work from home.

You are concerned with the recent progression in back pain and are even more concerned with regards to recent development of breathlessness. You are concerned you may be developing rheumatoid arthritis like your mother.

You will ask the doctor:

(a) Do I have rheumatoid arthritis?
(b) What is the cause of breathlessness?

C. Examiners' information

A good candidate will be able to:

- *Obtain history of back pain and breathlessness.*
- *Enquire about other rheumatological symptoms.*
- *Recognize ankylosing spondylitis and examine for associated clinical features.*
- *Be aware of the systemic associations of ankylosing spondylitis, and look for features that may cause breathlessness (heart block, aortic regurgitation, lung fibrosis).*
- *Examine the pulse for bradycardia (heart block)*
- *Assess JVP*
- *Auscultate the heart (aortic regurgitation)*
- *Auscultate the lung fields (apical fibrosis)*
- *Address patient's concerns*
- *Explain the need for further investigations: bloods, ECG, CXR, X-ray of pelvis and spine, echocardiogram, 24hr holter monitor, lung function tests, and high resolution CT (HRCT) chest*
- *Explain the need for up-titrating analgesic medications, physiotherapy, and exercise with referral to rheumatologist for specialist input.*

D. Focused history

History of presenting complaint

- Back pain:
  - How long has the back pain been present? (onset, duration, and progression)
  - Is it constant or intermittent?
  - Is there any radiation?
  - Are there any exacerbating or relieving factors?
  - Is there associated stiffness?
  - Is it worse in the mornings or evenings?
  - Does exercise or movement make it worse?
  - Are any other joints affected?
- Breathlessness:
  - How long has the breathlessness been present for?
  - Is it constant or intermittent?
  - Are there any exacerbating or relieving factors?
  - Is it related to exertion? Is it present at rest?
  - Any associated symptoms:
    - Chest pain?
    - Dizziness?
    - Ankle swelling?
    - Orthopnoea?
    - Paroxysmal nocturnal dyspnoea?
  - Ask about reduction in exercise tolerance.

Previous medical history

- Rheumatological history (rheumatoid arthritis and seronegative arthritis*)

Drug history

- Enquire about medications, side-effects, and compliance
- Review the analgesic medications.

Patients concerns

- What concerns does the patient have?
- Does the patient have any thoughts as to what this could be?

E. Focused examination

The diagnosis to recognize early in the consultation is ankylosing spondylitis. The focus of the examination is to demonstrate the clinical signs of ankylosing spondylitis and look for related pathology that may potentially account for breathlessness.

Examine for musculoskeletal features of ankylosing spondylitis

- Kyphosis (question-mark posture)
- Decreased spinal movements
- Tenderness over sacroiliac joints (check with patient and examiner)

---

* Psoriatic arthritis, enteropathic arthritis, ankylosing spondylitis, and reactive arthritis

- Flesche's test (increased occiput–wall distance)
- Modified Schober's test (do not need to perform in examination)
- Reduced chest expansion
- Arthritis of other joints (knees and hips)

Examine pulse
- Bradycardia (heart block)

Check blood pressure
- Wide pulse pressure (aortic regurgitation)

Examine the heart
- Assess JVP (elevated in cardiac failure)*
- Auscultate for aortic regurgitation (mitral regurgitation can also occur)
- Check for ankle oedema**

Examine chest
- Apical lung fibrosis

F. Diagnosis
- Ankylosing spondylitis

The differential diagnosis of morning back pain with stiffness that improves with exercise is:

(a) Ankylosing spondylitis (seronegative arthritis)
(b) Rheumatoid arthritis

In this patient, the clinical signs favour a diagnosis of ankylosing spondylitis.

The differential diagnosis for exertional breathlessness in a patient with ankylosing spondylitis is:

(a) Chest wall deformity and reduced chest expansion
(b) Aortic regurgitation
(c) Heart block
(d) Apical pulmonary fibrosis
(e) Amyloidosis with nephrotic syndrome (pleural effusions)
(f) Amyloidosis with restrictive cardiomyopathy

G. Feedback to the patient

Explain diagnosis
- 'The most likely cause for the back pain is ankylosing spondylitis. This condition is seen in young people and affects the spine.'

Address patient concerns
- The symptoms do not suggest rheumatoid arthritis, as other features of rheumatoid arthritis are not present on examination.
- The deformity of the chest wall can cause breathlessness. However, ankylosing spondylitis can affect other organs such as the heart and lung, and this may cause breathlessness. Although the exact cause of breathlessness is not clear, this warrants further investigation.

---

* Cardiac failure could be due to severe aortic regurgitation or restrictive cardiomyopathy (secondary to amyloidosis).

** Ankle oedema could be caused by congestive cardiac failure or amyloidosis (nephrotic syndrome).

H. Feedback to the examiner

Further investigations

- Blood tests
  - ◆ FBC
  - ◆ Inflammatory markers (CRP and ESR)
  - ◆ β-natiuretic peptide*
  - ◆ Rheumatoid factor
- X-ray of the sacroiliac joints**
- CXR
  - ◆ ECG (heart block)
  - ◆ Echocardiogram
  - ◆ Urinalysis***
  - ◆ Lung function tests (restrictive defect)
  - ◆ High resolution CT chest (pulmonary fibrosis)

Further management

- Patient education
- Exercise and physiotherapy
- Uptitrate analgesia
- Disease modifying anti-rheumatic drugs (DMARDS) (methotrexate and sulphasalazine) have no role in spinal disease, but can be used for peripheral disease
- Biological therapy—anti-TNFα therapy (adalimumab and etanercept) can be used for active spinal disease not responding to ≥2 NSAIDs (NICE guidelines)

I. Additional reading

Volume 1

Volume 2

---

* Normal levels are less than 100pg/mL. It has a negative predictive value of at least 96%, so cardiac failure (due to systolic or diastolic dysfunction) can be confidently ruled out for patients in the normal range.

** A plain X-ray is usually sensitive enough to demonstrate sacroilitis, and severity is graded from 0 (normal) to IV (fused). If this is normal but suspicion remains high, MRI is warranted, since it is the most sensitive and specific investigation for sacroilitis.

*** Proteinuria may indicate amyloidosis (nephrotic syndrome). If proteinuria is present, this can formally be quantified with a 24 hour urine collection.

Case 93 ◆ **Facial Rash**

A. Candidate information

Role: *On-call medical registrar*

This lady has been admitted with a swollen left calf. A diagnosis of deep vein thrombosis has been confirmed on doppler ultrasound scan. There is a previous history of migraines. She takes the oral contraceptive pill. She is currently therapeutically anticoagulated with low molecular weight heparin and warfarin has been initiated. She was noted to have a facial rash. A dermatology doctor has reviewed the patient and has requested a medical review.

Task: *Assess the patient and determine the cause of the rash. Advise on further investigation and treatment.*

B. Patient information

Age: 38 years

Problem: Facial rash

You have been admitted to the medical ward with a swollen left calf. A doppler ultrasound scan has confirmed deep vein thrombosis. You have been told that will require warfarin therapy for 6 months and you are currently receiving injections to thin the blood whilst the warfarin takes its effect. This morning on the ward round, the ward house officer noticed a rash on your face and requested a dermatology review. The dermatology doctor told you this morning that you will need further blood tests. You have had this rash on your face for some time now (>3 years) and have never really taken much notice of it. You frequently go on holidays and enjoy sun-bathing and found that this rash would get worse when exposed to the sun. It tends to improve on return from holidays, but does leave some degree of permanent scarring. You tend to get sun burnt very easily and application of sun block creams have helped. You feel that generally you are a photosensitive person, and attribute this as the cause of rash.

You have no other symptoms. You do not complain of cold hands or joint aches and pains. You have a history of frequent migraines and self medicate as and when you need with paracetamol. You have a strong family history of migraines. You have been using the contraceptive pill for the last 6 months.

You do not smoke and consume a glass of wine occasionally on the weekends. You work as a primary school mathematics teacher.

You are concerned that the dermatology doctor felt that you needed further blood tests.

You will ask the doctor:

(a) Why was the dermatology doctor concerned?
(b) Will I need further tests?

C. Examiners' information

A good candidate will be able to:

- Obtain a history of facial rash, and establish its photosensitive nature.
- Enquire about thrombotic risk factors—oral contraceptive pill.
- Establish that the rash has been present before oral contraceptive pill use.
- Recognize the rash of systemic lupus erythematosus.
- Enquire about other systemic symptoms of SLE (arthropathy and Raynaud's phenomenon).
- Examine the rash and look for other associations of SLE (conjunctival pallor for anaemia, hands and joints for arthropathy, mouth ulcers, and scalp for scarring alopecia).
- Look for other rheumatological conditions, e.g. scleroderma, rheumatoid arthritis, and dermatomyositis (mixed connective tissue disorders).
- Recognize the potential association between DVT, migraines, and SLE and the need to exclude antiphospholipid syndrome
- Address patient's concerns.
- Explain the need to stop the oral contraceptive pill and for further tests (auto-antibodies).
- If anti-phospholipid syndrome is confirmed, then this will require life-long warfarin anticoagulation.

D. Focused history

History of presenting complaint

- Establish the specifics of the current admission.
- How long has the rash been present?
- Was there a gradual or sudden onset?
- Are there any potential precipitants?
- Is it intermittent or persistent? Have there been periods of complete recovery?
- Are there any exacerbating or relieving factors? (photosensitivity)
- Are there associated symptoms:
  - ◆ Pain?
  - ◆ Itching?
- Are any other areas affected? (skin and scalp)
- Is there a history of joint aches and pains? If so, which joints are affected?
- What happens when your hands are exposed to the cold? Establish triphasic response with characteristic colour changes of Raynaud's.

Previous medical history

- Rheumatological disease
  - ◆ SLE
  - ◆ Rheumatoid arthritis
  - ◆ Systemic sclerosis
  - ◆ Dermatomyositis
- Anti-phospholipid syndrome
  - ◆ Previous thrombotic complications
  - ◆ Migraines
  - ◆ Miscarriages (females)
- Establish thromboembolic risk factors

Drug history

- Enquire complete drug history (drug-induced lupus)
- Oral contraceptive pill (as a cause of drug-induced lupus and increased thromboembolic risk)

Patients concerns

- What concerns does the patient have?
- Does the patient have any thoughts as to what this could be?

E. Focused examination

The key is to recognize SLE from the outset of the consultation and to look for clinical findings associated with this condition.

Examine the skin

- Facial rash*
- Palmar erythema
- Photosensitivity
- Vasculitic lesions
- Purpura
- Urticaria
- Livedo reticularis
- Telangiectasia
- Alopecia
- Raynaud's phenomenon

Examine for other rheumatological disease

- Inspect hands, arms, face, and feet. Look for the following:
  - Rheumatoid arthritis
  - Systemic sclerosis
  - Dermatomyositis

If present this will constitute a diagnosis of mixed connective tissue disease.

Look for other associations of SLE

There are many systemic associations of SLE. Due to time constraints in the MRCP (PACES) examination, the following can be easily looked for:

- Conjunctival pallor (anaemia)
- Arthropathy
- Mouth ulcers (seen in a third of patients)

Tell the examiner you would like to look for other systemic associations:

- **Respiratory**: interstitial lung disease, pleural effusions, and pleurisy (pleural rub)
- **Cardiovascular**: pericarditis, murmurs (Libman-Sacks endocarditis), pulmonary hypertension
- **Nervous system**: hemiparesis, cranial nerve lesions, mononeuritis multiplex, and polyneuropathy

---

* Erythematous, maculopapular rash in a butterfly distribution affecting the cheeks and the bridge of the nose, sparing the nasolabial folds with scaling and follicular plugging.

- **Renal**: hypertension, oedema, urinalysis for proteinuria and haematuria
- **Haematological**: lymphadenopathy, splenomegaly
- **Eyes**: Sjogren syndrome, cytoid bodies (retinal infarcts), roth spots, and papilloedema

F. Diagnosis

- Systemic lupus erythematosus*
- Anti-phospholipid syndrome (this must be excluded)

The clinical features of the rash suggest systemic lupus erythematosus. This patient is taking the oral contraceptive pill, and this raises the possibility of drug-induced lupus. However, it is clear from the history that the rash has been present before the use of the oral contraceptive pill, which supports a diagnosis of SLE rather than drug-induced lupus. The presence of a thrombotic complication and a history of migraines strongly raises the suspicion of antiphospholipid syndrome. It is possible that this is not anti-phospholipid syndrome, and the thrombotic complication may simply reflect oral contraceptive pill use. However, anti-phospholipid syndrome must be excluded, as it has long-term implications (the need for life-long anticoagulation).

G. Feedback to the patient

Explain diagnosis

- 'The examination findings suggest that you may have a condition called systemic lupus erythematosus or SLE. This is a condition that affects the skin and different organs in the body. The oral contraceptive pill can sometimes cause a similar rash, but this is unlikely to be the cause, as the rash was present before starting this.'
- 'There is an association between systemic lupus erythematosus, thrombosis, and migraines—a condition called anti-phospholipid syndrome.'

Address patient concerns

- Further tests will be necessary to diagnose systemic lupus erythematosus and anti-phospholipid syndrome.
- If systemic lupus erythematosus is diagnosed, then there are a number of drugs that help the skin rash. Furthermore, one would need further tests to look for other organs that may be involved.
- The oral contraceptive pill does increase the risk of thrombosis, and this must be discontinued. Alternative forms of contraceptives need to be considered.
- If anti-phospholipid syndrome is diagnosed, given the fact deep vein thrombosis has been diagnosed on this admission, the subsequent life-long risk of thrombosis is high, and therefore life-long anticoagulation will be necessary.

H. Feedback to the examiner

Further investigations

- Blood tests
  - ◆ FBC (anaemia and thrombocytopenia)
  - ◆ U&E (lupus nephritis)

---

* The diagnosis criteria for SLE is any four of the following 11 criteria (1) Malar rash, (2) Discoid rash, (3) Photosensitivity, (4) Oral ulcers, (5) Arthritis, (6) Serositis, (7) Renal involvement, (8) Neurological involvement, (9) Haematological involvement, (10) Immunological disorder, and (11) Positive antinuclear antibody.

- ♦ Clotting ($\uparrow$ APTT in antiphospholipid syndrome)
- ♦ Auto-antibodies*
- Urine tests**
  - ♦ Urinalysis
  - ♦ 24 hour urine collection for protein

Further management
- Request above investigations (blood tests and urinalysis)
- Stop oral contraceptive pill

If SLE is confirmed:

- Avoidance of over-exposure to sunlight (sunscreens with a protection factor>25)
- Anti-malarial agents and corticosteroids can be used for skin disease
- Screen for other organ involvement

If anti-phospholipid syndrome confirmed:

- Life-long anticoagulation with warfarin

I. Additional reading

Volume 1
Supplementary Skin Case 131 Systemic Lupus Erythematosus

Case 94 ♦ Painful Joints

A. Candidate information

Role: *Medical registrar (outpatient clinic)*

This man has been complaining of painful joints affecting both hands for the last 8 months. He has been using paracetamol and ibuprofen initially with good effect. He now complains of worsening symptoms despite regular use of these analgesic medications. He has no other previous medical history. Thank you for your assessment.

Task: *Assess the patient and determine the causes of painful joints. Advise on further investigation and treatment if necessary.*

B. Patient information

Age: 58 years

---

* Antinuclear antibodies, Anti-histone antibodies, Anti-dsDNA antibodies, Anti-Sm antibodies, Anti-Ro *and* anti-La antibodies, anti-phospholipid antibodies.

** These may be requested to look for renal involvement, as renal involvement is one of the 11 diagnostic criteria that can be used to diagnose SLE.

Problem: Painful joints

You have been referred to the rheumatology outpatient clinic with painful joints affecting both of your hands. This started approximately 8 months ago affecting the small joints of both hands. The joints are affected in a symmetrical pattern. Your GP had prescribed paracetamol and ibuprofen which you initially used on an as needed basis. This provided considerable relief of symptoms. Over the last month the joint pains have flared up, and you are finding that despite regular use of the tablets this is not improving. Your symptoms persist throughout the day, and there is no particular time throughout the day where your symptoms are better. Movement of the joints increases the pain. At times the joints can feel warm to touch. Others joints in the body are not affected. You have noticed increasing stiffness associated with the joints with difficulty making a closed fist and straightening your fingers. It has affected your ability to write and type.

You have no significant medical history. You smoke 5 cigarettes per day and consume 4 units of alcohol per week. You work in an office, which involves using computers. Over the last month you have not been able to work due to your debilitating symptoms. Your mother has rheumatoid arthritis and is left with considerable deformity of the hands.

You have been particularly concerned that this may be rheumatoid arthritis and you too will be left with a permanent disability.

You will ask the doctor:

(a) Is this rheumatoid arthritis?
(b) Are there any treatments available for this?
(c) Will I be able to return to work?

C. Examiners' information

A good candidate will be able to:

- Take a careful history of joint pain.
- Establish the distribution of affected joints with an appropriate differential diagnosis in mind.
- Enquire about previous history of rheumatological disease.
- Enquire about current therapy and its adequacy in controlling symptoms.
- Recognize the features of psoriatic arthropathy.
- Examine the hands and look carefully for nail changes.
- Look for evidence of involvement of other joints.
- Examine the skin for psoriasis (extensor surfaces, scalp, navel, and behind the ears).
- Address patient's concerns.
- Explain the need for further tests (X-rays and blood tests).
- Explain the need to initiate other drugs, particularly DMARDs.

D. Focused history

History of presenting complaint

- How long has the joint discomfort been present?
- Clarify the exact nature of the symptoms. Is there joint pain, stiffness and/or swelling?
- Which joints are affected? (symmetrical versus asymmetrical involvement)
- Enquire about the onset of symptoms. Was it over hours or over weeks?
- Have symptoms been constant or intermittent?

- Are there any exacerbating or relieving factors?
  - Are the symptoms worse in the morning or evening?
  - What is the effect of joint movement and exercise?
- Enquire about other associated symptoms (rheumatological disease):
  - Rash (vasculitis, SLE, psoriasis)
  - Back pain (ankylosing spondylitis)
  - Eye symptoms (rheumatoid arthritis)
  - Orogenital ulcers (SLE, Behcets disease, reactive arthritis)
  - Genitourinary symptoms? (reactive or gonococcal arthritis)
  - Gastrointestinal symptoms? (seronegative arthritis with inflammatory bowel disease)

Previous medical history

- Previous history of rheumatological disease
  - Rheumatoid arthritis
  - Osteoarthritis
  - Psoriatic arthropathy
  - Ankylosing spondylitis
  - SLE
  - Gout
  - Pseudogout (enquire about related conditions*)
- Other associated diseases (seronegative arthritis):
  - Psoriasis
  - Inflammatory bowel disease

Drug history

- Review the analgesic medications.
- Enquire about compliance

Social history

- How have the symptoms affected the patient?

Patients concerns

- What concerns does the patient have?
- Does the patient have any thoughts as to what this could be?

E. Focused examination

The key is to recognize psoriatic arthropathy early in the examination and to proceed with a focused examination, looking particularly for evidence of psoriasis.

Examine the joints

- Establish the distribution of joint involvement
  - Symmetrical versus asymmetrical joint involvement
  - Pattern of joint involvement
- Look for deformities
- Inspect overlying skin. Erythema suggests active inflammation or infection.

---

* Haemochromatosis, hypothyroidism, hyperparathyroidism, acromegaly, diabetes.

- Are the joints warm to touch? Warmth suggests active inflammation.
- Examine functional status

Examine the nails
- Look for the nail changes associated with psoriatic arthropathy:
  - Nail pitting
  - Onycholysis
  - Transverse ridging

Examine for psoriasis
Once a diagnosis of psoriatic arthropathy is apparent, proceed to look for psoriasis:

- Examine the extensor surfaces, scalp, and behind the ears.

If the diagnosis is not clear, then proceed to look for evidence of other rheumatological and/or associated diseases. Conduct a general examination and inspect hands, arms, face, and feet. See the differential diagnosis listed below.

F. Diagnosis
- Psoriatic arthropathy

There is a wide differential diagnosis for arthropathy of the small joints of the hands:

(a) Rheumatoid arthritis
(b) Seronegative arthropathies:
  - Psoriatic arthropathy
  - Ankylosing spondylitis
  - Reactive arthritis
  - Enteropathic arthritis
(c) Arthropathy related to other rheumatological diseases:
  - Scleroderma
  - SLE
  - Sarcoidosis
  - Vasculitis
(d) Osteoarthritis
(e) Gout
(f) Pseudogout
(g) Viral infections
(h) Malignancy

The pattern of joint involvement with nail changes will help make a diagnosis of psoriatic arthropathy, which is the focus of this station. It is important to look for evidence of psoriasis. Remember, that psoriatic arthropathy can occur with minimal skin involvement. In 20% of cases, the arthropathy precedes the onset of psoriasis, in some cases by up to 20 years.

G. Feedback to the patient
Explain diagnosis
- 'From the examination, I think that the most likely cause for the joint symptoms is psoriatic arthropathy, a joint condition related to psoriasis.'

Address patient concerns
- Psoriatic arthropathy is different to rheumatoid arthritis, and is often not associated with severe joint deformities and disability that can otherwise occur in rheumatoid arthritis.

- Further tests including blood tests and X-rays of the hands will be arranged.
- The mainstay of the treatment is symptom control with analgesic medications in the first instance.
- Other specific therapies are available if these measures do not control symptoms.

H. Feedback to the examiner

Further investigations

- Blood tests
  - FBC
  - liver function test (LFT)*
  - Inflammatory markers (CRP and ESR)
  - Rheumatoid factor
  - Autoimmune profile (if suspecting autoimmune disease)
- X-ray of the joint(s)

Further management

- Simple analgesics
- NSAIDs (in some patients NSAIDs may worsen psoriasis)
- Corticosteroids—intra-articular steroid injections for single troublesome joints.
- DMARDs—methotrexate, sulphasalazine, and cyclosporin**
- Biological therapy—anti-TNFα therapy (etanercept, infliximab, and adalimumab)***

I. Additional reading

Volume 1

Supplementary Locomotor Case 109 Psoriatic Arthropathy

Supplementary Skin Case 120 Psoriasis

Volume 2

Station 2 Case 23 Joint Pains

Case 95 ◆ Recurrent Nose Bleeds

A. Candidate information

Role: On-call medical registrar

This lady has been admitted with recurrent epistaxis. She has been seen by the ear, nose, and throat (ENT) surgeons and has undergone successful cauterization. She has a history of hypertension.

---

* This is important to establish base-line LFTs before starting DMARDs, e.g. methotrexate.

** They are effective in treating skin symptoms, and the symptoms of peripheral arthritis, but not axial symptoms.

*** Anti-TNFα therapy has been shown to improve skin disease, joint disease and disability in psoriatic arthritis. They are indicated if there is poor response to ≥2 DMARDs (NICE guidelines)

Her medications include aspirin 75mg OD and bendroflumethiazide 2.5mg OD. Her blood pressure on admission was 190/100. The ENT surgeons are concerned that it may be her poor blood pressure control that is accounting for recurrent epistaxis. They have requested a medical review.

Task: Assess the patient and determine the cause of recurrent epistaxis. Advise on further investigation and treatment if necessary.

B. Patient information

Age: 62 years

Problem: Recurrent nose bleeds

You have been admitted to the surgical ward with a large nose bleed. This is the third admission this year. Previously, the bleeding has been small and simply required packing the nose. However, on this admission you have required cauterization. The blood pressure on admission was high and has remained high throughout your admission. The blood pressure reading taken this morning was 170/100.

You have always suffered with trivial nose bleeds since your teens. You have never really taken any notice of it. You had consulted your GP about 6 months ago after a large nose bleed and were diagnosed with hypertension and initiated on bendroflumethiazide. You were told that poor blood pressure control was the likely cause of the nose bleeds. You are troubled by bendroflumethiazide with need to urinate frequently, and as a result of this admit that you do not take you blood pressure medication daily. You were also started on aspirin, as there is a strong family history of ischaemic heart disease.

Your medications include aspirin and bendrofluazide.

You have a strong family history of ischaemic heart disease. You have strong family history of nose bleeds affecting your mother, sister, and brother. They too have hypertension. You do not smoke and consume minimal alcohol.

You have been particularly concerned about your recurrent nose bleeds, especially as this episode was large. You are also concerned about your blood pressure control, especially as you find taking the bendrofluazide difficult.

You will ask the doctor:

(a) Is high blood pressure the cause of the recurrent nose bleeds?
(b) If my blood pressure is well controlled, will it completely stop the nose bleeds?

C. Examiners' information

A good candidate will be able to:

- Establish specifics of current admission
- Establish a history and family history of recurrent epistaxis
- Establish poor compliance to anti-hypertensive therapy
- Recognize hereditary haemmorhagic telangiectasia
- Enquire about other complications of hereditary haemmorhagic telangiectasia
- Look for clinical signs of anaemia
- Inspect oral cavity and nasal mucosa for telangiectasia
- Look for other systemic manifestations of hereditary haemmorhagic telangiectasia

- *Address patient's concern and explain diagnosis*
- *Suggest stopping the aspirin (if no strong indication).*
- *Suggest switching to an alternative anti-hypertensive agent.*

D. Focused history

It is important to recognize hereditary haemmorhagic telangiectasia early in the consultation and focus the history around this condition and associated complications. Furthermore, it is important to recognize that poor blood pressure control will be contributory and to explore why this may be, i.e. poor compliance to therapy.

History of presenting complaint
- Establish the specifics of the current admission.
- How long have you suffered with nose bleeds?
- How often do they occur?
- Are they increasing in frequency?
- How severe are the nose bleeds? (quantity of blood loss)
- Are they increasing in severity?
- Are there any precipitating factors?
- Is there a history of trauma?
- Enquire about symptoms of anaemia:
  - Pallor?
  - Lethargy?
  - Chest pain?
  - Breathlessness?
- Is there a history of gastro-intestinal blood loss?
- Is there a history of haemoptysis?
- Is there a generalized increased bruising or bleeding tendency?

Previous medical history
- Hereditary haemmorhagic telangiectasia
- Bleeding disorders
- Hypertension (ask about control)

Drug history
- Review patient's drug chart
- Is the patient on anti-thrombotic or anticoagulation therapy?
- Enquire about medications, side-effects, and compliance

Family history
- Is there a history of epistaxis or bleeding tendencies?

Patients concerns
- What concerns does the patient have?
- Does the patient have any thoughts as to what this could be?

E. Focused examination

The key in this scenario is to recognize hereditary haemmorhagic telangiectasia as the primary cause of epistaxis and to demonstrate the clinical signs associated with this condition.

Review observation chart

*   Check heart rate and blood pressure
*   Is the blood pressure control adequate?

Examine the skin

*   Telangiectasia (face, lips, tongue, buccal and nasal mucosa)
*   Cyanosis*

Examine for anaemia

*   Conjuctival pallor
*   Koilonychia

Look for evidence of coagulopathy

*   Purpura and echymoses
*   Evidence of prolonged bleeding (recent venepuncture sites)

Look for other associations of hereditary haemmorhagic telangiectasia

Tell the examiner you would like to look for the following associations (if time allows):

*   **Respiratory**: pulmonary arteriovenous malformation (clubbing, cyanosis, bruits)
*   **Cardiovascular**: high-output cardiac failure
*   **Gastrointestinal**: hepatosplenomegaly, cirrhosis, and portal hypertension
*   **Eyes**: retinal haemorrhage and detachment (fundoscopy)
*   **Neurological**: ischaemic stroke and subarachnoid haemorrhage

F. Diagnosis

*   Hereditary haemmorhagic telangiectasia
*   Uncontrolled hypertension (secondary to poor drug compliance)

The primary cause of epistaxis is hereditary haemmorhagic telangiectasia. This should be clear from a history of recurrent epistaxis, a family history, and findings of telangiectasia on examination (Shovlin criteria). Poor hypertension control is contributory, and from the history it should be clear that this is due to poor compliance to bendroflumethiazide therapy.

G. Feedback to the patient

Explain diagnosis

*   'The most likely cause of your recurrent nose bleeds is hereditary haemmorhagic telangiectasia (termed 'HHT'). This is an inherited condition that results in dilatation of small blood vessels in the skin and different organs of the body. Depending on their location, it can result in differing symptoms. These abnormal dilated vessels frequently affect the lining of the nose in 90% of patients. This predisposes to nose bleeds.'
*   'Poor blood pressure control is a significant contributory factor, which in itself can cause nose bleeds. It is important to control this, and this will reduce the frequency of nose bleeds.'

Address patient concerns

*   The most likely reason for poor blood pressure control is the side-effect of bendroflumethiazide therapy which has led to poor compliance. It is important to initiate an alternative blood pressure tablet, as poor blood pressure control will increase the frequency of nose bleeds.

---

* Cyanosis reflects the degree of arterio-venous shunting.

- Good blood pressure control will not completely eliminate the risk of nose bleeds, as it will not affect the presence of the abnormally dilated vessels in the nose. Different treatments are available for this, but in the first instance, you would like to assess the response to cauterization and adequate blood pressure control. The need for further therapies can be assessed in the future.
- It is important to check the full blood count as chronic blood loss can lead to anaemia.
- Aspirin increases bleeding tendency, and this will be stopped. This may be re-introduced later if the nose bleeds are controlled.

H. Feedback to the examiner

Further investigations
- Blood tests
  - FBC
  - Clotting
  - Iron studies
  - U&Es (if considering initiation of ACE inhibitor therapy)

Further management

General measures
- Stop aspirin*
- Stop bendroflumethiazide and initiate alternative antihypertensive therapy

Treatment of anaemia
- Iron supplementation
- Blood transfusion (severe anaemia)

Treatment of skin telangiectases
- Cosmetic therapy
- Laser ablation

Treatment of epistaxis
- Cauterization
- Laser ablation
- Septal dermatoplasty
- Oestrogen therapy (induces squamous metaplasia)
- Low-dose aminocaproic acid (anti-fibrinolytic agent)

I. Additional reading

Volume 1

Supplementary Skin Case 122 Hereditary Haemmorhagic Telangiectasia

Volume 2

Station 2 Case 1 Hypertension

---

* There is no strong indication for aspirin therapy in this patient. Given the cardiovascular risk profile, aspirin will be beneficial for cardiovascular protection, but one must weigh the benefits and the risks. In the setting of recurrent epistaxis and poorly controlled hypertension, it would be advisable to discontinue this. Aspirin may be re-introduced in the future if the epistaxis remains controlled.

Supplementary Cases
A. Endocrine

Case 96 ◆ Acromegaly

CASE PRESENTATION

This patient has **large, sweaty hands** *with broad palms and spatulate fingers.*[1] *The skin over the dorsum of the hands is thickened.*[2] *The face*[3] *has* **prominent supraorbital ridges, enlarged nose and lips,** *and* **prognathism.**[4] *There is* **interdental separation** *and the tongue is enlarged (***macroglossia**).[5] *There is evidence of* **hypertrichosis**[6] *and there is* **gynaecomastia.**[7]

The diagnosis is **acromegaly.**[8]

Clinical notes

1. The skin over the face and extremities has a doughy-feeling. One of the earliest sign in acromegaly is enlargement of the hands and feet. The presence of sweatiness is an important feature, as this indicates the disease is active.

2. The skin is generally thickened. This can be specifically looked for on the dorsum of the hands. The skin pores may become noticeably large. Skin tags (molluscum fibrosum) may develop, often in the axillae. The presence of skin tags has been shown to correlate with the presence of colonic polyps. Hyperpigmentation occurs in 40% of patients. Examine the neck and axillae carefully for acanthosis nigricans. The nails may become thick and hard. Hypertrichosis occurs in up to 40% of patients with acromegaly.

3. Patients with acromegaly have coarse facial features. The facial wrinkles may be exaggerated with deepening of forehead and nasolabial creases. Enlargement of the nose occurs, and often gives this a triangular configuration. The lower lip is affected more than the upper lip. Terms such as "coarse features' are not likely to endear you to the patient, and should not be used!

4. Look from the side for prognathism. Ask the patient to clench his teeth. Prognathism is malocclusion of the teeth where the lower teeth overbite the upper teeth.

5. Other causes for macroglossia include hypothyroidism, amyloidosis, and Down's syndrome.

6. Hypertrichosis or hirsutism (often mild) is seen in up to 50% of patients.

7. Look for gynaecomastia in males.

8. Tell the examiner you would like to proceed to look for other associated features:
   (a) **Bitemporal hemianopia** (seen in 10% of patients)
   (b) **Optic atrophy** (due to parasellar extension)
   (c) **Carpal tunnel syndrome** (examine the wrists carefully for scars indicating previous carpal tunnel surgery)
   (d) **Hypertension**
   (e) **Cardiomegaly**
   (f) **Diabetes** (finger pricks for glucose testing, diabetic retinopathy, glycosuria)
   (g) **Arthropathy** (knees, ankles and spine are affected; look for kyphosis)

(h) **Goitre** (may be diffuse or multinodular; thyroid function is usually normal)

(i) **Proximal myopathy**

Tell the examiner that would like to ask the patient some questions:

(a) Is there a history of headaches?

(b) Has there been a change in shoe or ring size?

Questions commonly asked by examiners

What is the pathophysiology of acromegaly?

The most common cause is a growth hormone (GH) secreting adenoma of the anterior pituitary. At diagnosis, 75% are macroadenomas (>10mm diameter), and these account for one-third of all functional pituitary adenomas. Other rare causes include growth hormone-releasing hormone (GHRH) hypothalamic tumours or ectopic GH production from carcinoid or small-cell tumours.

What are the complications of acromegaly?

- Hypertension (43%)
- Cardiomegaly
- Arthritis
- Impaired glucose tolerance (50%) and diabetes mellitus (10%)
- Visual field defects
- Cranial nerve palsies
- Tumours (uterine leiomyomata and colonic polyps are common; 10% develop malignant tumours)

What is the mortality of acromegaly?

The mortality is two to three times the expected rate, mostly from cardiovascular disease and cancer. This is proportional to the degree of GH excess.

How would you investigate this patient?

Document GH excess

- To determine GH excess, random GH measurements are usually not helpful since GH levels fluctuate considerably. In acromegaly, GH secretion does not respond to normal stimuli. In patients without acromegaly, an oral glucose tolerance test suppresses GH to less than 1.0 ng/mL within two 2 hours of a 75g oral glucose load. Over 85% of acromegalics have a value greater than 2.0ng/mL. A paradoxical rise in GH concentration is seen in 15–20% of patients.
- Serum insulin-like growth factor-I (IGF-1) does not vary diurnally, and is elevated in virtually all subjects with acromegaly. It also provides a measure of disease activity during follow-up.

Determine source of excess GH

- MRI (magnetic resonance imaging)of the pituitary detects tumours greater than 2mm. Three-quarters are macroadenomas >10mm). However, MRI does not determine if the pituitary tumour is functional, and 10–20% of normal subjects will have an incidental pituitary tumour.
- Ectopic GH secretion accounts for only 0.5% of cases.

What is the management of acormegaly?

Surgical

- Transsphenoidal hypophysectomy is curative in 90% of microadenomas, and in 50–60% of macroadenomas, with preserved pituitary function. Complications occur in 8%.

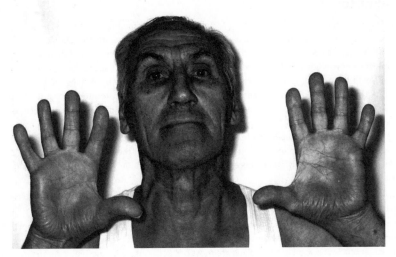

Figure 96.1 Coarsening of facial features and growth of hands in acromegaly.

Medical

* Pharmacological treatment is used as an adjunct, or where surgery is contraindicated or declined.
    * Somatostatin analogues (octreotide, lanreotide) inhibit GH release. These drugs are administered subcutaneously, and normalize IGF-1 in 75%. Side effects include gallstones from gallbladder stasis.
    * Dopamine agonists (cabergoline, bromocriptine) also inhibit GH secretion, and are administered orally.

Radiotherapy

* Decreases GH secretion, but very slowly. Deficiency of other pituitary hormones is common. Cranial nerve palsies, loss of vision and memory deficits may also occur.

Case 97 ◆ **Goitre**

CASE PRESENTATION

*This patient has **bilateral, multinodular enlargement of the thyroid gland**.[1] The thyroid gland is **not tender**,[2] and there **is no single, dominant nodule**.[3] The thyroid mass **moves on swallowing**,[4] but **does not move on tongue protrusion**.[5] There is no **lymphadenopathy**,[3] **retrosternal extension**,[6] or **bruit**.[7] The patient is clinically **euthyroid**.[8] There are no features of Graves' disease.[9]*

*The diagnosis is **multinodular goitre**.*

Clinical notes

1. Initially inspect the thyroid from the front and the side. Inspect the thyroid gland with the neck slightly flexed, which relaxes the strap muscles, and then slightly extended, which stretches overlying tissues. From the side, the contour from the cricoid cartilage to the suprasternal notch should be smooth. Any prominence beyond this contour is likely to be thyroid enlargement. Palpate the thyroid gland from behind, with the neck slightly flexed to relax the strap muscles. Begin by locating the thyroid isthmus (frequently impalpable unless enlarged). The thyroid isthmus is usually located at or just below the level of the cricoid cartilage of the trachea. The lobes of the thyroid extend laterally and, if enlarged, may extend posterior to the sternocleidomastoid muscles. Up to 80% of thyroid glands may have a pyramidal lobe extending superiorly from the isthmus. Place the tips of the fingers of each hand medial to the sternocleidomastoid muscle, and palpate for each lobe of the thyroid gland. Take care not to begin palpating too laterally, and compress the thyroid between the sternocleidomastoid and the trachea.

2. A painful thyroid gland is characteristic of thyroiditis. Causes of this pattern of thyroid inflammation are subacute granulomatous, infectious, traumatic and radiation thyroiditis.

3. If nodules are present, one must assess the number, size, consistency, fixation, and tenderness, and examine for regional lymphadenopathy. A fixed hard mass, obstructive symptoms, cervical lymphadenopathy, or vocal cord paralysis are most predictive of malignancy. Pemberton's manoeuvre demonstrates obstructive symptoms by holding the patient's arms above the head for 60 seconds, and forcing the thyroid into the thoracic inlet. The test is positive if the patient's neck veins become distended, or if the patient develops facial plethora, cyanosis, dyspnoea, or dysphagia. We do not recommend performing this manoeuvre in the MRCP (PACES) clinical examination setting. The differential diagnosis for a solitary nodule is listed below.

4. Usually, the patient will have a glass of water to hand. Ask the patient to hold the glass, and ask to 'take a sip and hold' and then 'swallow', during both inspection and palpation.

5. Cysts in the thyroglossal duct typically occur in the midline, and those in the upper tract may move on tongue protrusion. The thyroglossal duct is an embryological remnant of the migration of the thyroid gland from the pharynx to the anterior neck. The duct normally disappears, but persistence of the duct can give rise to cystic masses. Most lesions present during childhood, but some can present in adulthood.

6. One should percuss over the sternum for retrosternal extension of the goitre if the inferior border cannot be palpated. However, if the inferior border is clearly palpable, then this manoeuvre is not essential.

7. Auscultation should be performed over both lobes of the thyroid for a bruit. The presence of a bruit suggests Graves' disease. This occurs due to hypertrophy of the thyroid gland and accelerated blood flow through tortuous thyroid arteries. However, if heard, a thyroid bruit must be distinguished from a carotid bruit or an aortic murmur. A further precordial sign of thyrotoxicosis is the *Means-Lerman scratch*, which is a scratching sound heard over the precordium thought to result from rubbing of the hyperdynamic pericardium against pleura, mimicking pericarditis.

8. It is important to establish thyroid status in all patients with goitre:
   (a) Hyperthyroidism: tachycardia, sweaty palms, tremor, and lid lag
   (b) Hypothyroidism: bradycardia, slow-relaxing reflexes

9. In patients with a diffusely enlarged goitre, it is important to consider Graves' disease. In Graves' disease, the goitre can be diffuse or nodular. Look for the associated eye signs, thyroid acropachy and pretibial myxoedema.

10. A goitre can be classified according to its physical characteristics into one of the following:

MULTINODULAR **DIFFUSE**	Simple goitre (iodine deficiency) Iodine deficiency Physiological goitre (puberty and pregnancy) Grave's disease Hashimoto's disease De Quervain's thyroiditis Goitrogens Dyshormonogenesis
SOLITARY NODULE	Thyroid adenoma Toxic adenoma (Plummer's disease) Thyroid cysts Thyroid cancer A single palpable nodule in a multinodular goitre

Questions commonly asked by examiners

What is the differential diagnosis of a neck mass?

There are many causes for a mass in the neck. An accurate medical history greatly narrows this list of differentials. The causes of a neck mass in adults can be broadly categorized as follows:

- **Congenital**
  - Thyroglossal cyst—remnant of the embryological thyroglossal duct, typically present in the midline and moves on tongue protrusion.
  - Branchial anomalies—including cysts, sinuses, and fistulae, may present anywhere along the sternocleidomastoid muscle.
- **Lymphadenopathy**
  - Bacterial
  - Viral—including HIV
  - Granulomatous—including sarcoidosis and tuberculosis
  - Malignant—primary or metastatic
- **Vascular**
  - Carotid artery aneurysm / carotid body tumour
  - Jugular vein thrombosis / haemangioma
- **Salivary**
  - Sialadenitis
  - Salivary gland tumour
- **Neurogenic**
  - From neural crest derivatives, including schwannoma, neurofibroma, and malignant peripheral nerve sheath tumours. Increased incidence in neurofibromatosis syndromes.

What is the differential diagnosis of a retrosternal mass?

- Retrosternal goitre
- Thymoma
- Lymphoma
- Germ cell tumours (e.g. teratoma, seminoma)
- Mediastinal cysts (e.g. pericardial, bronchogenic)
- Parathyroid mass

Tell me about the causes of thyroiditis?

Painful thyroid swelling

- *Subacute granulomatous thyroiditis*—is characterized by an initial hyperthyroid phase, with neck pain, a tender diffuse goitre, and elevated thyroid hormones. The hyperthyroidism typically subsides after two to six weeks, and is followed by a period of hypothyroidism due to depletion of thyroid stores. Thyroid hormone levels return to normal as thyroid gland function is restored. Other names for this condition include de Quervain's thyroiditis, or subacute thyroiditis. The aetiology is thought to be viral, or a post-viral inflammatory process.

- *Infectious thyroiditis*—may occur with acute or chronic infections. Acute infections, due to gram-positive or gram-negative infections, may cause abscess formation. The mechanism of infection may be haematogenous spread, or direct spread from the piriform fossa. The most common organisms in immunocompetent individuals are streptococcal or staphylococcal species. Chronic infections, such as mycobacterial and fungal, may occur due to haematogenous spread in the immunocompromised. Patients with infectious thyroiditis are euthyroid, but present with neck pain and fever. The management involves needle aspiration of the thyroid mass for microbiological analysis, followed by drainage and antibiotic therapy.

- *Radiation thyroiditis*—may occasionally occur following treatment for Graves' disease with radioiodine.

Painless thyroid swelling

- *Painless thyroiditis*—is a variant of autoimmune (Hashimoto's) thyroiditis (termed Hashitoxicosis), which is characterized by transient hyperthyroidism, followed by hypothyroidism, then recovery.

- *Postpartum thyroiditis*—is similar to painless thyroiditis, but by definition occurs in women within one year of parturition. Generally, this is mild subclinical hyperthyroidism at 3 months postpartum followed by a hypothyroid phase at 6–9 months. Approximately 80% recover and 20% need long-term thyroxine. If thyroxine replacement is started at 6 months, it should be stopped at 12 months to see if condition has resolved. Biochemically, this occurs after 8–10% of pregnancies, but the proportion of women with symptomatic thyroid disease is lower. The major differential diagnosis in postpartum women is a postpartum exacerbation of Graves' disease, which may be a *de novo* diagnosis. However, these patients will have more severe disease, anti-TSH (thyroid-stimulating hormone) receptor antibodies, and elevated thyroid radioiodine uptake, unlike postpartum thyroiditis.

What is the diagnostic and therapeutic approach to a thyroid nodule?

The approach to the investigation of a thyroid nodule involves thyroid function testing, thyroid scintigraphy, thyroid ultrasound, and fine-needle aspiration (FNA).

The initial step is to establish if the nodule is functioning or non-functioning, since virtually all malignant nodules are non-functioning. Therefore, the initial test is serum TSH testing:

- If the serum TSH is low, suggesting overt or sub-clinical hyperthyroidism, then thyroid scintigraphy is indicated to delineate the functioning, or 'warm' nodule.

- If the TSH is normal or elevated, then FNA, with or without ultrasound, is indicated for cytological analysis of the nodule. With an experienced cytopathologist, the diagnostic accuracy of FNA is >95%. Of the non-functioning, 'cold' nodules, 5% will be malignant, 70% will be benign, and 25% will be indeterminate or non-diagnostic.

A proportion of the non-diagnostic FNAs will be due to the finding of follicular lesions, since follicular cancers cannot be distinguished cytologically from follicular adenomas, and vascular or capsular invasion is required for a follicular lesion to be described as malignant. Therefore, the indications for surgery following FNA cytology are:

- Malignant nodules
- Follicular neoplasms diagnosed using cytology
- Lesions with an atypical pattern on cytology
- When the clinical index of suspicion for malignancy is high despite benign cytology

What are the different types of thyroid cancer?

Thyroid cancer is a rare malignancy, accounting for less than 1% of all neoplasms, although the incidence appears to be rising. The major risk factor is head and neck irradiation, particularly early in life. Indeed, the rising incidence may be partially due to the use of radiation therapy to the head and neck for the treatment of benign childhood conditions between 1910 and 1960.

The histological subtypes are:

- **Papillary carcinoma**—this is the most common of the thyroid cancers, and has the most favourable prognosis. The spectrum of disease ranges from small microcarcinomas (<1cm diameter), to aggressive disease with regional lymph node metastases. Papillary thyroid cancer may also be a feature of rare inherited syndromes such as familial adenomatous poylposis and Gardner's syndrome.
- **Follicular carcinoma**—this is the second most common type of thyroid cancer. Diagnosis requires differentiation of adenoma from carcinoma, by demonstration of vascular or capsular invasion.

Both papillary and follicular cancers are considered differentiated thyroid cancers, and hence are treated similarly. Management involves surgery, with radioiodine as the major adjuvant therapy (combined with doses of thyroxine, which suppress TSH levels below the assay detection limit).

- **Anaplastic carcinoma**—this is a highly aggressive, undifferentiated thyroid cancer. The disease typically affects elderly patients, and is almost universally fatal. A proportion arises in patients with a history of differentiated thyroid cancer.
- **Medullary thyroid carcinoma**—this is a neuroendocrine tumour of the parafollicular, or C cells, of the thyroid. These tumours are characterized by the production of calcitonin, which is used as a serum tumour marker. Most medullary carcinomas are sporadic, but familial cases can occur as part of the multiple endocrine neoplasia type 2 syndrome (MEN2).
    - MEN2a is an autosomal dominant syndrome of medullary thyroid cancer, phaeochromocytoma, and primary hyperparathyroidism. Medullary carcinomas occur in almost all patients, whereas the penetrance of other features is variable.
    - MEN2b is also autosomal dominant, and is characterized by medullary thyroid cancer, phaechromocytoma, mucosal neuromas typically involving the lips and tongue, and a Marfanoid body habitus. These patients do not develop hyperparathyroidism, and also do not suffer with complications associated with Marfan's syndrome.

Genetic testing for MEN2 is possible, by detecting mutations in the *RET* gene (chromosome 10). Genetic testing should be offered to family members of affected individuals, since early diagnosis provides long-term benefit through prophylactic thyroidectomy and preventing medullary thyroid carcinoma.

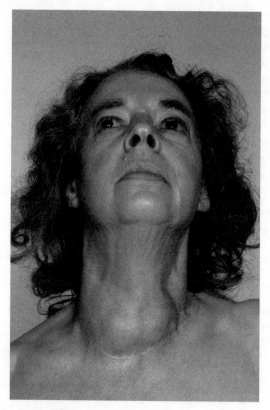

Figure 97.1 A large multinodular goitre.

What are the complications of large goitres?

- Dyspnoea and upper airway obstruction
- Dysphagia
- Recurrent laryngeal nerve paralysis and hoarseness
- Horner's syndrome
- Jugular vein compression and thrombosis
- Cerebrovascular steal syndromes

Case 98 ◆ Assessment of Thyroid State

Examiner's note

Assessment of thyroid state is very straightforward and candidates often pass this station. When assessing thyroid status, there are many other features that can be looked for, and if incorporated into the examination routine, will convert this into a robust and comprehensive assessment (and extra marks!). Often this will be the focus of the station, but assessing thyroid status is necessary when examining a patient with a goitre or Graves' disease.

CASE PRESENTATION 1

This patient is **thin**[1] and appears **fidgety** (with an air of restlessness).[2] The hands are **sweaty**[3] with **palmar erythema**[3] and a **fine tremor**[4] of the outstretched hands. The pulse is…beats per minute (**tachycardic**) and irregular (suggestive of atrial fibrillation (AF)).[5] There is **lid lag** and **lid retraction**.[6] There is evidence of a **proximal myopathy**.[7] There is no palpable goitre and there is no evidence of previous thyroidectomy.[8] There are no features of Graves' disease.[9]

This patient has **hyperthyroidism**.

I would like to ask for a history of weight loss, diarrhoea, palpitations, and heat intolerance.[10]

CASE PRESENTATION 2

This patient has an **elevated body mass index**.[1] There is **generalized slowness** of movement and speech.[2] There is **dry hair** and **dry skin** with **cool peripheries**.[3] The pulse is… beats per minute (**bradycardic**).[5] There is no evidence of **lid lag** or **lid retraction**.[6] There is **periorbital swelling** and **generalized, non-pitting oedema**.[6] There is evidence of a **proximal myopathy**.[7] There is no palpable goitre and there is no evidence of previous thyroidectomy.[8] There are no features of Graves' disease.[9]

This patient has **hypothyroidism**.

I would like to enquire about a history of weight gain, constipation, tiredness, and cold intolerance.[10]

I would like to examine for slow-relaxing deep tendon reflexes[11] and for associated autoimmune disease.[12]

Clinical notes

1. Often in thyrotoxicosis the patients are thin, but it is important to remember that obese or overweight individuals can present with thyrotoxicosis. Likewise, patients with hypothyroidism are usually obese or overweight. The term 'elevated body mass index' is preferable to 'overweight' or 'obese'. Similar to the phrase 'coarse features', these terms may be technically correct, but will not endear you to the patient!

2. Thyrotoxicosis is associated with anxiety, nervousness, hyperactivity, and a feeling of restlessness. Very rarely, choreiform movements can occur in thyrotoxicosis. Conversely, hypothyroidism is associated with slowness of movement and speech. The voice in hypothyroidism often has a hoarse and croaking character. The slowness in movement, speech, heart rate, and the gain in weight, are due to a generalized slowing of metabolic processes. The most extreme presentation of this is *myxoedema coma*, characterized by an altered level of consciousness, bradycardia, hypothermia, and hypercapnia. This most commonly occurs in untreated individuals who are exposed to an external stress such as surgery, sedatives, or infection.

2. Begin by shaking the patient's hand, and note the degree of warmth and sweat. In hyperthyroidism, palmar erythema reflects a hyperdynamic circulation. Briefly examine the nails for onycholysis (Plummer's nails). These are typically found bilaterally on the fourth finger in hyperthyroidism. In hypothyroidism, the skin is often dry and cold with cool peripheries.

3. Look for tremor, accentuated by placing a sheet of paper over outstretched hands. Now look for thyroid acropachy (with the hands outstretched, the nails and nail beds can be easily examined from the side to look for the appearances of digital clubbing).

5. Examine the pulse carefully. A tachycardia is often associated with hyperthyroidism, whilst a bradycardia is associated with hypothyroidism. AF is present in 10–20% of patients with hyperthyroidism. Most patients convert spontaneously to sinus rhythm when the hyperthyroidism is treated. However, anticoagulation is recommended whilst in AF.

6. After having felt the pulse, now examine the face. Look for the following:

    (a) **Lid retraction** (hyperthyroidism)—this is present if the sclera is visible above the iris with the eyes in the neutral (forward looking) position.

    (b) **Lid lag** (hyperthyroidism)—this is present if sclera can be seen above the iris as the patient looks downward. This may give the *appearance* of proptosis from the front, but proptosis is characterized by protrusion of the eyeball from the orbit as and is best assessed by inspecting from above the patient's head.

    (c) **Subcutaneous oedema** (hypothyroidism)—non-pitting oedema, or *myxoedema*, is a consequence of infiltration of the skin with glycosaminoglycans. This should not be confused *pretibial myxoedema*, which is an infiltrative dermopathy characteristic of Graves' disease. Periorbital swelling is a typical manifestation of myxoedema, but may also occur in Graves' ophthalmopathy. The differential diagnosis of periorbital oedema includes infective disorders such as orbital and periorbital cellulitis, allergic disorders such as conjunctivitis, local conditions such as blepharitis, and systemic conditions such as dermatomyositits, nephrotic syndrome (hypoalbuminaemia), and cardiac failure.

    (d) **Features of Graves' disease** (can be seen in hyperthyroidism, hypothyroidism and euthyroid state)—these include exophthalmos, chemosis, and ophthalmoplegia.

7. Proximal myopathy can be assessed in the abducted upper limbs, or by asking the patient to stand from sitting without using their arms. Proximal myopathy is present in most thyrotoxic patients, and may be the presenting feature. Thyrotoxic myopathy is believed to be secondary to a disturbance in the function of the muscle fibres from increased mitochondrial respiration, accelerated protein degradation and lipid oxidation, and enhanced beta-adrenergic sensitivity due to excessive amounts of thyroid hormone. Muscle weakness and proximal myopathy can also occur in hypothyroidism.

8. Look carefully for the absence or presence of a thyroidectomy scar. It is important to note the absence or presence of goitre. A small goitre or a small solitary nodule may not be easily seen, but easily felt. In certain cases, asking the patient to swallow whilst palpating may be the only way to reveal a small goitre.

9. Look for the associated features of Graves' disease—eye signs, thyroid acropachy, and pretibial myxoedema. It is important to comment on the absence or presence of features of Graves' disease.

10. After having assessed the thyroid status, tell the examiner you would like to enquire about associated symptoms of thyroid dysfunction.

11. Since there is poor correlation between the presence of this sign and thyroid status, do not perform this test routinely but ask the examiner for permission to examine for slow-relaxing reflexes. To perform this test, examine the ankle reflex with the patient kneeling on the chair, facing away from you. Other neurological manifestations of hypothyroidism include carpal tunnel syndrome and cerebellar ataxia. If neurological manifestations are present then vitamin B_{12} deficiency must be excluded, since autoimmune hypothyroidism is associated with pernicious anaemia.

12. The most common cause of hypothyroidism in developed countries is chronic autoimmune (Hashimoto's) thyroiditis. Similarly, the most common cause of hyperthyroidism is Graves' disease (an autoimmune condition). Thus in patients with hypothyroidism and hyperthyroidism, it is important to look for other autoimmune conditions.

    - **Type 1 diabetes**: finger tip skin pricks (regular glucose testing), fundoscopy to look for retinopathy
    - **Addison's disease**: pigmentation, postural hypotension
    - **Pernicious anaemia**: pallor, splenomegaly, polyneuropathy
    - **Hypoparathyroidism**: Chvostek's and Trousseau's sign, cataracts
    - **Alopecia areata**: areas of hair loss in scalp with white, short, tapering exclamation mark hairs
    - **Vitiligo**: areas of skin depigmentation
    - **Rheumatoid arthritis**: symmetrical arthropathy of small joints of the hands
    - **Systemic lupus erythematosus (SLE)**: butterfly rash, arthropathy
    - **Sjogren's syndrome**: dry mouth and eyes

Questions commonly asked by examiners

What are the causes of hyperthyrodism?

Increased hormone synthesis:

*   Graves' disease*
*   Hashimoto's disease (thyrotoxicosis prior to hypothyroidism)—termed 'Hashitoxicosis'
*   Toxic adenoma
*   Toxic multinodular goitre
*   Iodine-induced hyperthyroidism (contrast agents, amiodarone)
*   Trophoblastic disease and germ-cell tumours (human chorionic gonadotrophin (hCG) stimulates the TSH receptor)
*   TSH secreting pituitary tumour (rare)

Gland inflammation (thyroiditis) and release of preformed hormone:

*   de Quervain's thyroiditis (associated with coxsackie virus)
*   Infective thyroiditis (bacterial, tuberculous, fungal)
*   Radiation thyroiditis
*   Postpartum thyroiditis
*   Drug-induced thyroiditis (interferon-alpha, amiodarone, lithium)

What do you understand by the term 'apathetic hyperthyroidism'?

This is seen in elderly individuals, where there is a lack of signs indicating hyperthyroidism. The only presenting features may be unexplained weight loss or cardiac symptoms such as development of AF and congestive cardiac failure.

What are the causes of hypothyroidism?

Primary thyroid failure:

*   Autoimmune (Hashimoto's) thyroiditis**
*   Idiopathic atrophy**
*   Previous radioiodine treatment or thyroidectomy**
*   Iodine deficiency
*   Antithyroid drugs
*   Other drugs (see below)
*   Subacute, painless, and postpartum thyroiditis (all cause *transient* hypothyroidism)
*   Infiltrative conditions (eg. systemic sclerosis, sarcoidosis, Reidel's thyroiditis)

Secondary thyroid failure

*   Hypothalamic or pituitary disease

What is the effect of iodine on the thyroid gland?

Iodine deficiency, less than 100mcg/day, is the most common cause of hypothyroidism worldwide.

Iodine excess can cause hypothyroidism, by preventing organification of iodide and inhibiting thyroid hormone synthesis (the Wolff-Chaikoff effect). Patients with undiagnosed autoimmune thyroid disease are particularly at risk. This is the mechanism whereby iodine-containing drugs, such as amiodarone, cause hypothyroidism.

---

* Accounts for 60–80% of hyperthyroidism

** These three account for 90% of hypothyroidism in developed countries

Iodine excess can also induce hyperthyroidism in populations with iodide deficiency (the Jod-Basdeow phenomenon), or in patients with nodular goitres and autonomously functioning tissue. Similarly, patients with undiagnosed thyroid nodules are at risk from iodine-containing drugs or radiographic contrast agents.

Which drugs can cause hypothyroidism?

Iodine-containing supplements, tonics, and drugs such as amiodarone can cause both hypothyroidism and hyperthyroidism.

Lithium carbonate and thionamides (e.g. propylthiouracil) inhibit thyroid hormone synthesis. Interferon-alfa may induce autoimmune thyroid disease. Sunitinib is a tyrosine-kinase inhibitor, used for renal cell carcinoma and gastrointestinal stromal tumours, which is associated with hypothyroidism in one-third of cases.

Cytochrome P450 enzyme-inducing drugs, such as phenytoin, rifampicin, and carbamezapine, will increase thyroxine requirements in patients with treated hypothyroidism.

Which autoantibodies are required to diagnose hypothyroidism?

Antithyroid antibodies (anti-thyroglobulin and anti-thyroid peroxidase) are unhelpful for the diagnosis of hypothyroidism, but are commonly measured to define the cause of hypothyroidism, i.e. Hashimoto's disease. They may predict the progression of subclinical hypothyroidism (see below).

What is meant by the term 'subclinical hypothyroidism'?

This state is characterized by an elevated TSH, and normal T4, and is most common in patients who have been treated for hyperthyroidism, or in the elderly. Previous treatment with radioiodine, or the presence of antithyroid antibodies, predict progression to overt hypothyroidism. If the TSH is greater than 10mU/L then thyroxine treatment should be commenced to prevent overt hypothyroidism. Patients with a TSH 5–10mU/L should have repeat testing every six months.

What is the relevance of hypothyroidism in pregnancy?

Maternal iodine deficiency leading to goitre and hypothyroidism is associated with neurological damage and mental retardation in the offspring, termed 'neurological cretinism'. Iodine deficiency in later pregnancy causes neonatal hypothyroidism, which affects growth and development. This is termed 'myxoedematous cretinism', and unlike neurological cretinism is treatable with iodine and thyroxine replacement.

Hypothyroidism is associated with an increased risk of obstetric complications including preeclampsia, placental abruption, preterm delivery, and caesarean section. Patients also have greater requirements for thyroid replacement during pregnancy.

Is there any benefit in replacing triiodothyronine (T3) and thyroxine(T4)?

The thyroid gland is the only source of T4, but the majority of T3 is generated by peripheral conversion of T4 in extraglandular tissues. Since some patients with adequate thyroxine replacement have persistent symptoms, it has been suggested that combination therapy with T3 and T4 may be of benefit. However, several randomized studies have concluded that there is no benefit of combined therapy.

What is Riedel's thyroiditis?

Riedel's thyroiditis is a rare chronic inflammatory condition of the thyroid gland, with replacement of the thyroid parenchyma by dense fibrous tissue. Fibrosis may extend beyond the thyroid capsule, affecting local structures such as the parathyroid glands and recurrent laryngeal nerve.

Case 99 ♦ **Graves' Disease**

CASE PRESENTATION

*This patient has bilateral **exophthalmos** with **opthlamoplegia** (and resultant diplopia). There is no evidence of chemosis, exposure keratitis, or corneal ulceration. The visual acuity is normal, and there is no evidence of relative afferent pupillary defect.[1] There is evidence of **pretibial myxoedema**[2] and there is digital clubbing consistent with **thyroid acropachy**.[3] There is a **thyroidectomy scar** and there is no palpable goitre.[4] The patient is **euthyroid**.[5]*

*The diagnosis is **Graves' disease**. This patient has previously had a thyroidectomy and has a euthyroid status (on thyroxine replacement therapy). I would like to look for evidence of autoimmune disease.[6]*

Clinical notes

1. Graves' ophthalmopathy is a hallmark of Graves' disease. Up to 30% of patients have clinical evidence of Graves' ophthalmopathy. Involvement is always bilateral, and apparent unilateral cases reflect an asymmetrical involvement of the eyes. The features of Graves ophthalmopathy include:

    (a) **Oedema**: Deposition of glycoasaminoglycans and influx of water into the extra-ocular muscles increases orbital pressure and consequent obstruction of the superior ophthalmic vein. This leads to congestion and subsequent oedema of the eyelids (**periorbital oedema**) and conjuctival oedema (**chemosis**).

    (b) **Exophthalmos**: Proptosis occurs because the orbital contents are confined within the bony orbit, and decompression can only occur anteriorly. Exophthalmos is defined as protrusion of the eyeball such that the sclera is visible above the lower eyelid with eyes in the neutral position. Look for proptosis by assessing from the side and whilst standing behind the patient and looking from above (this can be done whilst palpating for a goitre).

    (c) **Ophthalmoplegia**: This is due to infiltration, oedema, and fibrosis of the extra-ocular muscles. It is important to examine the eye movements, and enquire about diplopia. The most common finding is diplopia on upward gaze due to early involvement of the inferior rectus muscle. If there is diplopia in multiple directions of gaze, then it is best not to confuse matters in the examination by trying to ascertain the individual muscle groups that are affected. In such cases it is best to describe and present as 'complex ophthalmoplegia'.

    (d) **Exposure keratitis and corneal ulceration**: This is secondary to severe exophthalmos and corneal exposure. Look for evidence of lateral tarsorrhaphy, which is used to protect the cornea. Determine the extent to which the eyelids will close, by asking the patient to close their eyes.

    (e) **Optic nerve compression**: This may occur even with mild proptosis, and it is important to assess visual acuity, colour vision, and look for relative afferent pupillary defects (RAPD).

    (f) **Glaucoma**: This can occur due decreased episcleral venous flow.

    At the end of the examination routine, it would be reasonable to tell the examiner you would like to perform fundoscopy to look for optic atrophy and glaucoma.

2. Pretibial myxoedema is a feature of Graves' disease (occurring in 5% of patients). It is a late manifestation of Grave's disease and usually occurs 1–2 years after the diagnosis and treatment of hyperthyroidism. Almost all patients with dermopathy have ophthalmopathy, with dermopathy usually following the onset of ophthalmopathy by 6–12 months. It is characterized by bilateral (although asymmetrical), firm, non-pitting plaques or nodules that may have a pink, purple, or brown appearance. They usually appear on the anterolateral aspects of the lower legs, but may appear on the thighs,

shoulders, hands, or the forehead. They often occur in areas of recent or prior trauma or skin graft donor sites. The lesions are often tender and they may be pruritic. In its extreme form, pretibial myxoedema can resemble lymphoedema. (See Case 143 Pretibial Myxoedema).

3. Thyroid acropachy occurs in 1% of patients with Graves' disease, and if present, it usually occurs after the dermopathy. The appearance is that of digital clubbing, but it is caused by subperiosteal new bone formation. Remember, severe thyroid acropachy can be disabling and can lead to total loss of hand function.

4. It is important to examine the neck for goitre. Note the presence of thyroidectomy scar. In Graves' disease the thyroid gland is usually diffusely enlarged, but may have a nodular enlargement. If a goitre is present, then auscultate for a bruit, which is associated with Graves' disease.

5. It is important to carefully examine the thyroid status (see Case 98 Assessment of Thyroid State). Patients with Graves' disease can be:

   (a) **Euthyroid**: naturally; following radioiodine therapy; following thyroidectomy with adequate thyroxine replacement

   (b) **Hypothyroid**: naturally*; following radioiodine therapy; following thyroidectomy with inadequate thyroxine replacement

   (c) **Hyperthyroid**: naturally; following thyroidectomy and radioiodine therapy with excess thyroxine replacement

6. After having presented the diagnosis of Graves' disease, it is important to mention evidence of previous therapy and current thyroid status. Given that Graves' disease is an autoimmune disorder, tell the examiner you would like to look for evidence of other autoimmune diseases.

Questions commonly asked by examiners

What is the pathophysiology of Graves' disease?

This is an autoimmune disease characterized by hyperthyroidism due to circulating autoantibodies. Thyroid-stimulating antibodies bind to and activate the TSH receptors. This causes the thyroid gland to enlarge and the thyroid follicles to increase synthesis of thyroid hormone. The B- and T-lymphocyte–mediated autoimmunity is directed at four thyroid antigens: thyroglobulin, thyroperoxidase, sodium-iodide symporter, and the TSH receptor. The TSH receptor is the primary autoantigen of Graves' disease and is responsible for hyperthyroidism.

What are the features of Graves' disease, independent of hyperthyroidism?

- Goitre
- Graves' ophthalmopathy
- Thyroid acropachy
- Pretibial myxoedema

What are the causes of proptosis?

- Graves' disease
- Cavernous sinus thrombosis
- Carotico-cavernous fistula
- Orbital cellulitis
- Retro-orbital tumour (lymphoma, leukaemia, meningioma, and metastases)
- Retro-orbital granuloma (Wegner's granulomatosis, histiocytosis X, sarcoidosis)
- Trauma

---

* Occasionally a patient with Graves' disease may progress spontaneously to hypothyroidism.

What eponymous signs are associated with Graves' ophthalmopathy?

- **Stellwag sign**: incomplete and infrequent blinking
- **Kocher's sign**: fixed staring look
- **Dalrympole sign**: lid retraction
- **Goffroy sign**: absent creases in the forehead on upward gaze
- **Mobius sign**: poor convergence
- **Von Graeffe sign**: lid lag
- **Ballet sign**: restriction of ≥1 extra-ocular muscles
- **Grove sign**: resistance to pulling down the retracted eyelid

What are the possible mechanisms of lid retraction in Graves' ophthalmopathy?

- Increased sympathetic tone of the Müller muscle (thyrotoxicosis)
- Proptosis
- Fibrosis of the levator muscle
- Cogan lid twitch sign (myasthenia gravis)*

How would you manage a patient with Grave's disease?

Symptomatic management

- Beta blockers treat the symptoms that are caused by increased beta-adrenergic tone. These include palpitations, tachycardia, tremor, anxiety, and heat intolerance. Often the use of a non-selective beta-blocker, i.e. propanolol, is appropriate in this setting.

Thionamides

- Carbimazole and propylthiouracil (PTU) are the primary drugs used to treat Graves' hyperthyroidism. Carbimazole has slightly greater efficacy, although PTU is preferred during pregnancy.
- Both drugs may cause the rare but serious side-effect of agranulocytosis in 0.5%. anti-neutrophil cytoplasmic antibody (ANCA)-positive vasculitis has also been reported with PTU.
- Monitoring of thyroid function occurs at 4–6 weekly intervals. A suppressed TSH after 18 months of treatment predicts long-term treatment failure.

Radioiodine ablation

- Radioiodine is administered as an oral solution of sodium $Na^{131}I$, which is rapidly concentrated in thyroid tissue. This causes tissue destruction and gland ablation over 6–18 weeks.
- Graves' ophthalmopathy may *worsen* with radioiodine therapy. There is some evidence that steroid therapy may help reduce this complication. Cigarette smoking also worsens eye disease, and should be counselled against.

Surgery

- Thyroidectomy is rarely indicated for Graves' disease. The most common indications are a large goitre or co-existing thyroid nodule.
- A randomized trial comparing thionamides, radioiodine, and surgery demonstrated that all were equally effective as initial treatment, although the relapse rate was highest amongst patients receiving thionamides (approximately 40%), as compared with radioiodine (20%), and surgery (5%).

What would you advise a patient who had recently received radioiodine?

- Patients must avoid contact with children or pregnant women for two weeks.

---

* Due to association of Graves' disease with other autoimmune diseases.

- Pregnancy is an absolute contraindication, and must be delayed for four months following therapy.
- The risk of developing hypothyroidism is 2–3% per year.

What protective measures should be taken in a patient with exophthalmos?

- Eyedrops and lubrication
- Sleep upright (with the eyes taped closed)—reduces lid oedema
- Lateral tarsorrhaphy to protect the cornea
- Smoking cessation—smoking increase the risk of oedema and congestion
- Prism glasses can help with diplopia

What is Graves' malignant exophthalmos?

This is severe inflammation and congestion that causes severe pain and the patient is at risk of blindness due to optic nerve compression.

What treatment options are available for Graves' malignant exophthalmos?

- Systemic steroids
- Orbital decompression
- Radiotherapy

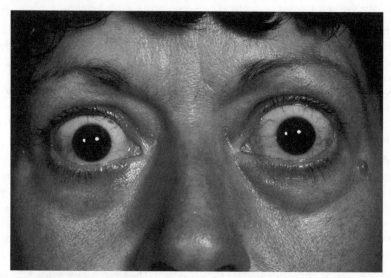

Figure 99.1 Thyroid eye disease. Note the exophthalmos (sclera visible above the lower eyelid), lid retraction (sclera visible below the upper eyelid), and a fixed staring appearance (Kocher's sign).

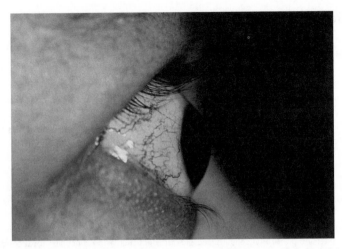

Figure 99.2 In thyroid eye disease, inflammation of the orbital tissue results in protrusion of the eyeball such that the sclera is visible above the lower eyelid with the eyes in the neutral position. Reproduced from Warrell et al. Oxford Textbook of Medicine, Volume 3, 4th edn. 2003, with permission from Oxford University Press.

Case 100 ◆ **Hypothyroidism**

CASE PRESENTATION 1

*This patient has an **elevated body mass index**,[1] **slow movement**, and **slow speech**.[2] There is **dry hair** and **dry skin**, with **cool peripheries**.[3] There is **periorbital swelling** and **generalized, non-pitting oedema**.[4] The pulse rate is **slow**[5] (mention heart rate). There is no evidence of **Graves' disease**.[6]*

*The diagnosis is **hypothyroidism**.*

I would like to examine for slow-relaxing deep tendon reflexes,[7] and for associated autoimmune disease.[8]

CASE PRESENTATION 2

*This patient has **exophthalmos** and **opthalmoplegia**. There is a **thyroidectomy scar**.[6] The patient is hypothyroid, as evidenced by the **bradycardia**,[5] **elevated body mass index**,[1] **slow movement** and **slow speech**.[2]*

*The diagnosis is treated **Graves' disease**, and resultant **hypothyroidism**.*

Clinical notes

1. This term is preferable to 'overweight' or 'obese'. Similar to the phrase 'coarse features', these terms may be technically correct, but will not endear you to the patient!

2. The slowness in movement, speech, heart rate, and the gain in weight, are due to a generalized slowing of metabolic processes. The most extreme presentation of this is *myxoedema coma*, characterized by an altered level of consciousness, bradycardia, hypothermia, and hypercapnia. This most commonly occurs in untreated individuals who are exposed to an external stress such as surgery, sedatives, or infection.

3. The skin is cool and pale in hypothyroidism due to decreased blood flow. Hair becomes dry, and hair loss may occur. However, in elderly patients these signs may be interpreted as normal features of ageing, and may be overlooked. Nail changes include longitudinal ridging and onycholysis. Associated cutaneous findings include autoimmune conditions such as vitiligo and alopecia areata (see clinical note 8).

4. Non-pitting oedema, or *myxoedema*, is a consequence of infiltration of the skin with glycosaminoglycans. This should not be confused with *pretibial myxoedema*, which is an infiltrative dermopathy characteristic of Graves' disease. Periorbital swelling is a typical manifestation of myxoedema, but may also occur in Graves' ophthalmopathy. The differential diagnosis of periorbital oedema includes infective disorders such as orbital and periorbital cellulitis, allergic disorders such as conjunctivitis, local conditions such as blepharitis, and systemic conditions such as dermatomyositis, nephrotic syndrome, and cardiac failure.

5. Bradycardia and pericardial effusions are the cardiac manifestation of hypothyroidism.

6. In the PACES examination, the finding of signs of Graves' disease is likely to be associated with a hypothyroid or euthyroid state, rather then a symptomatic hyperthyroid state. Signs of Graves disease include

   (a) Goitre (or previous thyroidectomy)

   (b) Signs of thyroid eye disease

   (c) Thyroid acropachy

   (d) Pretibial myxoedema

   Look carefully for a thyroidectomy scar, since patients who have been treated with thyroidectomy or radioiodine will inevitably require thyroid replacement. Patients on thionamide drugs may also require thyroxine, since a 'block-replace' regimen is occasionally used, although this regimen has not been proven to be more effective than anithyroid drugs alone.

7. Since there is poor correlation between the presence of this sign and thyroid status, do not perform this test routinely but ask the examiner for permission to examine for slow-relaxing reflexes. To perform this test, examine the ankle reflex with the patient kneeling on the chair, facing away from you. Other neurological manifestations of hypothyroidism include carpal tunnel syndrome and cerebellar ataxia. If neurological manifestations are present then vitamin B12 deficiency must be excluded, since autoimmune hypothyroidism is associated with pernicious anaemia (see below).

8. The most common cause of hypothyroidism in developed countries is chronic autoimmune (Hashimoto's) thyroiditis. It is important to look for evidence of other autoimmune disease.

Questions commonly asked by examiners

What are the causes of hypothyroidism?

Primary thyroid failure

- Autoimmune (Hashimoto's) thyroiditis*
- Idiopathic atrophy*
- Previous radioiodine treatment or thyroidectomy*
- Iodine deficiency
- Antithyroid drugs

---

* Accounts for 90% of hypothyroidism in developed countries.

- Other drugs (see below)
- Subacute, painless, and postpartum thyroiditis (all cause *transient* hypothyroidism–see case—)
- Infiltrative conditions (e.g. systemic sclerosis, sarcoidosis, Reidel's thyroiditis)

Secondary thyroid failure
- Hypothalamic or pituitary disease

What is the effect of iodine on the thyroid gland?

Iodine deficiency, less than 100mcg/day, is the most common cause of hypothyroidism worldwide.

Iodine excess can cause hypothyroidism, by preventing organification of iodide and inhibiting thyroid hormone synthesis (the Wolff-Chaikoff effect). Patients with undiagnosed autoimmune thyroid disease are particularly at risk. This is the mechanism whereby iodine-containing drugs, such as amiodarone, cause hypothyroidism.

Iodine excess can also induce hyperthyroidism in populations with iodide deficiency (the Jod-Basdeow phenomenon), or in patients with nodular goitres and autonomously functioning tissue. Similarly, patients with undiagnosed thyroid nodules are at risk from iodine-containing drugs or radiographic contrast agents.

Which drugs can cause hypothyroidism?

Iodine-containing supplements, tonics, and drugs such as amiodarone can cause both hypothyroidism and hyperthyroidism.

Lithium carbonate and thionamides (e.g. PTU) inhibit thyroid hormone synthesis. Interferon-alfa may induce autoimmune thyroid disease. Sunitinib is a tyrosine-kinase inhibitor, used for renal cell carcinoma and gastrointestinal stromal tumours, which is associated with hypothyroidism in one-third of cases.

Cytochrome P450 enzyme-inducing drugs, such as phenytoin, rifampicin, and carbamezapine, will increase thyroxine requirements in patients with treated hypothyroidism.

Which autoantibodies would you request to define the cause of hypothyroidism?

Antithyroid antibodies (anti-thyroglobulin and anti-thyroid peroxidase) are helpful for the diagnosis of Hashimoto's disease as a cause.

What is meant by the term 'subclinical hypothyroidism'?

This state is characterized by an elevated TSH, and normal T4, and is most common in patients who have been treated for hyperthyroidism, or in the elderly. Previous treatment with radioiodine, or the presence of antithyroid antibodies, predict progression to overt hypothyroidism. If the TSH is greater than 10mU/L then thyroxine treatment should be commenced to prevent overt hypothyroidism. Patients with a TSH 5—10mU/L should have repeat testing every six months.

What is the relevance of hypothyroidism in pregnancy?

Maternal iodine deficiency leading to goitre and hypothyroidism is associated with neurological damage and mental retardation in the offspring, termed 'neurological cretinism'. Iodine deficiency in later pregnancy causes neonatal hypothyroidism, which affects growth and development. This is termed 'myxoedematous cretinism', and unlike neurological cretinism is treatable with iodine and thyroxine replacement.

Hypothyroidism is associated with an increased risk of obstetric complications including preeclampsia, placental abruption, preterm delivery, and caesarean section. Patients also have greater requirements for thyroid replacement during pregnancy.

Is there any benefit in replacing triiodothyronine (T3) and thyroxine (T4)?

The thyroid gland is the only source of T4, but the majority of T3 is generated by peripheral conversion of T4 in extraglandular tissues. Since some patients with adequate thyroxine replacement have persistent symptoms, it has been suggested that combination therapy with T3 and T4 may be of benefit. However, several randomized studies have concluded that there is no benefit of combined therapy.

What is Riedel's thyroiditis?

Riedel's thyroiditis is a rare chronic inflammatory condition of the thyroid gland, with replacement of the thyroid parenchyma by dense fibrous tissue. Fibrosis may extend beyond the thyroid capsule, affecting local structures such as the parathyroid glands and recurrent laryngeal nerve.

Case 101 ◆ Cushing's Syndrome

CASE PRESENTATION

*This patient has **cushingoid facies**,[1,2] with **centripetal obesity, interscapular and supraclavicular fat pads**.[1,3] There is **acne vulgaris** on the face and trunk, and there are purpuric and petechial rashes consistent with **bruising and thin skin**.[4] There are **violaceous striae**[4] on the abdomen, and there is evidence of **proximal myopathy**.[5] There are no **adrenalectomy scars**.[6]*

*The diagnosis is **Cushing's syndrome**.[7]*

Clinical notes

1. Avoid terms such as 'moon face' and 'buffalo hump'—these are not likely to endear you to the patient!
2. Cushingoid facies are due to fat deposition in the cheeks. When examining the patient from the front, one should look to see if the cheeks obscure the ears, since this is part of the classical description of the cushingoid appearance. Fat deposition in the temporal fossae also contributes to a rounded facial appearance.
3. Fat deposition in the dorsocervical and supraclavicular fat pads is common, and usually consistent with the degree of centripetal obesity. Supraclavicular fat pads make the neck appear shortened and thickened.
4. The dermatological manifestations of Cushing's syndrome include:
    *   **Skin atrophy:** thinning of the stratum corneum
    *   **Poor wound healing:** secondary to skin atrophy
    *   **Purpura:** easy bruising due to loss of subcutaneous connective tissue
    *   **Violaceous striae:** consequence of skin stretching due to weight gain and impaired collagen synthesis
    *   **Fungal infections:** skin folds and nails
    *   **Acne:** due to increased androgens
    *   **Hirsutism:** increased hair in androgen-dependent regions of the body (presenting feature in females)

- **Hyperpigmentation**: if very prominent, consider Nelson's syndrome or ectopic adrenocorticotrophic hormone (ACTH) production
- **Acanthosis nigricans**: velvety and hyper-pigmented skin in axillae, neck, and groin
- **Telangiectasia**: this may be seen as a complication of topical steroid use

5. Proximal myopathy is almost universal in Cushing's syndrome, but is not typically present is pseudo-Cushing states, and is therefore a good discriminatory sign. Muscle weakness occurs due to the catabolic effect of excess glucocorticoids on skeletal muscle. Initially ask the patient to maintain their arms in an abducted position, and 'don't let me move them'. If there is no discernible muscle weakness in the upper limbs, ask the patient to rise from a seated position without assistance, looking for proximal muscle weakness in the lower limbs.

6. Bilateral adrenalectomy is a largely historical treatment for Cushing's disease following the advent of transphenoidal pituitary surgery. Whilst bilateral adrenalaectomy is a definitive cure for hypercortisolism, the adverse consequences of adrenal surgery are lifelong mineralocorticoid and glucocorticoid replacement, and the risk of Nelson's syndrome (see below). Since the retroperitoneal approach is the most common, look for scars on the back. If bilateral adrenalectomy scars are present, look for skin pigmentation and ask to examine the visual fields (looking for bitemporal hemianopia).

7. Glucose intolerance occurs due to gluconeogenesis from glucocorticoid excess, and insulin resistance from obesity. Hypertension occurs in all causes of Cushing's syndrome, but is most marked in ectopic ACTH syndromes where the high serum cortisol concentrations result in both mineralocorticoid and glucocorticoid effects. Marked pigmentation is typically seen in patients with ectopic ACTH syndromes. The mineralocorticoid effects also cause hypokalemia which may exacerbate proximal muscle weakness.

Tell the examiner you would like to look for complications, evidence of steroid-responsive conditions and ectopic ACTH secreting tumours:

- Complications:
    - **Diabetes**: finger pricks for glucose testing, diabetic retinopathy, glycosuria
    - **Hypertension**: measure blood pressure, hypertensive retinopathy
    - **Osteoporosis**: vertebral collapse (Kyphosis)
    - **Cataracts**: secondary to exogenous steroids (not usually seen in endogenous steroid excess, except in children)
- Steroid-responsive conditions:
    - **Asthma/COPD**: wheeze, hyper-inflated chest
    - **Interstitial lung disease**: clubbing, bibasal lung crepitations
    - **Rheumatoid arthritis**: symmetrical arthropathy of small joints of the hands
    - **SLE**: butterfly rash, arthropathy
- Ectopic ACTH secreting tumours:
    - **Small cell carcinoma of lung**: clubbing, nicotine staining, respiratory signs
    - **Carcinoid tumour**
    - **Carcinoma of the pancreas**

Questions commonly asked by examiners

What do you understand by the terms 'Cushing's syndrome' and 'Cushing's disease'?

- *Cushing's syndrome* refers to the symptoms and signs caused by states of cortisol excess.
- *Cushing's disease* refers to hypersecretion of ACTH by a pituitary adenoma, which is one of the causes of Cushing's syndrome.

Determining the cause of the excess cortisol requires an understanding of the different types of Cushing's syndrome, which may be *ACTH-dependent* or *ACTH-independent*.

- *ACTH-dependent Cushing's syndrome* is associated with bilateral adrenal hyperplasia:
  - Cushing's disease (ACTH hypersecretion by a pituitary adenoma)
  - Ectopic secretion of ACTH by a non-pituitary tumour (small-cell lung tumors, carcinoid tumours)
- *ACTH-independent Cushing's syndrome:*
  - Exogenous steroid administration (iatrogenic or factitious Cushing's syndrome)
  - Adrenocortical adenomas and carcinomas

The most common cause of Cushing's syndrome is exogenous steroid use. Ectopic ACTH syndrome occurs in 10% of patients with small-cell lung tumours, which is the most common cause of ectopic ACTH secretion. When it is not iatrogenic, i.e. due to exogenous steroid use, Cushing's disease accounts for 80% of cases of Cushing's syndrome, ectopic ACTH production accounts for 10% (of which half are benign and half malignant ACTH sources), and adrenal tumours account for 10% (of which half are benign and half malignant ACTH sources).

How would you assess this patient?

History

- Ensure there is no history of glucocorticoid use, including oral, inhaled, and topical.
  - Exclude pseudo-Cushing's, which is a state of cortisol excess complicating conditions such as chronic infection, severe obesity, depression, and chronic alcoholism. These patients have elevated cortisol levels, and may have some clinical features of Cushing's, but do not develop the cutaneous manifestations or muscle weakness.
  - Enquire about complications of Cushing's syndrome: diabetes (polyuria and polydipsia), osteoporosis (back and bone pain), avascular necross of femoral head (restricted and painful hip movements), proximal myopathy, and hypertension.

Demonstrate cortisol excess

- To determine cortisol excess, random serum cortisol measurement is useless, since cortisol secretion is pulsatile throughout the day, even in Cushing's syndrome.
  - *24 hour urinary free cortisol* is a reliable method of demonstrating cortisol excess. The test is typically repeated three times, since three normal values exclude endogenous Cushing's syndrome. A value greater than three times the upper limit of normal is suggestive of Cushing's syndrome. Mildly elevated values may represent Cushing's syndrome or pseudo-Cushing's, and require further assessment.
  - *Midnight serum cortisol* is an alternative screening tool for Cushing's syndrome, since the nocturnal nadir of serum cortisol is preserved in physiological states of cortisol excess, but the midnight cortisol is elevated in Cushing's syndrome. However, this test does not reliably distinguish Cushing's from pseudo-Cushing states.
- *Dexamethasone suppression tests* are dynamic endocrine tests, which rely on the physiological suppression of pituitary ACTH and serum cortisol by exogenous dexamethasone in physiological states, but not in Cushing's syndrome. The dose of dexamathasone required to suppress ACTH and cortisol will aid in determining the source of ACTH, and differentiating ACTH-dependent and ACTH-independent Cushing's syndrome. Relative contraindications to these tests include diabetes mellitus, psychological disease, and patients on enzyme-inducing agents such as anti-convulsants who may rapidly metabolize dexamethasone and decrease the sensitivity of the test. Furthermore, artificial oestrogens should be stopped prior to the test, since they may induce cortisol-binding protein and artificially increase total cortisol levels.
- *Overnight dexamethasone suppression test* is an alternative screening tool for Cushing's syndrome, although it does not reliably differentiate between Cushing's and pseudo-Cushing

states, or the source of ACTH. The test involves administration of 1mg of dexamthasone at 11pm, and measurement of serum cortisol at 8am.

Distinguish Cushing's syndrome from pseudo-Cushing states

- *Low dose dexamethasone suppression test* has greater specificity than the overnight test, and hence distinguishes Cushing's and pseudo-Cushing states, but is more cumbersome than the overnight test. An abnormal test, suggesting Cushing's syndrome, involves the failure to suppress serum cortisol after 0.5mg dexamethasone administered every 6 hours for 48 hours.

Determine the cause of Cushing's syndrome

- In a patient with confirmed Cushing's syndrome, an undetectable serum ACTH with a simultaneously elevated serum cortisol is diagnostic of ACTH-*independent* Cushing's syndrome. If this combination s found, then other tests such as CRH test and high dose dexamethsone suppression tests are not necessary, and one needs to proceed to imaging the adrenal glands.
- *CRH test* can be performed immediately after the low dose dexamethasone suppression test, to distinguish pituitary and ectopic ACTH production. The basis of the test is the principle that pituitary tumours are responsive to exogenous corticotrophin releasing hormone (CRH), whereas adrenal and ectopic tumours are not. In pituitary Cushing's disease, the suppressed serum ACTH and cortisol at the end of low dose dexamethasone suppression should *rise* following CRH administration (conventionally by more than 20% of baseline). However, in adrenal Cushing's, the low ACTH and high cortisol levels at baseline are not affected by CRH. Similarly, in ectopic Cushing's, the high ACTH and high cortisol levels at baseline are not affected by ACTH.
- *High dose dexamethasone suppression test* is an alternative method of differentiating pituitary Cushing's disease from ectopic Cushing's syndrome. The test involves measuring serum cortisol after 2mg of dexamethasone every 6 hours for 48 hours. Suppression of serum cortisol (conventionally by more than 50% of baseline) occurs in 75% of patients with Cushing's disease, although suppression also occurs in 10–25% of ectopic ACTH-secreting tumours, limiting sensitivity.
- *Inferior Petrosal Sinus Sampling* is carried out in patients with Cushing's syndrome and elevated ACTH, in whom there is no clear pituitary source. The test involves sampling blood peripherally and from each inferior petrosal sinus under X-ray guidance, and measuring ACTH in response to CRH administration. The aim of the test is to differentiate a pituitary and non-pituitary source of ACTH, and lateralize a corticotroph adenoma. If the petrosal sinus ACTH is greater than peripheral ACTH, this indicates a pituitary source of ACTH. Additionally, if the ACTH level is greater in one petrosal sinus than the contralateral side, this localizes the pituitary tumour to the ipsilateral side.

Assess for complications

- *Glucose intolerance*: fasting glucose and oral glucose tolerance test
- *Osteoporosis*: bone density measurements

What is the management of Cushing's syndrome?

The management of choice for endogenous Cushing's syndrome is surgical resection of the causative tumour, with transphenoidal hypophysectomy for Cushing's disease, and adrenalectomy for adrenal tumours.

If surgery is unsuccessful, or if symptoms require control whilst waiting for surgery, medications that inhibit steroidogenesis may be used. Ketoconazole is the first-line agent used, followed by the addition of metyrapone if symptoms persist.

Adjuvant radiotherapy is used for Cushing's disease if transphenoidal surgery is unsuccessful or impossible. The efficacy of radiotherapy is less than surgery, and the cortisol-lowering effect takes several months or years, so anti-adrenocortical medications may also be required. Adverse effects of radiotherapy include deficiency of other pituitary hormones, and cranial nerve palsies.

Immediately following removal of pituitary, adrenal, or ectopic tumours, patients require glucocorticoid replacement at 'stress' doses, which can be slowly tapered. Bilateral adrenalectomy is only used for refractory cases of Cushing's syndrome, where surgery, radiotherapy, and medical therapy have failed. These patients require lifelong glucocorticoid and mineralocorticoid replacement, and are at risk of Nelson's syndrome.

Tell me about Nelson's syndrome

Nelson's syndrome was first described by Nelson and colleagues in 1958, and represents the enlargement of a pituitary corticotroph adenoma due to the absence of negative feedback by adrenal cortisol production, following bilateral adrenalectomy. The defining clinical features are an enlarging pituitary tumour, in the presence of an elevated serum ACTH and hyperpigmentation. The pituitary corticotroph cells also produce melanocyte stimulating hormone (MSH), which is responsible for the hyperpigmentation. Patients may also develop bitemporal hemianopia due to the rapidly enlarging pituitary tumour.

Why is biochemical evaluation of Cushing's syndrome performed before imaging of the pituitary or adrenal glands?

Most cases of Cushing's disease are due to pituitary microadenomas (<1cm), and hence may not be clearly visible on MRI (50% are seen on MRI). Furthermore, the incidence of incidental, non-functioning adrenal or pituitary adenomas is 10%, which may mislead subsequent investigation and treatment.

What is the relevance of elevated serum calcium in a patient with a pituitary adenoma?

This may represent multiple endocrine neoplasia type 1 (MEN1). This is an autosomal dominant disorder characterized by hyperparathyroidism, pituitary adenomas, and pancreatic islet cell tumours. (see Case 97 Goitre for discussion of MEN2).

Almost all patients develop hyperparathyroidism, although pituitary and pancreatic lesions only affect 60%. The most common pancreatic lesion is a gastrinoma, which may cause the Zollinger-Ellison syndrome.

The MEN1 gene has been identified, and the gene product 'menin'. However, unlike MEN2, routine genetic screening of family members is not currently practised since there is little evidence that early diagnosis improves morbidity or mortality in the absence of symptoms.

Approach to the patient with suspected Cushing's syndrome:

1. Low clinical suspicion of Cushing's syndrome:
   Screening tests: Urinary free cortisol ×3, or midnight serum cortisol, or overnight dexamethasone suppression test
2. High clinical suspicion of Cushing's syndrome:
   Low dose dexamethasone suppression test
3. If low ACTH and high cortisol:
   Adrenal imaging
4. To differentiate ectopic and pituitary ACTH:
   High dose dexamethasone suppression test, CRH test, and MRI pituitary, or inferior petrosal sinus sampling

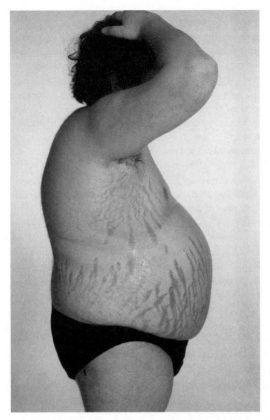

Figure 101.1 Centripetal obesity, interscapular and supraclavicular fat pads, and abdominal striae in Cushing's syndrome.

Case 102 ◆ **Addison's Disease**

CASE PRESENTATION

*This male[1] patient has evidence of **widespread pigmentation**,[2] most marked in the **buccal mucosa, skin creases**, and **pressure areas**. There is also **calcification of the auricular cartilage**.[3]*

*The diagnosis is **Addison's disease**. There are no **adrenalectomy scars**[4] to suggest Nelson's syndrome. I would like to examine for **postural hypotension**,[5] and look for evidence of other **autoimmune disease**[6] and **previous tuberculosis infection**.[7]*

Clinical notes

1. Comment of the sex of the patient. The sex of the patient has bearing on the clinical signs one encounters in Addison's disease. In females, look specifically for loss of axillary and pubic hair (androgen-dependent hair). This is not affected in males, as the testes are the main source of androgens, whereas in females the androgens are produced in the adrenal cortex.

2. Hyperpigmentation of the skin is present in 95% of patients with chronic primary hypoadrenalism. However, the presence of normal skin does not exclude the diagnosis. Look for pigmentation in light-exposed areas such as the face and neck, and pressure areas such as the elbows, knuckles, and shoulders (brassiere straps), as well as palmar creases. Hyperpigmentation also affects the buccal mucosa, nipples, axillae, perineum, and old surgical scars. Remember, pigmentation of the palmar creases may be a normal finding in dark-skinned individuals.

3. Calcification of the auricular cartilage occurs exclusively in males with longstanding primary or secondary adrenal insufficiency. It is thought to be a consequence of longstanding glucocorticoid deficiency, and does not resolve with steroid replacement.

4. Bilateral adrenalectomy scars may suggest previous surgical treatment for Cushing's disease, and consequent Nelson's syndrome (see Case 101 Cushing's Syndrome). If this is present, then examine the visual fields (bitemporal hemianopia).

5. Most patients are relatively hypotensive, but not all demonstrate postural hypotension. However, *hypertension* is rare in untreated hypoadrenalism, and if present makes a diagnosis of Addison's disease unlikely.

6. Autoimmune primary adrenal failure is associated with several autoimmune conditions, and is part of polyglandular autoimmune syndromes type I and II. The most frequent clinical sign of associated autoimmune disease is vitiligo, which is found in 10–20% of patients with autoimmune adrenalitis.
   - **Vitiligo**: areas of skin depigmentation
   - **Type 1 diabetes**: finger tip skin pricks (regular glucose testing), fundoscopy to look for retinopathy
   - **Autoimmune thyroiditis**: goitre (?thyroidectomy), features of Graves' disease, assess thyroid status
   - **Pernicious anaemia**: pallor, splenomegaly, polyneuropathy
   - **Hypoparathyroidism**: Chvostek's and Trousseau's sign, cataracts
   - **Alopecia areata**: areas of hair loss in scalp with white, short, tapering exclamation mark hairs
   - **Rheumatoid arthritis**: symmetrical arthropathy of small joints of the hands
   - **SLE**: butterfly rash, arthropathy
   - **Sjogren's syndrome**: dry mouth and eyes

7. The second most common cause of primary adrenal failure is tuberculosis. Tell the examiner you would like to examine the lung fields to look for evidence of old tuberculosis (?apical lung signs).

Questions commonly asked by examiners

What are the causes of primary adrenal failure?
- **Autoimmune** (70-90%)
- **Tuberculosis** (10-20%)
- **Bilateral adrenalectomy**—usually for Cushing's syndrome or malignant disease
- **Amyloidosis**
- **Haemochromatosis**
- **HIV**—due to associated CMV adrenalitis.
- **Disseminated fungal infection**—e.g. histoplasmosis (common in the USA) and cryptococcus
- **Haemorrhagic infarction**—associated with meningococcal septicaemia (Waterhouse-Friedrichsen syndrome), other bacterial sepsis, anticoagulation, thromboembolic disease, and thrombophilia (anti-phospholipid syndrome)

- **Adrenal metastases**—most commonly lung, breast, gastrointestinal, and melanoma
- **Congenital adrenal hyperplasia**

What other autoimmune endocrine disorders are associated with Addison's disease?

Half of patients with autoimmune adrenal failure have an associated autoimmune endocrine disorder. By contrast, patients with type 1 diabetes mellitus, or Graves' disease, rarely develop adrenal disease.

Polyglandular autoimmune syndrome type 1

This is a rare autosomal recessive disorder, characterized by hypoparathyroidism and mucocutaneous candida infection in childhood. Adrenal insufficiency and primary hypogonadism develop during adolescence.

Polyglandular autoimmune syndrome type 2

This autoimmune condition is more prevalent than type 1, and is almost universally associated with adrenal insufficiency. Half of the cases are familial. Autoimmune thyroid disease and type 1 diabetes mellitus are also associated with this condition. Hypoparathyroidism does not occur with this disorder.

What autoantibodies are present in primary autoimmune adrenal insufficiency?

There are 3 antibodies that have been described:

- Antibodies to 21-hydroxylase (the most common and specific)
- Antibodies to 17-hydroxylase*
- Antibodies to cytochrome P-450 (P-450 side chain–cleaving [P-450$_{scc}$] antibodies)*

What is the diagnostic test for adrenal insufficiency?

Single measurements of serum cortisol may be useful in excluding adrenal insufficiency, but are not as sensitive as dynamic adrenal tests. A 9am measurement of serum cortisol greater than 500 nmol/L effectively excludes adrenal insufficiency.

Dynamic testing is performed if the 9am cortisol is equivocal. This involves the administration of 250mcg of synthetic ACTH (*synacthen*), and the measurement of ACTH and cortiol before, and at 30 and 60 minutes after the intravenous administration of ACTH. If the test is performed at 9am, a normal response at 30 minutes is a rise in cortisol over 550nmol/L

Interpretation of an abnormal synacthen test:

- Impaired cortisol response and ACTH >200ng/L—primary adrenal failure
- ACTH <10ng/L—secondary (pituitary) adrenal failure

What is the treatment of adrenal insufficiency?
Adrenal crisis

The management of acute hypoadrenalism involves rapid steroid and fluid replacement, and reversal of electrolyte abnormalities.

- If the patient is not known to have adrenal insufficiency, previously, dexamethasone was considered the preferred steroid, since it is not measured in cortisol assays and will therefore not hinder subsequent diagnostic tests. However, hydrocortisone is the preferred steroid since it has both gluco- and mineralocorticoid actions—subsequent diagnostic tests are not affected if done more than 12 hours after the last dose of hydrocortisone.

---

* These are not as specific as antibodies to 21-hydroxylase because they are found in other tissues.

- Large volumes of 0.9% saline are the preferred fluid, to correct hypovolaemia and hyponatraemia.

Long-term management

Once the patient is stable, the diagnosis of adrenal failure can be confirmed with a synacthen test, and the cause can be sought.

The long-term management of primary adrenal insufficiency involves glucocorticoid replacement with hydrocortisone, and mineralocorticoid replacement with fludrocortisone. Secondary adrenal failure does not require replacement with mineralocorticoid. The patient must also be advised of the serious nature of the condition, the need for compliance with therapy, and the need to increase dosing of hydrocortisone (ant not fludrocortisone) during illness and stress. The patient should also be provided with a 'medic-alert' bracelet.

Why does pigmentation occur in primary adrenal failure?

ACTH is synthesized from a precursor called *proopiomelanocortin* (POMC). POMC undergoes post-translational processing to form either ACTH, MSHs or lipotropins (LPHs). As a consequence of the similarity in structure between ACTH and MSH, abnormally high concentrations of ACTH stimulate the melanocortin receptor, causing melanin deposition in skin by melanocytes.

What is the differential diagnosis of skin pigmentation?

- Addison's disease
- Nelson's syndrome
- Ectopic ACTH syndromes
- Haemachromatosis
- Jaundice
- Uraemia
- Pregancy (melasma)
- Solar purpura
- Café au lait spots
- Venous eczema
- Porphyria cutanea tarda
- Fixed drug eruption (tetracyclines, barbiturates, sulphonamides, NSAIDs)

What is the differential diagnosis of buccal pigmentation?

- Addison's disease
- Melanoma
- Peutz-Jehger's syndrome
- Leukoplakia
- Lichen planus
- Amalgam tattoo (from adjacent amalgam dental fillings)

How common is adrenal insufficiency in HIV disease?

Adrenal insufficiency is common in HIV and AIDS, affecting up to 15% of patients. This is most often due to CMV-related necrotizing adrenalitis, but may also be caused by infection with *Mycobacterium avium complex* and *Cryptococcus neoformans*, or infiltration by Kaposi's sarcoma.

Drugs used to treat opportunistic infection in HIV disease may also cause adrenal insufficiency. Ketoconazole inhibits cortisol synthesis, and rifampicin increases cortisol metabolism through enzyme induction.

How common is adrenal insufficiency in septic shock?

Almost half of patients with septic shock have an abnormal response to synacthen, and these patients seem to have a worse outcome than those with preserved adrenal function. However, there is conflicting evidence regarding the benefit of treating these patients with low dose hydrocortisone.[1]

Reference

1. Sprung CL, Annane D, Keh D et al. Hydrocortisone therapy for patients with septic shock. N Eng J Med. 2008; 358:111–24.

Case 103 ◆ **Hypopituitarism**

CASE PRESENTATION

*This male patient has evidence of **pallor** and the **skin is soft, dry, and wrinkled**.[1] There is **decreased facial and body hair**.[2] There is also **gynaecomastia**.[3]*

*The differential diagnosis is **primary hypogonadism**,[4] or **pituitary failure with treated secondary hypogonadism**.*

*I would like to assess **testicular volume**,[5] and examine for **postural hypotension**[6] and a **bitemporal hemianopia**.[7]*

Clinical notes

1. The skin in panhypopituitarism is described as *alabaster skin*, since it is pale and dry, with an inability to tan due to MSH and ACTH deficiency.

2. In males, pituitary gonadotropin deficiency causes testicular hypofunction, and loss of secondary sexual characteristics, i.e. loss of facial, axillary, and pubic hair.

3. Gynaecomastia is more common in primary hypogonadism, due to a compensatory rise in pituitary luteinising hormone (LH). However, secondary hypogonadism due to pituitary failure may be associated with gynaecomastia if treated with gonadotropin replacement. Remember to *palpate* for breast tissue, and to differentiate adipose tissue from gynaecomastia.

4. Primary hypogonadism is more common than hypopituitarism, and hence is the most likely diagnosis with these signs. Look carefully for signs of congenital conditions causing primary hypogonadism, such as Klinefelter's syndrome (see Case 105).

5. In adults, testicular size should be 4–7cm in length, or 20–25ml volume. You will *not* be expected to perform this test in the examination, but you should assess secondary sexual characteristics such as facial hair, body hair, and body musculature.

6. Unlike primary adrenal failure, ACTH deficiency does not cause salt wasting, hypovolaemia, hyponatraemia, or hyperkalemia, since there is no deficiency in mineralocorticoid which is controlled by the *renin-angiotensin* system. However, glucocortioids are required to maintain vascular tone; therefore hypotension may still occur in hypopituitarism.

7. The neurological manifestations of hypopituitarism are due to local effects of the pituitary disease. Headaches and visual field defects may occur if the lesion extends to the suprasellar region. Lateral

extension to the cavernous sinus may affect oculomotor nerves, and superior extension may damage the hypothalamus or cause hydrocephalus by occluding the Foramen of Munro.

Questions commonly asked by examiners

What are the causes of pituitary failure?

- **Pituitary mass**—adenoma, craniopharyngioma, cyst, metastasis.
- **Pituitary surgery or radiotherapy**
- **Infiltrative disease**—sarcoidosis, haemochromatosis, histiocytosis X
- **Lymphocytic hypophysitis**—lymphocytic infiltration of pituitary during late pregnancy/postpartum.
- **Pituitary infarction (Sheehan's syndrome)**—typically following postpartum haemorrhage and consequent hypovolemia.
- **Pituitary apoplexy**—sudden haemorrhage into the pituitary gland, most commonly into a pituitary adenoma.
- **Empty sella syndrome**
- **Trauma / subarachnoid haemorrhage**

What do you understand by the term 'empty sella syndrome'?

This refers to an enlarged sella turcica, which is not entirely filled with pituitary tissue. This may be secondary to surgery, radiotherapy, or infarction, and may cause hypopituitarism. However, primary empty sella syndrome is not associated with hypopituitarism, since the sella is enlarged by cerebrospinal-fluid (CSF) pressure through a defect in the sella membrane, and there is no deficit of pituitary tissue.

What are the clinical presentations of hypopituitarism?

The presentation depends on the *onset* of the condition, *which* pituitary hormones are deficient, and whether there are *local* symptoms such as headache or visual loss. As a general rule, in progressive pituitary disease, the secretion of GH and gonadotropins is affected *before* ACTH and TSH.

Sudden insults to the pituitary gland, such as infarction or apoplexy, may cause rapid life-threatening ACTH deficiency and hypotension. Slowly progressive disease, due to radiotherapy or infiltrative conditions, may present initially with hypogonadism.

- **GH deficiency**—in children, GH deficiency causes short stature. In adults, this causes decreased bone density and muscle mass, and possible diminished sense of well-being. GH replacement is licensed in adults with severe deficiency.
- **Gonadotropin deficiency**—in males, this causes testicular hypofunction, erectile dysfunction, and infertility. Testicular atrophy and gynaecomastia are usually clinically detectable. In adults, this may present with decreased libido, decreased facial hair affecting shaving, and eventually loss of body hair and muscle mass. In adult females, this causes similar symptoms to menopausal ovarian failure, such as infertility, amenorrhoea, and hot flushes, but there are few consistent clinical signs.
- **TSH deficiency**—this causes similar symptoms and signs to primary hypothyroidism. However, signs such as weight gain and myxoedema may be obscured by the signs of concomitant ACTH deficiency (weight loss, pallor).
- **ACTH deficiency**—this is similar to primary adrenal failure, apart from the lack of pigmentation, and the preservation of mineralocorticoid activity by the *renin-angiotensin* system.
- **Prolactin deficiency**—the only manifestation of prolactin deficiency is the inability to lactate following delivery. However, prolactin may be *elevated* if there is pituitary stalk compression and viable pituitary tissue.

What is the medical management of patients undergoing pituitary surgery?

* All patients undergoing pituitary surgery should undergo pituitary function and visual field testing pre-operatively. Check baseline: Free T4, TSH, prolactin, oestradiol (females), testosterone (males), FSH, LH, morning cortisol.
* Commence high dose steroid replacement on the day of surgery, with IV hydrocortisone.
* Convert to oral steroid replacement after 72 hours, if there are no post-operative complications.
* Monitor fluid balance and urine osmolality post-operatively, looking for diabetes insipidus (DI). This causes high serum osmolality and low urine osmolality. DI may be transient, but if persists is treated with desmopressin acetate (synthetic analogue of vasopressin) (DDAVP).
* Discharge *all* patients on oral hydrocortisone, and provide a steroid card and 'medic-alert' bracelet.
* After 3–4 weeks, perform a pituitary stimulation test (insulin tolerance test, metyrapone test, or short synacthen test [preferred test]), following the cessation of steroids the night before. Both metyrapone and insulin-induced hypoglycaemia should stimulate ACTH secretion, and therefore test pituitary ACTH reserve. In the short synacthen test, although directly stimulating the adrenal tissues, a normal result in this clinical context will only result if the adrenals have been stimulated by sufficient endogenous ACTH from the patients pituitary gland. If patients fail this test, they require long-term steroid replacement. However, some patients recover pituitary ACTH function, therefore patients on steroid replacement should have a further test in two years.
* Measure free T4 post-operatively (the TSH may be normal post-operatively), and replace if deficient. Aim to increase the free T4 within the upper half of normal limit (TSH levels are not a useful guide to the adequacy of replacement)
* If sex hormones are low, then replacement with testosterone or oestrogens in men and women respectively.

Case 104 ◆ **Gynaecomastia**

CASE PRESENTATION

This middle-aged male patient has bilateral increased **glandular tissue** *palpable beneath the nipple-areolar complex. This disc of tissue is* **firm**, **concentric**, *and* **mobile**.[1]

This patient has **gynaecomastia**.[2]

Clinical notes

1. If the examiner has not indicated that you should palpate the breasts, then ask for permission before doing so. Palpation of glandular tissue differentiates gynaecomastia from 'pseudogynaecomastia' due to adioposity. Place your thumb and forefinger on opposite sides of the areola, and feel for the presence of firm disc of mobile glandular tissue. Breast carcinoma is a further differential of a breast mass, and typically presents with a hard mass, which may be outside the nipple–areolar complex.

2. Making a diagnosis of gynaecomastia is very straightforward. It is important to be able to demonstrate your understanding of possible causes. Tell the examiner that you would like to look for possible causes:

   (a) **Hypogonadism**: lack of facial and body hair, reduced testicular volume*

   (b) **Testicular tumour**: examine the testes for masses*

   (c) **Chronic liver disease**: stigmata of chronic liver disease**

   (d) **Chronic renal failure**: evidence of renal replacement therapy

   (e) **Klinefelter's syndrome**: tall male patient, small firm testes

   (f) **Thyrotoxicosis**: assess thyroid status, goitre, eye signs

   (g) **Carcinoma of the lung**: clubbing, nicotine staining, cachexia

   (h) **Hepatocellular carcinoma**: hepatomegaly (tender irregular liver edge), cachexia

   (i) **Drugs**: enquire about a full drug history and look for specific diseases relating to specific drugs:***

   - **DIGOXIN**: Irregular pulse of AF
   - **SPIRONOLACTONE**: signs of cardiac failure; chronic liver disease with ascites

Questions commonly asked by examiners

What are the common causes of gynaecomastia?

- **Puberty**—during puberty, the serum oestradiol rises to adult levels before testosterone, causing transient gynaecomastia. This normally resolves within six months to two years.
- **Drugs** (see below).
- **Cirrhosis**—gynaecomastia occurs due to altered sex hormone metabolism, and an increase in the oestradiol:free testosterone ratio.
- **Hypogonadism**
  - *Primary* hypogonadism causes a compensatory rise in LH, in turn causing increased peripheral aromatization of testosterone to oestradiol (see diagram 1).
  - *Secondary* hypogonadism, due to pituitary or hypothalamic disease (e.g. prolactin excess, Kallman's syndrome, haemachromatosis), may also cause gynaecomastia despite LH deficiency, since the adrenal cortex continues to produce oestrogen precursors, which are converted to oestrogens in peripheral tissues.
- **Tumours**
  - *Testicular tumours:*
    - *Germ cell tumours* account for over 95% testicular tumours. Gynaecomastia occurs in 5% of patients, due to hCG secretion stimulating oestradiol production by the testes.
    - *Leydig cell tumours* cause gynaecomastia in 20–30% of cases. These tumours present with precocious puberty in boys, or poor libido and gynaecomastia in young males. Approximately 10% of these tumours are malignant.
    - *Sertoli cell tumours* cause gynaecomastia through excess aromatization of androgens to oestrogens. These tumours may occur in Peutz-Jeger's syndrome.
  - *Adrenocortical tumours* may cause gynaecomastia through overproduction of androgens such as androstenedione, which are converted to oestrogens in peripheral tissues.

---

* Examining the testes in the MRCP (PACES) examination will not be expected, but it is important to mention in a patient with gynaecomastia.

** Almost half of male patients with cirrhosis have gynaecomastia. This may be due to liver disease, or due to the use of spironolactone.

*** Drug-induced is the most common cause of gynaecomastia.

◆ *Ectopic hCG-secreting tumours* include lung, gastric, renal, and hepatocellular carcinomas.

◆ *Hypogonadism* from chemotherapy or radiotherapy may also cause gynaecomastia in patients with testicular tumours.

• **Graves' disease**—gynaecomastia may occur due to increased sex hormone-binding globulin (SHBG), and decreased free testosterone levels.

◆ **Chronic renal failure**—half of patients receiving haemodialysis develop gynaecomastia due to decreased Leydig cell function. Gynaecomastia may also occur following kidney transplantation due to ciclosporin use.

◆ **Androgen insensitivity syndromes**—complete androgen insensitivity, formerly termed 'testicular feminization syndrome', causes a female phenotype in patients who are genotypic males. These patients are regarded as female, and therefore present with infertility and amenorrhoea rather gynaecomastia. Partial androgen receptor defects may cause gynaecomastia in phenotypic males.

What drugs cause gynaecomastia?

• Anti-androgens
  ◆ Cyproterone acetate
  ◆ Finasteride / dutasteride
• Gastrointestinal drugs
  ◆ Cimetidine / ranitidine
• Cancer chemotherapy
  ◆ Alkylating agents / vinca alkaloids (due to testicular damage and hypogonadism)
  ◆ Imatinib (tyrosine kinase inhibitor used for chronic myeloid leukaemia (CML) and gastrointestinal stromal tumour (GIST))
• Cardiovascular drugs
  ◆ Spironolactone (displaces oestrogen from SHBG, increasing free oestrogen:testosterone ratio)
  ◆ Digoxin
  ◆ Amiodarone
  ◆ Methyl-dopa
• Antimicobial drugs
  ◆ Isoniazid
  ◆ Ketoconazole
  ◆ Metronodazole
• Anti-viral drugs
  ◆ highly active anti-retroviral (HAART) therapy (especially protease inhibitors)
• Neurological drugs
  ◆ Phenothiazines
  ◆ Metoclopramide
  ◆ Tricyclic anti-depressants
  ◆ Opiates

Does prolactin excess cause gynaecomastia?

Men with an elevated serum prolactin may develop gynaecomastia due to the effect of prolactin on reducing the secretion of gonadotropins, leading to secondary hypogonadism. However, prolactin does not directly cause gynaecomastia, but stimulates milk production in breast tissue that has been primed by oestrogen and progesterone.

Why is gynaecomastia more common with age?

Aromatase activity converts androgens to oestrogens in peripheral tissue. Aromatase activity increases with age, and with increased body fat. Therefore, a physiological increase in aromatase activity is likely to be responsible for the increase in gynaecomastia with age. Moreover, older men are more likely to be treated with medications which are associated with gynaecomastia.

How would you investigate this patient?

Clinical examination is usually sufficient to differentiate gynaecomastia from breast carcinoma, since malignant masses are usually unilateral, hard or firm, and may extend beyond the nipple–areola complex. Additionally, skin dimpling and nipple inversion may be seen in breast carcinoma. If there is any doubt, the patient should undergo mammography, which has a diagnostic sensitivity and specificity of 90%.

Once gynaecomastia has been confirmed, the initial step is to review the patient's medications, including herbal and over-the-counter remedies. Clinical examination should concentrate on testicular and adrenal tumours (possible co-existing Cushing's syndrome or mineralocorticoid excess), hyperthyroidism, liver disease, Klinefelter's syndrome, and androgen insensitivity.

If the patient has unilateral gynaecomastia, or painful bilateral gynaecomastia, and history and examination do not reveal a cause, then hCG, LH, testosterone, and oestradiol should be measured. These tests may identify primary or secondary hypogonadism, or excess hCG production. In asymptomatic patients with bilateral gynaecomastia, endocrine investigations are likely to be normal and are not generally required.

How would you assess a patient with testicular enlargement?

The initial investigation is an ultrasound examination, since it is able to characterize the lesion and specifically identify a mass. If the presentation suggests orchitis (acute onset, fever, risk factors for sexually acquired infection) then a trial of antibiotics may be considered with close monitoring for resolution of the lesion. If the mass is suspicious for cancer, then tumour markers should be measured (β-hCG, lactate dehydrogenase (LDH), αFP), and orchidectomy is indicated with subsequent histological evaluation. Patients with equivocal ultrasound findings may require further imaging with MRI. Patients with malignant disease require further axial imaging of the thorax, abdomen, and pelvis for staging. The initial site of metastasis is the para-aortic lymph nodes.

Almost all testicular cancers are germ cell tumours. These are further categorized as seminomas and non-seminomas. The tumour markers suggest the type of testicular cancer. β-hCG may be elevated in both seminomas and non-seminomas. Elevated αFP levels are not usually associated with pure seminomas. Tumours which are histologically seminomas but have an elevated αFP should be treated as nonseminomas.

Case 105 ◆ Klinefelter's Syndrome

CASE PRESENTATION

*This male patient is **tall**,[1] with **gynaecomastia**[2] and **decreased facial and body hair**.[3]*

The differential diagnosis includes causes of primary hypogonadism,[4] but the tall stature favours **Klinefelter's syndrome**.

I would like to examine the testes,[5] and look for associated conditions.[6]

Clinical notes

1. Begin by asking the patient to stand, to assess height. Patients with Klinefelter's syndrome usually have a disproportionate increase in lower limb bones compared to upper limb bones.

2. Remember that gynaecomastia must be distinguished from pseudogynaecomastia by palpation for breast tissue. This should be done routinely for liver cases in the abdominal station (Station 1), although in shorter endocrine cases (Station 5), one should ask the examiner for permission to palpate the breasts. Gynaecomastia is only present in 30–50% of patients with Klinefelter's syndrome. This is secondary to elevated oestradiol levels and an increased oestradiol-to-testosterone ratio. Look for the presence of breast masses, as the risk of breast cancer is increased 20–50 fold in men with Klinefelter's syndrome.

3. Patients have secondary sexual characteristics due to a decrease in androgen production. This results in decreased facial, axillary, and pubic hair; a high-pitched voice; and fat distribution as observed in females, i.e. broad hips.

4. Secondary hypogonadism is not associated with gynaecomastia, unless they have been treated with gonadotrophins therapy.

5. Although you will not be expected to examine the testes in the MRCP (PACES) clinical examination, it is important to be aware of the characteristic findings of small firm testes in Klinefelter's syndrome.

6. In Klinefelter's syndrome, there is an increased incidence of:

- **Autoimmune disease**:
  - ◆ SLE
  - ◆ Rheumatoid arthritis
  - ◆ Sjogren's syndrome
  - ◆ Hashimoto's thyroiditis
  - ◆ Diabetes
- **Mitral valve prolapse** (seen in 55% of patients)
- **Varicose veins** (seen in 20% of patients)

Although this is a short case, you will not be expected to look for all the associations. Certain associations may clearly be evident from gross inspection. To be able to list a few associations in the final case presentation will impress examiners!

Questions commonly asked by examiners

What do you understand by primary and secondary hypogonadism?

- **Primary hypogonadism**: hypogonadism secondary to a defect in the gonads ($\downarrow$ androgens and $\uparrow$ gonadotrophins)
- **Secondary hypogonadism**: hypogonadism secondary to defect in hypothalamic-pituitary function ($\downarrow$ androgens and $\downarrow$ gonadotrophins)

What is the karyotype in Klinefelter's syndrome?

The most common karyotype is 47XXY, which accounts for 80–90% of all cases. Mosaicism (46XY/47XXY) is observed in about 10% of cases. Other variant karyotypes, including 48XXYY; 48XXXY; 49XXXYY; and 49XXXXY, are rare. The mosaic forms of Klinefelter's syndrome are due to mitotic non-disjunction after fertilization of the zygote. These forms can arise from a

46XY zygote or a 47XXY zygote. Variant forms of Klinefelter's syndrome include 48XXXY; 49XXXXY; 48XXYY; and 49XXXYY.

What are the manifestations of Klinefelter's syndrome?

- Manifestations of testosterone deficiency
  - Infertility
  - Small testes and penis
  - Decreased facial, pubic, and body hair
  - Gynaecomastia
  - Long limbs and tall stature (testosterone deficiency delays growth plate fusion in long bones)
  - Decreased muscle tone
  - Osteoporosis
- Manifestations of XXY genotype
  - Cognitive deficits in language and motor function
  - Mental retardation, cryptorchidism, hypospadias, and radioulnar synostosis (if >2 X chromosomes)
  - Very tall stature and aggressive behaviour (if >2 Y chromosomes)

What are the common causes of primary hypogonadism in males?

- **Infection**—such as mumps orchitis, may cause infertility and hypogonadism.
- **Testicular torsion**—this is one of the most common reasons for orchidectomy before puberty. Even if torsion only affects one testis, hypogonadism may result for reasons which are unclear.
- **Cryptorchidism**—this refers to testes that are undescended, and remain in the abdominal cavity or inguinal canal by the age of one year. Bilateral cryptorchidism is required for hypogonadism to be clinically apparent, however even unilateral cryptorchidism is associated with a markedly increased risk of testicular cancer.
- **Klinefelter's syndrome**—this is the most common congenital abnormality causing primary hypogonadism, affecting 1 in 1000 live male births. The most frequent karyotype is an extra X chromosome, 47XXY, although 48XXY and mosaics have also been reported.
- **Noonan's syndrome**—short stature, webbed neck, right-sided cardiac defects, and primary testicular failure.
- **Varicocele**—this refers to varicosities within the venous plexus within the scrotum, which may damage the seminiferous tubules and cause hypogonadism and infertility.
- **Myotonic dystrophy**—causes hypogonadism along with muscle weakness, myotonia, cardiac, and ocular abnormalities (see Case 47 Myotonic Dystrophy).
- **Radiation**—radiotherapy for conditions such as leukaemia may cause testicular damage and hypogonadism.
- **Chemotherapeutic agents**—alkylating agents (e.g. cyclophoshamide) and platinum-containing drugs (e.g. cisplatin) may cause azoospermia and infertility.
- **Drugs**—which inhibit testosterone synthesis, such as ketoconazole, spironolactone, and cimetidine.

What are causes of secondary hypogonadism?

- Kallmann's syndrome
- Prader-Willi syndrome
- Dandy-Walker malformation
- Isolated LH deficiency

- Hypopituitarism
- Hyperprolactinemia
- Haemochromatosis
- Morbid obesity
- Malnutrition

Why is gynaecomastia not seen in secondary hypogonadism?

This is because serum FSH and LH concentrations are not high and therefore do not stimulate testicular aromatase to increase the conversion of testosterone to oestradiol.

What are the causes of tall stature?

- Familial tall stature
- Klinefelter's syndrome
- Marfan's syndrome
- Homocystinuria
- Mulitple endocrine neoplasia (MEN) 2B
- Precocoius puberty
- Hyperthyroidism

Case 106 ◆ **Turner's Syndrome**

CASE PRESENTATION

*This lady[1] has **short stature**,[2] with a **square chest** and **widely-spaced nipples**.[3] Other dysmorphic signs are a **webbed neck**,[4] **nail dysplasia**,[5] cubitus valgus,[6] a **high arched palate**[7] and **short fourth metacarpals**.[8] There numerous **naevi** present.[9]*

*The diagnosis is **Turner's syndrome**.[10]*

Clinical notes

1. Turner's syndrome is seen in females. Noonan's syndrome is where a Turner's phenotype is present with normal chromosomes (46XX or 46XY) occurring in both males and females. Fertility is normal in Turner's syndrome.
2. If the patient is seated, initially ask the patient to stand to be able to comment on height.
3. The prominent 'shield-like' chest deformity is a manifestation of an abnormal upper:lower body segment ratio, caused by a short sternum. The nipples are typically inverted and widely-spaced.
4. Proceed to seat the patient, and look at the neck, palate, and hands. The webbed neck is usually seen in infancy, as a result of cystic hygromas in utero. It may not be present in adult patients. However, Turner's patients may also have a short neck due to hypoplasia of cervical vertebrae. A short webbed neck may be associated with low posterior hair-line.
5. Nail dysplasia is a developmental abnormality due to peripheral lymphoedema. Nails are small, hyper-convex and inserted at an acute angle. Nail dysplasia is most marked in the feet, with some patients having complete absence of toenails.

6. Cubitus valgus (increased carrying angle): This is a common skeletal anomaly in girls due to abnormal development of the trochlear head.

7. Turner's syndrome is a cause of a high-arched palate.

8. Short fourth (and sometimes fifth) metacarpals and metatarsals may be seen. To demonstrate short metacarpals, ask the patient to make a fist—the absence of the fourth knuckle, with dimpling of skin over the knuckles, is a useful clue to a short fourth metacarpal. This is known as the Archibald sign.

9. A large number of naevi may be noted.

10. Tell the examiner you would like to look for associated features:

   (a) **Cardiovascular**: bicuspid aortic valve, coarctation of the aorta, hypertension (look for sternotomy scars)

   (b) **Eyes**: ptosis, strabismus, cataracts, nystagmus

   (c) **Thyroid**: hypothyroidism (assess thyroid status), goitre

   (d) **Diabetes**: finger pricks (glucose testing), diabetic retinopathy

   (e) **Legs**: lymphoedema

   (f) **Musculoskeletal**: osteoporosis (look for scoliosis and evidence of fractures)

Questions commonly asked by examiners

What are the medical complications of Turner's syndrome?

Hypogonadism

Primary ovarian failure occurs in most patients, and hormone replacement therapy is generally required to initiate puberty and complete growth. A minority of patients will have enough residual ovarian function for breast budding and vaginal spotting to occur, but secondary amenorrhoea will develop. Even in patients with some ovarian function, spontaneous fertility is rare.

Hypothyroidism

Hypothyroidism occurs in 15–30% of patients, with up to 50% of patients having anti-thyroid antibodies.

Diabetes

Women with Turner's syndrome are at a moderately increased risk of developing type 1 diabetes in childhood and a substantially increased risk of developing type 2 diabetes by adult years. The risk of developing type 2 diabetes can be substantially reduced by maintaining a normal weight.

Cardiovascular disease

Congenital heart disease affects one-third of patients. Coarctation and bicuspid aortic valve are the most common abnormalities, followed by other left-sided cardiac lesions. Hypertension and conduction defects also occur, however there is no increase in coronary heart disease. Aortic dissection is also more common in Turner's syndrome.

Musculoskeletal

Osteoporosis is common with increased incidence of bone fractures.

Renal malformations

Horseshoe kidney is the most common structural abnormality, followed by abnormalities in vascular supply. Patients should have a renal ultrasound at diagnosis, and patients with structural abnormalities should be monitored for infection and hydronephrosis.

Ocular abnormalities

Strabismus, cataracts, ptosis, and nystagmus are more common in Turner's syndrome.

Developmental and behavioural abnormalities

Most patients with Turner's syndrome have normal intelligence. However, 10% of patients have developmental delays, and require educational assistance.

What do you understand by the term 'mosaicism'?

Turner's syndrome is characterized by the karyotype 45XO, which is usually established from lymphocytes in a peripheral blood smear. Mosaicism implies the presence of two or more cell lines within the body, with either a 46XX or 46XY karyotype. Girls with a 45XO/46XX mosaic karyotype may have a less sever phenotype of Turner's syndrome, and may have some residual ovarian function. Girls with a cell population with the Y chromosome are at increased risk of gonadoblastoma tumours in their streak gonads.

How can short stature be prevented?

In childhood, GH therapy prevents short stature as an adult. Oestrogen replacement therapy is usually required, but if given too early can compromise adult height. Therefore, it is usually is started from age 12–15 years.

What are the causes of a webbed neck?

- Turner's syndrome
- Noonan's syndrome
- Klippel-Fleil syndrome
- Diamond-Blackfan anaemia
- Watson's syndrome

Case 107 ◆ **Pseudohypoparathyroidism**

(Albright's Hereditary Osteodystrophy)

CASE PRESENTATION

*On examination this patient has a **round face**,[1] **obesity**,[2] **short stature**,[3] **shortening of the fourth metacarpal**,[4] and **distal phalanx of the thumb**.[5] There are also **palpable subcutaneous calcifications**.[6]*

*The likely diagnosis is **pseudohypoparathyroidism**.[7]*

Clinical notes

1. The differential diagnosis of round facies includes the 'moon face' of Cushing's syndrome, 'chipmunk facies' (due to the skeletal changes of beta thalassaemia), myxoedema, and peri-orbital swelling due to nephrotic syndrome.

2. Obesity is a common feature of this condition. It may be best to term this as 'increased body mass index' in the final case presentation.

3. In any Station 5 'short case' where you are unsure how to proceed, begin by looking for facial, skeletal, and dermatological abnormalities, and then ask the patient to stand. These manoeuvres may reveal a

diagnosis such as short stature or ankylosing spondylitis, which would otherwise not be apparent. In this case, the facial abnormality and short stature should prompt the candidate to examine for the interscapular fat pad and proximal myopathy of Cushing's, and the skeletal abnormalities of Albright's hereditary osteodystrophy.

4. This is the most reliable sign in the diagnosis of this condition. It may be symmetrical or asymmetrical and may involve one or both hands or feet. Ask the patient to make a fist and look for the Archibald sign (see Case 106 Turner's Syndrome).

5. Shortening of the distal phalanx of the thumb is evident as a thumb in which the ratio of the width of the nail to its length is increased (murderer's thumb or potter's thumb).

6. The differential diagnosis of subcutaneous calcification includes gouty tophi, calcified nodules in systemic sclerosis, Ehlers-Danlos syndrome, pseudoxanthoma elasticum, dermatomyositis, and soft tissue tumours such as sarcomas.

7. Tell the examiner you would like to look for other associated features:

   (a) **Hypocalcaemia**: Chvostek sign and Trousseau sign

   (b) **Hypothyroidism**: assess thyroid status (NB: goitre is not present)

Questions commonly asked by examiners

What are the physiological actions of parathyroid hormone?

Secretion of parathyroid hormone (PTH) is stimulated by the detection of hypocalcaemia by the calcium-sensing receptor on parathyroid glands.

The effects of PTH on calcium and phosphate metabolism are via the type 1 PTH receptor:

- **Bone**—continuously elevated PTH levels cause release of calcium stores, and bone resorption. However, intermittent administration of PTH stimulates bone formation. This action is the basis for the recent use of recombinant PTH in the treatment of osteoporosis.

- **Kidneys**—PTH *stimulates* calcium reabsorption from the distal tubules, but *inhibits* reabsorption of phosphate. This is unlike vitamin D, which promotes the retention of both calcium and phosphate.

- **Vitamin D metabolism**—PTH stimulates the renal synthesis of 1-α hydroxylase, and thus the conversion of calcidiol to calcitriol, the active form of vitamin D. Calcitriol subsequently *decreases PTH release* by negative feedback.

What is meant by the term 'pseudohypoparathyroidism'?

Pseudohypoparathyroidism refers to defective PTH signalling by the type 1 PTH receptor, causing end-organ resistance.

- *Pseudohypoparathyroidism Type 1a*—is characterized by the skeletal abnormalities described above, collectively known as Albright's hereditary osteodystrophy, as well as hypocalcaemia and elevated serum PTH levels. The deficiency is in the α-subunit of the Gs protein that couples PTH receptor to adenylcyclase, that limits normal cyclic adenosine monophosphate (cAMP) production. Several other peptide hormones, including TSH, antidiuretic hormone (ADH), LH, follicle stimulating hormone (FSH), ACTH, GHRH, use the α-subunit of the Gs protein to increase cAMP production. Therefore, patients can present with resistance to the effects of any of these hormones, although in most patients, responses to ACTH and glucagon are clinically unaffected.

- *Pseudohypoparathyroidism Type 1b*—is characterized by end-organ PTH resistance, *without* the skeletal abnormalities of Albright's hereditary osteodystrophy. The expression of Gs protein is normal, but a defect in the PTH receptor is though to result in end-organ resistance to PTH.

- *Pseudo-pseudohypoparathyroidism*—occurs in first-degree relatives of patients with pseudohypoparathyroidism type 1a. Patients have the skeletal features of Albright's hereditary osteodystrophy, but do not have end-organ resistance to PTH or hypocalcaemia. This is because of genetic imprinting with a normal maternal allele.

What are the other causes of hypocalcaemia in adults?

- **Hypoalbumaemia**—causing a decrease in albumin-bound calcium, although the ionized calcium remains constant, hence there are no symptoms of hypocalcaemia.
- **Vitamin D deficiency**—due to liver or renal disease, or malabsorptive conditions such as coeliac disease.
- **Hypoparathyroidism**—due to peri-operative trauma, or autoimmune disease.
- **Acute pancreatitis**—due to the precipitation of calcium soaps by the inflammatory process in the retroperitoneum.
- **Hypomagnesaemia**—causes resistance to PTH, and hence hypocalcaemia results. Correction requires the administration of magnesium as well as calcium.
- **Acute hyperphosphataemia**—due to renal failure or tissue breakdown (e.g. rhabdomyolysis, tumour lysis syndrome), causes acute hypocalcaemia through extravascular precipitation of calcium phosphate. By contrast, chronic hyperphosphataemia is usually associated with chronic renal failure and normal calcium levels, since the parathyroid gland has time to compensate for vitamin D deficiency and hypocalcaemia.
- **Drugs**—chemotherapeutic agents (e.g. cisplatin), bisphosphonates, and anti-virals (e.g. foscarnet)
- **Autosomal dominant hypercalciuric hypocalcaemia**—is caused by an activating mutation of the parathyroid and renal calcium-sensing receptor. Therefore, there is constant inhibition of PTH release, causing mild hypocalcaemia. The hypercalciuria may cause nephrocalcinosis. Mutations of the calcium-sensing receptor that have the *opposite* effect (constitutive activation) cause *Familial Hypocalciuric Hypercalcaemia,* with elevated PTH levels and hypercalcaemia.

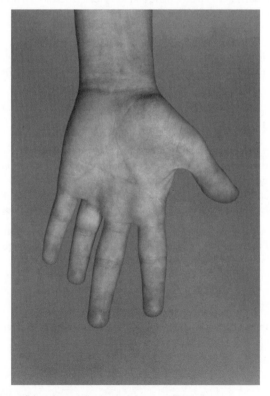

Figure 107.1 Short 4th and 5th metacarpals in pseudohypoparathyroidism.

B. Locomotor

Case 108 ◆ **Rheumatoid Arthritis**

Examiner's note

Rheumatoid arthritis (RA) is the most common case in the locomotor station of the MRCP (PACES) examination, and thus extra detail and notes have been provided below. The diagnosis is often clear at the outset, and obtaining a pass at this station is easy. However, extra marks can easily be gained at this station transforming a 'pass' into a 'clear pass'. Therefore to distinguish oneself from other candidates it is important to:

(a) Be aware of all the skin and joint changes associated with rheumatoid arthritis.
(b) Comment on whether the inflammation is active.
(c) Comment on functional status.
(d) Look for features of other connective tissue diseases such as systemic sclerosis, dermatomyositis, and systemic lupus erythematosus (SLE). This would suggest a mixed connective tissue disorder.
(e) Be aware of the multisystem involvement, and look for associations. This is a short station, and it may be appropriate to tell the examiner that you would like to look for other manifestations of the disease.

Therefore, an examination routine for this station must include the articular and (some) extra-articular features of RA, the features of differential diagnoses such as gout, psoriatic arthropathy and other connective tissue diseases, as well as an assessment of function.

CASE PRESENTATION

There is a **symmetrical deforming arthropathy** of the small joints of the hands involving the **proximal interphalangeal** and **metacarpophalangeal** joints with **sparing of the distal interphalangeal** joints.[1] There is **spindling** of the fingers due to soft tissue swelling at the PIP and MCP joints. There is **palmar subluxation** at the MCP joints and **ulnar deviation** of the fingers.[2] The deformities present include **swan-neck deformities**, **Boutonniere's deformities**, and **Z deformity of the thumb**.[3,4]

There are **nodules** present on the extensor surface of the forearm.[5,6] There is **palmar erythema** and generalized **wasting of the small muscles of the hand**.[7] There are **nail fold infarcts** and **vasculitic skin lesions**.[8] There is a palpable **flexor tendon nodule** (say where) with resultant **triggering of the finger**.[9] The skin is thin and atrophic with **purpura** on the hands and arms.[10] There is no evidence of entrapment neuropathy.[11] The affected joints are warm, erythematous, and tender.[12] The patient is unable to unbutton his/her clothes.[13]

The diagnosis is **rheumatoid arthritis**. There is evidence of active inflammation and associated disability. I would like to examine for extra-articular manifestations of disease.[14]

Clinical notes

1. Ask about joint pain before shaking the patient's hand or examining. Before touching the patient, spend some time making general observations. Look for walking aids or carpal tunnel splints. Now, gently place the patient's hands on a pillow, and look carefully at the pattern of joint involvement. Remember that rheumatoid arthritis is a symmetrical arthropathy, unlike gout or osteoarthritis, which are typically asymmetrical or seronegative arthropathies, which may also affect the knees, ankles, and spine. If there is DIP joint involvement, look for Heberden's nodes (DIP bony swelling) and Bouchard's nodes (PIP bony swelling) suggesting osteoarthritis, and consider seronegative arthropathies (e.g. psoriatic arthropathy). Remember that psoriatic arthropathy can mimic rheumatoid arthritis, thus look carefully for nail changes and psoriatic plaques. The hairline and extensor surfaces of the forearms will be examined later during the routine.

2. Disease activity should be differentiated from structural deformity. Fusiform swelling of the fingers is due to PIP and MCP synovitis. However, palmar subluxation and ulnar deviation of the MCP joints is due to structural damage to the palmar arches. In advanced disease, joint stiffness, swelling, and effusion can occur due to active inflammation *and* as a consequence of mechanical and degenerative change.

3. When describing deformities, it is best to name the deformities and avoid description, since this may cause confusion when presenting. Examiners may ask about details of the deformities, in which case the following descriptions may be given:

   (a) **Swan-neck deformity**: hyperextension at PIP joint and flexion at MCP and DIP joints

   (b) **Boutonniere's deformity**: flexion at PIP joint and hyperextension (contractures) at MCP and DIP joints

   (c) **Z deformity**: flexion at IP joint and hyperextension at the MCP joint

4. At this stage, proceed to feel the DIP, PIP, and MCP joints with the dorsum of your hand, and compare the warmth of the joints with the patient's forearm. Now palpate each DIP and PIP joint in turn, between your thumb and forefingers. The MCP joints can be palpated together. Finally, palpate the dorsum of the wrist for synovitis with both hands, and palpate the ulnar styloid, which may be 'floating' due to destruction of the ulnar collateral ligament (piano-key sign). Occasionally the elevated ulnar styloid may compress the extensor tendons of the 4th and 5th digits, leading to tendon rupture and inability to extend the 4th and 5th digits (pseudobenediction sign).

5. Now ask the patient to perform active movements. Initially test hand function by asking the patient to 'squeeze my fingers', and now 'open your hand and spread your fingers apart'. Test wrist dorsifelxion with the 'prayer' sign, and palmarflexion with the 'reverse prayer' sign. Now ask the patient to 'put one hand on each shoulder, folding your arms across your chest'. Look at the foreams for rheumatoid nodules, olecranon bursae, and psoriatic plaques. Assess shoulder mobility by asking the patient to 'put both hands behind your head'. Finally, palpate the earlobe for gouty tophi, and inspect the hairline for psoriasis. Finish by examining the hands for entrapment neuropathy, and assessing for functional impairment (see below).

6. Rheumatoid nodules are firm, non-tender lesions, unlike olcranon bursae, which are fluid-filled, tender, and may transilluminate. The differential diagnosis of a rheumatoid nodule includes gouty tophi, cutaneous sarcoidosis, granuloma annulare, and tendon xanthomata if the lesion occurs over a tendon. Nodules occur in 25% of patients with rheumatoid arthritis, and are almost always associated with seropositive disease. Common sites are bony prominences and juxta-articular regions.

7. Generalized wasting of the small muscles of the hands may be due to disuse atrophy. During inspection, kneel down to examine the palm from the side, looking specifically for wasting of the thenar or hypothenar eminence suggesting median or ulnar nerve entrapment respectively.

8. Vasculitis may be a feature of rheumatoid arthritis, but also a feature of other causes of polyarthritis such as polyarthritis nodosum, ANCA-associated vasculitides (Wegener's granulomatosis, Churg-Strauss syndrome and microscopic polyangiitis), and cryoglobulinaemia.

9. Tenosynovitis is one of the most common abnormalities of the hand in rheumatoid arthritis. Inflammation of the tendon and tendon sheath causes thickening and nodule formation on the flexor tendon sheath, resulting in trapping of the tendon in a fixed position—'triggering'. This should not be confused with deQuervain's disease, which is tenosynovitis of the tendons of the thumb causing pain

over the radial wrist. Reproduction of pain with Finkelstein's test is diagnostic for deQuervain's disease. This is performed by flexion of the thumb into the palm, followed by ulnar deviation of the wrist.

10. Purpura may reflect underlying vasculitis or steroid use. Look for other features of steroid use, such as atrophic skin, cushingoid appearance, and proximal myopathy.

11. Entrapment neuropathies may occur due to synovitis around the flexor tendons. Test for median, ulnar, and radial nerve function (see Cases 60 Ulnar Nerve Palsy, 61 Radial Nerve Palsy, and 62 Medial Nerve Palsy). Look for a scar over the wrist suggesting previous carpal tunnel decompression.

    (a) **Median nerve**: wasting of the thenar eminence, weakness of abductor pollicis brevis, decreased sensation over median border of hand

    (b) **Ulnar nerve**: wasting of the hypothenar eminence, weakness of finger abduction, decreased sensation over ulnar border of hand

    (c) **Radial nerve**: wrist drop, weakness of wrist dorsiflexion, decreased sensation over first dorsal interosseous.

12. Joint tenderness, swelling, stiffness, and pain on movement are features of active inflammation in rheumatoid arthritis.

13. Assessment of functional state is *essential*. Ask the patient to perform simple hand tasks, i.e. unbuttoning clothes, writing, or picking up coins from your outstretched palm.

14. Having made the diagnosis, it is important to comment on the degree of active inflammation and functional impairment. State the presence or absence of signs of other connective tissue disease (systemic sclerosis, dermatomyositis, SLE). Tell the examiner, that you would like to look for other manifestations of the disease:

    (a) **Musculoskeletal**: examine other joints (shoulder, elbows, knees, and feet)

    (b) **Cervical spine**: atlantoaxial subluxation (cervical myelopathy)

    (c) **Eyes**: episcleritis, scleritis, scleromalacia perforans, cataracts, Sjogren's syndrome

    (d) **Anaemia**: conjunctival pallor (the causes of anaemia in rheumatoid arthritis are listed below)

    (e) **Lungs**: pleural effusions, pulmonary fibrosis, Caplan's syndrome, bronchiectasis

    (f) **Heart**: pericarditis

    (g) **Skin**: pyoderma gangrenosum

    (h) **Abdomen**: splenomegaly (Felty's syndrome), hepatosplenomegaly (secondary amyloidosis)

    (i) **Kidneys**: nephrotic syndrome (oedema and proteinuria)

    (j) **Nervous system**: mononeuritis multiplex, polyneuropathy

Questions commonly asked by examiners?

Do you know of any diagnostic criteria for rheumatoid arthritis?

The American College of Rheumatology (ACR) have developed diagnostic criteria, primarily for the purposes of categorizing research rather than clinical use. Indeed, most patients have an insidious onset of fever, malaise, and arthralgia before the onset of joint swelling, and do not fulfil these criteria until they have advanced disease. A small proportion of patients (approximately 10%) have rapidly progressive disease, with an acute onset of synovitis and extra-articular manifestations.

The American College of Rheumatology criteria (1987) require at least 4 of the following to be present for the classification of RA:

- Morning stiffness >1 hour*
- Symmetrical joint involvement*
- Arthritis affecting ≥3 joints*
- Involvement of small joints of the hands*

---

* present for ≥6 weeks

- Positive rheumatoid factor
- Rheumatoid nodules
- Radiographic evidence

What do you know about rheumatoid factor?

Rheumatoid factor is an antibody, typically IgM, against the constant portion (Fc) of the body's own IgG. It is present in 70–75% of patients with RA, but also occurs in other connective tissue diseases such as Sjogren's syndrome and SLE, in chronic bacterial infections, malignancy in almost all patients with mixed essential cryoglobulinaemia due to hepatitis C. Up to 5% of normal individuals also have rheumatoid factor, hence the positive predictive value of the test is low in an unselected population.

Seropositive RA has a different clinical course to seronegative RA, characterzed by aggressive joint disease and extra-articular manifestations such as rheumatoid nodules and vasculitis.

Do you know of any other serological tests for rheumatoid arthritis?

Anti-cyclic citrullinated peptide (anti-CCP) antibodies are more specific for RA than rheumatoid factor (90% specificity), and may be more sensitive in early RA (60% sensitivity) preceding the development of overt arthritis and rheumatoid factor. Neither rheumatoid factor nor anti-CCP antibodies vary with disease activity, and hence are only useful diagnostically and not for disease monitoring.

Do you know of any poor prognostic markers in rheumatoid arthritis?

Poor prognostic factors in RA include a positive serum test for rheumatoid factor, the presence of anti-CCP antibodies, early radiographic evidence of erosive disease, impaired functional status, and persistently active synovitis with high levels of disease activity. These patients may be considered for early use of biological agents (see below).

What are the possible causes of anaemia in a patient with rheumatoid arthritis?

- Anaemia of chronic disease
- Iron-deficiency (gastro-intestinal blood loss due to NSAIDs)
- Folate deficiency secondary to methotrexate
- Pernicious anaemia (associated autoimmune disease)
- Bone marrow suppression (gold, sulphasalzine, methotrexate, and penicillamine)
- Felty's syndrome
- Autoimmune haemolytic anaemia
- Anaemia of renal disease

How can the eyes be affected be rheumatoid arthritis?

- Episcleritis
- Scleritis
- Scleromalacia (perforans)
- Keratoconjunctivitis sicca
- Sjogren's syndrome
- Extra-ocular muscle tenosynovitis, or paralysis due to mononeuritis multiplex
- Penicillamine-induced myasthenia gravis
- Steroid-induced cataracts
- Chloroquine-induced corneal deposits or retinopathy

How do you differentiate between scleritis and episcleritis?

Episcleritis is painless, whereas scleritis is painful.

What are the causes of renal involvement in rheumatoid arthritis?

Renal disease secondary to disease process

- Membranous glomerulonephritis
- Mesangioproliferative glomerulonephritis
- Mesangiocapillary glomerulonephritis
- Chronic tubulointerstitial nephritis
- Renal amyloidosis

Renal disease secondary to drug therapy

- Membranous glomerulonephritis (gold or penicillamine)
- Renal amyloidosis
- Acute tubulointerstitial nephritis (NSAIDs)
- Renal papillary necrosis (analgesic abuse)
- Minimal change disease (NSAIDs)

What are the principles of management of rheumatoid arthritis?

Treatment for RA is commenced *early* to suppress inflammation and prevent the development of deformity and disability. Therefore, most patients should receive treatment *before* they meet the ACR diagnostic criteria for RA. Early treatment relies on early diagnosis, which requires specific tests (e.g. anti-CCP antibodies) and skilled clinical assessment of synovitis.

Life expectancy for patients with RA is shortened by 5–10 years, although patients that respond to therapy may have lower mortality rates. The excess mortality is due to complications of the disease (e.g. vasculitis, amyloidosis, cardiovascular disease) as well as adverse effects of therapy (e.g. infection, gastrointestinal (GI) bleeding).

General measures

- **Patient education**—improves psychological symptoms, and may improve disability and pain scores.
- **Physiotherapy**—pain and stiffness may lead to disuse, with consequent loss of joint mobility, contractures, and muscle atrophy. Both aerobic exercises and exercises to increase muscle strength are of benefit in preserving joint function and preventing complications such as cardiovascular disease and osteoporosis.
- **Occupational therapy**—upper limb function may be optimized by the use of splints or assistive devices. Gait may be improved by appropriate footwear.
- **Bone protection**—RA causes loss of bone density *independent* of corticosteroid use. All patients should receive 1000mg of calcium and 800 units of vitamin D daily, with dietary supplementation if necessary. The Royal College of Physicians recommend osteoporosis prophylaxis with an anti-resorptive agent for high-risk patients (e.g. aged 65 or over, or a previous fragility fracture), and bone density measurement for patients who are likely to remain on steroids for at least 3 months.[1]
- **Vaccination**—Patients on immunosuppressive drugs should receive annual pneumococcal and influenza vaccines. Live vaccines should be avoided.

Pharmacological treament

Drugs used in the treatment of RA include analgesics, NSAIDs, corticosteroids, disease modifying anti-rheumatic drugs (DMARDs), and biological agents. DMARDs are the mainstay of management of early RA, since early intervention has been shown to delay disease progression and disability.

An initial treatment regimen may include an NSAID, short-course corticosteroids, and methotrexate either alone or in combination with another DMARD, with escalation to biological therapy if there is an inadequate response at 3 months.

- **Corticosteroids**—These are used to induce remission in symptomatic patients, whilst awaiting a clinical response to slower-acting DMARDs. Short-term may use may induce remission for up to six months, although prolonged use is associated with decreased efficacy and glucocorticoid side-effects. If the disease is mono/oligo-articular then intra-articular steroid injection may be used. However, patients with polyarthritis require either depot intra-muscular injection or oral therapy.

- **DMARDs**—Several DMARDs are used in the treatment of rheumatic disease. There is little evidence for the superiority of one agent over another, aside from combination regimens in which methotrexate-containing combinations have greater efficacy. For this reason methotrexate, either alone or in combination, is the first-line therapy. As well as decreasing disease progression and disability, methotrexate has also been shown to decrease overall mortality and cardiovascular death in RA. DMARDs for rheumatoid arthritis can be summarized as follows:

Drug	Side-effects	Monitoring
Sulphasalazine	Nausea, rash, neutropenia, thrombocytopenia, liver function abnormalities	Three-monthly blood count and liver function
Methotrexate	Nausea, mouth ulcers, neutropenia, thrombocytopenia, abnormal liver function, pneumonitis	Baseline CXR, monthly cell count and liver function
Leflunomide	Abnormal liver function, neutropenia, thrombocytopenia, diarrhoea, hypertension, alopecia	Blood pressure monitoring, two-monthly cell count and liver function
Azathioprine	Nausea, neutropenia, thrombocytopenia, abnormal liver function,	Check thiopurine methyltranserase level before starting—predicts bone marrow toxicity. Monthly cell count and liver function.
Sodium Aurothiomalate (gold)	Skin rash, mouth ulcers, neutropenia, proteinuria (membranous glomerulonephritis (GN))	Initial test dose. Cell count and renal function with each injection.
Hydroxychloroquine	Nausea, corneal deposits, retinopathy, skin rash	Annual visual acuity
Ciclosporin	Renal impairment, hypertension, abnormal liver function	Blood pressure monitoring, therapeutic drug level monitoring.

- **Biological therapy**—Agents are available which antagonize TNF-α (tumour necrosis factor-α), either as monoclonal antibodies against the cytokine (infliximab, adaluminab), or as a recombinant soluble TNF receptor (etanercept). Other agents used for RA include an IL-1 receptor antagonist (anakinra), and a B-cell depleting monoclonal antibody (rituximab). Anti-TNF drugs are similar in efficacy to methotrexate alone, although combination therapy with methotrexate is more effective than monotherapy. The drugs are generally well-tolerated and are more rapid in onset than DMARDs, but disadvantages include cost, risk of tuberculosis and other opportunistic infections, and a possible association with hepatosplenic T-cell lymphoma (see Case 109 Psoriatic Arthropathy). Currently, approximately 5% of RA patients receive biological therapy.

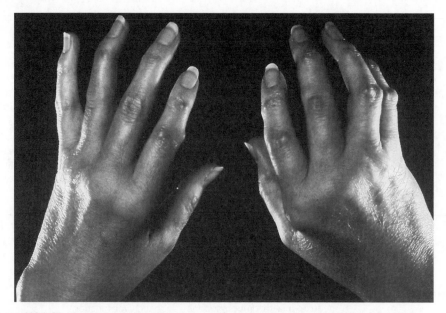

Figure 108.1 Rheumatoid hands. Note the symmetrical soft tissue swelling of the 2nd and 3rd metacarpophalangeal joints. There is a swan neck deformity of the left ring finger and ulnar deviation at the metacarpophalageal joints. There is wasting of the small muscles of the hand and several rheumatoid nodules can be seen.
Reproduced from Warrell et al. Oxford Textbook of Medicine, Volume 3, 4th edn. 2003, with permission from Oxford University Press.

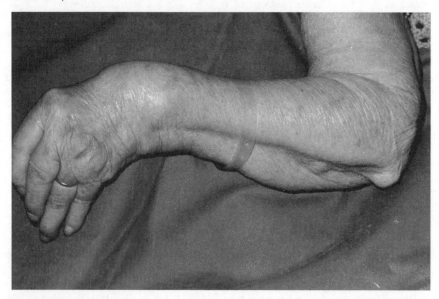

Figure 108.2 Ulnar deviation at the metacarpophalangeal joints and rheumatoid nodule at the elbow.

Case 109 ◆ **Psoriatic Arthropathy**

CASE PRESENTATION

There is an **asymmetrical arthropathy** *of the hands mainly involving the* **distal interphalangeal joints**.[1] *There is* **nail pitting, onycholysis, transverse ridging**, *and* **subungual hyperkeratosis**.[2] *In addition, there are well-defined* **erythematous plaques** *with* **silvery white scales** *over the* **extensor surfaces**.[3]

The diagnosis is **psoriatic arthropathy** *and* **psoriasis**.[4,5]

Clinical notes

1. Psoriatic arthropathy can present in 5 distinct patterns (see below). Asymmetrical, distal, oligoarthropathy was thought to be the most common presentation until recently. However, the most common presentation is now recognized to be a symmetrical polyarthropathy, similar to rheumatoid arthritis.

2. Examine carefully for nail changes that occur in 80% of patients with psoriatic arthropathy. Nail pitting, onycholysis, and transverse ridging are three features of nail involvement that should be noted. A direct correlation exists between the number of pits and the diagnosis of psoriatic arthropathy. Onycholysis is the separation of the nail plate from the nail bed. When skin and joint involvement begin simultaneously, nail changes are often present at the onset.

3. If psoriasis is not obvious over the extensor surfaces, it is important to examine at the scalp, navel, and behind the ears. Look carefully for plaques over sites of trauma (**Koebner phenomenon**). Inverse psoriasis is a variant of psoriasis that appears on the flexor surfaces and affects intertriginous areas, i.e. axillae, inguinal folds, infra-mammary creases, with minimal scaling.

4. Psoriatic arthropathy can occur with minimal skin involvement. In 20% of cases, the arthropathy precedes the onset of psoriasis, in some cases by up to 20 years. Similarly, psoriasis may be present without evidence of arthropathy, as only 5–8% of patients with psoriasis develop psoriatic arthropathy.

5. If time allows, ask the examiner whether other systems may be examined to demonstrate other systemic associations of psoriasis:

   (a) Musculoskeletal: gout (psoriasis is associated with hyperuricaemia)

   (b) Cardiovascular: aortitis and aortic regurgitation

   (c) Respiratory: apical lung fibrosis (rare)

   (d) Eyes: conjunctivitis, uveitis

Questions commonly asked by examiners

What is the link between psoriasis and psoriatic arthropathy?

There is no evidence to suggest a link between any particular subtype psoriasis or severity of psoriasis with psoriatic arthropathy. Psoriatic arthropathy can occur with minimal skin involvement. In 20% of cases, the arthropathy precedes the onset of psoriasis, in some cases by up to 20 years. Similarly, psoriasis may be present without evidence of arthropathy, as only 5–8% of patients with psoriasis develop psoriatic arthropathy.

What are the patterns of joint involvement in psoriatic arthropathy?

Pattern of joint involvement	Notes
Asymmetrical oligoarthritis, involving mainly the DIP joints	• Occurs in 25% of cases, although most patients progress to a polyarticular arthritis with time • Usually affects the hands and feet first, and may cause inflammation of both the flexor tendon and synovium leading to the 'sausage' appearance of dactylitis
Symmetrical polyarthritis, involving the PIP and MCP joints with sparing of DIP joints, i.e. rheumatoid pattern	• The most common form, occurs in 60–80% of cases • This can be clinically indistinguishable from RA, but rheumatoid factor and anti-CCP antibodies are typically *absent* • Other differentiating features from RA are absence of subcutaneous nodules, and some degree of asymmetry • Can affect hands, wrists, feet, and ankles
DIP arthritis	• Although considered a classical presentation of psoriatic arthropathy, this form only affects 5–10% of patients, mostly males • Associated nail involvement and nail bed swelling (paronychia) may make appreciation of distal joint arthritis difficult
Arthritis mutilans	• Aggressive, deforming arthritis, affecting 1–5% of patients • Resorption of bone with dissolution of joint leads to 'telescoping' of digits within redundant overlying skin.
Spondylitis +/– sacroiliitis	• This occurs in 20–40% of patients, mostly males • Spondylitis may occur with or without sacroiliitis. Vertebral involvement is asymmetrical (symmetrical in ankylosing spondylitis)

What do you know about the genetics of psoriatic arthropathy?

Patients with psoriatic arthropathy have an increased frequency of HLA-B27 and HLA-B7 antigens, although the association is not as strong as with ankylosing spondylitis or reactive arthritis. However, in the presence of spondylitis associated with psoriasis, 60–70% of cases are HLA-B27 positive.

Aside from the skin lesions, which features distinguish rheumatoid arthritis from psoriatic arthropathy?

	Rheumatoid arthritis	Psoriatic arthropathy
Epidemiology Clinical features	• More common in women • Sparing of distal joints • Symmetrical • Tenderness *precedes* deformity • No enthesopathy	• Equal sex distribution • Distal joints commonly involved • Asymmetry, even in polyarthritis • Less tender, so may *present* with deformity • Enthesitis, spinal involvement and dactylitis may occur

	Rheumatoid arthritis	Psoriatic arthropathy
Radiology	• Periarticular swelling, joint erosions, juxtaarticular osteoporosis, and uniform joint space narrowing	• Early deformity, with bone lysis and telescoping of digits, causing the 'pencil in cup' appearance
Serology	• Rheumatoid factor in 70% • Anti-CCP antibodies in 60%	• Rheumatoid factor in 10% • Anti-CCP antibodies in 15%
Extra-articular manifestations	• Rheumatoid nodules in seropositive disease	• Rheumatoid nodules typically absent
Genetics	• Weak association with HLA-DR4 and TNF-α polymorphisms	• Strong association of psoriatic spondylitis with HLA-B27

Aside from the skin lesions, which features distinguish the other spondyloarthropathies from psoriatic arthropathy?

Psoriatic arthropathy is classified with the spondyloarthropathies because of the presence of spondylitis in up to 40% of patients, the occurrence of extra-articular features common to the spondyloarthropathies (iritis, colitis, aortic root inflammation), and the association with HLA-B27. However, psoriatic arthropathy can be distinguished from the other spondyloarthropathies by the presence of peripheral arthritis, the asymmetry of spinal involvement, and a lesser degree of pain.

What do you understand by the term 'enthesitis'?

Enthesitis refers to inflammation of the site of insertion of ligaments, tendons, joint capsule, or fascia to bone. Enthesitis is relatively specific for spondyloarthropathy, and the most common sites of inflammation are the insertion of the Achilles tendon (Achilles tendonitis) and the insertion of the plantar fascia ligament to the calcaneus (plantar fasciitis).

And by the term 'dactylitis'?

Dactylitis is characterized by 'sausage-like' swelling of the finger or toe, due to inflammation of the tendon sheath and soft tissues. Dactylitis is a feature of spondyloarthropathy, but is not specific and may also be caused by tuberculosis, syphilis, sarcoidosis, and sickle-cell disease. Fusiform swelling of the digits may also occur due to soft tissue swelling in gout.

What are the principles of management of psoriatic arthropathy?

General measures
- Patient education
- Physiotherapy
- Occupational therapy

Pharmacological treatment
- Analgesics
- NSAIDs (in some patients NSAIDs may worsen psoriasis)
- Corticosteroids—Intra-articular steroid injections for single troublesome joints. Avoid systemic steroids, since skin disease may flare on steroid withdrawal.
- DMARDs—methotrexate, sulphasalazine, and cyclosporin are the most commonly used DMARDs. They are effective in treating skin symptoms, and the symptoms of peripheral arthritis, but not axial symptoms. Moreover, no studies have evaluated their efficacy in preventing or retarding progression of joint damage.

- *Biological therapy*—anti-TNF-α therapy with etanercept, infliximab, and adalimumab has been shown to improve skin disease, joint disease, and disability in psoriatic arthropathy.
- *Antimalarials*—Chloroquine and hydroxychloroquine were previously avoided due to concerns about worsening psoriasis and precipitating exfoliative dermatitis. Recent case-controlled studies have not confirmed this association, although these agents are still rarely used.

What are the indications for anti-TNFα drug therapy?

Condition	Drug(s)	Indication for therapy
Rheumatoid arthritis*	Infliximab Etanercept Adalimumab	Active rheumatoid arthritis not responding to methotrexate and one other DMARD
Juvenile idiopathic arthritis*	Etanercept	Children aged 4–-17 years with at least 5 joints affected Poor response to, or cannot tolerate methotrexate
Psoriatic arthropathy*	Etanercept (1st line) Infliximab	≥3 tender joints *and* ≥3 swollen joints Poor response to ≥2 disease modifying anti-rheumatic drugs
Psoriasis*	Infliximab Adalimumab Etanercept	Severe psoriasis refractory to ≥2 systemic treatments and photochemotherapy
Ankylosing spondylitis*	Adalimumab Etanercept (Infliximab is no longer recommended)	Active spinal disease not responding to ≥2 NSAIDs
Crohn's Disease**	Infliximab	Severe and active Crohn's disease, or fistulating Crohn's disease, in patients unable to tolerate or refractory to immunomodulators, and in whom surgical intervention is inappropriate.

* Currently recommended by NICE guidelines
** Unlicensed indication, but evidence of benefit. NICE has *not* approved the use of infliximab in subacute ulcerative colitis

What are the adverse effects of anti-TNFα drug therapy?

- **Serious infections (e.g. tuberculosis)**—incidence 3.6%, odds ratio 2.0[1]
- **Haematological malignancy**—incidence 0.9%, odds ratio 3.3[1]
- Nausea
- Hypersensitivity
- Worsening heart failure
- Haematological abnormalities (anaemia, leucopenia, thrombocytopenia, aplastic anaemia)

What are the contra-indications for anti-TNF-α drug therapy?

- Pregnancy and breast-feeding
- Active bacterial infection
- Active tuberculosis (requires 2 months of anti-tuberculous therapy before anti-TNF-α therapy.

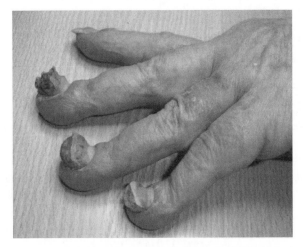

Figure 109.1 Nail changes in psoriasis. Note the gross onycholysis and subungual hyperkeratosis. Reproduced from Longmore et al. Oxford Handbook of Clinical Medicine 7th edn. 2007, with permission from Oxford University Press.

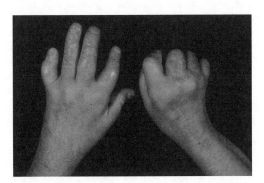

Figure 109.2 Severe psoriatic arthropathy (arthritis mutilans). Reproduced from Warrell et al. Oxford Textbook of Medicine, Volume 3, 4th edn. 2003, with permission from Oxford University Press.

• Latent tuberculosis (tuberculin testing may be falsely negative due to immunosuppression, so patients with risk factors should receive isoniazid for 6 months alongside anti-TNF-α therapy).[2]

• Septic arthritis in previous 12 months

• Congestive cardiac failure

• Demyelinating disease

References

1. T Bongartz et al. Anti-TNF antibody therapy in rheumatoid arthritis and the risk of serious infections and malignancies. JAMA. 2006; 295: 2275–85.

2. Ormerod LP et al. BTS recommendations for assessing risk, and for managing M tuberculosis infection and disease in patients due to start anti-TNF alpha treatment. Thorax. 2005; 60(10): 800–5.

Case 110 ◆ **Ankylosing Spondylitis**

CASE PRESENTATION

*This patient has a **protuberant abdomen**,[1] and **severe kyphosis**[2] with a 'question mark' posture. There is **decreased cervical movement**[3] in all directions. There is also **decreased spinal movement**, as evidenced by an **increased occiput to wall distance**,[4] and decreased chest expansion.[5] There is no evidence of psoriasis.[6]*

*The diagnosis is **ankylosing spondylitis**.[7] I would like to perform the **modified Schober's test** to further assess spinal mobility.[8] I would also like to examine for aortic valve disease and lung fibrosis, and ask about heel pain.[9]*

Clinical notes

1. The patient may be seated initially, making the underlying kyphosis and deformity difficult to spot! In any Station 5 'short case' where you are unsure how to proceed, begin by looking for facial, skeletal, and dermatological abnormalities, and then ask the patient to stand. These manoeuvres may reveal a sign such as short stature or kyphosis, which would otherwise not be apparent (see Case 107 Pseudohypoparathyroidism). In this case, the only clue with the patient seated may be the protuberant abdomen, which is a consequence of kyphosis (be careful how you present this!).

2. Having asked the patient to stand, look from the side to assess the degree of kyphosis. The question mark posture is due to loss of the cervical and lumbar lordosis, with increased thoracic kyphosis.

3. Now assess cervical movement, by asking the patient to 'look up, and down, and now to the left and the right'. Unlike mechanical spinal disease, mobility is decreased symmetrically in both anterior and lateral planes.

4. Proceed to ask the patient to stand with their back to the wall (Flesche's test). Assess the distance from the wall to the patient's occiput. Healthy patients should be able to touch the wall with their occiput. The distance between the wall and the occiput is a measure of flexion deformity of the upper spine.

5. Chest expansion is measured at the level of the 4th intercostal space with the patient's hands behind their head. Whilst the candidate is not expected to quantitatively measure chest expansion in the examination, a normal expansion is usually greater than 5cm, and less than 2.5cm is considered abnormal. However, this test has poor sensitivity for spinal disease, and is limited by pleuritic pain due to enthesitis of intercostal tendon insertions.

6. Finish by briefly looking at the nails and the hairline for evidence of psoriasis, which can present with spinal disease, although unlike ankylosing spondylitis the distribution is usually asymmetrical.

7. Sacroiliitis can be demonstrated by eliciting tenderness on palpation of the sacroiliac joints, although you will not be expected to perform this in the examination.

8. Again, you will not be expected to perform the modified Schober's test in the examination, but you should be aware of the details of the test. The test is performed by marking the level of the posterior iliac spines, at the level of the 'dimples of Venus'. Additional marks are made 10cm above and 5cm below this point, and the patient is asked to bend maximally forwards. The distance between the upper and lower marks should increase by at least 5cm in healthy adults.

9. The systemic manifestations of ankylosing spondylitis include anterior uveitis, aortic regurgitation, apical lung fibrosis, and atrioventricular conduction disease (see below). Look carefully in the infraclavicular regions for permanent pacemaker scars. Mention the possibility of anterior uveitis if the patient clearly has a red eye during the examination.

Questions commonly asked by examiners?

What is the definition of ankylosing spondylitis?

Ankylosing spondylitis is defined as symptomatic sacroiliitis (persistent pain and stiffness for >3 months) associated with morning stiffness and improvement on exercise or worsening with rest.

What are the systemic manifestations of ankylosing spondylitis?

The complications of ankylosing spondylitis can be remembered as the six 'A's.

- **Anterior uveitis**—affects up to 40% of patients
- **Aortic regurgitation**—mitral valve prolapse can also occur
- **Atrioventricular conduction defects**—affects up to 10% of patients
- **Apical pulmonary fibrosis**—costovertebral rigidity also contributes to a restrictive lung defect
- **Atlanto-axial subluxation**—neurological sequelae may result from atlanto-axial subluxation, fractures of ankylosed spine, or cauda equina syndrome
- **Achilles tendonitis**—enthesitis is a feature of the disease, particularly Achilles tendonitis and plantar fasciitis
- **Amyloidosis**—ankylosing spondylitis is a rare cause of secondary amyloidosis

Are the peripheral joints involved in ankylosing spondylitis?

Peripheral joint involvement occurs in at some stage in 20–30% of patients, particularly in patients with juvenile-onset disease. The knees and hips are most commonly affected.

What do you know about the genetics of ankylosing spondylitis?

The HLA-B27 antigen is present in 95% of Caucasian patients with ankylosing spondylitis. By contrast, HLA-B27 is present in 8% of healthy adults, and only 6% of patients with HLA-B27 develop ankylosing spondylitis, implying that the allele confers an 80-fold increased relative risk. The mechanism by which HLA-B27 confers an increased risk of disease remains unclear.

Testing for HLA-B27 is unnecessary, since the diagnosis is usually clinically and radiologically apparent.

How does one diagnose ankylosing spondylitis?

The hallmark of the disease is sacroiliitis. Patients with a history of back pain and morning stiffness, which is relieved by exercise or worsed with rest, should undergo plain radiography of the sacroiliac joints. Plain radiography is usually sensitive enough to demonstrate sacroiliitis, and severity is graded from 0 (normal) to IV (fused). If plain radiography is normal but suspicion remains high, MRI is warranted, since it is the most sensitive and specific investigation for sacroiliitis.

Inflammatory markers, such as erythrocyte sedimentation rate (ESR) and C-reactive protein (CRP), are only elevated in 50% of patients.

What do you understand by the term 'seronegative arthritis'?

Seronegative arthritis refers to a group of overlapping conditions, such as psoriatic arthropathy, enteropathic arthritis, ankylosing spondylitis, and reactive arthritis (remembered by the pneumonic PEAR). The conditions are characterized by:

- Asymmetric oligoarthritis, particularly affecting the spine
- Association with HLA-B27 and anterior uveitis
- Absence of rheumatoid factor

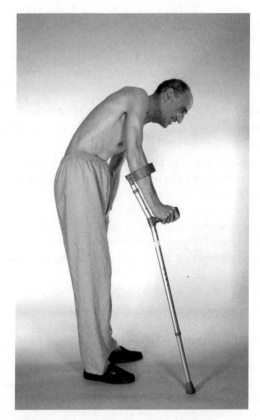

Figure 110.1 Question mark posture in ankylosing spondylitis.

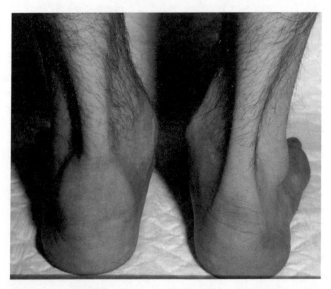

Figure 110.2 Left Achille's enthesitis in a patient with ankylosing spondylitis. Reproduced from Watts et al. Oxford Desk Reference Rheumatology. 2009, with permission from Oxford University Press.

What is the management strategy for ankylosing spondylitis?

General measures

- *Patient education*—genetic counselling is relevant, since the risk of transmitting the HLA-B27 antigen to offspring is 50%, and these children have a 1:3 risk of developing the disease, hence the overall risk is 1:6.
- *Physiotherapy*—is the cornerstone of management, by preserving spinal mobility.
- *Occupational therapy*

Pharmacological treatment

- *Analgesics*
- *NSAIDs*
- *Corticosteroids*—only pulsed intravenous steroids are occasionally used. Oral corticosteroids have no role in the management of ankylosing spondylitis.
- *DMARDs*—gold and penecillamine have no role in the treatment of ankylosing spondylitis. Methotrexate and sulphasalazine have some effect on peripheral disease, but not on the spine.
- *Biological therapy*—anti-TNF-α therapy adalimumab and etanercept is approved by NICE (see Case 109 Psoriatic Arthropathy).

Case 111 ◆ **Gout**

CASE PRESENTATION

*There is **asymmetrical deformity and swelling**[1] of the small joints of the hand. There are **tophi**[2] present in the hands (and feet), and also the ear. There is also an **olecranon bursa**.[3]*

*The diagnosis is **tophaceous gout**.[4,5]*

Clinical notes

1. Gout may cause inflammation of the soft tissues resembling dactylitis, and hence suggesting spondyloarthropathy or sarcoidosis. These can be differentiated by the presence of tophi and olecranon bursae.

2. Look and feel for tophi in the hands, forearms, and the ears. Tophi are an accumulation of uric acid crystals, surrounded by histiocytes, giant cells, and fibrosis. They are visible or palpable, but are not usually tender. Typical sites are the ear helix, Achilles tendon, olecranon bursa, or prepatellar bursa. Rarely, tophi have been reported to cause carpal tunnel syndrome and cardiac conduction and valvular abnormalities.

3. The most common causes of bursitis are repetitive use and trauma. Systemic causes include gout, pseudogout, rheumatoid arthritis, uraemia, hypertrophic pulmonary osteoarthropathy, and infections such as tuberculosis. Joint mobility is usually preserved, since the bursae are not continuous with the joint space. Aspiration and analysis of bursal fluid will distinguish septic and crystal bursitis.

4. Gout may present as an acute mono/oligo-arthritis, or as chronic tophaceous gout. Acute gout is unlikely to occur in the MRCP (PACES) examination, since the condition is extremely painful!

However, acute gout is more common than tophaceous gout in clinical practice, hence the candidate must be familiar with the investigation and management of mono/oligo-arthritis.

5. Remember to include an assessment of the degree of active inflammation and functional state in your presentation.

Questions commonly asked by examiners?

What is the differential diagnosis of a single, inflamed joint?

* Septic arthritis—gonococcal or non-gonococcal
* Crystal arthritis—gout or pseudogout
* Spondyloarthritis
* Mycobacterial or fungal infection
* Osteoarthritis
* Systemic conditions e.g. Still's disease, rheumatic fever
* Lyme disease

How would you assess a patient with monoarthritis?

Septic arthritis must be considered in every patient with monoarthritis. The history does not reliably distinguish between causes of monoarthritis, however the following features must be asked about:

* **Onset**—an insidious onset is inconsistent with acute gout or bacterial arthritis, but atypical infection, chronic gout, and spondyloarthropathy must be considered.
* **Fever**—may occur in infection, crystal arthritis, and systemic conditions such as Still's disease and rheumatic fever.
* **Previous joint disease**—may suggest the diagnosis, but chronic injury leaves the joint susceptible to infection. Recent steroid injection is also a risk factor for infection.
* **History of trauma.**
* **Distribution**—gout typically affects the great toe, whereas pseudogout affects the knee, wrist, and shoulder. However, infection and systemic conditions may affect any joint.
* **Symptoms of systemic rheumatic disease**—fatigue, rash, sicca symptoms, alopecia, oral ulceration, eye symptoms, Raynaud's phenomenon.
* **Associated features**—genitourinary symptoms or recent sexual exposures may suggest a reactive or gonococcal arthritis. Gastrointestinal symptoms suggest arthritis due to recent enteric infection or inflammatory bowel disease.
* **Recent travel**—to areas endemic for Lyme disease (New Forest, Northeastern United States) and for tuberculosis.
* **Predisposing factors**—for gout (renal failure, recent chemotherapy, hypertension treatment) and pseudogout (haemochromatosis, hypothyroidism, hyperparathyroidism).

Patients with a clinical suspicion of septic arthritis must have urgent joint aspiration performed for diagnosis. Septic arthritis typically causes a large effusion and decreased range of movement, although these may be absent if the patient is immunosuppressed or the joint is prosthetic. Investigations for monoarthritis include:

* **Joint aspiration:**
  * Leucocyte count, gram stain, and culture are performed for infection (the sensitivity of gram stain is only 60%, so empirical antimicrobial treatment may be required until culture results are known)
  * Polarized light microscopy is performed for crystal arthropathy
* **Blood cultures** (if septic arthritis is suspected)
* **Rectal, cervical, urethral, pharyngeal, and skin lesion cultures** (may reveal gonococcus)

What is the role of serum uric acid levels in the diagnosis of acute gout?

Measurement of serum uric acid levels are of little use to diagnose acute gout, since values may be normal in an acute attack, and conversely asymptomatic hyperuricaemia is relatively common and may co-exist with other causes of monoarthritis.

What is the pathophysiology of gout?

Uric acid is produced by the breakdown of purines in the liver by the enzyme *xanthine oxidase*. The plasma concentration of uric acid is determined by purine concentration (from diet, breakdown of cellular nucleoproteins, and *de novo* synthesis), *xanthine oxidase* activity, and uric acid elimination by the kidneys and gastrointestinal tract. Hyperuricaemia may occur due to decreased renal uric acid elimination or increased purine production:

Decreased uric acid excretion	Increased purine production
Idiopathic (primary hyperuricaemia)	Idiopathic
Hypertension	Lymphoproliferative and myeloproliferative disorders
Increased levels of organic acids	Chemotherapeutic drugs
(exercise, alcohol, starvation, ketoacidosis)	
Chronic renal disease	Secondary polycythaemia
Dehydration	Severe exfoliative dermatitis
Drugs:	Glycogen storage diseases
Diuretics	
ACE inhibitors	
Aspirin (low dose)	
Ciclosporin, tacrolimus	
Pyrazinamide	

The serum uric acid concentration is the major determinant of the risk of developing gout. Diets rich in meat and seafood increase the risk of developing gout by 50%, although diets containing purine-rich vegetables do not carry the same risk, and diets containing dairy products are associated with a reduced risk of gout due to the uricosuric effect of dairy proteins.

Acute attacks may be provoked by dietary excess, alcohol, systemic illness, physical exercise, drugs (see table above), or the initiation of uricosuric therapy or a xanthine oxidase inhibitor (since acute changes in serum urate can cause arthritis). The precipitation of monosodium urate crystals in joints causes inflammation and arthritis.

What is the treatment of acute gout?

- Rest
- Rehydration
- NSAIDs
    - Aspirin should be avoided since it decreases uric acid elimination unless given in high dose
- Colchicine is an alternative if NSAIDs are contraindicated due to gastrointestinal or renal disease. However, nausea, diarrhoea, and abdominal pain are common side-effects.
- Intra-articular corticosteroid injection if symptoms persist

Avoid starting allopurinol or uricosuric drugs during an acute attack, and avoid diuretics if possible. If blood pressure treatment is required, losartan is the agent of choice since it has uricosuric effects.

What is the treatment for recurrent gout?

Patients with recurrent attacks of gout, tophaceous gout, or risk factors for recurrent attacks (renal failure, family history of gout, or metabolic disease) should receive drug therapy to lower serum urate. Asymptomatic hyperuricaemia does not require therapy in the absence of a history of gout.

- Lifestyle measures to reduce alcohol and meat intake, and lose weight if obese.
- Allopurinol, a xanthine oxidase inhibitor, is the drug of choice because of convenience and low incidence of side-effects. An NSAID or colchicine should be prescribed during initiation of allopurinol, for prophylaxis against an acute attack of gout. Allopurinol is relatively contraindicated in patients on azathioprine, due to the risk of serious bone marrow suppression. Dose reduction is required in renal disease.
- A uricosuric agent such as probenecid or benzbromarone may be used as an alternative to allopurinol.

What is 'pseudogout'?

Pseudogout is a crystal arthropathy, caused by calcium pyrophosphate crystal deposition. The crystals are *positively birefringent* in polarized light, unlike uric acid crystals which are *negatively birefringent*.

Similar to gout, the most common presentation is mono/oligo-arthritis. However, the knee is the most frequently involved joint in pseudogout, unlike gout which most commonly affects the great toe. The radiographic appearance of pseudogout is *chondrocalcinosis*, due to pyrophosphate crystal deposition on articular cartilage. Clinical associations are haemochromatosis, hypothyroidism, chronic renal failure, hyperparathyroidism, and familial hypocalciuric hypercalcaemia.

	Gout	Pseudogout
Crystals	Negatively birefringent urate crystals	Positively birefringent pyrophosphate crystals
Distribution	Monoarticular: 1st MTP, ankle, knee	Oligoarticular: knee, wrist
Associations	Hyperuricaemia, chronic renal failure, drugs	Haemochromatosis, hypothyroidism, chronic renal failure

What are the renal manifestations of hyperuricaemia?

- **Urolithiasis**—uric acid stones comprise less than 10% of all renal stones, and affect less than 10% of patients with gout. However, similar factors predispose to both gout and uric acid stones, such as increased purine production and decreased renal urate excretion. Uric acid stones are not radiopaque, hence plain X-rays are unhelpful in diagnosis. Treatment involves hydration, alkalinization of the urine with potassium bicarbonate or potassium citrate, to dissolve stones, and allopurinol.
- **Chronic urate nephropathy**—typically causes mild renal impairment due to renal tubular obstruction from uric acid crystals. Most patients also have other risk factors for renal disease such as hypertension, or the metabolic syndrome.
- **Acute crystal nephropathy**—is a form of acute renal failure, due to precipitation of uric acid crystals within the collecting ducts. The most common cause is *tumour lysis syndrome*, which describes the metabolic complications of cell lysis due to chemotherapy for leukaemias and lymphomas. Patients develop hyperphosphataemia, hyperuricaemia, hypocalcaemia (due to precipitation of calcium phosphate), and hyperkalaemia. Allopurinol is used for

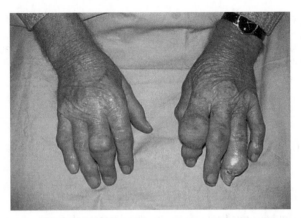

Figure 111.1 In chronic tophaceous gout, the tophi can sometimes be clinically indistinguishable from rheumatoid nodules, although they may appear as eccentric swellings. Reproduced from Hakim & Clunie. Oxford Handbook of Rheumatology. 2002, with permission from Oxford University Press.

prophylaxis during chemotherapy, along with hydration and alkalinization of the urine. Recombinant Aspergillus uricase (Rasburicase) is used for treatment.

Which are the common infective causes of arthritis?

- **Bacterial (non-gonococcal) arthritis:** The most common route of infection is through haematogenous spread. Predisposing factors are advanced age, prosthetic joints, pre-existing arthritis, intravenous drug use, indwelling venous catheters, and immunocompromised states.
- Staphylococci are the most common organism causing septic arthritis and osteomyelitis in adults. *Staph. aureus* typically infects native joints, whereas *Staph. epidermidis* infects prosthetic joints. Streptococci may cause joint infection in patients with splenic dysfunction, or with another source of streptococcal infection, such as infective endocarditis. Group A streptococci (eg. *Strep. pyogenes*, *Strep. pneumoniae*) are causative agents of rheumatic fever, although the associated arthritis is immune-mediated, polyarticular and migratory, rather than infective. *Chlamydia*
- **Gonococcal arthritis:** Arthritis is a manifestation of disseminated gonococcal infection. Patients typically present with purulent arthritis which may affect more than one joint, or a triad of dermatitis, tenosynovitis, and polyarthralgia without purulent arthritis. Gonococcus may be identified from blood cultures, from synovial fluid, or from skin, pharyngeal, cervical, urethral, and rectal swabs.
- **Mycobacterial arthritis:** *M. tuberculosis* and *M. leprae* can cause suppurative bone and joint infection. Furthermore, tuberculosis is associated with a reactive tenosynovitis and arthritis, termed Poncet's disease, developing in the presence of active tuberculosis elsewhere.
- **Lyme disease:** Arthritis is a late complication of Lyme disease. The initial infection with *Borrelia burgdorferi* is through a bite from an infected tick. Early disease is characterized by the rash of erythema chronicum migrans, followed by late cardiac, neurological, and

rheumatological manifestations. In the USA, 60% of patients develop acute monoarthritis or oligoarthritis, although Lyme arthritis is less common in Europe.

- **Viral arthritis:** Viral infections which may cause a reactive arthritis are parvovirus B19, rubella, hepatitis B, and HIV.

Case 112 ◆ **Osteoarthritis**

CASE PRESENTATION

*There is **asymmetrical bony swelling**[1] affecting the **distal interphalangeal**[2,3] and **proximal interphalangeal**[3] joints, with **squaring of the first metacarpophalangeal** joint.[4] There is no evidence of synovitis or rash.*

*There is **varus deformity of the knees**,[5] with associated **effusions** and **crepitus**.[6] The gait is **antalgic**,[7] and **Trendelenberg's sign**[8] is positive, suggesting proximal weakness of hip stabilizers.*

*The diagnosis is **osteoarthritis**.*

Clinical notes

Although there is less deformity and disability in osteoarthritis (OA), and fewer systemic signs, the candidate should adopt a similar routine for examination of the hands as outlined in Case 108 Rheumatoid Arthritis.

1. Remember to ask about joint pain before shaking the patient's hand or examining. Before touching the patient, look for walking aids or carpal tunnel splints. Now, gently place the patient's hands on a pillow, and look at the pattern of joint involvement.
2. DIP involvement suggests OA, psoriatic arthropathy, or gout. Remember to look for nail changes, and examine the hairline for rash and earlobes for tophi.
3. Bony swellings at the DIP (Heberden's nodes) and PIP (Bouchard's nodes) joints are characteristic of OA. These are tender osteophytic extensions of the joint, unlike tophi which are non-tender urate collections in the soft tissues, or rheumatoid nodules which are non-tender inflammatory lesions.
4. The first MCP joint is commonly involved in OA, particularly in females. Enlargement of this joint results in a 'squared' appearance of the hand. Remember to assess mobility of the hands, wrists, elbows, and shoulders (see Case 108 Rheumatoid Arthritis).
5. Now look briefly at the knees, noting any deformity. Varus deformity is more common in OA, since the medial compartment of the knee is most frequently affected. Palpate for warmth with the dorsum of your hand, and palpate for tenderness on the joint line. Now use the 'bulge test' to look for an effusion, since they are likely to be small in the MRCP (PACES) examination. Place your left hand above the knee, and 'milk' the suprapatella bursa towards the knee, looking for a bulge in the medial patella fossa.
6. Now place your palm on the knee joint, feeling for crepitus during passive movement of the knee.
7. An antalgic gait, or 'limp', implies a painful joint, whereby the phase of the gait is shortend to alleviate pain on the weight-bearing side. A waddling, or Trendelenberg, gait may also be present if there is bilateral weakness of hip stabilizers.
8. Trendelenberg's sign is positive if, when standing on one leg, the pelvis drops on the non-weight bearing leg, implying weakness of the hip stabilizers on the weight-bearing side.

Questions commonly asked by examiners

How would you distinguish osteoarthritis from rheumatoid arthritis?
Patients with OA have pain that is worse on movement and relieved by rest. Whilst they may have a degree of morning stiffness, this is typically less than an hour, unlike RA. Stiffness may occur following a period of activity ('gelling'), but this is less prominent than the stiffness seen in RA.

In OA, the disease is asymmetrical, and involves the DIP joints, unlike RA which is typically symmetrical and spares the DIP joints. Furthermore, OA has distinct radiological features.

What are the radiological features of osteoarthritis?
*   Joint space narrowing
*   Marginal osteophytes
*   Subchondral sclerosis
*   Subchondral cyst formation
Radiological findings are poor predictors of the degree of symptoms in a particular patient.

What are the principles of management of osteoarthritis?
General measures (see Case 108 Rheumatoid Arthritis)
*   *Patient education*—weight loss
*   *Physiotherapy*—to prevent disuse atrophy, particularly of the quadriceps
*   *Occupational therapy*

Pharmacological treatment
*   *Analgesics*
*   *NSAIDs*
*   *Corticosteroids*—Intra-articular steroid injections for single troublesome joints, although no more than 4 times per year. There is no role for systemic steroids.

Non-pharmacological treatment
*   *Arthroscopy*—this is only useful if there is a mechanical defect that can be debrided
*   *Surgery*—osteotomy for a malaligned hip or knee joint, or total joint replacement for end-stage disease

Case 113 ◆ Marfan's syndrome

CASE PRESENTATION

*This patient is **tall**,[1] with **disproportionately long limbs**[2] compared with the trunk. There is **kyphoscoliosis**[3] of the spine, and **pectus excavatum**[4] of the chest wall. The **thumb**[5] and **wrist**[6] signs are positive, confirming **arachnodactyly**. There is **hyperextensibility of the joints**.[7] There is a **high-arched palate**.[8] There are **blue sclerae**, there is **heterochromia of the irides** and **iridodonesis** (indicating lens dislocation).[9] There is **pes planus**.[10]*

*This patient has a **marfanoid body habitus**. The differential diagnosis is **Marfan's syndrome** or **homocystinuria**. I would like to assess mental status and examine for valvular heart disease.[11]*

Clinical notes

1. Start by asking the patient to stand, to demonstrate tall stature. This is a useful manoeuvre for any Station 5 case where the diagnosis is not apparent and you are unsure how to proceed. The differential diagnosis of tall stature includes endocrine conditions such as acromegaly and hyperthyroidism (before fusion of the growth plates in adolescence), and chromosomal disorders such as Klinefelter's syndrome.

2. Now ask the patient to hold their arms out to the sides, to compare arm span with height and trunk size (arm span > height). Disproportionately long limbs is termed dolichostenomelia. With long extremities the following measurements (although not expected to be objectively measured) are important to note: pubis–sole > pubis–vertex.

3. Kyphoscoliosis is common, occurring in 60% of patients.

4. Pectus excavatum or pectus carinatum may occur. Look for scars suggesting surgical correction, to preserve pulmonary and cardiac function.

5. The thumb (Steinberg) sign is positive when the thumb, when completely enclosed within the clenched hand, protrudes beyond the ulnar border.

6. The wrist (Walker) sign is positive if the 1st and 5th digits of one hand overlap when wrapped around the opposite wrist.

7. Although all joints can be hyperextensible, the digit joints are most commonly affected. One can use the Beighton's nine-point joint hypermobility scoring system to assess hyperextensibility (see Case 140 Ehlers-danlos Syndrome).

8. The high-arched palate is a consequence of the long, narrow facies of Marfan's syndrome, and a narrow maxilla. The presence of a *bifid uvula* with craniofacial abnormalities suggests Loeys-Dietz syndrome, which is associated with aortic dissection or rupture at an early age.

9. The ocular manifestations of Marfan's syndrome include blue sclerae, heterochromia of the irides, lens dislocation (usually upwards and outwards and affects 50% of patients), myopia, and retinal detachment. The first two may be easily detected, if present. Do not examine for lens displacement in the examination, since this requires pupil dilatation and slit lap examination. However, tremor of the iris (iridodonesis) indicates lens dislocation. Inspect closely for this.

10. Pes planus occurs due to the medial displacement of the medial malleolus.

11. Homocystinuria shares the skeletal and ocular features of Marfan's syndrome, although lens displacement is downwards in homocystinuria and upwards in Marfan's syndrome. Furthermore, homocystinuria is not associated with aortic root and valvular heart disease, but is associated with mental retardation, seizures, osteoporosis, livedo reticularis, and thromboembolic disease.

Questions commonly asked by examiners?

What do you know of the pathogenesis of Marfan's syndrome?

Marfan's syndrome occurs due to mutations in the fibrillin-1 gene, which is an extracellular matrix protein. Inheritance is autosomal dominant, although 25% of patients have no family history, suggesting that de novo mutations in the large fibrillin-1 gene account for these cases.

Do you know of any diagnostic criteria for Marfan's syndrome?

The Ghent criteria rely on 'major' and 'minor' clinical manifestations involving the skeletal, cardiovascular, and ocular systems. Major criteria include typical skeletal manifestations, lens displacement (by slit-lamp examination), aortic root dilatation or aortic dissection, and lumbosacral dural ectasia.

Genetic testing for fibrillin-1 mutations is possible, although a genetic abnormality alone is insufficient for diagnosis because the phenotype is variable, so major clinical manifestations are also required.

What are the main clinical features of Marfan's syndrome?

- **Cardiovascular:** Aortic root aneurysm, aortic regurgitation, and aortic dissection are the major causes of morbidity and mortality in Marfan's syndrome, and are the result of cystic medial necrosis. Aortic dilatation occurs in 70--80% of patients. The risk of aortic dissection increases when the diameter at the sinus of Valsalva exceeds 5cm, when the aortic dilatation is more extensive, when the rate of dilatation exceeds 1.5mm per year, and if there is a family history of aortic dissection. Annual surveillance and medical prophylaxis is offered to all patients (see below). Two-thirds of patients have mitral valve disease.
- **Ocular:** Lens displacement (upwards), myopia, heterochromia of the irides, blue sclerae, and retinal detachment may occur.
- **Musculoskeletal:** Joint hypermobility and kyphoscoliosis are common, leading to arthralgia and back pain in most patients. Dural ectasia is an enlargement of the neural canal (usually in the lumbosacral region), which is common in Marfan's syndrome and may contribute to back pain.
- **Respiratory:** Pectus excavatum occurs in most patients, and may cause a restrictive lung defect if severe. Spontaneous pneumothorax and apical bullae may also occur.
- **Other:** Inguinal, femoral, and incisional herniae are common. Stria atrophicae (stretch marks) often occur in the absence of marked weight change or pregnancy. Small nodules or papules can occur on the skin of the neck (Meischer's elastoma).

What are the causes of heterochromia of the irides?

- Marfan's syndrome
- Congenital Horner's syndrome
- Hirschsprung's disease
- Sturge-Webers syndrome
- Can be inherited as an autosomal dominant trait

What are the causes of a high-arched palate?

- Marfan's syndrome
- Turner's syndrome
- Friedreich's ataxia
- Tuberous sclerosis

What are the causes of lens dislocation (ectopia lentis)?

- Marfan's syndrome (up and out)
- Homocystinuria (down and in)
- Ehlers-Danlos syndrome
- Refsum's syndrome
- Weil-Marchesani syndrome
- Chronic uveitis
- Trauma

How would you assess and manage a patient with Marfan's syndrome?

Initially, all patients should undergo:

- Fibrillin-1 gene testing
- Echocardiography
- Ocular evaluation

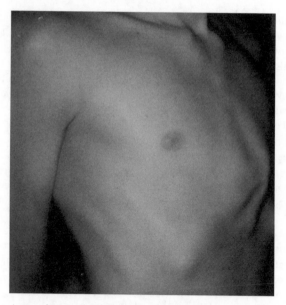

Figure 113.1 Pectus carinatum (pigeon chest). Reproduced from Longmore et al. Oxford Handbook of Clinical Medicine, 7th edn. 2007, with permission from Oxford University Press. Image courtesy of Professor Eric W. Fonkalsrud.

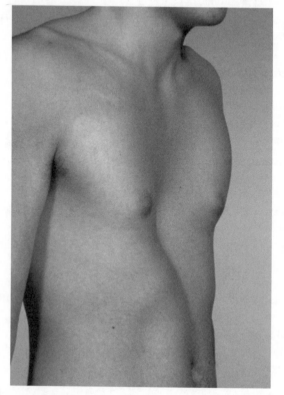

Figure 113.2 Pectus excavatum (funnel chest).

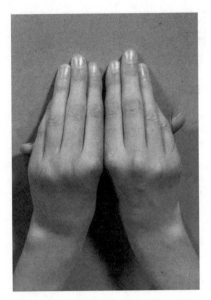

Figure 113.3 The thumb (Steinburg) sign. Reproduced from Watts et al. Oxford Desk Reference Rheumatology. 2009, with permission from Oxford University Press.

- X-ray for protrusio acetbulae*
- MRI for dural ectasia

What are the causes of dural ectasia?

- Marfan's syndrome
- Ehlers-Danlos syndrome
- Neurofibromatosis type 1
- Ankylosing spondylitis
- Trauma
- Scoliosis
- Tumours

What is the management of aortic disease in patients with Marfan's syndrome?

The European Society of Cardiology has proposed recommendations for the management of aortic disease:

1. Lifelong beta-blockade
2. Periodic routine imaging of the aorta
3. Prophylactic replacement of the aortic root before diameter exceeds 5.0cm in patients with family history of dissection
4. Prophylactic replacement of the aortic root before diameter exceeds 5.5cm
5. Moderate restriction of physical activity

---

* This is a deformity of the hip joint in which the medial wall of the acetabulum invades the pelvic cavity with medial displacement of the femoral head. The prevalence is about 50%.

Case 114 ◆ **Paget's disease**

CASE PRESENTATION

There is **enlargement of the skull**,[1] and **deformity of the long bones**,[2] particularly the **tibia**. There are scars consistent with **surgery for previous long bone fractures**.[3] This patient is also using a **hearing aid**.[4] The pulse character is normal, with no evidence of a **hyperdynamic circulation**.[5]

The diagnosis is **Paget's disease**.

Clinical notes

1. Skull enlargement occurs in the frontal and occipital areas, leading to the 'lion face' of Paget's disease, although this is another term that should be used with caution in the examination.

2. Deformities in the long bones are caused by enlargement, which leads to deformity and bowing. Typical abnormalities include anterior bowing of the tibia, and anterolateral bowing of the femur. These deformities can cause an abnormal gait, which predisposes to degenerative change in the spine. Enlargement of the long bones also leads to increased blood flow, which may be detectable by increased warmth over the long bones, although this is a subtle sign.

3. Traumatic and pathological fractures are common in Paget's disease, although they typically affect the long bones unlike other metabolic bone diseases, which more often affect the vertebrae.

4. Neurological complications may occur due to compression of cranial nerves in the skull. The 8th nerve is most commonly affected, causing sensorineural deafness in one-third of patients. Paget's disease may also affect the ossicles of the middle ear causing conductive deafness. Rarely, the 2nd, 5th and 7th nerves may be compressed in the skull, causing visual disturbance and facial weakness. Spinal disease may also cause neurological involvement by compression, or by a 'vascular steal' syndrome from the highly vascular bone causing spinal ischaemia.

5. Look for a collapsing pulse, which indicates a hyperdynamic circulation. High output heart failure can occur in Paget's disease, but is rare. Extensive skeletal involvement is required for heart failure to occur. A similar effect can occur in patients with extensive bone involvement in multiple myeloma. Other causes of high output heart failure include large arterio-venous fistulae, anaemia, thyrotoxicosis, beri-beri, and pregnancy.

Questions commonly asked by examiners?

What do you know about the epidemiology of Paget's disease?

Studies in the 1980s demonstrated a high prevalence of the disease in Lancashire towns, with markedly decreased rates in the rest of the United Kingdom and Western Europe. Furthermore, the incidence has fallen over recent years. Both of these factors suggest an environmental trigger for the disease, such as paramyxovirus infection, although the exact cause remains undetermined.

How does one diagnose Paget's disease?

Paget's disease is suspected on the basis of an elevated alkaline phosphatase, in the presence of normal vitamin D levels which exclude osteomalacia. Most patients are asymptomatic, or have chronic complaints which may not come to medical attention. An isotope bone scan is the most sensitive method of identifying pagetic bone lesions, which appear as areas of increased uptake.

What is the pathophysiology of Paget's disease?

This disorder is characterized by abnormal osseous remodelling and evolves through three stages:

- **Lytic (hot) phase:** increased osteoclastic activity (this starts at the end of the bones, except when it occurs in the tibia)
- **Intermediate (mixed) phase:** osteolytic and disorganized osteoblastic activity (the new bone is abnormal with coarsened trabeculae and cortical thickening in the cancellous and compact bone)
- **Final (cold) phase:** the woven bone is converted to dense lamellar bone

What are the causes of bowing of the tibia?

- Pseudoarthrosis of the tibia (neurofibromatosis)
- Rickets
- Fibrous dysplasia
- Fibular hemimelia
- Trauma
- Congenital

What is the treatment of Paget's disease?

Initial treatment is with analgesics and NSAIDs to treat pain. Calcitonin and bisphosphonates are used to decrease bone turnover in patients with refractory pain, or with deformity.

What is the significance of night pain in Paget's disease?

Bone tumours occur in 1% of patients with Paget's disease, most commonly osteosarcomas. These tumours present with increased pain and night pain at pagetic sites, with or without an enlarging mass. The prognosis from these lesions is poor, with a five-year survival of 10%.

What are the complications of Paget's disease?

- Cranial nerve compression
- Deafness
- High-output cardiac failure
- Pathological fractures
- Osteoarthritis
- Osteosarcoma

Case 115 ◆ Osteomalacia and Rickets

CASE PRESENTATION 1

*This patient has **kyphosis**[1] and a **waddling gait**.[2] There is evidence of a **proximal myopathy**[3] in the upper limbs. There are no features of Cushing's syndrome and there is no evidence of thyroid disease.[4] There are no features of dermatomyositis.[5]*

*This patient has a proximal myopathy. The presence of kyphosis suggests metabolic bone disease, i.e. **osteomalacia**.*

CASE PRESENTATION 2

*This patient has a **waddling gait**.[2] There is evidence of a **proximal myopathy**[3] in the upper limbs. There are **multiple skeletal deformities**, including **frontal bossing**[6] of the skull, enlargement of the costochondral junction causing **beading of the chest**,[7] and **bilateral symmetrical bowing deformities**[7] of the long bones.*

*The diagnosis is **old rickets**, with persistent skeletal abnormalities and proximal myopathy.[8]*

Clinical notes

1. Similar to other cases in Station 5, the major abnormalities may not be apparent with the patient seated. Begin by asking the patient to stand, and look from behind for scoliosis and from the side for kyphosis. The presence of kyphosis suggests metabolic bone disease or spondyloarthropathy. It is reasonable to assess cervical spine mobility to decide whether to proceed to a metabolic bone disease 'routine', or an ankylosing spondylitis 'routine'.

2. Now ask the patient to walk a short distance. A waddling gait suggests weakness of the proximal muscles that stabilize the weight-bearing hip. The pelvis drops, and the patient will lean to the weight-bearing side to maintain balance. This is the same as the Trendelenberg gait.

3. Osteomalacia causes a proximal myopathy and muscle tenderness. Elicit this by static testing of muscle power in the upper limbs, 'keep your elbows out to the sides, and don't let me move them'. The differential diagnosis of proximal myopathy includes:

    (a) Cushing's syndrome

    (b) Polymyalgia rheumatica

    (c) Hyperthyroidism

    (d) Polymyositis / dermatomyositis

    (e) Osteomalacia

    (f) Paraneoplastic syndrome

    (g) Alcohol

4. Cushing's syndrome and thyrotoxicosis can produce proximal myopathy. Although this is a musculoskeletal and not an endocrine station, it is still important to look for these endocrinopathies when assessing a patient with proximal myopathy. This can be rapidly assessed by looking for:

    (a) **Cushing's syndrome**: cushingoid facies, centripetal obesity, purpura, and striae

    (b) **Thyrotoxicosis**: goitre (thyroidectomy scar), thyroid eye disease, lid lag, tachycardia, and tremor

5. Look for Gottron papules on the hands and the characteristic heliotrope rash on the face (see Case 124 Dermatomyositis).

6. Parietal and frontal bossing of the skull occurs due to the deposition of unmineralized osteoid. Other causes of frontal bossing in adults include congenital syphilis, acromegaly, and osteopetrosis.

7. In long bones, the laying down of unmineralized osteoid at the metaphyses leads to a 'knobbly' deformity. In the chest wall this leads to the 'rachitic rosary' along the costochondral junctions, and in weight-bearing limbs this causes 'bowlegs' and 'knock knees'. Paget's disease is an important cause for bowing of the legs in the MRCP (PACES) examination. It is important to remember that Paget's disease results in unilateral bowing of the legs. Bilateral bowing can rarely occur, but even so, it will not be symmetrical. Rickets results in bilateral *and* symmetrical bowing of the legs. It is important to feel for warmth over the affected bones as, often, the affected bones in Paget's disease are warm due to increased blood flow.

8. Most of the skeletal abnormalities of rickets correct with growth, although they may persist into adulthood if the vitamin D deficiency is severe and uncorrected. Adults may have concomitant proximal myopathy if there is ongoing vitamin D deficiency.

Questions commonly asked by examiners

What is the aetiology of rickets and osteomalacia?

Bone is normally comprised of an organic *osteoid*, synthesized by osteoblasts, which is *mineralized* by the deposition of calcium and phosphate. Defective mineralization due to calcium and phosphate leads to osteomalacia and rickets.

Osteomalacia refers to unmineralized osteoid, whereas rickets refers to the consequent skeletal abnormalities. Rickets and osteomalacia occur together in childhood, causing deformity while the growth plates are open and long bones are still growing. Only osteomalacia occurs in adulthood, after the growth plates have fused.

- **Hypocalcaemic rickets**—is due to vitamin D deficiency, calcium deficiency, or rare defects in the enzymatic conversion of 25(OH)vitamin D to the active form 1,25(OH)vitamin D. Vitamin D and calcium deficiency may occur due to dietary deficiency, inadequate sunlight exposure, or malabsorption.

- **Hypophosphataemic rickets**—is almost always caused by renal phosphate wasting by renal tubular disorders such as Fanconi's syndrome. Hereditary causes of renal phosphate wasting include X-linked hypophosphataemic rickets (vitamin D-resistant rickets), which is a specific defect in tubular phosphate reabsorption.

- **Adult-onset osteomalacia**—the most common cause of osteomalacia in adults is vitamin D deficiency causing hypophosphataemia and secondary hyperparathyroidism. Drugs that inhibit mineralization, such as bisphosphonates (which are used to treat *osteoporosis*—see below) and aluminium, may cause osteomalacia. Barbiturates also interfere with vitamin D metabolism and may cause osteomalacia.

What are the radiological features of osteomalacia?

The characteristic radiological findings of osteomalacia are *Looser's zones*. These are narrow, radiolucent lines with sclerotic borders that occur in the pelvis or femoral neck, and are often termed 'pseudofractures'. They may represent stress fractures that have been repaired with inadequately mineralized osteoid. Reduced bone density, with thinning of the cortex, also occurs but is a non-specific finding. Vertebral compression fractures occur less frequently than in osteoporosis.

What is the difference between osteoporosis and osteomalacia?

	Osteoporosis	Osteomalacia
Pathology	Decreased bone mass due to loss of osteoid and mineralization	Decreased mineralization but preserved osteoid
Aetiology	Low peak bone mass and increased bone resorption	Calcium, phosphate, or vitamin D deficiency
Clinical features	No clinical manifestations until fracture	Proximal myopathy and bone pain
Diagnosis	Low bone density* as measured by dual energy X-ray absorptiometry	• Hypocalcaemia • Hypophosphataemia • Vitamin D deficiency • Secondary hyperparathyroidism

Disease associations	• Post-menopausal
	• Thyrotoxicosis
	• Hypogonadism
	• Corticosteroid excess
	• Cigarette smoking
		• Vitamin D deficiency
		  ◆ malabsorption
		  ◆ dietary deficiency
		  ◆ inadequate sun exposure
		• Renal tubular disease

	Osteoporosis	Osteomalacia
Treatment	• Calcium / vitamin D • Bisphosphonates • Hormonal therapies Parathyroid hormone (PTH)	• Calcium / phosphate / vitamin D

* Bone density 2.5 standard deviations or more *below* that of young, adult controls (T-score <−2.5)

Can you outline the management of postmenopausal osteoporosis?

Consider excluding secondary causes of osteoporosis. Less than 10% of patients have a secondary cause, however the following investigations may be indicated:

* Multiple myeloma—protein electrophoresis and urine Bence-Jones protein
* Osteomalacia—calcium, phosphate, alkaline phsophatase, vitamin D
* Thyrotoxicosis—thyroid function tests
* Hyperparathyroidism (primary or secondary)—serum PTH
* (Male) hypogonadism—serum testosterone

Therapeutic options for osteoporosis include:

* *Smoking cessation advice*
* *Calcium and vitamin D supplementation*—unless deficiency has been clearly excluded.
* *Bisphosphonates*—act on the osteoclast to prevent bone resorption. The most common side effect is oesophagitis, although osteonecrosis of the jaw has been reported with parenteral preparations.
* *Hormonal agents*—*hormone replacement therapy* increases bone density and treats menopausal symptoms, although there is an increased risk of breast and uterine cancer, and of venous thromboembolism. *Raloxifene* is a selective-oestrogen receptor modulator, with oestrogenic effects on bone, but anti-oestrogenic effects on the endometrium and breasts. Therefore, raloxifene improves bone density, without conferring any additional risk of breast or uterine cancer, although there remains an increased risk of venous thromboembolism.
* *Recombinant PTH*—although PTH is catabolic for bone when given continuously, in intermittent administration it has been shown to increase bone density. PTH is administered by daily subcutaneous injection.

NICE guidelines (2005) for the secondary prevention of osteoporosis in postmenopausal women suggest that bisphosphonates should be used initially for the secondary prevention of osteoporosis, with raloxifene reserved for patients who are intolerant of bisphosphonates.

How can one determine the source of an isolated, elevated serum alkaline phosphatase?

Most patients with an isolated rise in alkaline phosphatase have biliary disease rather than bone disease. The most immediate way to differentiate these is to measure the serum gamma glutamyl transpeptidase (GGT), which is usually elevated in biliary disease. Alternatively, the different biliary and bone isoenzymes can be differentiated by electrophoresis, although this test is not universally available. Remember that the alkaline phosphatase is physiologically elevated in the third trimester of pregnancy, due to placental production!

Case 116 ◆ Down's Syndrome

CASE PRESENTATION

This patient has **short stature,**[1] *with* **low-set, dysplastic ears**[2] *and a* **flattened nasal bridge.**[3] *The eyes have* **upslanting palpebral fissures,**[4] **epicanthal skin folds,**[5] *and there are* **brushfield spots**[6] *on the iris. The* **neck is short,**[7] *with redundant skin behind the neck. Peripherally, there is* **generalized hypotonia, a single transverse palmar crease,** *and* **clinodactlyly of the fifth finger.**[8]

The diagnosis is **Down's syndrome.**[9]

Clinical notes

1. The differential diagnosis of short stature includes Turner's syndrome, achondroplasia, hypothyroidism, hypopituitarism, or systemic illnesses such as chronic renal failure and malabsorption.

2. The ears are typically small, with an overfolded helix.

3. This is due to a hypoplastic nasal bone.

4. Avoid the terms 'slanting eyes' or 'slit eyes'.

5. Epicanthal folds are skin folds of the upper eyelid that cover the inner corner of the eye. They are a normal finding in individuals of East Asian descent.

6. Brushfield spots are collections of connective tissue, which manifest as white/grey spots in the periphery of the iris. They can be a normal finding in infants, but occur more frequently in Down's syndrome. Refractive errors, strabismus, and nystagmus may also occur.

7. A short neck also occurs in Turner's syndrome (see Case 106 Turner's Syndrome).

8. The hands are short and broad, with a short, curved fifth finger due to hypoplasia of the middle phalynx. Abnormalities of the feet also occur, such as the 'sandal gap deformity' between the first and second toes.

9. There are many conditions associated with Down's syndrome. Not all can be looked for at the bedside (especially in the MRCP (PACES) examination), but certain associations can easily be noted, and this will demonstrate your wider understanding and undoubtedly impress examiners! Tell the examiner that you would like to look for the following associated features:

   - **Congenital heart abnormalities**: cardiovascular examination*
   - **Hypothyroidism**: assess thyroid status
   - **Diabetes**: glucose finger prick (glucose testing), fundoscopy (diabetic retinopathy)

The congenital heart abnormalities are seen in 40–50% of patients and include atrio-ventricular septal defects, patent ductus arteriosus, and tetralogy of Fallot. The patient may be clubbed and cyanosed and this will be easy to detect. If present in a patient with Down's syndrome, then this should strongly raise the suspicion of underlying cyanotic congenital heart disease.

Questions commonly asked by examiners

What are the genetics of Down's syndrome?

Down' syndrome is caused by trisomy of chromosome 21, the most common autosomal trisomy in newborns. Three types of cytogenetic abnormality result in Down's syndrome:

- Trisomy 21 (94%)—an extra copy of chromosome 21.

- Robertsonian translocation involving chromosome 21 (3–4%)—this is an unbalanced, non-reciprocal translocation between two chromosomes (i.e. two long arms or two short arms), where the unbalanced exchange may result in the addition of genetic material, such as trisomy 21.
- Trisomy 21 mosaic (2–3%)—there are two cell lines within the body, one normal and another with trisomy 21

What are the major complications of Down's syndrome?

- *Cognitive impairment / learning disability (>95%)*
- *Congenital heart disease (40–50%)*—atrio-ventricular septal defect, patent ductus arteriosus, and tetralogy of Fallot.
- *Gastrointestinal (15%)*—duodenal atresia, Hirschprung's disease, Meckel's diverticulum, imperforate anus, coeliac disease.
- *Endocrine (15%)*—hypothyroidism, type 1 diabetes mellitus.
- *Haematological malignancy (1–2%)*—Acute myeloblastic leukaemia and acute lymphoblastic leukaemia.
- *Atlanto-axial instability (2%)*
- *Infertility*—almost all males, although females are fertile
- Early inset Alzhermer's disease affects 50% by the age of 35.

How is the prenatal diagnosis of Down's syndrome made?

The risk of Down's syndrome varies with maternal age:

- 1:1500 at 20 years
- 1:800 at 30 years
- 1:270 at 35 years
- 1:100 at 40 years
- >1:50 at >45 years

The risk is 1:100 after a previously affected pregnancy.

There is a national screening programme for Down's syndrome in the United Kingdom. Serum testing and ultrasound are used as screening tools, and the risk of Down's syndrome is calculated taking into account maternal age and gestation.

Serum tests include: pregnancy associated plasma protein A (PAPP-A), β-human chorionic gonadotrophin (β-hCG), α-fetoprotein (α-FP), unconjugated oestriol, and inhibin A. Only PAPP-A and β-hCG can be used in the first trimester.

Ultrasound examines fetal nuchal translucency, which reflects fetal heart failure, and is strongly associated with chromosomal abnormalities.

Mothers with a risk of Down's syndrome >1:250 are offered diagnostic testing, using either chorionic villus sampling (if less than 13 weeks gestation) or amniocentesis (if beyond 15 weeks gestation). These tests carry a risk of miscarriage: 1–2% for chorionic villus sampling, 0.5–1% for amniocentesis.

Case 117 ◆ Osteogenesis Imperfecta

CASE PRESENTATION

This patient has **kyphoscoliosis, short stature,**[1] *with* **blue sclerae,**[2] *and* **scars consistent with previous long bone fractures.**[3] *The patient is also wearing* **hearing aids.**[4] *There is evidence of* **joint hyperextensibility.**[5] *There is no evidence of dentinogenesis imperfecta.*[6]

The diagnosis is **osteogenesis imperfecta.**[7]

Clinical notes

1. Ask the patient to stand to demonstrate short stature, and look carefully for kyphoscoliosis. In a tall patient, kyphoscoliosis should lead you to consider Marfan's syndrome.

2. Blue sclerae are also found in Marfan's syndrome, Ehlers-Danlos syndrome, pseudoxanthoma elasticum, hypophosphatasia, Diamond-Blackfan anaemia, and alkaptonuria. However, this is often a subtle finding, and easily missed.

3. Scars and deformities occur due to previous fractures and poor wound healing. Patients with Osteogenesis imperfecta are prone to fracture. There may be evidence of corrective orthopaedic surgery. Long bone deformities include anterior bowing of the humerus, tibia, and fibula and lateral bowing of the femur, radius, and ulna.

4. Deafness occurs due to otosclerosis. Another cause of skeletal abnormalities and deafness is Paget's disease, although this typically manifests later in life.

5. Ligamentous laxity results in joint hyperextensibility and subluxation. This is seen in type I and IV osteogenesis imperfecta.

6. Dentinogenesis imperfecta (or defective brittle teeth) are seen in all types except type I osteogenesis imperfecta.

7. Although the most common type of osteogenesis imperfecta is type I, and most likely to be encountered in the MRCP (PACES) examination, it is best to avoid unnecessary confusion and trying to determine the sub-type.

Tell the examiner that you would like to examine the cardiovascular system due to the association with valvular heart disease. There may be evidence of sternotomy scars, indicating previous valvular heart surgery.

Questions commonly asked by examiners

What is the molecular defect in osteogenesis imperfecta?

This is caused by defects in synthesis of type 1 collagen. This defect in the extracellular matrix results in osteoporosis that results in an increased tendency to fracture. Mutations occur in one of two genes that encode type 1 collagen: COL1A1 and COL1A2.

What are the different types of osteogenesis imperfecta?

There are at least four types recognized, but type 1 is the most likely diagnosis in adults with the condition.

Type	Inheritance	Clinical features
Type I	AD	Limited bone fragility and deformity; blue sclerae, early hearing loss; joint hypermobility; no dentinogenesis imperfecta
Type II	AD	Stillbirth or neonatal death; multiple rib fractures at birth; dentinogenesis imperfecta
Type III	AD, AR	Severe bone fragility; multiple fractures and disability; sclerae may be white or blue; dentinogenesis imperfecta
Type IV	AD	Variable fragility and disability; sclerae usually white; joint hypermobility; dentinogenesis imperfecta; basilar impression of the skull is common (70%)

The syndrome of brittle bones, blue sclerae, and deafness was first described in 1918 by van der Hoeve and de Kleyn of Utrecht. More recently, Samuel L Jackson's character 'Mr Glass' in the film *Unbreakable* (2000) depicted the disability of type 1 osteogenesis imperfecta.

What is the management of osteogenesis imperfecta?

General measures

- Patient education
- Occupational therapy
- Genetic counselling

Pharmacological measures

- Analgesia
- Vitamin D and calcium supplements
- Bisphosphonates

Non-pharmacological measures

- Hearing aids
- Orthopaedic surgery for scoliosis and fractures

Case 118 ◆ **Polydactyly**

CASE PRESENTATION

*This patient has **polydactyly** of the hands. The extra digit contains bone without joints, and is non-functioning.*

The differential diagnosis for polydactyly includes

(a) **Bardet-Biedl syndrome (previously known as Laurence-Moon-Bardet-Biedl syndrome)**

(b) **Holt-Oram syndrome**

(c) *Carpenter syndrome*

(d) *Patau syndrome (Trisomy 13)*

(e) *Familial (inherited as an autosomal dominant trait)*

I would like to look for features of these conditions.

Clinical notes

1. Polydactyly is an extra digit, often a small piece of soft tissue, on the hands and/or feet. It is important to examine the digit and determine if it contains bone and joints and, if so, to determine its functional status. Rarely, it may present as a complete functioning digit.

2. It is important to be aware of simple descriptive terminology when describing polydactyly. This will impress examiners! The extra digits often arise from the fingers (sides of the hands) and may be classified as:
   (a) **Post-axial**: on the ulnar side (little finger) of the hand (most common)
   (b) **Central**: on the middle three fingers of the hand
   (c) **Pre-axial**: on the radial side (thumb) of the hand
   Occasionally, a fully functioning digit may originate at the wrist (as a normal digit does).

3. There are many conditions associated with polydactyly, and it important to remember a few causes and be aware of the associated features of these conditions. Tell the examiner you would like to look for features of underlying disease.

Condition	Clinical features
Bardet-Biedl syndrome	Short stature, hypogonadism, cognitive impairment, retinitis pigmentosa, truncal obesity, polydactyly
Holt-Oram syndrome	Atrial septal defect, hypoplastic limbs, polydactyly
Carpenter syndrome	Craniofacial deformities, craniosynostosis, high-arched palate, cognitive impairment, polydactyly, syndactyly, heart defects (transposition of the great vessels, narrow pulmonary artery)
Patau syndrome (trisomy 13)*	Cleft lip and palate, polydactyly, macrocephaly, rocker-bottom feet, microphthalmia, neural tube defects, heart defects (atrio-ventricular septal defects, patent ductus arteriosus, and dextrocardia)
Familial	Enquire about a family history

*Those with Patau syndrome frequently die in the neonatal period. Up to 5% survive beyond 6 months. There are reports of patients growing into adolescence. There are rare reports of adults with Patau syndrome.

4. Laurence-Moon-Bardet-Biedl syndome is associated with retinitis pigmentosa, truncal obesity, short stature, and mental retardation. (see Case 152 Retinitis Pigmetnosa).

5. Holt-Oram syndrome is associated with atrial and ventricular septal defects, and variable upper limb deformities including aplasia, hypoplasia, fusion, and anomalous development of upper limb bones (see Case 35 Atrial Septal Defect).

C. Skin

Case 119 ◆ **Scleroderma**

CASE PRESENTATION

This patient has **sclerotic skin over the face and fingers** *that appears* **smooth, shiny,** *and* **tight***. There is loss of facial wrinkles,* **perioral puckering** *with* **restrictive mouth opening***, and the* **nose appears pinched**.[1] *There is* **telangiectasia** *of the face.[2] On examination of the hands, there is* **sclerodactyly** *with* **flexion deformities***. There are* **dilated nail-fold capillaries** *with* **dystrophic nails***. There is* **atrophy of soft tissue***, in particular the finger pulps, with* **digital ulceration** *and* **gangrene***. There is evidence of* **Raynaud's phenomenon***. There are palpable nodules of* **calcinosis**.[3]

The diagnosis is **systemic sclerosis**.[4,5]

Clinical notes

1. Systemic sclerosis is characterized by thickening and fibrosis of the skin. Look carefully for the tight, shiny, and waxy skin over the face and hands. The loss of facial wrinkles, perioral puckering, and pinched appearance of the nose result from sclerotic skin process. If present, comment on them.

2. Telangiectasia commonly occurs over the face. They can be present on the hands.

3. The key examination findings in the hand are listed above. Other skin features that may be present include oedema, livedo reticularis, morphoea, pigmentation, scarring alopecia, and vitiligo. Raynaud's phenomenon is common and is the presenting feature in 70% of cases, and the fingers are cold and cyanosed. This is associated with a physiological response to cold resulting in arteriolar spasm to produce white fingers. With re-warming, the colour sequence is white → blue (cyanosis) → red (rebound hyperaemia). If allowed, ask the patient some questions to elicit this history. Often, patients with chronically impaired circulation have cyanotic hands even in warm environments, i.e. in the examination setting. Please see Case 127 for further discussion on Raynaud's phenomenon.

4. Systemic sclerosis may occur in the context of mixed connective tissue disease. There may be features of rheumatoid arthritis, systemic lupus erythematosus (SLE) or polymyositis. It is important to look for features of these conditions.

5. Systemic sclerosis is a multi-system disorder. If time allows, ask the examiner whether you may ask questions and to examine further systems to demonstrate the features of systemic sclerosis.

Questions:

(a) What happens to your hands when you go into the cold? (Raynaud's)
(b) Do you have any swallowing problems? (Dysphagia)

Examination:

(a) **Respiratory system**: interstitial lung disease
(b) **Cardiovascular system**: pulmonary hypertension, restrictive cardiomyopathy
(c) **Gastrointestinal system**: primary biliary cirrhosis

Questions commonly asked by examiners

What organ systems are involved in systemic sclerosis?

Organ system	Features
Skin	Raynaud's phenomenon; sclerodactyly; soft tissue atrophy; calcinosis; nail dystrophy; ulceration; gangrene; flexion deformities; calcinosis; oedema; telangiectasia; vitiligo; morphoea; pigmentation; pruritis
Musculoskeletal	Arthritis; myositis; myopathy; intra-articular calcification; osteopenia
Gastrointestinal	Dysphagia; gastro-oesophageal reflux; intestinal hypomotility → bacterial overgrowth → steatorrhoea and malabsorption; pneumatosis coli; colonic diverticulae; bowel obstruction; primary biliary cirrhosis
Renal	Malignant hypertension; glomerulonephritis; renal crises
Respiratory	Interstitial lung disease; restrictive lung defects; pleural effusions; atelectasis
Cardiovascular	Restrictive cardiomyopathy (myocardial fibrosis); pericarditis; pericardial effusions; pulmonary hypertension; conduction defects

How is systemic sclerosis classified?

Diffuse scleroderma

- Diffuse involvement of the skin: trunk and extremities
- Early involvement of the lungs, kidneys, gut and heart

Limited scleroderma

- Skin is affected only at the extremities and/or face
- CREST syndrome (see below)
- Late involvement of lungs
- Late development of pulmonary hypertension
- Renal crises are rare

Scleroderma sine scleroderma

- Organ involvement without skin involvement

Malignant scleroderma

- An accelerated course of scleroderma leading to death
- Often in elderly men

What are the American Rheumatism Association (ARA) diagnostic criteria for systemic sclerosis?

- MAJOR features: skin sclerosis affecting arms, face and/or neck
- MINOR features: sclerodactyly, finger pulp atrophy, bilateral pulmonary fibrosis

1 MAJOR *or* ≥2 MINOR criteria are required to make a diagnosis of systemic sclerosis.

What is the CREST syndrome?

- **C**alcinosis
- **R**aynaud's phenomenon
- **E**sophageal dysmotility
- **S**clerodactyly
- **T**elangiectasia

What is the most important cause of mortality in systemic sclerosis?

Renal failure is the major cause of death.

What autoantibodies are associated with the different subsets of systemic sclerosis?

Limited systemic sclerosis	Diffuse systemic sclerosis
Anti-centromere	Anti-ScL 70 (topoisomerase 1) Anti RNA polymerase I, II, and III
ANA Rheumatoid factor	

In mixed connective tissue disease, anti-ribonuclear protein (RNP) antibody is strongly positive, which is typically distributed in a speckled pattern.

What is the management of systemic sclerosis?

General management
- Patient education and counselling
- Physiotherapy and exercises for contractures and deformities
- Analgesia for arthritis or arthralgia
- A multidisciplinary approach to management

Raynaud's phenomenon
- Smoking cessation
- Hand-warmers, i.e. gloves
- Vasodilators (calcium antagonists, ACE inhibitors, prostacyclin analogues)
- Sympathectomy in severe cases

Gastrointestinal
- Low-residue diets and nutritional supplements for malabsorption
- Antibiotics for bacterial overgrowth
- Proton pump inhibitors for reflux symptoms
- Prokinetic drugs for dysmotility

Renal
- Aggressive management of hypertension (ACE inhibitors)
- ACE inhibitors for renal crises

Respiratory
- Vasodilator therapy for pulmonary hypertension
- Anti-fibrotic therapy for pulmonary fibrosis (D-penicillamine and interferon-γ)

Case 120 ◆ **Psoriasis**

CASE PRESENTATION

*There are well-defined **erythematous plaques** with **silvery white scales** over the **extensor surfaces, scalp, navel,** and **behind the ears**.[1] In addition, there is an **asymmetrical arthropathy** of the hands mainly involving the **distal interphalangeal joints**.[2] There is **nail pitting, onycholysis, transverse ridging,** and **subungual hyperkeratosis**.[3]*

The diagnosis is **psoriasis** *and* **psoriatic arthropathy**.[4,5]

Clinical notes

1. If psoriasis is not obvious over the extensor surfaces, it is important to examine at the scalp, navel, and behind the ears. Look carefully for plaques over sites of trauma (**Koebner phenomenon**). Inverse psoriasis is a variant of psoriasis that appears on the flexor surfaces and affects intertriginous areas, i.e. axillae, inguinal folds, infra-mammary creases, with minimal scaling. Psoriatic plaques tend to be symmetrically distributed over the body. There may tiny punctate bleeding points visible over the plaque surface. This results from bleeding from enlarged dermal capillaries after removal of individual scales (intense scratching). This is the **Auspitz sign**.

2. Psoriatic arthropathy can present in 5 distinct patterns (see Case 109 Psoriatic Arthropathy).

3. Examine carefully for nail changes. Although nail changes are associated with psoriatic arthropathy, nail pitting can occur in 20% of patients with uncomplicated psoriasis.

4. Psoriatic arthropathy can occur with minimal skin involvement. In 20% of cases, the arthropathy precedes the onset of psoriasis, in some cases by up to 20 years. Similarly, psoriasis may be present without evidence of arthropathy.

5. If time allows, ask the examiner whether other systems may be examined to demonstrate other systemic associations of psoriasis:

    (a) **Musculoskeletal**: gout (psoriasis is associated with hyperuricaemia due to increased cell turnover)

    (b) **Cardiovascular**: aortitis and aortic regurgitation

    (c) **Respiratory**: apical lung fibrosis (rare)

    (d) **Eyes**: conjunctivitis, uveitis

Questions commonly asked by examiners

How common is psoriasis?

This affects 1–2% of the UK population.

What is the pathophysiology of psoriasis?

This is an inflammatory skin condition with reactive abnormal epidermal proliferation. Current research shows that the inflammatory mechanisms are immune-mediated and initiated and maintained by dermal T cells. Antigen presenting cells in the skin migrate from the skin to regional lymph nodes, where they interact with T cells. The antigen which is presented to the T cells is yet unknown. This triggers an immune response leading to T cell activation and cytokine release. These activated T cells are released into the circulation, which traffic back to the skin. Re-activation of T cells in the dermis and epidermis and the local effects of cytokines such as tumour necrosis factor lead to inflammation and epidermal proliferation, up to 10 times the normal rate.

What do you know about the genetics of psoriasis?

*   HLA-B13, B17 and Cw6 are associated with psoriasis
*   Genetic susceptibility loci have been identified: *psoriasis susceptibility (PSOR) 1–6*
*   PSOR1 on chromosome 6 is associated with 50% of cases
*   Both genetics and environmental factors play an important role

What are the triggering or exacerbating factors in psoriasis?

*   Trauma
*   Sunburn

- Stress
- Alcohol
- Smoking
- β haemolytic streptococci (guttate psoriasis)
- Drugs (lithium, ACE inhibitors, beta-blockers, indomethacin, and anti-malarial drugs)
- Withdrawal of steroid drugs
- HIV

What are the cardinal histopathological features of psoriasis?

- Acanthosis (skin thickening)
- Parakeratosis (retention of nuclei in the horny layer)
- Absence of a granular cell layer
- Polymorphonuclear abscesses of Munro in the upper epidermis
- Dilated capillary loops in the upper epidermis

What are the variants of psoriasis?

- Chronic plaque psoriasis (most common)
- Pustular psoriasis*
- Guttate psoriasis**
- Palmoplantar psoriasis
- Erythrodermic psoriasis (most severe form and life threatening)

What skin conditions demonstrate Koebner phenomenon?

- Psoriasis
- Lichen planus
- Vitiligo
- Viral warts
- Molluscum contagiosum
- Pemphigus
- Pemphigoid
- Darier's disease
- Mycoses fungoides (cutaneous T-cell lymphoma)
- Necrobiosis lipoidica diabeticorum
- Pyoderma gangrenosum

What is the treatment of psoriasis?

General measures

- Patient education
- Avoidance of exacerbating factors

Topical therapy

- Emollients (aqueous cream or soft yellow paraffin)
- Keratolytic agents (salicylic acid)
- Topical steroids

---

* Can present as palmoplantar, localized, or generalized. Superficial pustules stud the plaques. These are not infected, and represent sterile collections of inflammatory cells.
** Rain-drop shaped plaques that occur 2 weeks after streptococcal throat infections, and often resolve after 1–2 months.

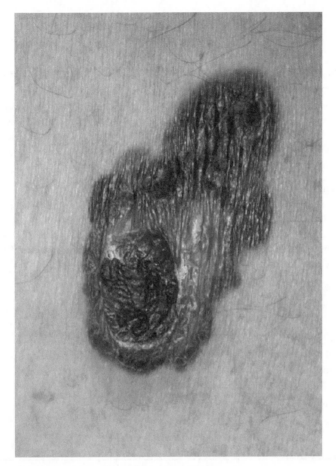

Figure 120.1 Chronic plaque psoriasis (see colour plate section).
Reproduced from Collier et al. Oxford Handbook of Clinical Specialties, 7th edn. 2006, with permission from
Oxford University Press.

- UVB phototherapy
- Tar (Goeckerman regime = tar + UVB phototherapy)
- Dithranol (Ingram regime = dithranol + UVB phototherapy)*
- Calcipotrol

Systemic therapy
- Photochemotherapy (PUVA)
- Steroids
- Methotrexate
- Azathioprine
- Cyclosporin

---

* Remember **I** in di**t**hranol, for **I**ngram regime

- Tacrolimus
- Retinoids
- Anti-TNFα therapy (etanercept)*

What do you know about (a) UVB phototherapy and (b) photochemotherapy?

(a) UVB phototherapy

This uses light with wavelengths of 290–320ms. This is often combined with tar (Goeckerman regime) or dithranol (Ingram regime). It can also be combined with other topical agents such as emollients, steroids, or calcipotrol. Narrow band UVB phototherapy uses a fluorescent bulb with a narrow emission spectrum that peaks at 311nm. This selective and relatively longer wavelength is more effective than broadband UVB for the treatment of chronic plaque psoriasis.

(b) Photochemotherapy

This uses UVA phototherapy (wavelengths of 320–400ms) with photosensitizing drugs (methoxsalen, 8-mothoxypsoralens). These agents form covalent bonds with DNA in ultraviolet light, thus reducing cell turnover. Short-term complications include nausea, pruritis, and burns. Long-term complications include squamous cell carcinoma and melanoma. More than 85% of patients report relief of disease after 20–30 treatments.

What are the side effects of retinoids?

- Dry lips
- Epistaxis
- Alopecia
- Deranged liver function tests (LFTs)
- Hyperlipidaemia
- Ligament ossification
- Teratogenesis

Case 121 ◆ **Neurofibromatosis**

CASE PRESENTATION

*This patient has multiple irregularly shaped, evenly pigmented brown macules (**café-au-lait spots**).[1] There are multiple **neurofibromata** along the course of peripheral nerves.[2] There is **axillary freckling**.[3]*

*The diagnosis is **neurofibromatosis**.[4]*

Clinical notes

1. Café-au-lait spots are irregularly-shaped, well-defined, and often present as brown macules. They tend to fade, and therefore may be less obvious on clinical examination. ≥6 café-au-lait spots are required

---

* NICE guidelines (2006) recommend therapy for severe psoriasis refractory to ≥2 systemic treatments and photochemotherapy. Etanercept should be withdrawn if no response after 12 weeks.

for a diagnosis of neurofibromatosis. Café-au-lait spots can be seen in healthy children (≥5 spots in children should lead one to suspect neurofibromatosis), and in pregnancy.

2. Neurofibromata are the most common benign tumours for NF-1, and can develop anywhere along the course of peripheral nerves. Thee are three subtypes of neurofibromata:

Subtype	Clinical features

Subcutaneous
Cutaneous
	Well circumscribed; brown, pink, or skin-coloured; soft or firm;
	    button-hole invagination when pressed (pathognomic feature);
	    not specific for NF-1

Plexiform	Non-circumscribed, thick and irregular; often an entire nerve trunk may be
	    involved with overgrowth, hyperpigmentation and hypertrichosis of
	    overlying tissues; can be locally invasive and quite deep; may be associated
	    with deformities (temporal and frontal scalp) and bony erosions;
	    specific for NF-1

3. Axillary and/or inguinal freckling (Crowe's sign) occurs in two-thirds of patients.
4. Neurofibromatosis is a multisystem disorder. Although it can be classified as NF-1 or NF-2 (see below), there may be overlap of clinical features. Once a diagnosis is presented, tell the examiner that you would like to examine further to demonstrate other associated features:
   (a) **Blood pressure**: hypertension (secondary to renal artery stenosis or phaeochromocytoma)
   (b) **Cranial nerves**: acoustic neuroma and cerebellopontine angle lesions; **don't miss the hearing aid**
   (c) **Eyes**: look for cataracts, test visual acuity (optic glioma), fundoscopy (optic glioma and retinal hamartoma), slit-lamp examination (Lisch nodules)
   (d) **Cardiovascular**: restrictive cardiomyopathy
   (e) **Respiratory**: pulmonary fibrosis, pneumothorax
   (f) **Musculoskeletal**: kyphoscoliosis, pseudoarthrosis (especially tibial), Charcot's joints, bowing of long bones

Questions commonly asked by examiners

What are the major subtypes of neurofibromatosis?
1. **Neurofibromatosis type 1 (NF-1)**—peripheral (von Recklinghausen's disease)—most common
2. **Neurofibromatosis type 2 (NF-2)**—central

These classifications are not completely accurate, as NF-1 often has central features.

What do you know about the genetics of neurofibromatosis?
NF-1: autosomal dominant, chromosome 17
This gene encodes the neurofibromin protein that has a GTPase region, which binds to Ras oncoprotein, thus down-regulating it. It therefore acts as a tumour suppressor.

NF-2: autosomal dominant, chromosome 22
Less is known about this gene, but this also encodes a tumour suppressor.

What are the different clinical features and associations with neurofibromatosis?
Neurofibromatosis is a neurocutaneous syndrome with multi-organ involvement. There is often overlap of clinical features, with patients having NF-1 often have central features.

NF-1 (peripheral):

Organ system	Features
Skin	• ≥6 café-au-lait spots
	• Axillary and/or inguinal freckling
	• Neurofibromata (can undergo malignant sarcomatous change)
Eyes	• Lisch nodules on the iris
	• Retinal hamartomata
Lungs	• Pulmonary fibrosis
	• Pneumothorax (lung cysts)
Heart	• Cardiomyopathy (often restrictive)
Musculoskeletal	• Kyphoscoliosis
	• Pseudoarthrosis (especially tibial)
	• Bowing of the legs
	• Rib notching
	• Subperiosteal bone cysts
	• Dysplasia of the skull (sphenoid)
	• Charcot's joints
Kidneys	• Renal artery stenosis
Endocrine	• Phaeochromocytoma

NF-2 (central):
- Acoustic neuroma
- Meningioma
- Optic glioma
- Ependymoma
- Cataracts/lens opacity

What is the histology of neufibromata?
These tumours are composed of Schwann cells, fibroblasts, mast cells, and vascular components.

What do you know about the diagnostic criteria for neurofibromatosis?
NF-1 (if ≥2 features are present):
- ≥6 café-au-lait spots (diameter >5mm (pre-pubertal) or >15mm (post-pubertal individuals)
- ≥2 neurofibromata of any type or 1 plexiform neurofibroma
- ≥2 Lisch nodules
- Axillary or inguinal freckling
- Optic glioma
- Distinct osseous lesion, i.e. sphenoid dysplasia and thinning of long bones (with or without pseudoarthrosis)
- First degree relative with NF-1 (according to above criteria)

NF-2 (if any one of the following feature is present):
- Bilateral VIII nerve involvement (confirmed by CT or MRI)
- First degree relative with NF-2, and either one of the following:
  - Unilateral VIII nerve involvement
  - Any two of the following: neurofibroma, meningioma, glioma, schwanonoma, or juvenile posterior subcapsular lenticular opacity

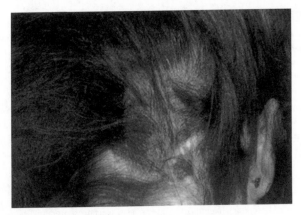

Figure 121.1 Multiple peripheral neurofibromata (see colour plate section).
Reproduced from Sybert, V.P., Genetic Skin Disorders, 1997, with permission from Oxford University Press.

What are Lisch nodules?

* These are hamartomata that appear on the iris
* Well-defined, dome-shaped
* Can be clear or yellow-brown in colour
* Incidence increases with age (100% of patients aged >20 years)
* If older patients do not have Lisch nodules, they are unlikely to have NF-1
* Usually require slit-lamp examination to be visualized

Case 122 ◆ **Hereditary Haemmorhagic Telangiectasia (HHT)**

CASE PRESENTATION

*There are multiple **telangiectases** on the **face**, **around the mouth**, on the **lips**, **tongue**, **buccal**, and **nasal mucosa**.[1] There are no other features of systemic sclerosis.[2] There is conjunctival pallor and koilonychia.[3] There is no evidence of cyanosis.[4]*

*The diagnosis is **hereditary haemmorhagic telangiectasia** (also known as **Osler-Weber-Rendu syndrome**). The clinical signs suggest **iron deficiency anaemia**, which is associated with this condition.[5]*

Clinical notes

1. Telangiectases in this condition represent dilatations of post-capillary venules. They are usually present on the face, particularly around the mouth. They are also present on the buccal and nasal mucosa, tongue (remember to look under the tongue), arms, hands, nail beds, feet, ears, conjunctiva, and trunk. They appear as small purplish stains that partially blanch with pressure. A typical telangiectasia is smaller than 5mm and may be macular, papular, or punctate lesions.

2. There are many causes of telangiectasia. Systemic sclerosis can cause telangiectasia in a similar distribution, and it is important to comment on the absence or presence of other features of this condition.

3. These lesions can be present anywhere. Often these patients present with epistaxis, haemoptysis, or gastrointestinal bleeding. Often these patients present with chronic iron deficiency anaemia (look for conjunctival pallor and koilonychia). It is important to comment on the absence or presence of anaemia.

4. It is important to comment on the absence or presence of cyanosis. The presence of cyanosis reflects the degree of arterio-venous shunting.

5. Once a diagnosis of hereditary haemmorhagic telangiectasia is presented, tell the examiner that you would like to examine further to demonstrate other features of this condition, as telangiectases and arteriovenous malformations can occur in many organ systems:

    (a) **Respiratory**: pulmonary arteriovenous malformation (look for clubbing and cyanosis and listen for bruits)

    (b) **Cardiovascular**: high-output cardiac failure (secondary to left-to-right shunts)

    (c) **Gastrointestinal**: iron-deficiency anaemia, hepatomegaly, splenomegaly, cirrhosis, and portal hypertension

    (d) **Eyes**: retinal haemorrhage and detachment (fundoscopy)

    (e) **Neurological**: central nervous vascular lesions, ischaemic stroke, and cerebral abscess (paradoxical embolism due to right-to-left pulmonary-arteriovenous shunts) and subarachnoid haemorrhage

Questions commonly asked by examiners

What is the definition of telangiectasia?

This refers to an enduring dilatation of small blood vessels. These can be capillaries or venules. In hereditary haemmorhagic telangiectasia, this represents dilatation of post-capillary venules.

What do you know about hereditary haemmorhagic telangiectasia?

This is an autosomal dominant disorder characterized by telangiectases of the skin and mucous membranes and arteriovenous malformations. A number of genes are implicated that include *endoglin* (chromosome 9), *ALK-1* (chromosome 12), *SMAD4* (chromosome 18), and a yet unidentified gene (chromosome 5). All encoded proteins are involved in the signalling of transforming growth factor (TGF-β) Telangiectases and arteriovenous malformations can affect the nasopharynx, central nervous system, lung, liver, spleen, urinary and gastrointestinal tracts. Epistaxis is the most common presentation and gastrointestinal bleeding is also common.

Skin

* Telangiectases are multiple and not associated with significant bleeding
* They are largely of cosmetic concern

Nose

* Recurrent epistaxis occurs in 90% of patients
* Bleeding occurs from telangiectases from nasal mucosa, and can be spontaneous and severe

Lungs

- Patients with the *endoglin* gene mutation have a higher risk of pulmonary arteriovenous malformations (often has a predilection for the lower lobes)
- Pulmonary arteriovenous malformations can lead to left-to-right shunting
- Complications include: ischaemic stroke (paradoxical embolism) and brain abscess formation, which account for 10% of the mortality in HHT
- Small arteriovenous malformations (shunt < 25% of pulmonary blood flow) show no cyanosis, but are associated with exertional breathlessness.
- Large arteriovenous malformations (shunt >25% of pulmonary blood flow) result in exertional breathlessness, fatigue, and haemoptysis. They are associated with clubbing, cyanosis, polycythaemia, and bruits over the lung fields.
- Cyanosis and clubbing is associated with increased risk of stroke and cerebral abscess

Nervous system

- Neurological manifestations are due to arteriovenous malformations (subarachnoid haemorrhage) and paradoxical embolism through right-to-left pulmonary arteriovenous malformations (ischaemic stroke and brain abscess)
- Migraine occurs in 50% of patients
- Approximately 7% of patients have mycotic aneurysms
- Spinal arteriovenous malformations can lead to paraparesis

Gastrointestinal tract

- Both telangiectases and arteriovenous malformations can occur
- Gastrointestinal bleeding occurs in 20–40% of patients and risk of bleeding increases with age

Liver

- Telangiectases and arteriovenous malformations can affect the liver in up to 30% of patients
- Many are patients are asymptomatic
- Complications include jaundice, right upper quadrant pain, high-output cardiac failure, hepatomegaly, cirrhosis, portal hypertension, and encephalopathy
- Mesenteric angina can occur (mesenteric arterial steal syndrome)
- Shunting from hepatic artery to hepatic vein, portal vein to hepatic vein, or both can result in high-output cardiac failure

What are other causes of telangiectasia?

- Systemic sclerosis
- Pregnancy
- Mitral stenosis
- Myxoedema
- Carcinoid syndrome
- Ataxia telangiectasia
- Hepatic failure
- Polycythaemia
- Dermatomyositis
- SLE
- Radiation therapy
- Necrobiosis lipoidica diabeticorum
- Grauloma annulare
- Lupus pernio

- Topical steroid therapy
- Essential telangiectasia
- Temperate/cold climates

What do you know about the Shovlin criteria for diagnosing hereditary haemmorhagic telangiectasia?

Any 3 of the following should be present to make a diagnosis:

- Recurrent epistaxis
- Telangiectasia at a site other than nasal mucosa
- Evidence of autosomal dominance inheritance
- Visceral involvement

How would you manage this patient?

- **Anaemia**: iron supplementation and blood transfusion
- **Skin telangiectases**: cosmetic therapy and laser ablation
- **Epistaxis**: cauterization, laser ablation, septal dermatoplasty, oestrogen therapy (induces squamous metaplasia), and low-dose aminocaproic acid (anti-fibrinolytic agent)
- **Pulmonary arteriovenous malformations**: embolization, surgical resection, and ligation of arterial blood supply
- **Gastrointestinal telangiectases**: blood transfusion and photocoagulation therapy

Case 123 ◆ Vitiligo

CASE PRESENTATION

This patient has **well-demarcated areas of depigmentation** *on the face (around the eyes and mouth), dorsal surfaces of the hands, extensor surfaces of the elbows and knees and dorsal surfaces of the feet.*[1,2]

The diagnosis is **vitiligo**.[3]

Clinical notes

1. Vitiligo can affect any part of the skin and/or mucous membranes. It has a predilection for hyperpigmented areas such as the face, neck, areolae, groin, and genitalia. It can also develop in areas that are subjected to repeated trauma or friction (Koebner phenomenon): bony prominences (extensor surfaces of elbows and knees), extensor surface of the forearms, dorsal surfaces of the hands and feet and digital phalanges. Mucosal involvement often occurs with generalized vitiligo.
2. Hairs in the affected areas are depigmented.
3. The diagnosis can be rapidly made, and it is important to remember the spectrum of autoimmune diseases that occur in association with vitiligo. There are many associations with vitiligo, but the following conditions can be sought for during clinical examination:
   (a) **Alopecia areata**: areas of hair loss in scalp with white, short, tapering exclamation mark hairs
   (b) **Hashimoto's disease**: goitre (? previous thyroidectomy scar), features of hypothyroidism

(c) **Grave's disease**: goitre (? previous thyroidectomy scar), eye signs, thyroid acropachy, pretibial myxoedema, features of hypo- or hyperthyroidism

(d) **Addison's disease**: pigmentation, postural hypotension

(e) **Hypoparathyroidism**: Chvostek's and Trousseau's sign, cataracts

(f) **Diabetes**: finger tip skin pricks (regular glucose testing), fundoscopy to look for retinopathy

(g) **Idiopathic pulmonary fibrosis**: bibasal crepitations

(h) **Primary biliary cirrhosis**: scratch marks, pigmentation, icterus, xanthelesma, signs of chronic liver disease

(i) **Pernicious anaemia**: pallor, splenomegaly, polyneuropathy

(j) **Atrophic gastritis**: pallor, koilonychia-iron deficiency anaemia

Questions commonly asked by examiners

What do you know about the epidemiology of vitiligo?

This occurs worldwide with an overall prevalence of 1%. Both sexes are equally affected, although threr is greater reporting in females due to the cosmetic concern. It affects adults and children equally.

What is the differential diagnosis for localized loss of pigmentation?

- Pityriasis versicolor
- Naevus depigmentosus
- Leprosy (tuberculoid)
- Tuberous sclerosis (ash-leaf spots)
- Discoid lupus
- Morphoea
- Lichen sclerosis
- Melanoma-associated leukoderma
- Chemical leukoderma*
- Pityriasis alba

Is there a genetic cause of vitiligo?

There is a family history of vitiligo in up to 40% of patients. The mode of transmission is complex, and is probably polygenic with variable penetrance.

What is the histological finding in vitiligo?

Partial or complete loss of melanocytes.

What is the management of vitiligo?

The key aims are to (a) arrest disease progression and (b) repigmentation.

General measures

- Sunscreens (tanning of surrounding skin exaggerates the appearance of vitiligo)
- Cosmetic camouflage

Medical therapy

- Corticosteroids (topical and systemic)
- Topical tacrolimus ointments
- Photochemotherapy (PUVA)
- Narrow-band UVB (311nm) phototherapy

---

* Industrial exposure to hydroxyquinones, catechols, phenols, or mercaptoamines.

Surgical therapy
- Punch grafts
- Minigrafts

Other measures
- Micro-pigmentation (tattooing to repigment skin)
- Depigmentation of normal skin (if vitiligo is widespread)

Case 124 ◆ **Dermatomyositis**

CASE PRESENTATION

There is a symmetrical **heliotrope rash** *around the* **eyes**.[1] *There are flat-topped, violaceous, scaly papules and plaques over the knuckles, elbows, and knees (***Gottron papules***).[2] There are dilated nail-fold capillaries (***periungual telangiectases***).[3] There is* **erythema** *and* **poikiloderma** *in a* **photosensitive distribution** *(extensor surfaces of the arm, V-shaped distribution over the anterior neck, upper chest and back).[4,5] There is* **proximal muscle weakness** *and tenderness.[6]*

The diagnosis is **dermatomyositis**.[7,8]

Clinical notes

1. Heliotrope is derived from *heliotropium* that has purple flowers. The heliotrope rash has a purple or violet colour and is a characteristic and pathognomic feature of dermatomyositis. It often has a symmetrical distribution involving the periorbital skin. There may be subcutaneous oedema around the eyes due to increased capillary permeability.

2. Gottron papules are also characteristic of dermatomyositis. The lesions consist of flat-topped violaceous papules and plaques. There is often a slight scale over them, and in some cases a thick psoriasiform scale may be present. They are found over bony prominences, particularly the MCP, proximal, and DIP joints, elbows, knees, and feet.

3. Nail changes include periungual telangiectases and hypertrophy of the cuticle.

4. Poikiloderma (hyperpigmentation and telangiectases) may occur on sun-exposed skin. The V-shaped distribution over the neck and upper chest is known to as the **shawl sign**.

5. It is important to remember, that there are many cutaneous manifestations of dermatomyositis. If present they should be commented on:
   (a) Heliotrope rash
   (b) Gottron papules
   (c) Subcutaneous oedema (increased capillary permeability)
   (d) Violaceous rash on extensor surfaces
   (e) Malar erythema (photosensitive distribution)
   (f) Telangiectasia (photosensitive distribution)
   (g) Hyperpigmentation (photosensitive distribution)
   (h) Poikiloderma (photosensitive distribution)
   (i) Periungual telangiectases

(j)   Hypertrophy of the cuticles

(k)   Raynaud's phenomenon

(l)   Scalp involvement with non-scarring alopecia

(m) Ichthyosis

(n)   White plaques on the buccal mucosa

(o)   Cutaneous vasculitis

(p)   Hyperkeratosis of the palms (known as mechanic's hands)

(q)   Calcinosis (unusual in adults, commoner in children and adolescents)

6.   Proximal muscle weakness may be present with muscle involvement. Muscle tenderness is a variable finding.

7.   Dermatomyositis is associated with underlying respiratory, gastrointestinal, breast, ovarian, and prostatic malignancy. In patients aged >40 years, a search for underlying malignancy should be made. Tell the examiner that you would like to conduct a thorough clinical examination.

8.   In addition to skin and muscle involvement, dermatomyositis frequently affects the joints, oesophagus, and the lungs. Tell the examiner, you would like to look for these additional features:

(a)   **Joints**: look for arthritis

(b)   **Oesophagus**: ask about dysphagia

(c)   **Lungs**: bibasal crepitations (interstitial lung disease)

Questions commonly asked by examiners?

What is dermatomyositis?

This is an idiopathic inflammatory myopathy with characteristic cutaneous features. It frequently affects the joints, oesophagus (dysphagia), and lungs (interstitial lung disease). Patients often present with skin disease. Muscle involvement may occur concurrently, precede the skin disease, or follow the skin disease by weeks to years. Malignancy is possible in any patient with dermatomyositis, and should be sought for in adults aged >40 years.

What is dermatomyositis-sine myositis?

Patients have cutaneous manifestations without clinical evidence of muscle weakness (normal serum muscle enzyme levels for at least 2 years).

What drugs can induce dermatomyositis-like skin changes?

* Hydoxyurea
* Penicillamine
* Statin
* Quinidine
* Phenylbutazone

What other skins lesions may resemble the appearance of Gottron papules?

* SLE
* Psoriasis
* Lichen planus

What would muscle enzymes demonstrate in a typical patient with dermatomyositis?

Muscle enzyme levels are often abnormal except in patients with no muscle involvement. The most sensitive/specific enzyme is creatine kinase. Sometimes, elevation of the muscle enzymes precedes clinical evidence of myositis.

How would you investigate this patient?

* Serum creatine kinase

- EMG*
- Muscle biopsy**

What is the treatment for dermatomyositis?

General measures

- Patient education
- Bed rest for patients with severe muscle inflammation
- Physiotherapy for muscle weakness (prevents contractures)

Skin disease

- Avoidance of sunlight or use of sunscreens
- Hydroxychloroquine
- Methotrexate and myocfenolate mofetil may be useful

Muscle disease

- High dose steroid therapy
- Methotrexate, azathioprine, and mycofenolate mofetil can be used as steroid-sparing agents
- High dose intravenous immunoglobulins (often for 6 months) in refractory cases

---

* Myopathic changes: spontaneous fibrillation, salvos of repetitive potentials, and short duration of low amplitude polyphasic potentials.
** Muscle biopsy will show necrosis and phagocytosis of muscle fibres with perivascular and interstitial inflammatory cells.

Case 125 ◆ **Purpura**

CASE PRESENTATION

This patient has **red-brown coloured macular lesions** *over the hands and upper limbs. They* **do not blanch under pressure**.

In addition there is a symmetrical deforming arthropathy of the small joints of the hands mainly involving the metacarpophalangeal and proximal interphalangeal joints, with subcutaneous nodules over the extensor surfaces of the upper limb (inkeeping with rheumatoid arthritis).

The diagnosis is **purpura**. *This patient has rheumatoid arthritis, and the purpura is most likely to be drug-induced (steroid or gold therapy)*

Clinical notes

1. Purpura is caused by bleeding from capillaries into the skin. These lesions are painless and non-blanching and can be palpable or non-palpable. Purpuric lesions include petechiae and echymoses.

   (a) **Petechiae**: round pin-point lesions, 1–3mm in diameter, often red-brown in colour and usually develop on dependent portions of the body

   (b) **Echymoses** are larger than petechiae, and often present as red-purple, blue, or yellow-green bruises and can arise anywhere on the body as a result of trauma.

2. Purpura has a vast differential diagnosis. Once the diagnosis of purpura is established, it is important to look for a possible cause. The cause may be evident on general examination (as in the above case). The causes of purpura (differential diagnosis) are discussed in detail below. Tell the examiner you would like for underlying systemic disease and take a detailed drug history.

If unable to find a cause for the purpura, then it is best to give a diagnosis of purpura, and provide a list of differential diagnoses (see below).

Questions commonly asked by examiners

What are the causes of purpura?

Platelet defect

*   Thrombocytopenia*
*   Uraemia
*   Chronic liver disease
*   Insecticides

Capillary defect

*   Age
*   Corticosteroids (endogenous or exogenous)
*   Drugs
*   Vasculitis**
*   Cholesterol embolism
*   Ehlers-Danlos syndrome
*   Pseudoxanthoma elasticum
*   Hereditary haemmorhagic telangiectasia
*   Scurvy
*   Amyloidosis
*   Venous stasis

Coagulation defect

*   Antithrombotic therapy (aspirin, warfarin, and heparin)
*   Von-Willebrand's disease
*   Haemophilia
*   Disseminated intravascular coagulation
*   Amyloidosis (capillary fragility and factor X deficiency)

How would you investigate a patient with purpura?

Often the cause of purpura may be clear, i.e. steroid therapy. If the cause is not clear, then the following investigations can be requested (some will be dependent on clinical suspicion):

*   Full blood count (FBC)
*   Blood film
*   Clotting profile
*   Fibrin degradation products
*   Autoimmune profile

---

* Drugs, disseminated intravascular coagulation, bone marrow replacement (malignancy and myeloproliferative disorders), hypersplenism, immune thrombocytopenic purpura, thrombotic thrombocytopenic purpura, haemolytic uraemic syndrome, aplastic anaemia.
* Henoch Schonlein purpura, polyarteritis nodosa, Churg-Strauss syndrome, Wegner's granulomatosis, SLE, infective endocarditis, Sjogren's syndrome, cryoglobulinaemia, Waldenstrom's macroglobulinaemia.

- Serum protein electrophoresis
- Bone marrow biopsy
- Skin biopsy

What drugs can cause purpura?

- Aspirin
- Warfarin
- Heparin
- NSAIDs
- Thiazide diuretics
- Phenytoin
- Sulphonamides
- Penicillins
- Tetracyclines
- Quinine
- Gold

Case 126 ◆ Lichen Planus

CASE PRESENTATION

*There are **flat-topped, violaceous, polygonal papules** on the **flexor surfaces** of the wrist, forearms, and legs. There are **fine white striae (Wickham's striae)** visible on the surfaces of these lesions.[1] They are also present along scratch marks and scars, thus exhibiting **Koebner phenomenon**.[2] There is **scalp involvement** with scarring alopecia.[3] There is a **lace-like pattern of white lines** on the **buccal mucosa**.[4] The **nails** are **dystrophic** with **longitudinal ridging**.[5]*

*The diagnosis is **lichen planus**.*

Clinical notes

1. The papules are violaceous, shiny, and polygonal. They vary in size (1mm to 1cm in diameter). They most commonly affect the flexor surfaces (especially the upper limbs), mucous membranes, genitalia, scalp, palms, and soles. They can be solitary lesions or can occur in groups of lines or circles. There is often a fine white scale over these lesions (Wickham's striae). The typical rash of lichen planus can be remembered with the 6 Ps: Pruritic, Polygonal, Planar, Purple, Papules, and Plaques.

2. Lichen planus exhibits Koebner phenomenon, and thus it is important to look at sites of trauma and scars. This is pruritic condition, and often these lesions will be noted in a liner pattern over scratch marks.

3. It is important to examine the scalp. Lichen planus causes follicular and perifollicular violaceous polygonal scaly papules, follicular plugging, bottlebrush hair formation (multiple hair shafts emerge from a single follicular orifice), and lead to scarring alopecia with permanent hair loss. Lichen planus lesions that occur on the scalp are known as lichen planopilaris.

4. Mucosal membrane involvement is common and may occur without skin involvement. Lesions are most commonly found on the tongue and buccal mucosa. Often the lesions are bilateral. They are

characterized by a white-lacy streaking pattern on a violaceous background. Lesions may also be found on the conjunctivae, larynx, and tonsils.

5. Nail involvement occurs in 10% of affected individuals. Nail changes include: nail pitting, thinning of the nail plate, onychorrhexis (longitudinal grooving and ridging), subungual hyperkeratosis, onycholysis (separation of the nail plate from the bed), onychoschizia (distal splitting), anonychia (permanent nail loss), and pterygium formation.

Questions commonly asked by examiners

What is the epidemiology of lichen planus?

The exact prevalence is unknown, but it affects less than 1% of the population. It affects middle-aged adults of both sexes, with slight female preponderance.

What are the different forms of lichen planus?

Variant of lichen planus	Notes
Annular	These lesions have atrophic centres; found on buccal mucosa and male genitalia
Linear	Develop as a Koebner phenomenon
Hypertrophic	Plaque-like lesions; thick and warty appearance; extensor surfaces of legs, especially around ankles; more common in Afro-Caribbean patients
Erosive	Often develop on mucosal surfaces. Assocaited with an increased risk of oral squamous cell carcinoma formation
Bullous	Often develop in the mouth or the legs; lichen planus pemphigodes is a rare combination of lichen planus and bullous pemphigoid

What are the causes of lichen planus?

* Idiopathic
* Drugs*
* Hepatitis C**

What is the prognosis?

* This is a benign condition that often resolves in 6–24 months
* Mucosal lesions, annular and hypertrophic forms may be chronic and persistent
* Oral lichen planus (erosive) in the mouth is associated with malignant transformation (squamous cell carcinoma)

What is the treatment?

Treatment must be individualized, and it is important to remember that spontaneous remission can occur in the majority of patients.

General measures

* Alteration of pharmacotherapy (if a potential offending medication is prescribed)
* Patient education and measures to reduce physical and local trauma (Koebner phenomenon)

---

* The following drugs are assocaited with the development of a lichen planus like eruption: β-blockers, thiazides, ACE inhibitors, NSAIDs, gold, phenothiazines, quinidine, and anti-malarial drugs
** There is evidence to suggest that hepatitis C virus (HCV) infection predisposes to the development of lichen planus. The exact mechanism for this is unknown.

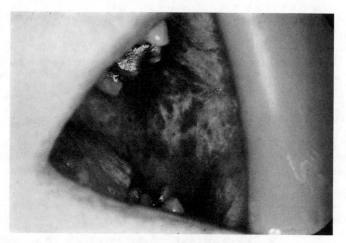

Figure 126.1 Wickham's striae seen on the buccal mucosa and tongue.
Reproduced from Warrell et al. Oxford Textbook of Medicine, Volume 2, 4th edn. 2003, with permission from Oxford University Press.

- Those with oral lesions should have good oral hygiene and scaling of teeth to remove calculous deposits and reduce sharp edges (Koebner phenomenon)
- Inform patients with oral lesions, the risk of squamous cell carcinoma (smoking cessation and reducing alcohol intake reduces this risk)

Local therapy
- Topical steroids
- Intralesional steroids
- Cyclosporin mouthwash (oral lichen planus)

Systemic therapy
- Systemic steroids
- Retinoids
- PUVA photochemotherapy
- Cyclosporin

Case 127 ◆ Raynaud's Phenomenon

CASE PRESENTATION

The fingers of both hands[1,2] are **cold** *and* **cyanosed**.[3] *There is* **finger pulp atrophy** *and* **gangrenous fingertips**.[4] *There are* **dilated nail-fold capillaries**.[5]

The diagnosis is **Raynaud's phenomenon**.[6]

Clinical notes

1. Raynaud's disease demonstrates symmetrical involvement. Raynaud's phenomenon, however, may have asymmetrical involvement. It is a good idea, to mention the presence of symmetrical or asymmetrical involvement. Symmetrical involvement may indicate both Raynaud's disease or phenomenon, but asymmetrical involvement strongly suggests Raynaud's phenomenon, in which case, the candidate should look carefully for an underlying association. In most cases this will be systemic sclerosis.

2. The hands are almost always involved. Other sites that may be involved include the tip of the nose, earlobes, and the toes.

3. In the examination setting, the room is often warm. There is evidence to suggest that patients with Raynaud's disease and phenomenon have abnormal blood flow even in normal conditions. This chronic impairment of circulation will often result in cold cyanosed hands even in the examination setting. On the other hand, the hands may be warm and red.

4. Tissue necrosis is a feature of Raynaud's phenomenon.

5. Abnormal large nail-fold capillaries are a feature of Raynaud's phenomenon. They may not be clearly evident, and warrant careful examination. Usually this is done by capillaroscopy, but in the examination setting, the nail-folds may be inspected carefully using a magnifying glass or an ophthalmoscope.

6. After presenting the diagnosis of Raynaud's phenomenon, tell the examiner that you would like to look for associated underlying diseases. The most common association is systemic sclerosis and this may be evident on gross inspection. Look for:

   (a) **Systemic sclerosis**: tight sclerotic facial skin, telangiectases, sclerodactyly, and calcinosis

   (b) **SLE**: butterfly skin rash and arthropathy

   (c) **Rheumatoid arthritis**: arthropathy, subcutaneous nodules, episcleritis, and scleritis

   (d) **Dermatomyositis**: heliotrope rash, Gottron papules, proximal weakness, and tenderness

   (e) **Polymyositis**: proximal weakness and tenderness

   (f) **Myeloproliferative disorders**: lymphadenopathy and hepatosplenomegaly

   (g) **Hepatitis B and C**: may have signs of chronic liver disease

   (h) **Thoracic outlet syndrome (cervical rib)**: supraclavicular bruit, reduced upper limb pulses on the affected side, reduced blood pressure in upper limb on affected side, wasting of small muscles of hand, C8/T1 sensory impairment

   (i) **Atherosclerosis**: diminished pulses on the affected side(s)

   (j) **Carpal tunnel syndrome**: wasting of thenar eminence, loss of sensation in the median nerve distribution, Tinel's and Phalen's sign

   (k) **Hypothyroidism**: myxoedematous facies, bradycardia, slow relaxing ankle jerks

   (l) **Drugs**: β-blockers (bradycardia), cyclosporin (gingival hyperplasia)

   Tell the examiner you would like to take a detailed drug history and occupational history (vibration injury).

Questions commonly asked by examiners

What is the pathophysiology of Raynaud's?

This is reversible ischaemia of the peripheral arterioles secondary to an abnormal exaggerated response to cold or stress. There is a triphasic response with characteristic colour changes:

- **White** (pallor due to intense vasospasm)
- **Blue** (as tissues get colder and with stasis of blood, cyanosis develops)
- **Red** (the attack end with rapid reflow of blood and hyperaemia)

Patients with Raynaud's (primary and secondary) have abnormal blood flow, even in normal conditions. The decreased blood flow may be due to increased blood viscosity, abnormal vasculature, or intense vasoconstriction.

What is the difference between Raynaud's disease and Raynaud's phenomenon?

Raynaud's disease (primary Raynaud's) is an idiopathic condition, whereas Raynaud's phenomenon (secondary Raynaud's) is associated with other conditions, most commonly an autoimmune disease.

How can you differentiate between Raynaud's disease and Raynaud's phenomenon?

	Raynaud's disease	Raynaud's phenomenon
Age	Usually <40 years	Usually >40 years
Associated conditions	None	Many systemic diseases (see below)
Symmetrical involvement	Yes	No (can involve one hand)
Nail fold capillaries	Normal	Abnormal
Tissue necrosis or gangrene	Never occurs	Can occur
ESR	Normal	Elevated
Serological findings (ANA)	Negative	Positive

What drugs are associated with Raynaud's phenomenon (secondary Raynaud's)?

- Bromocriptine
- β-blockers
- Oral contraceptive pill
- Ciclosporin
- Clonidine
- Chemotherapeutic agents (bleomycin, cisplatin)
- Interferon-α

What toxins are associated with Raynaud's phenomenon (secondary Raynaud's)?

- Vinyl chloride exposure
- Arsenic exposure
- Lead exposure

What investigations would you request in a patient with Raynaud's phenomenon?

Investigations	Rationale
FBC	Haematological and autoimmune disorders
Urea and electrolytes (U&Es)	Renal impairment and/or dehydration
LFTs	Chronic liver disease (hepatitis B and C)
Creatine kinase (CK)	Polymyositis, dermatomyositis
Clotting	Antiphospholipid syndrome (elevated activated partial thromboplastin time (APTT))
Glucose (fasting glucose)	Diabetes
Thyroid function tests	Hypothyroidism
ESR	Auto-immune disease
Full autoimmune profile	Auto-immune disease
Rheumatoid factor	Rheumatoid arthritis
C3 and C4 complement	Auto-immune disease, cryoglobinaemia
Cryoglobulins	Cryoglobinaemia

Investigations	Rationale
Cold agglutinins	Cold agglutinin diseases, i.e. Mycoplasma
Serum protein electrophoresis	Paraproteinaemia
CXR	Cervical rib

What is the management of Raynaud's phenomenon?

General measures
- Patient education
- Avoiding vasoconstrictor drugs
- Remove occupational or toxic exposure
- Hand warmers (electrically heated gloves are available)
- Smoking cessation

Pharmacological treatment
- Calcium antagonists
- ACE inhibitors or angiotensin-II receptor blockers
- Nitrates
- Prostacyclin analogues (parenteral)
- Calcitonin gene related peptide (parenteral)

Surgical treatment
- Digital sympathectomy

Case 128 ◆ **Erythema Nodosum**

CASE PRESENTATION

There are **poorly defined, red, tender,** *and* **nodular lesions** *of varying sizes (2–6cm in diameter) over the anterior surface of the lower legs.*[1,2]

The diagnosis is **erythema nodosum**.[3]

Clinical notes

1. The primary skin lesions are red and tender nodules. They are often poorly defined, and although they can affect any part of the skin, they are often limited to the extensor surface of the lower legs. In the first week, the lesions become tense, hard, and painful. In the second week, they may become fluctuant but do not suppurate or ulcerate. Individual lesions last for approximately 2 weeks, although new lesions may appear for up to 6 weeks. The colour of the lesions alters with time. Initially, they are red, becoming red-blue in the second week. As the lesions heal, they fade to give an appearance of a bruise. This eventually disappears as the overlying skin desquamates.

2. Joint involvement occurs in 50% of cases, and it is important to comment on joint involvement. Arthralgia occurs in the eruptive skin phase, or may precede this by 4 weeks. The joints commonly implicated are the ankles, knees, and wrists. Erythema, tenderness, and swelling occur, sometimes with an effusion. The synovial fluid is acellular and the rheumatoid factor is negative.

3. Erythema nodosum is a delayed hypersensitivity reaction and occurs in association with several systemic diseases and drugs. Tell the examiner that you would like to look for possible causes:

    (a) **Streptococcal throat infection**

    (b) **Tuberculosis**: productive cough, apical chest signs

    (c) **Sarcoidosis**: lupus pernio, interstitial lung disease

    (d) **Myeloproliferative disorders:** lymphadenopathy, hepatosplenomegaly

    (e) **Inflammatory bowels disease**: clubbing, laparotomy scars

    (f) **Behcet's disease**: orogenital ulceration

    (g) **Drugs**: take a detailed drug history (see below)

Questions commonly asked by examiners

What infections are associated with erythema nodosum?

*   **Bacterial infections**
    *   Streptococcal throat infections (Group A β-haemolytic streptococci)
    *   Tuberculosis
    *   Leprosy
    *   Mycoplasma
    *   Chlamydia
    *   Syphilis
*   **Viral infections**
    *   CMV
    *   EBV

- **Gastrointestinal infections**
  - ◆ Salmonella
  - ◆ Campylobacter
  - ◆ Yersinia
- **Fungal infections**
  - ◆ Coccidiomycosis
  - ◆ Histoplasmosis
  - ◆ Blastomycosis

What drugs are associated with erythema nodosum?

- Oral contraceptive pill
- Penicillins
- Tetracyclines
- Sulphonamides
- Sulphonylureas
- Gold

What is Lofgren syndrome?

This is a form of acute sarcoidosis that presents with fever, arthritis, hilar lymphadenopathy, erythema nodosum, and uveitis. It has a good prognosis with complete resolution within months.

NB. The most common cutaneous manifestation of sarcoidosis is erythema nodosum.

What is the histology of such lesions?

The classic features are septal panniculitis with perivascular inflammatory lymphocytic infiltrate. The septa of the subcutaneous fat are thickened. As the lesions evolve, periseptal fibrosis, giant cells, and granulation tissue appears. The hallmark feature of erythema nodosum is the presence of Meischer granulomas.

What initial investigations would you request?

The investigations will reflect clinical suspicion of the underlying diagnosis. Specific tests may be ordered, but preliminary tests should include:

- FBC
- Inflammatory markers
- Throat swabs
- Anti-streptolysin titre
- Blood cultures
- CXR
- Stool microscopy and culture

How would you treat erythema nodosum?

- Identify and treat underlying cause
- NSAIDs are often helpful
- Potassium iodide (a short course 400–900mg/day)
- Systemic steroid therapy may be required

Case 129 ◆ Erythema Multiforme

CASE PRESENTATION

*There are **target lesions** present on the palms and soles.[1] These **maculopapular** lesions are* **symmetrically distributed** *and comprise of* **three concentric zones**: *a central dark red-purple area, surrounded by a pale oedematous ring, which in turn is surrounded by a rim of erythema.[2] There is no eye or mucosal involvement.[3]*

The diagnosis is **erythema multiforme**.[4]

Clinical notes

1. Target lesions can occur anywhere, but commonly favour the palms and soles. Other common sites include the face, dorsum surface of the hands, and extensor surfaces of the limbs. Koebner phenomenon may be observed.

2. Target lesions comprise of three concentric zones, thus giving them their characteristic name and appearance. They are expanding macules or papules that start off as a dull red macule or urticarial plaque reaching a diameter of up to 2cm in 24–48 hours. In the centre a small papule, vesicle develops, flattens and may clear. The intermediate ring then develops that is raised, pale, and oedematous. This ring then becomes surrounded by a rim of erythema to form a concentric target lesion. Some lesions may be atypical comprising of only 2 rings.

3. Mucosal involvement occurs in 25% of cases of erythema multiforme and is often mild, limited to the oral cavity. Eye involvement occurs in 10% of cases of erythema multiforme, manifesting as bilateral purulent conjunctivitis and increased lacrimation. In Stevens-Johnson syndrome there is greater mucosal involvement most commonly the mouth, lips, conjunctivae, nasopharynx, respiratory, gastrointestinal, and genitourinary tract (a minimum of 2 mucosal surfaces must be involved, and 3 mucosal surfaces are involved in 40% of patients). Eye involvement occurs in 85% of cases of Stevens-Johnson syndrome.

4. When presenting the diagnosis of erythema multiforme, it is important to mention whether is mucosal involvement. **Erythema multiforme is idiopathic in 50% of cases** but can occur in association with several systemic diseases and drugs. Tell the examiner that you would like to look for possible causes:

    (a) **Tuberculosis**: productive cough, apical chest signs

    (b) **Streptococcal throat infection**

    (c) **Sarcoidosis** : lupus pernio, interstitial lung disease

    (d) **SLE**: butterfly skin rash, arthritis

    (e) **Polyarteritis nodosa**: vasculitic skin lesions

    (f) **Wegners granulomatosis**: nasal deformities, respiratory involvement

    (g) **Malignancy**: cachexia

    (h) **Myeloproliferative disorders**: lymphadenopathy, hepatosplenomegaly

    (i) **Drugs** : take a detailed drug history (see below)

Questions commonly asked by examiners

What infections are associated with erythema multiforme?

- **Bacterial infections**
    - Streptococcal throat infections (Group A β-haemolytic streptococci)
    - Tuberculosis

- ◆ Mycoplasma
- ◆ Rickettsiae
- ◆ Syphilis
- **Viral infections**
  - ◆ Herpes simplex virus (HSV)
  - ◆ Epstein-Barr virus (EBV)
  - ◆ Cytomegalovirus (CMV)
  - ◆ Human immunodeficiency virus (HIV)
  - ◆ Varicella zoster virus (VZV)
  - ◆ Hepatitis (A, B and C)
- **Gastrointestinal infections**
  - ◆ Campylobacter
  - ◆ Salmonella
  - ◆ Campylobacter
  - ◆ Yersinia
- **Fungal infections**
  - ◆ Coccidiomycosis
  - ◆ Histoplasmosis
  - ◆ Blastomycosis
- **Parasitic infection**
  - ◆ Toxocara
  - ◆ Toxoplasma

What drugs are associated with erythema multiform?

- Penicillins
- Tetracyclines
- Sulphonamides
- Sulphonylureas
- Barbiturates
- Phenytoin
- Carbamazepine
- NSAIDs
- Salicylates
- Oral contraceptive pill

What is Stevens-Johnson syndrome?

This is a variant of erythema multiforme (erythema multiforme major) that is characterized by fever and mucosal membrane involvement. The skin findings are similar to erythema multiforme but more severe, with target lesions often being larger and more confluent. Typically there are vesiculobullous lesions, often with haemorrhage and necrosis. Blistering of the skin (epidermal detachment) can occur involving less than 10% of the body surface area. It is associated with a 5% mortality risk.

What is the treatment?

Erythema multiforme

- Identify and treat underlying cause
- Prompt withdrawal of possible causative drug

- Symptomatic treatment for mild cases:
  - Analgesics as needed
  - Cold compresses with saline or Burow solution
  - Soothing oral treatments (saline gargles)

Stevens-Johnson syndrome
- Identify and treat underlying cause
- Prompt withdrawal of possible causative drug
- Analgesics as needed
- Anti-pyretics
- Intravenous fluids and replacement of electrolytes
- Antibiotics (for secondary infection)
- Meticulous wound care (sterile dressings; Burow or Domeboro solution dressings)
- Eye care (artificial tears)

Case 130 ◆ Livedo Reticularis

1. Livedo reticularis

CASE PRESENTATION

*There is **reticular pattern** of **red-brown erythema**[1] present bilaterally over the anterior aspect of the lower legs.[2]*

*The diagnosis is **livedo reticularis**.[3]*

Clinical notes

1. A reticular or arborescent pattern of red-brown erythema (a macular rash comprising of red-brown or violaceous rings forming a net-like pattern) is the classical appearance of livedo reticularis.
2. It is often present bilaterally, and commonly affects the legs.
3. Livedo reticularis is associated with many systemic conditions. Tell the examiner you would like to look for associated conditions (see below).

2. Erythema ab igne

CASE PRESENTATION

*There is **reticular pattern** of **red-brown erythema**[1] over the **lateral aspect** of the **right leg**.[2]*

*The diagnosis is **erythema ab igne**.[3]*

Clinical notes

1. This reticular pattern of red-brown erythema is similar to that seen in livedo reticularis. Erythema ab igne, however, is the discoloration of skin that is associated with repeated exposure to heat that is not painful and does not burn the skin.

2. It may be difficult to differentiate this from livedo reticularis clinically, but the feature that may help is unilateral involvement of the lateral aspect of one leg (often elderly people may sit by the fire). It may result form local heat due to a hot-water bottle, in which case it may not simply present unilaterally. If such a rash is present on the anterior abdominal wall or lumbar region, this may imply a chronic pain state, i.e. chronic pancreatitis, abdominal malignancy or chronic back pain (often the use of a hot-water bottle helps with alleviating the pain).

3. Once the diagnosis of erythema ab igne is presented, look for possible underlying causes for repeated exposure to heat. Often in the elderly, there may be no cause other than sitting by a fire, but tell the examiner that you would like to exclude:

    (a) **Hypothyroidism**: assess thyroid state (myxoedematous facies, hoarse voice, bradycardia, slow relaxing ankle jerks)

    (b) **Chronic pancreatitis**: features of alcoholic liver disease

    (c) **Abdominal malignancy**: cachexia, previous laparotomy scars, stoma bag, lymphadenopathy, masses, organomegaly

    (d) **Chronic back pain**: presence of arthritis, kyphoscoliosis, previous spinal surgery

NB. If you are not sure that the rash represents erythema ab igne, it may be best to present it as livedo reticularis, whilst giving your reasoning for and against a diagnosis of erythema ab igne.

Questions commonly asked by examiners

What are the causes of livedo reticularis?

Livedo reticularis (without systemic association)
- Physiological (cutis marmorata)
- Primary livedo reticularis
- Idiopathic livedo reticularis

Livedo reticularis (with systemic associations)
- Antiphospholipid syndrome
- Cryoglobulinaemia
- Polycythaemia rubra vera
- Essential thrombocythaemia
- Waldenstrom's macroglobulinaemia
- Cold agglutinins
- SLE
- Polyarteritis nodosa
- Wegners granulomatosis
- Churg-Strauss syndrome
- Cholesterol embolization
- Septic embolization

What is the pathophysiology of livedo reticularis?

The appearance of livedo reticularis is easily explained by the physiology of the cutaneous microvasculature. Arteriolar inflow comprises a series of ascending arterioles that rise perpendicularly to the skin surface, and form a capillary bed with the arteriole at the centre.

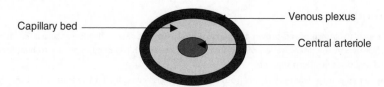

Figure 130.1

These drain into a venous plexus at the periphery of the capillary bed. Thus anything that increases the visibility of the venous plexus can result in the appearance of livedo reticularis (Figure 130.1).

Potential causes for this include:

- **Increased venodilatation**: hypoxia, venodilators, autonomic dysfunction
- **Decreased arteriolar inflow**: vasospasm (cold), arterial thrombosis, increased blood viscosity
- **Increased resistance of venous outflow**: venous thrombosis, increased blood viscosity

What is the difference between primary and idiopathic livedo reticularis?

Both conditions are not associated with any systemic disease and are independent of the ambient temperature. The main difference is whether the skin rash is persistent or intermittent:

- **Primary livedo reticularis:** appears and resolves, i.e. intermittent and not persistent
- **Idiopathic livedo reticularis**: persistent

What is the pathogenesis of erythema ab igne?

Erythema ab igne is caused by chronic repeated exposure to heat from an external source. The resulting cutaneous hyperthermia (43–45°C) results in similar changes that are seen in solar-damaged skin, resulting in a reticular pattern of pigmentation. When the skin is exposed to heat, there is a mild, transient, and often reticular erythema. With repeated exposure, the reticular erythema persists, and with time becomes hyperpigmented. The exact mechanism is unknown, but experimental evidence suggests that this may denature the DNA in squamous cells.

At what sites does erythema ab igne develop?

Erythema ab igne can develop at any site that is chronically exposed to heat. Examples include:

- Anterior shins (often elderly patients sitting in front of an open fire)
- Anterior abdomen (hot water bottle for chronic abdominal pain)
- Lower back (hot water bottle or heated seats for chronic back pain)
- Face and palms (cooks who work over an open fire)
- Anterior thighs (laptop users; laptops can generate significant heat when used for prolonged periods)

What are the complications of erythema ab igne?

- Epitheliomas
- Premalignant keratosis
- Squamous cell carcinoma

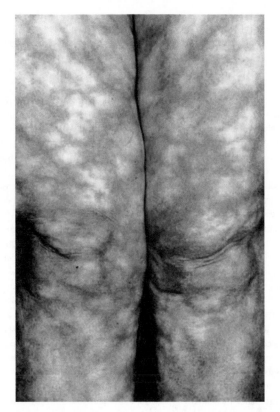

Figure 130.2 A 'net-like' pattern of discoloration gives the classical appearance of livedo reticularis (see colour plate section).
Reproduced from Longmore et al. Oxford Hanbook of Clinical Medicine, 7th edn. 2007, with permission from Oxford University Press

Case 131 ♦ Systemic Lupus Erythematosus (SLE)

CASE PRESENTATION

*There is an **erythematous, maculopapular** rash in a **butterfly distribution** over the cheeks and the bridge of the nose, sparing the nasolabial folds,[1] with **scaling** and **follicular plugging**.[2,3]*

There is also a symmetrical arthropathy of the small joints of the hands affecting the proximal interphalangeal joints and metacarpophalangeal joints as well as the wrists and the knees. There is evidence of Raynaud's phenomenon.[4]

*The diagnosis is **systemic lupus erythematosus**.[5]*

Clinical notes

1. The rash in lupus erythematosus is photosensitive and occurs in sun-exposed areas. It commonly occurs on the face in a butterfly distribution over the cheeks and bridge of the nose. The nasolabial folds are often spared. The chin and ears are often involved. The rash may be macular, papular, or maculopapular.

2. The rash is associated with some degree of scaling. Closer examination reveals the scales to comprise of tiny white dots, where the scales have plugged the skin follicles (follicular plugging or patulous follicles). If the scale where to be removed, a tiny spicule would project from the undersurface of the scaly mass, a finding unique to this condition. As the lesion progresses, the scaling may thicken and become adherent. As the lesions heal, there is atrophy, scarring with hyper- or hypopigmentation. The scalp may be involved, and this may lead to scarring alopecia.

3. Look for other skin features of lupus erythematosus: palmar erythema, photosensitivity, vasculitic lesions, purpura, urticaria, livedo reticularis, telangiectasia, alopecia, Raynaud's phenomenon, and subcutaneous nodules (similar to those in rheumatoid arthritis).

4. Once having established the rash of lupus erythematosus, it is important to establish whether or not other systems are involved. A quick examination of the hands will demonstrate the absence or presence of arthritis. Joint involvement occurs in 90% of patients with SLE. Tenderness, oedema, and effusions are present with a symmetrical, non-erosive polyarthritis that often involves the small joints of the hands affecting the PIP joints and MCP joints as well as the wrists and the knees. It is usually non-deforming, although a severe non-erosive deforming arthropathy is recognized (Jaccoud's arthropathy). Raynauds phenomenon occurs in 20% of cases. Look for features of rheumatoid arthritis, systemic sclerosis, and dermatomyositis that may occur as art of a mixed connective tissue disorder.

5. If the findings are confined to the skin, the diagnosis is discoid lupus erythematosus. If there is evidence of multisystem involvement, then the diagnosis is SLE. Look for rheumatoid arthritis, systemic sclerosis, or dermatomyositis, to make a diagnosis of mixed connective tissue disease. Tell the examiner that you would like to examine further to look for multisystem involvement:

    (a) **Conjunctivae**: pallor (anaemia)
    (b) **Hands**: palmar erythema, arthritis, Raynaud's phenomenon, dermatomyositis
    (c) **Nails**: splinter haemorrhages, nail-fold capillaries, periungual infarcts
    (d) **Mouth**: mouth ulcers (present in a third of patients)
    (e) **Scalp**: scarring alopecia
    (f) **Respiratory**: interstitial lung disease, pleural effusions, and pleurisy (pleural rub)
    (g) **Cardiovascular**: pericarditis (pericardial rub), murmurs (Libman-Sacks endocarditis), pulmonary hypertension
    (h) **Nervous system**: hemiparesis, cranial nerve lesions, mononeuritis multiplex, and polyneuropathy
    (i) **Renal**: hypertension, oedema, urinalysis for proteinuria, and haematuria
    (j) **Haematological**: lymphadenopathy, splenomegaly
    (k) **Eyes**: Sjogren syndrome and fundoscopy for cytoid bodies (retinal infarcts), roth spots and papilloedema

It is important to be aware of drug-induced lupus, and it is important to exclude drugs as a cause of the condition. Tell the examiner that you would like to take a detailed drug history.

Questions commonly asked by examiners

What other organs systems can be affected in SLE?

Organ system	Features
Skin	Butterfly rash, photosensitivity, palmar erythema, vasculitic lesions, purpura, urticaria, livedo reticularis, telangiectasia, alopecia, subcutaneous nodules (5%), Raynaud's phenomenon (20%)

Organ system	Features
Musculoskeletal	Non-erosive polyarthritis of the small joints of the hands affecting the PIP joints and MCP joints as well as the wrists and the knees; Jaccoud's arthropathy; splinter haemorrhages, nail-fold capillaries, periungual infarcts; avascular necrosis (especially if on steroid therapy)
Respiratory	Restrictive lung defect, interstitial lung disease, pleural effusions, pleurisy
Cardiovascular	Pericarditis, myocarditis, heart failure, Libman-Sacks endocarditis, accelerated coronary atherosclerosis
Neurological	Seizures, hemiparesis, ataxia, cranial nerve lesions, aseptic meningitis, chorea, mononeuritis multiplex, polyneuropathy, neurosis and a syndrome resembling multiple sclerosis
Haematological	Normochromic normocytic anaemia, haemolytic anaemia, leucopoenia, thrombocytopenia, pancytopenia, lymphadenopathy, splenomegaly
Renal	Lupus nephritis (see below)
Eyes	Sjogren syndrome, cytoid bodies (retinal infarcts), roth spots, and papilloedema

What are the diagnostic criteria for SLE?

The American College of Rheumatology criteria require any 4 of the following 11 criteria to make a diagnosis:

1. Malar rash
2. Discoid rash
3. Photosensitivity
4. Oral ulcers
5. Arthritis
6. Serositis
7. Renal involvement
8. Neurological involvement
9. Haematological involvement
10. Immunological disorder
11. Positive ANA

What are the causes of drug-induced lupus?

- Procainamide (most common)
- Hydralazine
- Isoniazid
- Quinidine
- Chlorpromazine
- Methyldopa
- Phenytoin
- Carbamazepine
- Sulphonamides
- Oral contraceptive pill
- Tetracycline

NB. Patients are often taking the drug for months or years before developing drug-induced lupus, and should not be confused with short-term side effects.

How can you differentiate drug-induced lupus from SLE?

Differentiating features	Drug-induced lupus	SLE
Sex	Male:female = 1:1	Female:male = 9:1
Organ involvement	Renal and CNS involvement is rare Lung involvement is common	Renal and CNS involvement is common
Auto-antibodies	Positive anti-histone antibodies Negative anti-dsDNA antibodies	Positive anti-dsDNA antibodies
Drug discontinuation	Resolution of clinical manifestations (within days to weeks)	No effect on clinical manifestations

What autoantibodies are seen in lupus?

* *Antinuclear antibodies* are present in 95% of cases (diagnosis is unlikely if negative)
* *Anti-histone antibodies* are characteristic but not specific for drug-induced lupus
* *Anti-dsDNA antibodies* are very specific for SLE, but only seen in 60% of patients
* *Anti-Sm antibodies* are very specific for SLE, but only seen in 20% of cases
* *Anti-Ro and anti-La antibodies* are found in ANA negative subacute cutaneous lupus
* *Antiphospholipid antibodies* (false positive VDRL test) occur in 40% of cases

What is the WHO classification for lupus nephritis?

Class	Definition	Treatment
I	Normal	
II	Mesangial glomerulunephritis	Treat extrarenal manifestations. If proteinuria>1g/day, ↑ anti-dsDNA or ↓ C3 complement, then proliferative component must be present and steroids should be considered.
III	Focal proliferative glomerulunephritis	For proliferative component: cyclophosphamide, azathioprine or mycophenolate mofetil
IV	Diffuse proliferative glomerulunephritis	
V	Membranous glomerulunephritis	Steroid therapy. If proliferative component present, then immunosuppressive therapy (as above)
VI	Sclerosing glomerulunephritis	Unlikely to respond to medical therapy. Consider renal replacement therapy.

What do you know about Libman-Sacks endocarditis?

* This is the most characteristic cardiac manifestation of SLE, and first described by Libman and Sacks in 1924 as atypical, sterile, verrucous valvular masses
* The exact pathogenesis is unknown, but anti-phospholipid antibodies are frequently associated with valvular abnormalities. These lesions consist of immune complexes and mononuclear cells
* Valvular abnormalities include masses (Libman-Sacks vegetations), diffuse leaflet thickening, valvular regurgitation and stenosis (rare). The most commonly involved valves are the aortic and mitral

- Valvular abnormalities may be present in up to 75% of patients, and valve thickening is observed on echocardiography in 50% of patients. Libman-Sacks vegetations are post-mortem findings in 50% of patients
- Complications include congestive cardiac failure, embolic phenomena, and secondary infective endocarditis

What is Jaccoud's arthropathy?

This is a non-erosive deforming arthritis of the small joints of the hands, resembling rheumatoid arthritis. Whereas, in rheumatoid arthritis, loss of bone and joint stability is secondary to a synovitis, Jaccoud's arthropathy mainly involves ligaments and peri-articular soft tissue. The deformity is a result of loss of ligamentous constraint, as opposed to the destructive effect of synovitis. The causes of Jaccoud's arthropathy include:

- Rheumatic fever
- SLE
- Parkinson's disease
- Hypocomplementaemic urticarial vasculitis
- HIV

How would you manage a patient with SLE?

Non-pharmacological

- Avoidance of over-exposure to sunlight (sunscreens with a protection factor >25)
- Avoid high dose oestrogen contraceptive pill (use low dose oestrogen or progesterone only pill)
- Removal of offending drugs (drug-induced lupus)
- Smoking cessation and primary prevention for cardiovascular disease (accelerated coronary atherosclerosis)

Pharmacological

- There are four main classes of drugs in patients with SLE:
  1. NSAIDs
  2. Anti-malarial drugs (hydroxychloroquine)
  3. Corticosteroids
  4. Cytotoxic drugs (azathioprine, cyclophosphamide, mycophenolate mofetil, cyclosporin)
- Plasma exchange may be used in difficult cases with severe disease, but its limitations include rebound disease in days/weeks, technical difficulties, patient discomfort, and cost.

	NSAIDs	Anti-malarials	Corticosteroids	Cytotoxic drugs
Fever	•		•	
Malaise		•	•	
Arthritis	•	•	•	•
Skin rash		•	•	
Serositis	•		•	
Pneumonitis			•	•
Vasculitis			•	•
Nephritis			•	•
Neurological			•	
Haemolytic anaemia			•	•
Thrombocytopenia			•	•

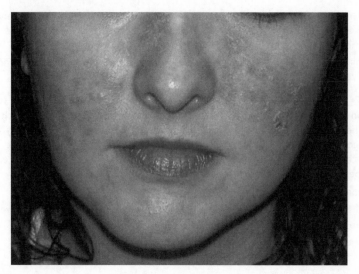

Figure 131.1 The characteristic malar 'butterfly' rash in systemic lupus erythematosus. Note sparing of the nasolabial folds (see colour plate section).
Reproduced from Longmore et al. Oxford Handbook of Clinical Medicine, 7th edn. 2007, with permission from Oxford University Press.

Case 132 ◆ **Alopecia**

CASE PRESENTATION

There are round (or oval) **patches of hair loss** *over the posterior aspect of scalp. They are* **well-circumscribed** *and have a* **distinctive border** *where normal hair demarcates the periphery.[1] The affected skin is normal, with no evidence of scarring.[2] There are* **exclamation point hairs** *visible within and around the patches.[3] The eyebrows, eyelashes, beard (in males), underarm, and body hair is not affected.[4] There is evidence of* **nail pitting**.[5]

The diagnosis is **alopecia areata**.[6]

Clinical notes

1. Alopecia areata manifests as sudden loss of hair with one (or more) well-circumscribed patches of hair loss. The patches have distinctive borders, with normal hairs demarcating the periphery. The scalp is the most common site affected by alopecia areata (90%). Hair loss progresses in a circumferential pattern and smaller patches may coalesce to form larger patches. With regrowth, the hair often lacks pigment resulting in blonde or white hairs.

2. The affected skin is usually normal, or in some cases may be slightly erythematous. In patients with alopecia, it is important to comment on scarring (see below).

3. The exclamation point hairs (or exclamation mark hairs) are characteristic, but not always seen. They may be seen in the patches (particularly in the peripheries) or around the patch. These are tapered towards the scalp and thickened at the distal end (resembling an exclamation mark).

4. Examine other hair-bearing body parts carefully, as other parts may be affected. Look carefully for involvement of eyebrows and eyelashes. If the entire body is involved, then this is termed alopecia universalis. Total loss of scalp hair is termed alopecia totalis.

5. Nail involvement occurs in up to 40% of patients, and is often seen in severe alopecia areata. Nail pitting is the most common finding. Other findings include trachyonychia, Beau's lines, koilonychia, leuconychia, and red-spotted lanulae.

6. Alopecia areata is an autoimmune disease. Look for evidence of other autoimmune diseases:

   (a) **Vitiligo**: hypopigmented patches
   (b) **Hashimoto's disease**: goitre (? previous thyroidectomy scar), features of hypothyroidism
   (c) **Grave's disease**: goitre (? previous thyroidectomy scar), eye signs, thyroid acropachy, pretibial myxoedema, features of hypo- or hyperthyroidism
   (d) **Addison's disease**: pigmentation, postural hypotension
   (e) **Hypoparathyroidism**: Chvostek's and Trousseau's sign, cataracts
   (f) **Diabetes**: finger tip skin pricks (regular glucose testing), fundoscopy to look for retinopathy
   (g) **Pernicious anaemia**: pallor, splenomegaly, polyneuropathy
   (h) **Myasthenia gravis**: myasthenic facies, ptosis, diplopia, proximal weakness, and fatigability
   (i) **SLE**: arthropathy, butterfly skin rash
   (j) **Idiopathic pulmonary fibrosis**: bibasal crepitations
   (k) **Primary biliary cirrhosis**: scratch marks, pigmentation, icterus, xanthelesma, signs of chronic liver disease
   (l) **Atrophic gastritis**: pallor, koilonychia-iron deficiency anaemia

      Other associated disorders include (that may be present):

      (a) **Atopic eczema**: look in flexural areas: dry skin, papulovesicular eruption, lichenification and excoriation
      (b) **Downs syndrome**: low-set ears, flattened nasal bridge, flat occiput, epicanthic folds, Brushfield spots on iris, small mouth that hangs with protruding tongue, single transverse palmar crease, fifth finger clinodactyly, wide sandal gap

Questions commonly asked by examiners

What are the causes of alopecia?

Non-scarring alopecia

- Alopecia areata
- Androgenic alopecia (male pattern baldness)
- Telogen effluvium
- Traction alopecia
- Endocrine disorders
  - Diabetes
  - Hyperthyroidism
  - Hypothyroidism
  - Hypopituitarism
  - Hypoparathyroidism
  - Pseudohypoparathyroidism
- Drugs (cause telogen effluvium)
  - Anti-thyroid drugs (carbimazole and propylthiouracil)
  - Anticoagulant drugs (warfarin and heparin)
  - Lithium

- ◆ Retinoids
- ◆ Oral contraceptive pill
- ◆ Anti-mitotic drugs (bleomycin, doxorubicin, vincristine, hydoxyurea and fluorouracil)

Scarring alopecia
- Radiotherapy
- Burns
- Tuberculosis (lupus vulgaris)
- Syphilis
- Lichen planus (lichen planopilaris)
- Morphoea
- Lupus erythematosus
- Tinea
- Sarcoidosis
- Necrobiosis lipoidica diabeticorum

What is telogen effluvium?

This is the diffuse hair loss (shedding of telogen hairs) that may occur 2–3 months after severe bodily stress. The stressful event causes premature and simultaneous shift of large number of follicles from the angen to the telogen phase. Examples of such stressful events include: febrile illnesses, childbirth, crash diets and psychological stress. Telogen effluvium is self-limiting and reversible. The drugs listed above cause telogen effluvium.

What is anagen effluvium?

This is also known as anagen arrest and is the diffuse hair breakage that follows the use of chemotherapeutic drugs. These drugs cause a temporary arrest of mitotic activity in the matrix region of anagen hair, resulting in constriction of the hair shaft and hair breakage. This occurs 1–3 weeks after commencing therapy, and 80–90% of the hair is affected. The hair follicle cycles out of the anagen phase and remains in the telogen phase, until a few months after the pharmacological effects of the drug have worn out.

What is trichotillomania?

A disorder where that patient compulsively pulls out or breaks his or her own hair. This is more common in females and children. There are often irregular patches of hair loss, and the scalp is the most common site, followed by eyebrows and eyelashes. The hairs in the affected areas are often short with a mixture of broken and tapered hairs. The patches are often unilateral, often on the same side as the dominant hand. Patients may be unaware of this habit. Other clues to the diagnosis are changing patterns of hair loss from visit to visit, and exclusive loss of hair from the upper eyelashes (hair pulling from lower eyelashes can be painful).

What is the treatment of alopecia areata?

Non-pharmacological
- Cosmetic camouflage
- Wigs or hairpieces
- Micro-tattooing

Pharmacological
- Corticosteroids (topical, intralesional, and systemic)
- Topical anthralin (20–30 minutes per day for 2 weeks)

- Topical minoxidil
- Topical immunotherapy*
- PUVA

---

* This is defined as the eliciting of an allergic contact dermatitis by applying potent contact allergens to the affected skin, resulting in immunomodulatory effects. Commonly used contact allergens include dinitrochlorobenzene (DNCB), squaric acid dinitryl ester (SADBE) and diphenylcyropropenone (DPCP).

Case 133 ◆ Tuberous Sclerosis

CASE PRESENTATION

*There are salmon-coloured papules and nodules over the face in a butterfly distribution, particularly in the nasolabial folds (**adenoma sebaceum**).[1] There are smooth, firm, nodular lesions adjacent to the nails, both in the fingers and toes (**periungual fibroma**).[2] There are irregularly shaped, green-brown, unevenly thickened plaques in the lumbosacral region with a cobble stone appearance (**shagreen patches**).[3] There are hypopigmented macules, in an ash leaf configuration, over the trunk and buttocks (**ash leaf macules**).[4] In the flexural areas (neck and axillae), there are large, soft, pedunculated, skin-coloured papules and nodules (**molluscum fibrosum pendulum**).[5] There are also multiple, irregularly shaped, evenly pigmented brown macules (**café-au-lait spots**).[6]*

*These cutaneous features together would suggest a diagnosis of **tuberous sclerosis**.*

Clinical notes

1. These lesions are angiofibromata composed of vascular and connective tissue elements. They are seen in 75% of cases. They often begin in childhood and early adolescence, and may be initially mistaken for freckles. They become paulonodular over time.

2. Both periungual and ungual fibromata occur in 20% of cases. They occur more commonly on the toes (don't miss examination of the toes).

3. The 'shagreen' or 'leather' patch is an accumulation of collagen, resulting in thickened plaques over the lumbosacral regions. These plaques have a cobble stone appearance, resembling studded leather.

4. This is the most common skin manifestation (seen in 90% of cases). These hypopigmented macules are rounded at one end, and tapered at the other—named after the European mountain ash tree. In fair-skinned individuals, these lesions may be difficult to visualize, requiring the aid of ultraviolet light (Wood's lamp). Sometimes, these lesions may have an irregular reticuloid appearance, as if white confetti paper had been strewn over the skin (confetti lesions)

5. These lesions resemble skin tags and may not be present in all patients.

6. Café-au-lait spots are seen in 30% of patients.

7. Tuberous sclerosis is a multisystem disorder, characterized by hamartomata formation in different organ systems. Tell the examiner, you would like to look for other manifestations of this disease:

   (a) **Ocular**: angiofibromata of the eyelids; fundoscopy for retinal hamartomata and hypopigmentation

   (b) **Oral**: gingival hamartomata; dental pitting; bifid uvula; high arched palate

   (c) **Respiratory**: pneumothorax; lung cysts

(d) **Abdomen**: hepatic or renal cysts

(e) **Neurological**: focal neurological findings depending on location of tubers

Epiloia is the classical triad of e̲pilepsy, l̲ow i̲ntelligence and a̲denoma sebaceum (seen in a third of patients). Tell the examiner you would like to test the IQ and ask about a history of epilepsy.

Questions commonly asked by examiners

What are the genetics of tuberous sclerosis?

This is inherited as an autosomal dominant condition, and two gene loci have been identified:

- Chromosome 9 (9q34): TSC1 gene that encodes hamartin
- Chromosome 16 (16p13): TSC2 gene that encodes tuberin

Approximately 65% of cases are caused by spontaneous mutation.

What is the pathophysiology of tuberous sclerosis?

Hamartin and tuberin have tumour suppressor activity. Mutations of these genes lead to uncontrolled cellular differentiation and development of hamartomata throughout the body.

What other organs may be involved?

Organ	Features
Eyes	Retinal hamartomata or phakomata (50%); retinal hypopigmentation; angiofibromata of the eyelids
Heart	Cardiac rhabdomyoma (often multiple and can cause outflow obstruction, valvular dysfunction, and arrhythmias)
Brain	Tubers; subependymal nodules; subependymal giant cell astrocytoma (may lead to obstructive hydrocephalus); mental retardation (50%); seizures (75%)
Lungs	Lung cysts; pneumothorax; multifocal multinodular pneumocyte hyperplasia; lymphangioleomyomatosis
Kidneys	Renal hamartoma or angiomyolipoma (80%); renal cysts (single or multiple)
Mouth	Gingival hamartoma; dental pits (seen in almost all patients); high-arched palate; bifid uvula
Bone	Bone cysts; sclerotic lesions; periosteal new bone lesions
Abdomen	Hamartomata and polyposis of stomach, intestine and colon; hamartomatous rectal polyps; hepatic cysts; hepatic angiomyolipoma
Vascular	Aneurysm formation may affect the aorta, carotid, renal, and intracranial arteries

Case 134 ◆ **Clubbing**

CASE PRESENTATION

There is bulbous, fusiform enlargement of the distal portions of the digit (giving them a **drumstick appearance**).[1] There is **thickening of the nail bed** with **loss of the obtuse angle between the proximal nail fold and nail plate**.[2] When the dorsum of two fingers from opposite hands are opposed, the diamond-shaped gap at the base of the nails is obliterated (**Shamroth's sign**).[3] There is **increased curvature of the nail**[4] and **increased sponginess of the nail bed**.[5]

These features are inkeeping with **clubbing**, that may be idiopathic or secondary to many systemic pathologies.[6]

Clinical notes

1. With marked swelling of the nail bed, they may have the classical drumstick appearance.
2. In the absence of clubbing, when the profile of the distal digit is viewed, the **Lovibond angle** (angle between the nail plate and nail fold) is usually ≤160°. In clubbing, this angle flattens out, and increases with severity of clubbing. An angle greater than 180° indicates definite clubbing. An angle between 160–180° is a grey area, and may represent early clubbing.
3. The Shamroth's sign reflects loss the obtuse Lovibond angle.
4. The curvature of the nails is increased both in a longitudinal and transverse direction.
5. As a result of increased fibrovascular tissue between the nail and the phalanx, there is increased sponginess and fluctuation of the nail and the nail bed.
6. Clubbing has many secondary causes. Tell the examiner you would like to look for associated systemic diseases (see below for a list of causes).

Questions commonly asked by examiners

What are the secondary causes of clubbing?

Respiratory

- Bronchogenic carcinoma
- Mesothelioma
- Interstitial lung disease
- Bronchiectasis
- Cystic fibrosis
- Empyema
- Tuberculosis
- Asbestosis
- Pulmonary arterio-venous malformations

Cardiovascular

- Cyanotic congenital heart disease
- Bacterial endocarditis
- Atrial myxoma

Gastrointestinal

- Chronic liver disease
- Inflammatory bowel disease
- Gastrointestinal lymphoma
- Coeliac disease
- Tropical sprue
- Whipples disease

Other

- Thyroid acropachy
- Thyroid cancers
- Thymus cancers
- Palmoplantar keratoderma
- POEMS syndrome*

What are the primary causes of clubbing?

- Idiopathic
- Familial clubbing (autosomal dominant)
- Primary hypertrophic osteoarthropathy (autosomal dominant)**

What are the causes of unilateral clubbing?

- Idiopathic
- Bronchial arteriovenous aneurysm
- Axillary artery aneurysm
- Subclavian artery aneurysm
- Ulnar artery aneurysm
- Arteriovenous fistula (dialysis fistula)
- Hempilegia
- Brachial plexus injury
- Trauma

What is pseudoclubbing?

This is defined as increased curvature (longitudinal and transverse) of the nails, with a normal Lovibond angle. This can involve only a single digit.

What do you know about the pathophysiology of clubbing?

There is increased blood flow in the clubbed portion of the finger, secondary to distal digital vasodilatation. Initially there is increased interstitial oedema, and as clubbing progresses, there is an increase in vascular connective tissue. The exact mechanism of vasodilatation is unclear, and many theories exist.

---

* POEMS: Polyneuropathy, Organomegaly, Endocrinopathy, Monoclonal gammopathy, and Skin changes; a paraneoplastic syndrome secondary to plasma cell dyscrasias; other features include clubbing, white nails, sclerotic bone lesions, Thrombocytosis, papilloedema, pleural effusions, and ascites.
** This is disorder is characterized by clubbing, periostosis, and skin manifestations (skin thickening, coarsening of facial features, hyperhidrosis, and seborrhoea).

Circulating vasodilators

Evidence for this derives from clubbing associated with cyanotic congenital heart disease, as many potential vasodilators that would otherwise be inactivated in the lungs bypass the lungs through right-to-left shunts. This would also explain the differential clubbing (clubbing of the feet, with sparing of the hands) seen in patients with right-to-left shunting through a patent ductus arteriosus, where the shunted blood passing into the descending aorta.

Hypoxia

This has been proposed as an alternative mechanism for clubbing in cyanotic heart diseases and pulmonary diseases. Hypoxia may activate local vasodilators, increasing blood flow to the distal portions of the digits. However, hypoxia is not always present in patients with clubbing, and many hypoxic conditions are not associated with clubbing.

Platelet precursors

Recent research shows that platelet precursors fail to fragment into platelets in the pulmonary circulation in patients with clubbing. These megakaryocytes or large platelet clumps, are easily trapped in the peripheral vasculature, and become lodged in the vascular beds of the digital digits. These release platelet-derived growth factor and vascular endothelial growth factor that increase vascular permeability and connective tissue formation.

Case 135 ◆ **Bullous Skin Eruptions**

---

1. Pemphigus Vulgaris

CASE PRESENTATION

*There are **flaccid blisters** filled with clear fluid that are present on normal skin and in some areas with an erythematous base. The blisters are **fragile**, and many blisters have burst leaving **red, denuded skin**.[1] In addition, there are poorly defined, irregularly shaped, **red**, **denuded erosions** in the **buccal cavity**, **pharynx**, and **conjunctivae**.[2]*

*The diagnosis is **pemphigus vulgaris**.[3]*

Clinical notes

1. The primary lesion of pemphigus vulgaris is a flaccid blister filled with clear fluid. The blisters are fragile and, therefore, intact blisters may not be present. The contents soon become turbid, or the blisters rupture leaving denuded areas of skin, that are extremely tender. These lesions are often large because they tend to extend peripherally with the shedding of the epithelium. Occasionally, the lesions may occur without initial blister formation.

2. Mucous membranes are usually affected first and may precede skin lesions by months (on average ~ 5 months). They are affected in 50–75% of patients. The mucous membranes often affected are those of the oral cavity, which is involved in almost all patients and sometimes is the only area involved. Intact bullae are rare in the mouth, leaving red denuded gingival, buccal, or palatine erosions. They can be quite extensive and may spread to involve the larynx. They are extremely tender, and the patient is

often unable to eat or drink. Other mucosal surfaces may be involved, including the conjunctiva, oesophagus, labia, vagina, penis, urethra, and anus.

3. There are certain signs associated with pemphigus vulgaris, which the candidate should be aware of. They should *not* be elicited in the examination, as they can cause significant discomfort:

   (a) **Nikolsky sign:** firm sliding pressure with a finger causes normal skin to slide off. This is invariably present, but is not specific for this condition. Other causes include toxic epidermal necrolysis and staphylococcal scalded skin syndrome.

   (b) **Asboe-Hansen sign:** Lateral pressure on the edge of a blister may spread the blister into clinically unaffected skin.

4. Although the exact cause of pemphigus vulgaris is unknown, there are many potential associations:

   (a) **Drugs:** Tell the examiner that you would like to take a detailed drug history

   (b) **Myasthenia gravis:** myasthenic facies, ptosis, diplopia, proximal weakness, and fatigability

2. Pemphigoid

CASE PRESENTATION

There are **tense blisters** *filled with clear (or haemorrhagic) fluid that are present on normal and erythematous skin, with a* **predilection for flexural areas.**[1] *There is* **no mucosal involvement.**[2]

The diagnosis is **pemphigoid.**

Clinical notes

1. The primary lesion of pemphigoid is the formation of tense bullae that can occur on any part of the skin, but commonly occur in flexural areas. Some patients may present with persistent urticarial lesions that convert to bullous eruptions, and in some, this may be the sole manifestation of the disease. The bullae tend to heal without scarring. Unlike pemphigus, the blisters are thicker, and unlikely to rupture. Pemphigoid primarily tends to occur in the elderly, but onset in younger individuals has been reported.

2. There is usually no mucosal involvement, but this can occur.

3. Dermatitis herpetiformis

CASE PRESENTATION

There are **groups** *of* **erythematous vesicles** *and* **papules** *present* **bilaterally** *and* **symmetrically** *on the* **extensor surfaces** *(elbows, knees, posterior neck, back, and buttocks). These are associated with widespread* **excoriation marks,** *suggesting these lesions are* **pruritic.**[1,2]

The characteristics and distribution of this rash suggests a diagnosis of **dermatitis herpetiformis.**[3]

Clinical notes

1. The primary lesion of dermatitis herpetiformis consists of erythematous vesicle or papules. Grouping of these lesions commonly occurs. As these lesions are intensely pruritic, vesicles have usually ruptured by scratching, and patients may present only with multiple erosions.

2. The hallmarks of the disease are grouping of these lesions, their symmetry, and characteristic distribution on the extensor surfaces.

3. This condition is usually associated with a gluten-sensitive enteropathy (Coeliac's disease). There may be no other features of Coeliac's disease on physical examination, but look for:
   (a) **Conjunctival pallor** (anaemia)
   (b) **Peripheral neuropathy** (B_{12} deficiency)
   (c) **Purpura** (poor vitamin K absorption leading to a bleeding diasthesis)
   (d) **Chvostek's** or **Trousseau sign** (hypocalcaemia)

Questions commonly asked by examiners

What are other causes of a bullous skin eruption?

- Burns
- Contact dermatitis
- Impetigo
- Chicken pox
- Pompholyx eczema
- Bullous erythema multiforme
- Staphylococcal scalded skin syndrome
- Porphyria cutanea tarda
- Epidermolysis bullosa congenital (and acquisita)
- Liner IgA disease
- Herpes gestionatis
- Barbiturates

What is the pathophysiology of pemphigus?

This is an autoimmune mucocutaneous bullous disease. Blistering occurs in the epidermis, and the IgG autoantibodies are directed at antigens on the surface of keratinocytes (desmogleins—these act as cell adhesion molecules). There are two forms of pemphigus—vulgaris and foliaceous—which affect different layers of the epidermis and have different target antigens (see below). In all forms of pemphigus, there is separation of the keratinocytes by dissolution of the intercellular substance and separation of desmosomes (acantholysis). Immunoflorescence biopsy shows intercellular epidermal deposits of IgG.

What are the differences between pemphigus vulgaris and foliaceous?

Features	Pemphigus vulgaris (deep)	Pemphigus foliaceous (superficial)
Site of blisters	Just above the basal cell layer	High in the epidermis, below stratum corneum
Antigen	Desmoglein-1	Desmoglein-3
Oral lesions	Common	Do not occur
Prognosis	Worse	Better

What drugs are implicated in pemphigus?

- Penicillamine
- Benzylpenicillin
- Cephalosporins
- ACE inhibitors (captopril, ramipril, fosinopril, and cilazapril)
- Phenylbutazone

- Phenobarbitone
- Aspirin
- NSAIDs
- Rifampicin
- Levodopa
- Propanolol
- Nifedipine

What is the treatment for pemphigus?

The morbidity and mortality from untreated pemphigus is significant. With medical therapies the mortality has fallen from 75% to 10%, and the main cause of morbidity and mortality is due to complications of therapy. The goals of therapy are to induce and maintain remission with the lowest possible doses of medication.

General measures
- Cessation of potentially offending drugs
- Avoid dehydration
- Treat secondary infection
- Barrier nursing

Specific therapies
- Corticosteroids (the mainstay of treatment)
- Other immunosuppressive drugs (corticosteroid-sparing drugs):
  - Azathioprine
  - Mycofenolate mofetil
  - Methotrexate
  - Cyclophosphamide
  - Cyclosporin
  - Dapsone
  - Gold
  - Tetracycline (with nicotinamide)

Others (investigational) therapies
- Rituximab (monoclonal anti-CD20 antibody)
- Infliximab (anti-TNF-α therapy)
- Cholinergic agonists

What is the role of plasmapharesis in the treatment of pemphigus?

Based on recent randomized controlled data, plasmapharesis has shown a lack of benefit and increased mortality. It is not recommended for the treatment of newly diagnosed pemphigus. The concurrent need for corticosteroid or immunosuppressive therapy is often needed to prevent rebound production of antibodies. Plasmapharesis with immunosuppressive therapy may have a role in the treatment of severe pemphigus.

What is the pathophysiology of pemphigoid?

This is an autoimmune bullous skin disease that rarely involves mucous membranes. Blistering occurs at the basement membrane (between the epidermis and dermis), and the IgG autoantibodies are specific for the hemidesmosomal antigens BP230 (BPAg1) and BP180 (BPAg2). Immunoflorescence biopsy shows a band of IgG at the level of the basement membrane.

What are the differences between pemphigus and pemphigoid?

Feature	Pemphigus	Pemphigoid
Blisters	Flaccid, tend to burst easily	Tense, less likely to burst
Site of blisters	Epidermal	Subepidermal (basement membrane)
Antigens	Desmoglein-1 and desmoglein-3	BPAg1 and BPAg2
Mucosal involvement	Present	Rare
Nikolsy sign	Positive	Negative
Prognosis	Fatal if untreated	A relatively benign condition

Remember, pemphigu**S** for **S**uperficial (epidermal) blisters and pemphigoi**D** for **D**eep (supepidermal) blisters.

What is the treatment for pemphigoid?

Corticosteroids
- Topical corticosteroids (localized mild disease)
- Systemic corticosteroids

Corticosteroid sparing drugs
- Azathioprine
- Mycofenolate mofetil
- Methotrexate
- Cyclophosphamide
- Cyclosporin
- Tetracycline (with nicotinamide)

What is the pathophysiology of dermatitis herpetiformis?

This is an autoimmune bullous skin disorder that is commonly associated with a gluten-sensitive enteropathy. This is caused by IgA deposits at the dermo–epidermal junction that results in neutrophil chemotaxis, cytokine, and complement activation. Metalloproteinases are released, that breakdown the connective tissue, and this results in vesicle formation at the dermo–epidermal junction.

What is the link between dermatitis herpetiformis and coeliac disease?

Dermatitis herpetiformis and coeliac disease share a unique intestinal sensitivity to gluten, with dermatitis herpetiformis representing a skin manifestation of intestinal gluten sensitivity resulting from cross-reactivity of autoantibodies to antigens in the skin (see above). Patients with dermatitis herpetiformis are unlikely to have malabsorption or gastrointestinal symptoms. However, nearly all patients have histological changes on small bowel biopsy. This may range from the classical complete villous atrophy to partial villous atrophy (more common).

What is the treatment for dermatitis herpetiformis?

- Gluten-free diet
- Dapsone (rash often clears within days, with complete clearance in 1 week)*

---

* Adverse effects include methaemoglobinaemia, haemolysis, and agranulocytosis.

Case 136 ◆ **Peutz-Jeghers Syndrome**

CASE PRESENTATION

There is cutaneous pigmentation characterized by **brown-black pigmented macules**[1] *affecting the* **peri-oral area**, **lips**, *and* **buccal mucosa** *(whilst* **sparing the tongue**).[2] *They are also present on the hands and feet.*[3]

These findings suggest a diagnosis of **Peutz-Jeghers syndrome**.[4]

Clinical notes

1. The characteristic findings are well-defined brown, black, or blue coloured pigmented macules (1–5mm). These macules may fade after puberty. In adult patients, who are frequently present in the examination, look carefully for fading pigmented macules. Remember, they do not fade in the buccal mucosa, so if in doubt, look in the mouth!

2. These lesions commonly affect the peri-oral and peri-nasal area. They are present on the lips, and usually cross the vermilion border. Mucosal membrane involvement occurs, most commonly the buccal mucosa. The tongue is NEVER affected.

3. Other sites that are involved include the hands, feet, peri-anal, and peri-genital areas.

4. This condition is characterized by mucocutaneous pigmented macules, intestinal polyposis (hamartomata), and an increased frequency of malignancies (both intestinal and extra-intestinal). Tell the examiner you would like to look for:

   (a) **Iron deficient anaemia**: conjunctival pallor and koilonychia

   (b) **Rectal polyps** : rectal masses may be found on rectal examination

   (c) **Breast malignancy** (in females): breast lumps (look for previous lumpectomy or mastectomy scars)

   (d) **Ovarian malignancy** (in females): ovarian masses

   (e) **Pancreatic malignancy**: pancreatic mass

   (f) **Sertoli cell tumours** (in males): tall (rapid growth) and gynaecomastia

Questions commonly asked by examiners

What are the genetics of Peutz-Jeghers syndrome?

This is inherited as an autosomal dominant condition. There is a germline mutation of the gene encoding serine threonine kinase (STK11) located on chromosome 19 (19p13.3).

What are the complications of this condition?

- Recurrent colicky abdominal pains
- Gastrointestinal haemorrhage
- Iron deficiency anaemia
- Intestinal obstruction
- Intestinal intussusception
- Malignancy (both intestinal and extra-intestinal)

Where are bowel polyps located in this condition?

The most common sites in descending order are small intestine (jejunum>ileum>duodenum), large intestine, and stomach.

What malignancies are associated with this condition?

- Gastrointestinal (oesophagus, stomach, small and large intestine)
- Pancreatic
- Breast tumours
- Ovarian (sex cord tumours)
- Uterine (adenocarcinomas)
- Testicular (Sertoli cell tumours)

Peutz-Jeghers syndrome is a cancer predisposing condition. There is a 9-fold greater risk of dying from cancer compared to the general population. In one registry 48% of patients developed cancer, from which 73% occurred outside the gastrointestinal tract.

What is the management for this condition?

- Genetic counselling
- Endoscopic polypectomy (polyps >5mm)
- Consider laparotomy and intraoperative endoscopy for larger polyps (>15mm)*
- Appropriate screening for intestinal and extra-intestinal tumours

Case 137 ◆ **Necrobiosis Lipoidica Diabeticorum**

CASE PRESENTATION

There are multiple, bilateral, **well-circumscribed, coalescing, oval plaques** *on the* **anterior surface of the lower legs**.[1] *They have a* **shiny surface** *with* **waxy yellow atrophic centres** *and* **red-brown margins**, *with* **telangiectasia** *over their surface.*[2]

The diagnosis is **necrobiosis lipoidica diabeticorum**, *which has a strong association with diabetes.*[3]

Clinical notes

1. Necrobiosis lipoidica diabeticorum commonly occurs on the pretibial area, but can occur on the face, trunk, and upper extremities.

2. The skin lesions are often multiple and bilateral. They comprise well-circumscribed coalescing plaques that expand with a red-brown border leaving a waxy yellow atrophic centre. Multiple telangiectases can be seen on the surface of the thinning epidermis. They often become painless because of cutaneous nerve damage, but can be extremely painful in 25% of cases. They exhibit the Koebner phenomenon, and thus it is important to look at sites of trauma and scars.

3. Necrobiosis lipoidica diabeticorum has a strong association with diabetes. Tell the examiner that you would like to further examine various systems to demonstrate other features and association of diabetes:

   (a) Finger tip skin pricks: confirm regular glucose testing to support a diagnosis of diabetes

   (b) Other cutaneous manifestations of diabetes (see below)

---

* Excision of affected bowel segments should be avoided, as the polyps tend to recur.

(c)   Visual acuity and fundoscopy: evidence of diabetic eye disease

(d)   Cardiovascular examination: measurement of blood pressure and peripheral pulses

(e)   Neurological examination: peripheral neuropathy

Questions commonly asked by examiners

What are the causes of necrobiosis lipoidica diabeticorum?

This is often associated with diabetes. It can occur in the pre-diabetic individual or on its own.

What is the histology of these skin lesions?

There is collagen necrosis with palisades of granulomatous epithelioid cells in the subcutaneous tissue and dermis.

What other skin lesions can be seen in diabetes?

- Infections (boils, carbuncles, cellulitis)
- Ulceration and gangrene
- Lipoatrophy
- Lipohypertrophy
- Eruptive xanthomata (hypertriglyceridaemia)
- Xanthalesmata
- Acanthosis nigricans
- Erythema nodosum (secondary to sulphonylureas)
- Erythema multiforme (secondary to sulphonylureas)
- Vitiligo (association with autoimmune disease)
- Alopecia (association with autoimmune disease)
- Granuloma annulare
- Diabetic dermopathy*
- Diabetic rubeosis**

What is granuloma annulare?

These are non-itchy, non-scaly, well–demarcated, circular papules that coalesce in rings (1–3cm in diameter). They are often present on the dorsal surfaces of the hands and feet.

What other skin conditions mimic necrobiosis lipoidica diabeticorum, both clinically and histologically?

- Cutaneous sarcoidosis
- Necrobiosis xanthogranuloma (paraproteinaemia and haematological malignancies)

What is the treatment for this condition?

- Skin protection (localized trauma can lead to ulceration)
- Good diabetic control (controversy exists whether this helps)
- Topical or intralesional steroids may help
- Pentoxifylline may have some beneficial effects
- Excision and skin grafting in severe cases
- Laser therapy (pulse dye lasers)

---

* Diabetic dermopathy is the presence of atrophic and pigmented lesions that often occur on the pretibial area.
** Diabetic rubeosis is the redness of the face, hands, and feet that is thought to be due to diabetic microangiopathy.

Case 138 ◆ **Skin Malignancies**

1. Basal cell carcinoma (BCC)

CASE PRESENTATION

There is a round, dome-shaped, skin-coloured (or erythematous), **well-circumscribed nodule** *on the face, measuring 1cm in diameter, just under the lateral aspect of the left eye.[1] It has a* **rolled, pearly edge** *that is* **not everted**.[2] *There is a* **necrotic, ulcerated centre** *with a* **sloughy coat**.[3] *It is confined to the skin and is freely mobile over the underlying tissues. The surrounding skin is normal[4] and there is* **no regional lymphadenopathy**.[5]

The diagnosis is **basal cell carcinoma (BCC)**.

Clinical notes

1. BCC presents as insidious painless nodules or ulcers on areas exposed to the sun. It has a predilection for the upper two-thirds of the face (90% occur above the line joining the angle of the mouth to external auditory meatus). Common sites affected are around the eye, nasolabial folds, and hairline of the scalp. It is important to provide some estimate of the size in the case presentation.

2. It has characteristic rolled pearly edges that are NOT everted-a feature that distinguishes it from squamous cell carcinoma (SCC).

3. Ulceration may not be present.

4. The surrounding skin may be normal or show evidence of sun-exposed damage.

5. Lymphatic and haematogenous spread is rare.

2. Squamous cell carcinoma (SCC)

CASE PRESENTATION

There is an irregular, round, **shallow ulcer** *with well-defined* **everted edges** *on the right cheek,[1] measuring 1.5cm in diameter.[2] There is a* **necrotic ulcer base** *covered with* **slough** *and* **granulation tissue**.[3] *It is confined to the skin and is freely mobile over the underlying tissues.[4] The surrounding skin is normal.[5] There is* **regional lymphadenopathy** *(say which nodes are enlarged).[6] There is no evidence of perineural invasion.[7]*

The diagnosis is **squamous cell carcinoma (SCC)**.

Clinical notes

1. SCC typically presents as a non-healing ulcer on sun-exposed areas of the skin. Approximately 70% occur on the head and neck. Common sites affected are the lower lip, external ear, periauricular region, forehead, and scalp. The everted edges help differentiate this from BCC. The presentation of SCC is preceded by precancerous lesions-actinic keratosis (scaly plaques and papules with an erythematous base).

2. It is important to give the size and location, as they have prognostic implications. A width >2mm, depth >4mm, location on the lip or the ear are associated with increased risk of recurrence and metastases.

3. Slough and unhealthy granulation tissue may be seen over the ulcer base. Often this becomes adherent and the ucler base is covered with a plaque.

4. It is important to establish depth of involvement. Advanced tumours may become fixed to underlying structures and immobile.

5. The surrounding skin may be normal or show evidence of sun-exposed damage.

6. Unlike BCC, where lymph node involvement is rare, metastases to local lymph nodes occur in 10% of cases, and all SCC lesions should be regarded as metastatic until proven otherwise. Most commonly affected are upper cervical lymph nodes or those within the parotid gland. However, in 30% of cases, palpable lymph nodes are reactive due to secondary infection. SCCs affecting the lip and ear have a high rate of lymphatic spread.

7. SCC can exhibit perineural invasion in up to 10% of cases. Look for evidence of cranial neuropathy (most commonly affected are V and VII). Assess facial movements (VII) and sensation (V).

3. Malignant melanoma

CASE PRESENTATION

*There is an **asymmetrical**, **dark brown/red-brown/blue-black** coloured **nodule** (unevenly pigmented and a **variegated appearance**) with **irregular edges**[1] on the leg.[2] It measures 9mm in diameter (**greater than 6mm**), and is **elevated** to 2mm above the skin.[3] There is no lymphadenopathy.[4] There is no evidence of bleeding or ulceration.[5]*

*The diagnosis is **malignant melanoma**.[6]*

Clinical notes

1. Melanomas often display a variation in colour, giving it an unevenly pigmented and variegated appearance. The ABCDE pneumonic helps differentiate melanomas form benign naevi:

   A: **A**symmetry

   B: **B**order irregularity

   C: **C**olour variation

   D: **D**iameter >6mm

   E: **E**levated above the skin

2. Melanomas can occur anywhere on the skin, often in sun-exposed areas. Different clinical subtypes have predilections for certain sites (see below).

3. An estimated of size and depth is important for prognosis.

4. Melanomas can spread via lymphatics to regional lymph nodes, or haematogenously to lymph nodes elsewhere in the body. It is important to examine all lymph nodes.

5. Comment on bleeding or ulceration if present (as these would distinguish it from a benign naevus).

6. Although this is typically a short case, tell the examiner that you would like to examine all lymph nodes and conduct a general examination to assess for metastatic spread.

3. Mycosis fungoides (cutaneous T-cell lymphoma)

CASE PRESENTATION

There are multiple, **well-defined, irregularly shaped, thickened, erythematous plaques**[1] *with* **fine scaling** *distributed asymmetrically over the hips, buttocks, and lower trunk.*[2] *There are also multiple erythematous* **nodules** *with* **ulceration.**[3]

The diagnosis is **mycosis fungoides.**[4]

Clinical notes

1. The plaques may be single or multiple. They initially appear as flat erythematous macules. In dark-skinned individuals they may be hypo- or hyper-pigmented. As the patches become more thickened, they evolve into palpable plaques with irregular borders. There is fine scaling over these lesions, and they may be confused with eczema or psoriasis.

2. Although they may affect any skin area, they tend to be confined to areas that would be covered by a bathing suit, i.e. hips, buttocks, genitals, lower trunk, axillae, and breast.

3. Some patients may also have nodules. They may have a violaceous or erythematous appearance, and physical findings for these are variable: they may be dome-shape, exophytic, or ulcerated.

4. Although mycoses fungoides is primarily a skin malignancy, extracutaneous involvement can occur. Lymph nodes are the most frequent site of extracutaneous involvement. Look for
   (a) **Scratch marks**: lesions can be pruritic; Koebner phenomenon
   (b) **Scalp involvement**: associated with scarring alopecia
   (c) **Erythroderma**: can occur as the disease advances; associated with profound scaling and pruritis
   (d) **Leonine facies**: extensive nodular infiltration of the face leading to thickening of skin folds
   (e) **Lymphadenopathy**: most frequent site of extracutaenous involvement
   (f) **Visceral involvement**: lungs, liver, and spleen

Questions commonly asked by examiners

What are the risk factors for (a) BCC, (b) SCC, and (c) malignant melanoma?

(a) Risk factors for BCC
- Sunlight exposure (particularly UVB radiation)
- Fair-skinned individuals
- Poor ability to tan (ability to tan is the most important protective factor)
- Basal cell naevus syndrome*
- Xeroderma pigmentosum**
- Epidermodysplastic verruciformis***

(b) Risk factors for SCC
- Sunlight exposure
- Fair-skinned individuals
- Immunosupression
- Carcinogens (arsenic, tar, soot, and polyaromatic hydrocarbons)

---

* Autosomal dominant condition, associated with multiple BCCs, odontogenic keratocysts, calcification of falx cerebri, and rib anomalies.
** Autosomal recessive condition, with hypersensitivity to ultraviolet light with defects in DNA repair and synthesis.
*** Autosomal recessive disorder characterized by development of BCC and SCC from warts.

- Chronic ulceration (Marjolin's ulcer)
- Xeroderma pigmentosum**
- Epidermodysplastic verruciformis***
- Bowen's disease****
- Solar keratosis
- Lupus vulgaris
- Erythema ab igne

(c) Risk factors for malignant melanoma
- Sunlight exposure
- Precursor lesions: dysplastic naevus, congenital naevus, and cellular blue naevus
- Familial (autosomal dominant)

What is the epidemiology of (a) BCC, (b) SCC, and (c) malignant melanoma?
(a) Epidemiology of BCC
- Most common skin cancer (80% of all non-melanoma skin cancers)
- More common in white people
- Male:female = 2:1
- Peak incidence in people aged 55–75 years

(b) Epidemiology of SCC
- The second most common skin cancer
- More common in white people
- Male:female = 2:1
- Peak incidence in people aged 70–80 years

(b) Epidemiology of malignant melanoma
- The sixth most common cancer in females and seventh most common cancer in males
- More common in white people
- Australia has the highest incidence of melanoma in the world
- Slightly more common in males

What are the different clinical subtypes of malignant melanoma?

Clinical subtype	Frequency	Clinical features
Superficial spreading	70%	Usually on the trunk (males) and legs (females)
Nodular	10–15%	Usually found on the trunk; male:female = 2:1; presents as a dome-shaped nodule characterized by vertical growth; carries a poor prognosis
Lentigo	10–15%	Usually on sun-exposed areas (most lesions occur on the face); males=females; usually in the elderly
Acral lentiginous	10%	The only type of melanoma that has an equal frequency in blacks and whites; occur on the palms, soles, and subungual areas
Mucosal lentiginous	3%	Develop from respiratory, gastrointestinal, or genitourinary mucosa; more aggressive than cutaneous melanoma

**** This is an intra-epidermal carcinoma in situ; appears as a slow growing thickened plaque; can occur anywhere on the body (usually the trunk); not assocaited with sun exposure.

What is the treatment for BCC?

- Surgical excision
- Radiotherapy for advanced tumours or locally invasive

What is the treatment for SCC?

- Surgical excision
- Radiotherapy

What is the treatment for malignant melanoma?

- Surgical excision is the mainstay of treatment (wide excision margins)
- Sentinel node biopsy and/or elective lymph node dissection
- Adjuvant interferon- therapy is recommended for those at high risk of recurrence
- Chemotherapy for advanced (metastatic) melanoma

What do you know about mycoses fungoides?

This is a malignant lymphoma characterized by clonal expansion of $CD4^+$ cells that have affinity for the skin. These cutaneous malignant T-cells enter the skin, and have a particular affinity for the epidermis, where they cluster around Langerhans cells (seen microscopically as Pautrier microabscesses). Mycosis fungoides usually doesn't show visceral involvement for many years. The malignant cells in the skin, however, retain the ability to exit the skin via the lymphatic system back into the blood. When this happens, it becomes a systemic disease, even though the disease is clinically limited to the skin.

What is Sezary syndrome?

This is a variant of mycosis fungoides, occurring in 5% of cases and characterized by generalized exfoliative erythroderma, lymphadenopathy, and a large number (>1000/mm^3) of atypical T lymphocytes with cerebriform nuclei in the blood (Sezary cells). This is associated with a poor prognosis.

What is the treatment for mycoses fungoides?

Topical therapy

- Corticosteroids
- Retinoids
- Nitrogen mustard
- PUVA
- Total body electron beam radiation

Systemic therapy

- Interferon-α
- Extracorporeal photophoresis*
- Retinoids

---

* Leucophoresis with PUVA therapy for the collected white cells, followed by re-infusion of these treated cells.

Case 139 ◆ **Pseudoxanthoma Elasticum**

CASE PRESENTATION

*There are **folds of loose skin** over the **neck, antecubital**, and **popliteal fossae, axillae, groin**, and the **peri-umbilical** region.[1,2] In these areas, there are **yellow-coloured papules** that coalesce to form larger **pseudoxanthomatous plaques** giving the skin a **'plucked chicken' appearance**.[3]*

*The diagnosis is **pseudoxanthoma elasticum**.[4]*

Clinical notes

1. The skin changes of pseudoxanthoma elasticum occur on the sides of the neck and in the flexural areas of the body. The skin is loose in these areas, and as the disease progresses, the skin becomes lax and wrinkled, hanging in folds. Generalized severe laxity of the skin is rare.

2. Facial involvement has an important clinical value, especially for diagnosing pseudoxanthoma elasticum in younger patients. The presence of horizontal and mental creases has a high specificity for diagnosis before the age of 30 years.

3. The primary initial skin lesions in this condition are yellowish papules (1–5mm in diameter). Typically, these lesions are present on the sides of the neck and in the flexural areas, and gradually coalesce to form plaques with a cobblestone appearance ('plucked chicken' appearance). The sides of the neck are affected first (8–12 years) and flexural involvement tends to start later (12–18 years). The most commonly affected flexural site is the axillae. At the point of maximal coalescence, the skin starts to lose its elasticity, and typical redundant folds develop.

4. Pseudoxanthoma is a systemic disease. Tell the examiner that you would like to look for other features:

    (a) **Eyes**: visual acuity, blue sclerae, angioid streaks, peau d'orange appearance of the fundus, optic nerve drusen, retinal haemorrhages, comet-like streaks, colloid bodies, and macular degeneration (the first ocular sign is the peau d'orange appearance—a yellow mottled hyperpigmentation of the retina temporal to the retina, and predates angioid streaks by up to 10 years)

    (b) **Mouth**: yellow-coloured papules and plaques (identical to skin lesions) are often present on the inner aspect of lower lip (look for this)

    (c) **Blood pressure**: hypertension is 3 times more common than the general population, and occurs at an early age (arterial wall thickening and narrowing and renovascular disease)

    (d) **Heart**: aortic regurgitation, mitral valve prolapse, mitral regurgitation, and coronary artery disease (may cause congestive cardiac failure); restrictive cardiomyopathy (can occur due to calcification of the atrial and ventricular endocardium)

    (e) **Peripheral pulses**: diminished or absent pulses

    (f) **Joints**: hyper-extensible joints

    (g) **Nervous system**: cerebral infarction (cerebrovascular disease) and cerebral haemorrhages (intracerebral aneurysms)

Questions commonly asked by examiners

What do you know about the genetics of pseudoxanthoma elasticum?

The genetic defect has been mapped to the ABCC6 gene on chromosome 16 (16p13). ABC proteins are active pumps that transport various substrates. The mode of inheritance is both autosomal dominant and autosomal recessive (autosomal dominant inheritance is more common).

What is the pathophysiology of pseudoxanthoma elasticum?

There is abnormal mineralization and calcification of elastic fibres that become secondarily fragmented. These fragmented elastic fibres and calcium deposits are found in the deep and middle dermis. Similar changes occur in the elastic fibres of blood vessels, eyes, and the endocardium.

What is the pathogenesis of angioid streaks?

These are irregular red-brown or grey lines that radiate form the optic disc, and occur in 85% of patients with pseudoxanthoma elasticum. They result from degeneration and calcification of the elastic fibres of the retina leading to breakdown in the Bruch's membrane.

Are angioid streaks pathognomic of pseudoxanthoma elasticum?

They are not pathognomic of pseudoxanthoma elasticum and can occur in other systemic disorders:

* Ehlers-Danlos syndrome
* Paget's disease
* Marfan's syndrome
* Sickle cell disease
* Lead poisoning
* Hyperphosphataemia

What is the Grönblad-Strandberg syndrome?

This is a triad of pseudoxanthomatous skin lesions, angioid streaks, and vascular abnormalities.

What are the cardiovascular manifestations of pseudoxanthoma elasticum?

* Aortic regurgitation
* Mitral regurgitation
* Mitral valve prolapse
* Peripheral vascular disease
* Accelerated coronary artery disease
* Restrictive cardiomyopathy
* Renovascular disease
* Hypertension
* Aneurysm formation

What are the gastrointestinal manifestations of pseudoxanthoma elasticum?

Gastrointestinal haemorrhage occurs in up to 15% of patients, and often occurs early in the course of the disease, when cutaneous and eye changes are minimal. This occurs secondary to degeneration of the elastic tissue in the arteries of the gastric wall.

What are other causes of loose or redundant skin?

* **Elastoderma**
* **Anetoderma***
    * Primary: idiopathic
    * Secondary: amyloidosis, cutaneous lymphoma, SLE, sarcoidosis, syphilis, lymphocytoma, acrodermatitis chronica atrophicans, and dermatofibroma

---

* Focal loss of dermal elastic tissue, resulting in localized areas of flaccid or herniated sac-like skin.

- **Cutis laxa***
  - Inherited—autosomal dominant, autosomal recessive, and X-linked recessive
  - Acquired—penicillamine, penicillin, complement deficiency (C3 and C4), SLE, sarcoidosis, multiple myeloma, and amyloidosis
- **Ehlers-Danlos syndrome**

---

* Connective tissue disorder where the skin becomes inelastic and hangs loosely in folds.

Case 140 ◆ **Ehlers-Danlos Syndrome**

CASE PRESENTATION

This patient has **epicanthal folds**, *a* **broad nasal bridge**, **widely spaced eyes**, *and* **kyphoscoliosis**.[1] *The skin is* **thin**, **hyperextensible**, *and* **elastic**.[2] *There is evidence of* **skin fragility** *and* **impaired wound healing** *with* **cigarette-paper scars** *and gaping* **fish-mouth wounds** *over sites of minor injury especially over the bony prominences*.[3] *There is evidence of a* **bleeding diasthesis** *with* **purpura**, **haematomas**, *and* **pseudotumours** *(over the bony prominences)*.[4] *The* **joints** *are* **hyperextensible**[5] *and this patient has* **hallus valgus**, **genu recurvatum**, *and* **pes planus**.

The diagnosis is **Ehlers-Danlos syndrome**.[6]

Clinical notes

1. Ehlers-Danlos patients may exhibit the above facial features. Although they may be present, they are not characteristic. Ask the patient to stand up and examine the back to look for kyphoscoliosis.

2. The skin is soft, velvety, and often has a doughy feel. It is thin, and often underlying vessels may be seen. It can easily be stretched (hyperextensible), and when released, it immediately returns to its original position (elastic)—this can be checked for at the back of the hand. Late in the disease, the skin may hang in loose folds.

3. Skin fragility is a characteristic feature with poor wound healing. Often there are skin lacerations present that heal slowly leaving scars: cigarette-paper scars and fish-mouth wounds. These are especially common over the knees and elbows. If there are old surgical scars, then the scars are often wide, and incisional hernias may form over abdominal surgical scars.

4. There is an increased tendency to bleed. Pseudotumours are small spongy tumours found over scars and bony prominences. They result from trauma, which leads to haematoma formation that subsequently undergoes fatty degeneration and calcification.

5. Although all joints can be hyperextensible, the digit joints are most commonly affected. One can use the Beighton's nine-point joint hypermobility scoring system for the following manoeuvres:
   (a) Hyperextension of 5th MCP joint to 90°
   (b) Apposition of thumb to volar aspect of the forearm
   (c) Hyperextension of the elbow (>10°)
   (d) Hyperextension of the knee (>10°)
   (e) Place palms of the hand on the floor with knees extended
   For (1)–(4), 2 points are assigned for each side (right and left); for (5), 1 point is assigned.

6. There are 11 variants of Ehlers-Danlos syndrome, each with different genetic and clinical features. There is a defect in collagen and connective tissue synthesis, which can affect many organ systems. Tell the examiner you would like to look for other manifestations of this condition:

    (a) **Eyes**: myopia (patient may be wearing glasses), blue sclerae, glaucoma, retinal haemorrhage and detachment (rupture of the globe can occur in some patients)

    (b) **Mouth**: gingival resorption and hypodontia (loss of teeth)

    (c) **Cardiovascular**: mitral valve prolapse, mitral and aortic regurgitation, arterial aneurysms

    (d) **Respiratory**: spontaneous pneumothorax

    (e) **Musculoskeletal**: osteoarthritis (long-term consequence of hyperextensibility)

    (f) **Gastrointestinal**: examine hernial orifices and look for conjunctival pallor and koilonychia (iron deficiency anaemia resulting from gastrointestinal blood loss)

Questions commonly asked by examiners

What do you know about Ehlers-Danlos syndrome?

There are 11 different forms of Ehlers-Danlos syndrome that are now recognized. They show different patterns of inheritance (AD and AR) and all involve a genetic defect in collagen or connective tissue synthesis.

What are the gastrointestinal complications?

*   Gastrointestinal bleeding
*   Diverticulae
*   Diaphragmatic herniation
*   Megacolon
*   Colonic rupture

What are the cardiovascular complications?

*   Mitral valve prolapse
*   Mitral regurgitation
*   Aortic regurgitation
*   Arterial aneurysms
*   Aortic dissection
*   Arterial rupture

What are the other causes of blue sclerae?

*   Pseudoxanthoma elasticum
*   Marfan's syndrome
*   Osteogenesis imperfecta
*   Diamond-Blackfan anaemia
*   Hypophosphatasia
*   Alkaptonuria

What are the other causes of joint hypermobility?

*   Pseudoxanthoma elasticum
*   Marfan's syndrome
*   Osteogenesis imperfecta
*   Turner's syndrome
*   Noonan's syndrome

- Fragile X syndrome
- Williams syndrome
- Downs syndrome
- Lowe syndrome (occulocerebrorenal dystrophy)

Case 141 ◆ Acanthosis Nigricans

CASE PRESENTATION

*There are **soft**, **velvety**, **hyperpigmented plaques** that are present on the intertriginous areas of the **axilla**, **groin**, and **posterior neck**.*[1,2]

*The diagnosis is **acanthosis nigricans**.*[3]

Clinical notes

1. Acanthosis nigricans is characterized by hyperpigmented, brown, velvety plaques appearing on the skin of the intertriginous areas. They often begin as hyperpigmented macules that progress to palpable plaques. They are often symmetrical, although a unilateral form is recognized that is inherited as an autosomal dominant trait. Often, there are skin tags that are found around the affected areas.

2. The vulva is most commonly affected in obese females who are hyperandrogenic (polycystic ovarian syndrome). Occasionally, these lesions may occur on the mucous membranes of the oropharynx, nose, and oesophagus. In up to 50% of cases associated with internal malignancy, there is involvement of the oral cavity—the tongue and the lips being most commonly affected with elongation of the filliform papillae on the dorsal and lateral surfaces of the tongue and multiple papillary lesions on the commissures of the lips. Oral lesions are often not pigmented. Papillomatous lesions may occur on the eyelids and/or conjunctivae.

3. Acanthosis nigricans is associated with many conditions. Tell the examiner, that you would like to examine further to look for possible associations:

   (a) **Obesity**: comment on the BMI of the patient

   (b) **Diabetes**: finger tip skin pricks (confirm regular glucose testing); fundoscopy for diabetic retinopathy

   (c) **Cushing's syndrome**: moon face, centripetal obesity, buffalo hump, purpura, proximal myopathy

   (d) **Acromegaly**: acromegalic facies, large hands, thickened skin, carpal tunnel syndrome, bitemporal hemianopia

   (e) **Thyroid disease**: assess thyroid status (hyper- or hypothyroidism), goitre (? previous thyroidectomy scar), thyroid eye disease, pretibial myxoedema, and thyroid acropachy

   (f) **Underlying malignancy**: gastrointestinal tract, uterus, ovary, prostate, breast, and lung

   (g) **Drugs**: tell the examiner that you would like to take a drug history (although drug-induced acanthosis nigricans is uncommon, it can be induced by several medications), see below

   Younger patients (<40 years) are most likely to have an underlying endocrinopathy, whereas older patients (>40years) are most likely have an underlying malignancy.

Questions commonly asked by examiners

What are the causes of acanthosis nigricans?

- Obesity (most common cause)
- Insulin resistance
- Diabetes
- Cushing's syndrome
- Acromegaly
- Hypothyroidism
- Hyperthyroidism
- Polycystic ovarian syndrome
- Familial (inherited as an autosomal dominant trait)
- Malignancy (most commonly an adenocarcinoma of the gastrointestinal tract)
- Drugs (see below)

What drugs have been reported to cause acanthosis nigricans?

- Insulin
- Nicotinic acid
- Steroids
- Oral contraceptives
- Fusidic acid

When acanthosis nigricans is associated with obesity, what happens to skin lesions with weight loss?

In the context of obesity, acanthosis nigricans is thought to be weight-dependent, and the lesions regress with weight reduction.

In the presence of internal malignancy, when does acanthosis nigricans appear?

Remember the rule of thirds:

- In one third of cases, the skin changes appear before any signs of cancer (up to 5 years)
- In one third of cases, the skin changes occur simultaneously with the cancer
- In one third of cases, the skin changes occur after the diagnosis of cancer

Regression of acanthosis nigricans can occur with treatment of the underlying malignancy, and reappearance suggests recurrence or metastases of the primary tumour.

Case 142 ◆ Pyoderma Gangrenosum

CASE PRESENTATION

There is a **necrotic ulcer** with a **ragged**, **violaceous border** that **overhangs** the ulcer bed.[1] The surrounding skin is indurated and erythematous. It is present over the lateral aspect of the left lower leg.[2]

This appearance is consistent with **pyoderma gangrenosum**.[3]

Clinical notes

1. Pyoderma gangrenosum is characterized by deep ulceration. The initial lesion starts as a small red papule or a collection of papules. These form small ulcers with a 'cats-paw' appearance and then coalesce with necrosis of the central area to form a single larger ulcerative lesion. It has a red-blue or violaceous overhanging edge. The surrounding skin is often indurated and erythematous. They develop rapidly, and can progress from a single papule to a large ulcer within 24–48 hours. These lesions are usually very painful.

2. This can occur anywhere on the body, but commonly occurs on the legs, with a predilection for the pre-tibial areas. It exhibits the Koebner phenomenon, so it is important to look at scars or sites of trauma. It may occur around stoma sites, and may be mistaken for a wound infection or irritation (peristomal pyoderma gangrenosum). It may occur on the genitalia (penile or vulval pyoderma gangrenosum). An intra-oral variant is recognized (pyostomatitis vegetans) that occurs primarily in patients with inflammatory bowel disease.

3. Pyoderma gangrenosum is associated with systemic diseases in 50% of cases. The cause may be apparent on gross inspection, but once making a diagnosis of pyoderma gangrenosum, tell the examiner that you would like to look for evidence of associated systemic diseases:

    (a) **Inflammatory disease**: clubbing, arthropathy, laparotomy scars, and stoma site

    (b) **Chronic active hepatitis**: signs of chronic liver disease

    (c) **Primary biliary cirrhosis**: scratch marks, xanthelesma, and signs of chronic liver disease

    (d) **Rheumatoid arthritis**: arthropathy, subcutaneous nodules, episcleritis, and scleritis

    (e) **Ankylosing spondylitis**: loss of lumber lordosis, kyphosis, stooped posture, and reduced chest expansion

    (f) **Psoriatic (and other seronegative) arthropathy**: arthropathy, nail changes, and psoriatic plaques

    (g) **Myeloproliferative disorders**: lymphadenopathy and hepatosplenomegaly

    (h) **Polycythaemia rubra vera:** facial plethora, dusky cyanosis, and splenomegaly

    (i) **Wegner's granulomatosis**: nasal deformities

    (j) **Sarcoidosis**: lupus pernio, erythema nodosum, and interstitial lung disease

    (k) **Thyroid disease**: assess thyroid status (hyper- or hypothyroidism), goitre (? previous thyroidectomy scar), thyroid eye disease, pretibial myxoedema, and thyroid acropathy

    (l) **Diabetes**: finger tip glucose testing skin pricks, fundoscopy for retinopathy

Questions commonly asked by the examiners

What is the histology of these lesions?

These findings are not specific, but help in the exclusion of other diseases. Microscopic features include massive neutrophilic infiltration, haemorrhage and necrosis of the epidermis. Granulation tissue may be present in the later stages, but granuloma formation is against a diagnosis of pyoderma gangrenosum.

What is the treatment for pyoderma gangrenosum?

Topical treatment

- Topical potent steroids, i.e. triamcinolone
- Topical tacrolimus

Systemic treatment

- High dose oral steroids
- Cyclosporin
- Azathioprine
- Anti-TNF-α (Infliximab)

What is the role of surgery in the management of pyoderma gangrenosum?
As these lesions exhibit Koebner phenomenon in up to 50% of cases, they tend to develop at sites of minor trauma or surgical scars. Thus surgery or debridement is contraindicated.

Case 143 ◆ **Pretibial Myxoedema**

CASE PRESENTATION

There are **bilateral, asymmetrical, firm, non-pitting,** *and* **pink** *to* **purple-brown** *coloured* **plaques** *with* **well-defined serpiginous margins**[1] *on the* **anterolateral aspects of the lower legs.**[2] *The lesions are* **tender** *to touch.*[3] *The skin is* **shiny** *and the* **prominent hair follicles** *give a* **peau d'orange texture.**[4] *There is overlying* **hyperhidrosis** *and* **hypertrichosis.**[5] *There is* **non-pitting ankle oedema.**[6]

In addition, there is **exophthalmos, thyroid acropachy,** *and an old* **thyroidectomy scar.** *On assessing the thyroid status, this patient is* **euthyroid.**[7]

The diagnosis is **pretibial myxoedema,** *which is associated with* **Graves' disease.** *The patient has previously had a thyroidectomy, and is currently euthyroid.*

Clinical notes

1. Pretibial myxoedema (thyroid dermopathy or infiltrative dermopathy) is characterized by bilateral (though asymmetrical), firm, non-pitting plaques or nodules that may have a pink, purple, or brown appearance.

2. Lesions characteristically appear on the anterolateral aspects of the lower legs. They may appear on the thighs, shoulders, hands, or the forehead. They often occur in areas of recent or prior trauma or skin graft donor sites.

3. The lesions are often tender and they may be pruritic.

4. Prominent hair follicles give the shiny skin an orange peel appearance.

5. This may be present.

6. The lesions may be associated with non-pitting ankle and feet oedema. This is due to mucin deposition in the dermis causing compression of the dermal lymphatics and resultant dermal oedema. In its extreme form, pretibial myxoedema can resemble lymphoedema.

7. Pretibial myxoedema is a feature of Graves' disease (occurring in 5% of patients). Thus it is important to look for other features of Graves' disease. Pretibial myxoedema is a late manifestation of Grave's disease and usually occurs 1–2 years after the diagnosis and treatment of hyperthyroidism. Almost all patients with dermopathy have ophthalmopathy, with dermopathy usually following the onset of ophthalmopathy by 6–12 months. Thyroid acropachy occurs in 1% of patients with Graves' disease, and if present, it usually occurs after the dermopathy. It is important to determine the thyroid status. Patients may be euthyroid as a result of previous thyroidectomy (look for a scar) or radioactive iodine treatment (absence of a scar).

Questions commonly asked by examiners

The questions asked for pretibial myxoedema will overlap with those asked for thyroid disease. It is important to revise this case in conjunction with the cases of thyroid disease. Please refer to Cases 97 Goitre, 98 Assessment of Thyroid State, 99, Graves' Disease, 100 Hypothyroidism.

What is the pathophysiology of pretibial myxoedema?

Pretibial myxoedema results from deposition of mucopolysaccharides (hyaluronic acid) in the dermis.

Case 144 ◆ Lupus Pernio

CASE PRESENTATION

*There are **purple-red, indurated plaques and nodules**[1] affecting the **nose, cheeks, ears**, and **lips**.[2] There is no evidence of scaling or scarring.[3]*

*These appearances are in keeping with a diagnosis of **lupus pernio**, a characteristic cutaneous manifestation of sarcoidosis.[4]*

Clinical notes

1. Lupus pernio is characterized by purple-red or violaceous plaques and nodules. In cases that have been treated, there may just be a faint purplish discoloration. The lesions are hard and indurated, which distinguishes it from lupus vulgaris.

2. Although it usually affects the nose, cheek, ears, and lips, it can appear on the forehead, dorsal surfaces of the hands and feet.

3. The absence of scales and scarring is important, as these features further help differentiate this from lupus pernio.

4. Lupus pernio is the most characteristic cutaneous manifestation of sarcoidosis, whilst erythema nodosum is the most common manifestation. Remembering that sarcoidosis is a multi-system disorder, tell the examiner that you would like to examine other systems to look for manifestations of sarcoidosis:

   (a) **Cutaneous**: erythema nodosum (see below for list of other cutaneous manifestations)

   (b) **Ocular**: anterior uveitis, chronic uveitis, glaucoma, cataracts, optic neuritis, and conjunctival nodules

   (c) **Parotids**: parotid gland swelling

   (d) **Respiratory**: interstitial lung disease

   (e) **Cardiovascular**: restrictive cardiomyopathy and pulmonary hypertension

   (f) **Abdomen**: hepatosplenomegaly and portal hypertension

   (g) **Lymphatic**: lymphadenopathy (cervical nodes are the second most common site)

   (h) **Neurological**: VII nerve palsy (common) and mononeuritis multiplex

   (i) **Musculoskeletal**: arthropathy

Questions commonly asked by examiners

What are the other cutaneous manifestations of sarcoidosis?

Cutaneous lesions	Clinical features
Erythema nodosum	Red, tender, and nodular lesions over the anterior surface of the lower legs (see Case 128 Erythema Nodosum)
Erythema multiforme	Target lesions most commonly present on the palms and soles (see Case 129 Erythema Multiforme)
Papules Maculopapules Plaques	Red-brown to purple papules (diameter <1cm); affect eyelids, periorbital areas, and nasolabial folds; can occur on mucous membranes; diascopy of sarcoid plaques reveals a yellowish-brown or apple-jelly colour
	Round or oval, red-brown in colour; bilateral and symmetrical involvement; tend to resolve with scarring; commonly affect the extensor surfaces, face, scalp, and back
Annular plaques	Plaques that clear in the centre giving a ring appearance
Subcutaneous nodules	Multiple, firm mobile, round nodules; skin coloured; commonly affect extremities, trunk and face; may be slightly tender; also known as *Darier-Roussy sarcoidosis*
Angiolupoid	These are sarcoid plaques or nodules that develop telangiectases on their surface
Infiltrative scars (scar sarcoid)	Red or purple-brown infiltration of old scars, tattoo, or venepuncture sites
Alopecia	Scarring or non-scarring alopecia may occur
Ulcers	Necrotic ulcers with a violaceous border and atrophic centre surrounded by yellow plaques with telangiectases; often affects the pretibial areas; may resemble necrobiosis lipoidica diabeticorum
Hypopigmentation	Commonly affects dark-skinned individuals; may appear as macules, papules, or nodules
Psoriasifrom lesions	Scaly plaques on elbows and knees; heal with a scar (this differentiates this from true psoriasis
Erythrodermic lesions	Erythematous, yellow-brown plaques with overlying desquamation

What are the other systemic manifestations of sarcoidosis?

In sarcoidosis, non-caseating epithelioid granulomas can affect many organ systems. As a result clinical presentation is variable.

Organ system	Features
General symptoms	Fever; fatigue; weight loss
Glands	Parotid swelling (uveoparotid fever); lacrimal and parotid gland enlargement (Mikulicz syndrome); parotid gland enlargement, acute uveitis and VII palsy (Heerfordt's syndrome)
Cutaneous	Erythema nodosum (most common), maculopapular lesions, papules, plaques, subcutaneous nodules, scar sarcoid, scarring alopecia; ichthyosiform sarcoidosis; ulceration
Eyes	Anterior uveitis (most common); posterior uveitis; chronic uveitis (can lead to adhesions, cataracts, and glaucoma); lacrimal gland involvement (keratoconjunctivitis sicca); optic nerve granulomata; choroidal granulomata; optic neuritis; conjunctival nodules

(continued)

Organ system	Features
Lungs	Bilateral hilar lymphadenopathy; interstitial lung disease; fibrotic bands; bronchiectasis; restrictive lung defect (65%); concurrent obstructive lung defect (50%).
Abdomen	Elevated ALT and ALP (10%); hepatic granulomata (60%); cholestasis; hepatosplenomegaly; cirrhosis (1%); portal hypertension; hepatopulmonary syndrome
Heart	Cardiac granulomata (commonly in the left ventricular free wall or interventricular septum); conduction defects; arrhythmias; sudden death; restrictive cardiomyopathy; pulmonary hypertension
Nervous system	Cranial nerve palsies (VII nerve palsy is most common); aseptic meningitis; ataxia; seizures; hypothalamic and pituitary involvement; mononeuritis multiplex; psychosis
Lymphatics	Lymphadenopathy (one-third of patients); mobile soft lymph nodes; right paratracheal lymph node involvement is the most common followed by the cervical nodes
Metabolic	Hypercalcaemia (40%); hypercalciuria (11%); diabetes insipidus
Musculoskeletal	Arthropathy; bone cysts (phalanges)
Renal	Nephrocalcinosis; urinary lithiasis; granulomatous interstitial nephritis (rare)

What investigations would you request?

Investigations	Notes
FBC	Lymphopenia (redistribution of T-cells to sites of disease)
U&Es	Renal impairment
ESR	Elevated
LFTs	Elevated alanine aminotransferase (ALT) and alkaline phosphatase (ALP) (10%)
Calcium	Elevated in 40% of patients
Serum ACE	Elevated in 60% of patients
CXR	Bilateral hilar lymphadenopathy; pulmonary infiltrates; bronchiectasis
ECG/24 hour Holter	Arrhythmias and heart block (unsuspected asymptomatic ECG changes are seen in 10% of patients)

Investigations	Notes
Mantoux test	Cutaneous anergy to tuberculin skin testing (70% of patients)
Lung function test	Restrictive and obstructive lung defects
Slit-lamp eye examination	For full ophthalmic evaluation
Kveim test	Most specific test for sarcoidosis; not performed due to risk of transmitting infection
Whole body Ga-67 scan	Lambda pattern: uptake by right paratracheal and bilateral hilar lymph nodes, and panda pattern: symmetrical uptake by lacrimal and parotid glands
Bronchoalveolar lavage	Increase in lymphocytes with an increased CD4: CD8 ratio; a CD4:CD8 >3.5 has a 94% specificity for sarcoidosis
Tissue biopsy	Lymph node, skin, or transbronchial lung biopsy to confirm non-caseating granulomata

What is the Kveim test?

This is also known as the Kveim-Siltzbach test. This involves an intradermal injection of human sarcoid tissue extract (usually from a lymph node of the spleen of a sarcoid patient). After 4–6 weeks a papule develops. The test is positive if the histological examination demonstrates non-caseating granuloma formation. This is the most specific test for sarcoidosis, but is not performed nowadays due to risk of transmitting infection.

What is the role of angiotensin converting enzyme (ACE) in diagnosing sarcoidosis?

- ACE levels are elevated in 60% of patients with sarcoidosis
- It is derived from the cell membranes of epithelioid cells in sarcoid granulomata, and thus reflects granuloma load
- As a diagnostic tool it lacks sensitivity and specificity
- Can be helpful in monitoring disease activity and treatment response (reflects granuloma load)

What are the other causes of raised serum ACE levels?

- Berylliosis
- Lymphoma
- Asbestosis
- Silicosis
- Tuberculosis
- Diabetes
- Gaucher's disease
- Histoplasmosis

What is the treatment for cutaneous sarcoidosis?

Topical therapy (mild localized disease)

- Topical steroids
- Intralesional steroids

Systemic therapy (moderate to severe disease)

- Oral steroids
- Methotrexate
- Hydroxychloroquine
- Chloroquine
- Minocycline
- Azathioprine
- Pentoxifylline
- Thalidomide
- Allopurinol

Case 145 ◆ **Lupus Vulgaris**

CASE PRESENTATION

There are **red-brown, sharply demarcated plaques** with **atrophic centres** and **thickened, hyperkeratotic margins**[1] on the face and neck.[2] They have a **soft gelatinous consistency**.[3] There is evidence of **scaling**.[4] There is associated **scarring**.[5]

These features would be inkeeping with **lupus vulgaris**, a chronic progressive from of cutaneous tuberculosis.

Clinical notes

1. The macroscopic appearance of lupus vulgaris is characteristic. These lesions start of as a small enlarging red-brown papule, which represents multiple coalescing micropapules (lupomes). These coalesce to form a slow growing plaque, with thickened and hyperkeratotic margins and central atrophy.

2. The face and neck are involved in 90% of cases, with a predilection for the face around the nose. Other common sites are the nose and earlobes. Direct extension from the nose along the mucous membranes can involve the palate, gums, and throat. They can affect arms and legs, with legs and buttock being a common site in developing world countries. They usually occur as solitary lesions (in more than 50% of cases) but can be multiple. A variant is lupus postexanthematicus, which usually follows an episode of measles, and is characterized by multiple lesions.

3. These lesions are soft, which differentiate this from lupus pernio. Diascopy (looking through a glass slide pressed against the lesion) reveals an apple-jelly coloured infiltrate.

4. Scaling usually occurs over the central areas. It is important to look for this, as this can further help differentiate these lesions from lupus pernio.

5. Scarring is a characteristic feature.

Questions commonly asked by examiners

What are the other cutaneous manifestations of tuberculosis?

Cutaneous manifestation	Notes
Tuberculoid chancre	Primary inoculation of mycobacteria into skin or mucosa in a patient not previously infected with tuberculosis or received BCG vaccination. An inflammatory papule develops in 2–4 weeks, which breaks down into an ulcer with a granulomatous base and undermined edges. Regional adenopathy occurs in 3–8 weeks. The primary lesion usually heals by 3 months (healing can be delayed for up to 12 months, if poor host-immune response). The ulcer-lymphadenopathy complex is analogous to the Ghon complex.
Tuberculosis verrucosa cutis	Direct inoculation of mycobacteria into the skin in a patient previously infected with tuberculosis. This results in a solitary verrucous plaque usually on the hands and feet. Regional lymph nodes are not infected. Lesions may evolve and persist for years. Spontaneous resolution with scarring can occur.

Cutaneous manifestation	Notes
Scrufulodema	This is caused by continuous propagation of infection from an underlying tuberculous focus (lymph node, infected bone or joint). Firm, painless subcutaneous nodules that gradually enlarge and suppurate and then form ulcers and sinus tracts in overlying skin. The most commonly affected areas are the neck, axillae, chest wall, and groin. Spontaneous healing can occur, but this takes years and often results in a hypertrophic scar.
Tuberculosis periorificalis	This is caused by continuous propagation of infection from an active underlying tuberculous focus from the deep tissue. Oral lesions result from active tuberculosis affecting the upper airways or lungs. The tips and lateral margins of the tongue, the hard and soft palate are common sites. Perineal lesions result from intestinal or genitourinary disease. Lesions start as red papules that develop into painful shallow ulcers with a pseudomembranous fibrinous base. Perianal skin, vulva, and penis are common sites.
Tuberculosis cutis miliaris disseminanata	Acute miliary tuberculosis of the skin occurs in the context of advanced pulmonary or disseminated tuberculosis. There is haematogenous spread of mycobacteria to multiple organs including the skin. Lesions can occur anywhere on the body, but the trunk is most commonly affected. Multiple erythematous macule and papules occur with central necrosis.
Gummas	These are cold abscesses that develop on the hands, feet, or trunk. They result from reactivation of latent mycobacteria at one or multiple skin sites. They occur as single or multiple non-tender subcutaneous nodules that may become fluctuant and break down the overlying skin to form sinuses.
Tuberculids	These are symmetrical generalized skin eruptions that result from hypersensitivity reactions to the mycobacterium bacillus: • Erythema induratum (Bazin disease): tender nodules and plaques that may ulcerate or scar in the posterior aspect of the calves; usually affects women. • Papulonecrotic tuberculid: clusters of small plaques with necrotic centres; usually found on extensor surfaces, buttock, and lower abdomen; usually present in patients with active tuberculosis. • Lichen scrufulosum: multiple small follicular or parafollicular lichenoid papules; commonly arranged in clusters; almost always affect the trunk; occurs mostly in children.

What are the clinical variants of lupus vulgaris?

Plaque form

- Enlarging plaque with thickened and hyperkeratotic active edge and area of central atrophy
- Scaling occurs (can give the impression of psoriasis)
- Irregular scarring occurs

Ulcerative form

- Scarring and ulceration are the predominant features
- Crusts form over the areas of necrosis
- Erosion of deeper tissue and cartilage can produce deformities and contractures

Nodular form

- Relative absence of ulceration and scarring
- Large nodular masses that frequently occur on earlobes

Vegetative form

- Characterized by necrosis, ulceration, and proliferative and papillomatous granulation tissue
- Associated with minimal scarring

What are the complications of lupus vulgaris?

- SCC
- BCC

D. Eyes

Case 146 ◆ Diabetic Retinopathy

Examiner's note

Diabetic retinopathy accounts for almost 50% of the cases encountered in the short eye cases. These predominantly comprise of background retinopathy and proliferative retinopathy treated with photocoagulation. Diabetic retinopathy has many features on fundoscopy, and it is important for candidates to be aware of the different subtypes and characteristic features. This is reflected in the cases presented below.

CASE PRESENTATION 1

*There are **microaneurysms**,[1] **dot haemorrhages**, **blot haemorrhages**[2] and **hard exudates**.[3] There is no macular involvement.[4]*

*The diagnosis is **background diabetic retinopathy**.*

Clinical notes

1. Microaneurysms are the earliest sign of diabetic retinopathy. These are outpoachings of capillary walls due to pericyte loss. They appear as small red dots.
2. Microaneurysm rupture can result in dot and blot haemorrhages (deep retinal layers) and flame-shaped haemorrhages (superficial retinal layer). Blood in the deeper retina is relatively confined by vertical arrangement of the Muller fibres. Dot haemorrhages are smaller than blot haemorrhages. Flame shaped haemorrhages occur with blood tracking more superficially along the nerve fibre layer.
3. Increased permeability of retinal capillaries leads to leakage of proteins and lipoproteins into the retina. Hard exudates are well defined and have a yellow-white colour.
4. When describing the above changes, it is important to state where they are, especially in relation to the macula, as macular involvement indicates diabetic maculopathy. The macula is a small red-yellow central portion of the retina.

CASE PRESENTATION 2

*There are microaneurysms, dot haemorrhages, blot haemorrhages, and hard exudates.[1] There are haemorrhages with a **circinate formation of hard exudates** near but encroaching upon the **right macula** (indicating **macular oedema**).[2]*

*The diagnosis is **background diabetic retinopathy** with maculopathy affecting the right eye (which is associated with reduced visual acuity).[3]*

Clinical notes

1. Look for features of background retinopathy throughout the retina, and if present comment on them.

2. The macula is a small red-yellow central portion of the retina. When someone looks directly at an object, the light from the object forms an image on the macula. Therefore to assess the macula, use a tiny spotlight of the ophthalmoscope and ask the patient to look at the light. You will be looking at the macula, and this will help determine if there are haemorrhages or hard exudates involving the macula. The presence of hard exudates, often in rings, indicates oedema.

3. Diabetic maculopathy is the most common cause of loss of vision in patients with non-proliferative diabetic retinopathy. Tell the examiner that you would like to test visual acuity.

CASE PRESENTATION 3

*There are microaneurysms, dot haemorrhages, and hard exudates.[1] In particular, there are **multiple large blot haemorrhages**[2] and **cotton wool spots**.[3] There are venous irregularities with **venous dilatation, venous beading**, and **venous loops**.[4]*

*The diagnosis is **preproliferative diabetic retinopathy**.[5]*

Clinical notes

1. Look for features of background retinopathy throughout the retina, and if present comment on them.

2. Multiple large blot haemorrhages are a feature of preproliferative diabetic retinopathy.

3. Cotton wool spots, as the name suggests, are less well defined, when compared to hard exudates. They are also known as 'soft exudates'. These represent nerve fibre layer infarction from occlusion of precapillary arterioles (microvascular ischaemia). This is associated with stasis in axonoplasmic flow.

4. Venous irregularities include venous dilatation, venous loops, and venous beading, and reflect increasing retinal ischaemia.

5. Lesions in preproliferative retinopathy suggesting microvascular ischaemia and imminent neovascularization include:

    (a) Multiple large blot haemorrhages

    (b) Multiple cotton wool spots

    (c) Venous dilatation*

    (d) Venous beading*

    (e) Venous loops*

    (f) Arteriolar narrowing

CASE PRESENTATION 4

*There are microaneurysms, dot haemorrhages, blot haemorrhages, and hard exudates.[1] In addition, there are cotton wool spots, large blot haemorrhages with venous beading, and venous loops.[2] There is neovascularization with **leashes of new vessels**[3] and with evidence of **vitreous haemorrhage**.[4] **Photocoagulation scars** are present.[5]*

---

* These are the most significant predictors of progression to proliferative retinopathy.

*The diagnosis is **proliferative diabetic retinopathy** and the patient has been treated with* **photocoagulation therapy**.

Clinical notes

1. Look for features of background retinopathy throughout the retina, and if present comment on them.
2. Comment on features of preproliferative retinopathy, which will invariably be present.
3. It is important to remember, new vessels protrude into the vitreous, and when focusing on these using the ophthalmoscope, the retina will be further away, and therefore appear out of focus. The most common site of new vessel growth is on and around the optic disc The new vessels may be associated with a small amount of white fibroglial tissue. The new vessels may regress leaving only networks of avascular fibrous tissue adherent to the retina and vitreous. As the vitreous contracts, traction forces may be exerted along these fibroglial connections that can result in retinal detachment.
4. The new vessels are fragile, highly permeable and disrupted easily by vitreous traction. This leads to haemorrhage into the vitreous.
5. Look carefully for photocoagulation scars on the retina. Remember, when you see these, the leash of new vessels will not be seen, as they will be out of focus. Do not miss them if present!

Questions commonly asked by examiners

What are the other ocular manifestations of diabetes?

- Cataracts
- Rubeosis iridis
- Glaucoma (complicating rubeosis iridis)
- Visual changes (secondary to osmotic changes in the lens)
- Extra-ocular muscle paralysis secondary to mononeuritis multiplex
- Increased external eye infections (e.g. conjunctivitis or styes)
- Retinal vein occlusion
- Hypertensive retinopathy (co-existent hypertension)
- Retinal artery occlusion (co-existent atherosclerosis)

What is the prevalence of diabetic retinopathy?

- Diabetic retinopathy is related to the duration and control of disease
- The overall prevalence is 25% (type 1 diabetes: 40% and type 2 diabetes: 20%)
- It is unusual in type 1 diabetes, until 5 years after diagnosis, but eventually occurs in nearly all patients (50% at 15 years and 100% at 30 years)
- In type 2 diabetes, it is present in 10% at diagnosis, 50% after 10 years, and 80% after 20 years

What is the pathophysiology of diabetic retinopathy?

- The hyperglycaemia has a structural and physiological effect on retinal capillaries. Persistently elevated glucose levels shunt glucose into the aldose reductase pathway, which converts sugars to alcohol (glucose → sorbitol and galactose → dulcitol). The pericytes of retinal capillaries are affected by the increased level of sorbitol, resulting in loss of pericyte function, i.e. autoregulation of the retinal capillaries. This results in increased permeability and weakness of retinal capillaries.
- Diabetes is associated with increased red blood cell (RBC) aggregation, decreased RBC deformability and increased platelet aggregation all of which predispose to a sluggish circulation, endothelial damage, capillary occlusion, and retinal ischaemia.

- Retinal ischaemia triggers the production of vasoproliferative factors, in particular VEGF (vascular endothelial growth factor) that lead to new vessel formation.

Which factors worsen diabetic retinopathy?
- Poor glycaemic control
- Hypertension
- Anaemia
- Diabetic nephropathy (proteinuria)
- Hyperlipidaemia (increased risk of leakage and hard exudates)
- Pregnancy (5% with background retinopathy develop proliferative retinopathy)
- Tight glycaemic control in a patient previously with poor glycaemic control*

What is the main cause of visual loss in a patient with non-proliferative diabetic retinopathy?
Macular oedema remains the principal cause. Focal laser photocoagulation reduces the risk of visual loss by 50% and increases the chance of visual improvement. Photocoagulation therapy is most effective when initiated before visual acuity is lost.

What are the signs of macular oedema?
- Retinal thickening at 500µm or less from the centre of the macula
- Hard exudates at 500µm or less from the centre of the macula
- Retinal thickening of 1 disc area or larger in size located within 1 disc diameter from the centre of the macula

What are the indications for referral to an ophthalmologist?
- Non-proliferative retinopathy: Macular involvement
- Pre-proliferative retinopathy: See above for features
- Proliferative retinopathy: See above for features
- Advanced eye disease: Vitreous haemorrhage, retinal detachment, and rubeosis iridis

What is the association with glycaemic control and diabetic retinopathy?
There is evidence that tight glycaemic control reduces the incidence and progression of diabetic retinopathy. In the DCCT study, for type 1 diabetes, each 10% decrease in HbA_{1C} level reduces the risk of diabetic retinopathy by 39%. In the UKPDS study, for type 2 diabetes, each 10% decrease in HbA_{1C} level reduces the risk of microvascular events (including diabetic retinopathy) by 25%.

What is the association with hypertension and diabetic retinopathy?
There is strong evidence that tight blood pressure control in patients with hypertension and diabetes reduces visual loss resulting from diabetic retinopathy. The UK Prospective Diabetes Study (UKPDS) study showed that each 10mmHg reduction in systolic blood pressure is assocaited with a 13% reduction in the risk of microvascular complications, independent of glycaemic control.

What do you know about laser photocoagulation therapy for diabetic retinopathy?
Retinal laser photocoagulation therapy is an ablative treatment used for diabetic maculopathy (focal laser photocoagulation-macular grid therapy), pre-proliferative and proliferative diabetic

---

* In the Diabetes Control and Complications Trial (DCCT) study, tight glycaemic control was associated with early worsening of diabetic retinopathy, but this effect was reversed by 18 months. Those at risk had higher HbA_{1C} at baseline. It is important to avoid rapid reductions in HbA_{1C}, where possible.

retinopathy (panretinal photocoagulation). The technique involves producing numerous retinal burns (complete panretinal photocoagulation requires at least 1500 burns). Each burn is approximately 50–100µm in diameter.

In diabetic maculopathy, area(s) of leakage can be identified by examination (retinal thickening) or by fluorescein angiography. In those with diabetic maculopathy and proliferative retinopathy, focal laser therapy for maculopathy should precede panretinal photocoagulation by at least 6 weeks, because panretinal photocoagulation can worsen diabetic maculopathy. However, in patients with severe pre-proliferative of high-risk proliferative retinopathy, panretinal photocoagulation should not be delayed.

The laser therapy ablates a portion of the retina, and does not target and cauterize the new vessels. It aims to destroy the ischaemic and hypoxic retina, hoping to reduce the stimulus for neovascularization.

What are the complications of laser photocoagulation therapy?

- Vitreous haemorrhage can follow photocoagulation of retinal vessels
- Visual field constriction
- Headaches can follow photocoagulation therapy (usually relieved with rest and analgesia—glaucoma must be excluded if headache is severe or persistent)
- Retinal vein occlusion

What are the novel therapies for diabetic retinopathy?

There are a number of novel therapies in diabetic retinopathy that are showing considerable promise. At present, they are not licensed, and off-label treatment can be considered in patients unresponsive to traditional standard care. These include:

Intravitreal corticosteroids

In addition to anti-inflammatory effects, corticosteroids cause down-regulation of VEGF. Intravitreal triamcinolone acetonide (IVTA) is commonly used as an off-label adjunctive treatment

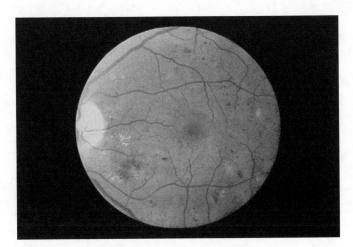

Figure 146.1 Background diabetic retinopathy (see colour plate section).
Reproduced from Warrell et al. Oxford Textbook of Medicine, Volume 3, 4th edn. 2003, with permission from Oxford University Press.

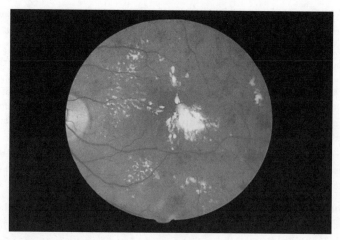

Figure 146.2 Diabetic maculopathy with hard exudates visible at the macula (see colour plate section). Reproduced from Warrell et al. Oxford Textbook of Medicine, Volume 3, 4th edn. 2003, with permission from Oxford University Press.

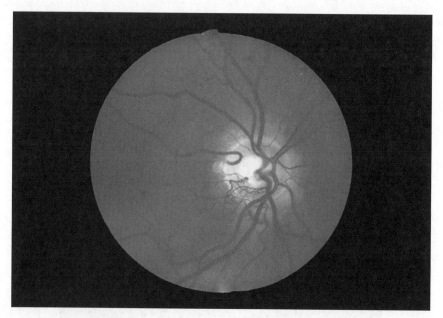

Figure 146.3 Proliferative diabetic retinopathy with new vessel formation on the inferior part of the optic disc (see colour plate section).
Reproduced from Warrell et al. Oxford Textbook of Medicine, Volume 3, 4th edn. 2003, with permission from Oxford University Press.

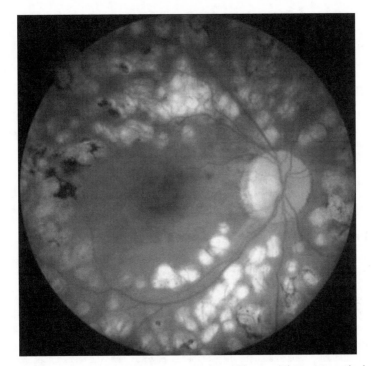

Figure 146.4 Pan-retinal photocoagulation laser treatment for proliferative diabetic retinopathy (see colour plate section).
Reproduced from Sundaram et al. Training in Ophthalmology. 2009, with permission from Oxford University Press.

in diabetic maculopathy. IVTA may be a useful adjunct to photocoagulation for proliferative diabetic retinopathy, by decreasing macular oedema, often worsened by panretinal photocoagulation therapy. Complications of IVTA include secondary glaucoma and cataract formation. Other intravitreal corticosteroids under evaluation include fluocinolone acetonide intravitreal implant and a biodegradable extended release dexamethasone implant.

VEGF inhibitors
Intravitreal anti-VEGF therapy is currently being evaluated in randomized controlled trials. There are 3 agents which are currently available: pegaptanib, bevacizumab, and ranibizumab.

Ruboxistaurin
VEGF activated protein kinase C (PKC-β), and there is some evidence, that ruboxistaurin, an orally administered PKC-β inhibitor, may be beneficial in diabetic maculopathy. Ruboxistaurin is currently being evaluated in randomized controlled trials.

Hyaluronidase
Intravitreal hyaluronidase was proposed to accelerate clearance of vitreous haemorrhage from proliferative diabetic retinopathy and other causes. A recent phase 3 trial has shown some favourable efficacy and safety.

Case 147 ◆ **Hypertensive Retinopathy**

CASE PRESENTATION

The retinal arterioles are **tortuous, thickened,** *and* **narrowed**[1] *with an* **enhanced light reflex ('copper wiring').**[2] *There is* **arterio-venous nipping** *at the arteriovenous junctions.*[3] *There are* **microaneurysms,**[4] **dot and blot haemorrhages,**[4] **flame-shaped haemorrhages,**[4] **cotton wool spots,**[5] *and* **hard exudates.**[6] *There is* **papilloedema.**[7]

The diagnosis is **grade 4 hypertensive retinopathy.**[8]

Clinical notes

1. Chronic hypertension is associated with thickening of the arteries and small arterioles. This response is initially beneficial, since it prevents the increase in pressure from being transmitted to the capillaries, thereby minimizing capillary damage. The initial response is diffuse vasospasm, which later becomes permanent with fibrosis. The arterioles may be tortuous and demonstrate a varying calibre (segments of localized arteriolar constriction followed by segments of arteriolar dilatation). This represents an initial focal followed later by more generalized arteriolar constriction.

2. The normal light reflex is formed by the reflection from the interface between the blood column and vessel wall. Initially, the increased thickness of the vessel walls causes the reflex to become more diffuse and less bright. Sclerosis and hyalinization causes the reflex to become more diffuse and the retinal arterioles to become red-brown. This is 'copper wiring'. With advanced sclerosis, the optical density of the arteriolar wall becomes increased—'sheathing' of the vessel on fundoscopy. When the anterior surface becomes involved, the entire vessel appears opaque (pipestem sheathing), however, the vessel is patent. This produces a silver-wire vessel (known as 'silver wiring').

3. At points where the retinal arteriole crosses over the retinal venule, compression of the vein by the thickened arteriole within the same sheath causes the appearance of arteriovenous nipping or nicking (the Gunn sign).

4. Disruption of the blood-retina barrier leads to an exudative stage, which is characterized by microaneurysms, dot/blot haemorrhages, flame-shaped haemorrhages, cotton wool spots, and hard exudates. The exudative signs are non-specific, as they are also seen in diabetes. Microaneurysms form at localized areas of capillary wall weakness. Microaneurysm rupture can result in dot and blot haemorrhages (deep retinal layers) and flame-shaped haemorrhages (superficial retinal layer).

5. Cotton wool spots represent nerve fibre layer infarction from occlusion of precapillary arterioles (microvascular ischaemia).

6. Hard exudates are well defined and have a yellow-white colour, which results from increased permeability of retinal capillaries that leads to leakage of proteins and lipoproteins into the retina.

7. Swelling of the optic disc usually indicates severe hypertension and can occur anytime. It can occur in the absence of exudative signs (microaneurysms, haemorrhages, cotton wool spots, and exudates) or sclerotic signs (arteriolar narrowing, thickening, and arteriovenous nipping).

8. See below for the classification of hypertensive retinopathy. The fundoscopic features of hypertensive retinopathy may not be sequential. For example, exudative signs may be seen in the absence of sclerotic signs, especially with acute rapid elevation in blood pressure. The sclerotic signs represent chronic hypertension.

Questions commonly asked by examiners

What is the Keith-Wagner-Barker classification of hypertensive retinopathy?

Grade 1	Arteriolar narrowing
Grade 2	Arteriovenous nipping
Grade 3	Microaneurysms, dot/blot haemorrhages, flame-shaped haemorrhages, cotton wool spots, and hard exudates
Grade 4	Papilloedema

What is malignant hypertension?

This is a syndrome that refers to an acute elevation of blood pressure associated with end-organ damage. The characteristic vascular lesion is fibrinoid necrosis of arterioles and small arteries, which results in end-organ damage. The red blood cells are damaged as they pass through vessels obstructed by fibrin deposition, resulting in microangiopathic haemolytic anaemia. The organ systems involved are the central nervous system (cerebral infarction or haemorrhage and encephalopathy), cardiovascular system (myocardial ischaemia), kidneys (renal failure), and eyes (grade 3 or 4 hypertensive retinopathy).

What are the other ocular manifestations of hypertension?

- Retinal vein occlusion
- Retinal artery occlusion (co-existent atherosclerosis)
- Extra-ocular muscle paralysis secondary to mononeuritis multiplex
- Hypertensive choroidopathy
- Hypertensive optic neuropathy

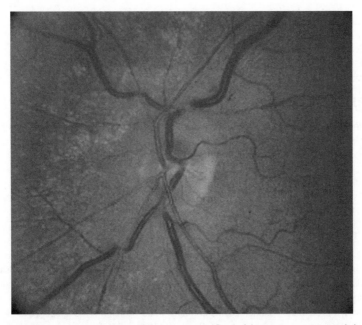

Figure 147.1 Arteriolar narrowing and arteriovenous nipping (Grade 2 hypertensive retinopathy) (see colour plate section).
Reproduced from Sundaram et al. Training in Ophthalmology. 2009, with permission from Oxford University Press.

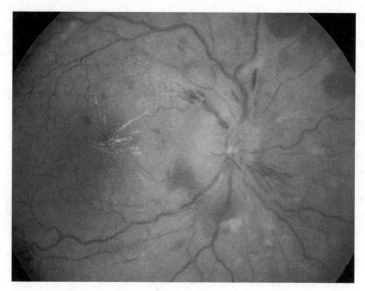

Figure 147.2 Arteriolar narrowing, cotton wool spots, blot haemmorhages, macular star, and papilloedema (Grade 4 hypertensive retinopathy) (see colour plate section).
Reproduced from Sundaram et al. Training in Ophthalmology. 2009, with permission from Oxford University Press.

Case 148 ◆ **Papilloedema**

CASE PRESENTATION

There is an **increase in venous calibre and tortuosity** *with* **loss of spontaneous venous pulsation.**[1] *The* **optic discs** *appear* **hyperaemic** *with* **blurred margins.**[2] *There are* **haemorrhages, cotton wool spots**, *and* **exudates** *around the discs.*[3] *These features are present* **bilaterally.**[4]

The diagnosis is **papilloedema.**[5]

Clinical notes

1. The earliest manifestations are increased venous calibre (venous engorgement) and tortuosity with loss of venous pulsations. Spontaneous venous pulsations are present in 80% of normal individuals. These are lost when the intracranial pressure rises above 20cm H_2O. Recognition of this sign requires practice and experience.

2. In the early stages, there is subtle oedema of the nerve fibre layer, which often begins in the area of the nasal disc. This obscures the fine peripapillary vessels in this area. At this stage, small haemorrhages of the nerve fibre layer may be detected using the green light of the ophthalmoscope. The optic disc initially becomes hyperaemic, and the nerve fibre layer oedema obscures the disc margins (initially the nasal side). As the papilloedema worsens, all the disc margins become obscured.

3. In the late stages, venous congestion develops, and the peripapillary haemorrhages become more obvious. Cotton wool spots and exudates may appear around the blurred optic disc. The peripapillary sensory retina may develop concentric or radial folds (Paton lines).

4. It is important to comment on whether the papilloedema is unilateral or bilateral. Most cases of papilloedema are bilateral. The causes of unilateral papilloedema are listed below in the questions.

5. Having diagnosed papilloedema, look for a possible cause. The causes of papilloedema are listed below in the questions, but the following can easily be looked for:

    (a) **Benign intracranial hypertension**: female; obese; and VI nerve palsy (false localizing sign)

    (b) **Malignant hypertension**: features of hypertensive retinopathy; and measure blood pressure

    (c) **Intracranial space occupying lesion**: tell the examiner you would like to look for localizing neurological signs; and check blood pressure and heart rate (Cushing's reflex)

    Tell the examiner, you would like to assess:

    (a) **Visual acuity**: usually preserved, but may be affected in late stages (chronic papilloedema)

    (b) **Blind spot**: enlarged

    (c) **Visual fields**: constriction of visual fields, especially inferiorly (chronic papilloedema); a pseudo-bitemporal hemianopia may be seen with marked disc oedema

Questions commonly asked by examiners

What is the definition of papilloedema?

Papilloedema is swelling of the optic nerve head as seen on fundoscopy.

What are the causes of papilloedema?

Raised intracranial pressure

*   Benign intracranial hypertension (see below)
*   Intracranial space occupying lesion
*   Intracranial haemorrhage
*   Venous sinus thrombosis*
*   Cerebral oedema
*   Hydrocephalus
*   Meningitis
*   Encephalitis

Metabolic disorders

*   Hypercapnoea
*   Hypocalcaemia
*   Severe anaemia
*   Graves' ophthalmopathy*
*   Hypervitaminosis A
*   Lead poisoning

Other

*   Malignant hypertension
*   Central retinal vein occlusion*
*   Guillain-Barré syndrome

---

* Can cause unilateral papilloedema.

What is the Foster-Kennedy syndrome?

This refers to tumours of the olfactory lobe, frontal lobe, or the pituitary body that press on the optic nerve to cause ipsilateral optic atrophy, whilst raising the intracranial pressure to cause contralateral papilloedema.

What is papillitis?

Papillitis refers to inflammation of the intraorbital portion of the optic nerve.

What are the differences between papillitis and papilloedema?

	Papillitis	Papilloedema
Unilateral/bilateral	Unilateral	Bilateral
Visual acuity	Reduced	Only affected in the late stages
Eye movements	Painful	Not painful
Visual fields	Central scotoma	Enlarged blind spot, constriction of fields
Marcus Gunn pupil	Present	Absent

What are the risk factors for developing benign intracranial hypertension?

Endocrine factors

- Female sex (can occur in males)
- Reproductive age group
- Menstrual irregularity
- Obesity
- Recent weight gain
- Adrenal insufficiency
- Cushing's disease
- Hypoparathyroidism
- Hypothyroidism

Pharmacological factors

- Tetracycline
- Penicillin
- Nitrofurantoin
- Minocycline
- Corticosteroids (topical and systemic)
- Cyclosporin
- Growth hormone (GH)
- Lithium
- Oral contraceptive pill
- Levonorgestrel implant
- Tamoxifen
- Danazol
- Levothyroxine
- Carbidopa
- Levodopa
- Amiodarone
- Indomethacin

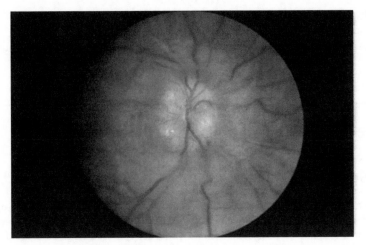

Figure 148.1 Chronic papilloedema (see colour plate section).
Reproduced from Sundaram et al. Training in Ophthalmology. 2009, with permission from
Oxford University Press.

- Vitamin A
- TrimeThoprim-sulphamethoxazole

Systemic diseases
- Chronic renal failure
- SLE
- Multiple sclerosis
- Reye syndrome

What is the treatment for benign intracranial hypertension?

General measures
- Weight loss*
- Cessation of potential offending drugs**
- Treatment of underlying systemic diseases
- Treatment of headache

Medical management
- Diuretics (acetazolamide)
- Corticosteroids***

Surgical management
- Optic nerve sheath fenestration

---

* This is an important factor in long-term management. A 6% reduction in weight loss can lead to a
resolution of papilloedema.
** In some cases, benign intracranial hypertension may continue despite discontinuation of the presumed
offending drug.
*** Corticosteroids are effective in those with an inflammatory cause for benign intracranial hypertension.
They can be used in conjunction with acetazolamide to improve recovery in patients with severe
papilloedema. However, adverse effects limit their long-term use.

- Lumbo-peritoneal shunting procedure
- Ventriculo-peritoneal shunting procedure

NB. The use of repeated lumbar punctures is now not considered as an effective therapeutic option.

Case 149 ◆ Optic Atrophy

CASE PRESENTATION

*The optic disc is **pale** and has **distinct margins**.[1] The pupil on the affected side exhibits a **loss of direct light reflex**, whereas, the **consensual light reflex is preserved**.[2] Visual field testing (using a red hat pin) reveals a **central scotoma** on the affected side.[3] The **visual acuity is reduced** on the affected side.[4]*

*The diagnosis is **optic atrophy**.[5]*

Clinical notes

1. The optic disc in acute optic neuritis may appear normal, as two-thirds of cases are retrobulbar, and only with time the optic disc becomes pale. One-third of patients with acute optic neuritis have papillitis, and the oedema of optic neuritis is often diffuse. This must be differentiated from papilloedema.

2. In advanced cases of optic atrophy, the pupil reacts consensually but not directly. However, in early stages, before the direct reflex is completely lost, a Marcus Gunn pupil (relative afferent papillary defect) may be demonstrated.

3. Central scotomas are most commonly detected in optic neuritis. Peripheral extension of a scotoma may result in a generalized reduction of the visual field in a particular direction.

4. Visual acuity may be affected to varying degrees, ranging from mild loss to complete loss of vision. Visual acuity may be normal with only a mild visual field defect. Patients with reduced visual acuity will have reduced colour vision, which can be tested using Ishihara plates.

5. Inflammation of the optic nerve is predominantly due to demyelination, and multiple sclerosis is the most common cause. Tell the examiner you would like to look for features of multiple sclerosis (cerebellar signs).

Questions commonly asked by examiners

What is the difference between optic neuritis and optic atrophy?

Optic neuritis is an acute inflammatory process the affects the optic nerve. Optic atrophy is often sequelae of optic neuritis.

What are the causes of optic atrophy?

Inherited
- Leber's hereditary optic neuropathy
- Friedreich's ataxia
- DIDMOAD syndrome (mitochondrial disease)*

Acquired
- **Post optic neuritis**: see below

---

* <u>D</u>iabetes <u>I</u>nsipidus <u>D</u>iabetes <u>M</u>ellitus <u>O</u>ptic <u>A</u>trophy <u>D</u>eafness

- **Compression**: tumours of the anterior visual pathways
- **Ischaemia**: temporal arteritis and central retinal artery occlusion
- **Toxic:** methanol, tobacco, cyanide, arsenic, lead
- **Drugs**: ethambutol, isoniazid, chloramphenicol, quinine
- **Metabolic:** vitamin B_1, B_2, B_6 and B_{12} deficiencies and diabetes
- **Infiltration:** syphilis, tuberculosis, sarcoidosis, carcinoma, leukaemia, and lymphoma
- **Others**: trauma, glaucoma, radiation, retinitis pigmentosa, and post papilloedema

What are the causes of optic neuritis/papillitis?

- **Demyelination**: multiple sclerosis and neuromyelitis optica (Devic disease)
- **Infections**: Lyme disease, HIV, viral encephalitis, and infection mononucleosis
- **Inflammation**: syphilis, tuberculosis, sarcoidosis, contiguous with orbital cellulitis, and meningitis

What is consecutive optic atrophy?

This a term that is used to describe optic atrophy that results form damage to the parent retinal ganglion cells, as that which occurs in retinitis pigmentosa, macular degeneration, choroidoretinitis, and retinal artery occlusion.

What do you understand by the term 'ischaemic optic neuropathy'?

This refers to infarction of the anterior portion of the optic nerve and results in acute severe loss of vision. The most common cause is temporal arteritis. Other causes include retinal artery occlusion, arteriosclerosis, or severe hypotensive episodes.

Case 150 ◆ **Retinal Vein Occlusion**

CASE PRESENTATION 1

The veins are **dilated** and **tortuous**.[1] There are **widespread haemorrhages** (both superficial and deep) throughout the retina, giving a **'blood and thunder' appearance**.[2] There are **cotton wool spots**.[3] The **optic disc is hyperaemic** with **blurred margins**.[4]

The diagnosis is **central retinal vein occlusion**.[6]

CASE PRESENTATION 2

The veins are **dilated** and **tortuous**[1] with **haemorrhages** (both superficial and deep) and **cotton wool spots** that are confined to sector **spreading distally from an arteriovenous crossing** (say where)[5].

The diagnosis is **branch retinal vein occlusion**.[6]

Clinical notes

1. Venous obstruction results in marked dilatation and tortuosity of the retinal veins, with loss of spontaneous venous pulsation (seen in 80% of normal individuals).

2. Retinal haemorrhages may be present after several days. Peripheral haemorrhages appear first. The appearance of the retina with widespread haemorrhages in central retinal vein occlusion has been classically described as a 'blood and thunder' appearance.

3. Cotton wool spots (soft exudates) have indistinct margins and represent retinal ischaemia.

4. Central retinal vein occlusion is a cause of papilloedema. This may not be present.

5. In branch retinal vein occlusion, the occlusion occurs at an arteriovenous crossing, and the changes of retinal vein occlusion are confined to a wedge centred upon the arteriovenous crossing, and spread distally. Up to two thirds of cases involve the superior temporal quadrant (higher number of arteriovenous crossings in this quadrant). They are often associated with quadrantic field defects.

6. There are many causes of retinal vein occlusion. The following may be easily looked for:

   (a) **Diabetes**: features of diabetic retinopathy (unaffected eye)

   (b) **Hypertension**: features of hypertensive retinopathy; measure blood pressure

   (c) **Polycythaemia rubra vera**: plethoric facies; splenomegaly

   (d) **Waldenstrom's macroglobulinaemia**: lymphadenopathy; purpura; hepatosplenomegaly

   (e) **Multiple myeloma**: urinary bence-jones protein

Questions commonly asked by examiners

What do you understand by the terms (a) 'non-ischaemic' and (b) 'ischaemic' retinal vein occlusion?

(a) 'Non-ischaemic' retinal vein occlusion

This is also known as 'venous stasis retinopathy', and a less severe fundoscopic appearance is seen usually with dilated and tortuous veins with minimal haemorrhage formation. It is the most common form of retinal vein occlusion, accounting for 75% of cases. Visual acuity is slightly reduced. This is potentially benign and the visual prognosis is good, unless the macula is involved. One third progress to 'ischaemic' retinal vein occlusion within 4 years.

(b) 'Ischaemic' retinal vein occlusion

This is also known as 'haemorrhagic retinopathy' and accounts for 25% of cases. The fundoscopic appearance includes widespread haemorrhages with cotton wool spots. It usually presents with an acute decrease in visual acuity and carries a poor visual prognosis.

What are the causes of retinal vein occlusion?

- Diabetes mellitus
- Hypertension
- Glaucoma
- Arteriosclerosis
- Hyperviscosity syndromes
  - Waldenstrom's macroglobulinaemia
  - Polycythaemia rubra vera
  - Multiple myeloma
  - Sickle cell anaemia

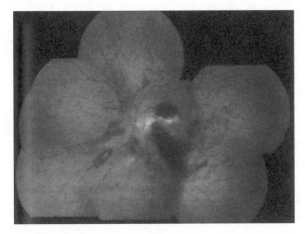

Figure 150.1 Central retinal vein occlusion.
Reproduced from Collier et al. Oxford Handbook of Clinical Specialties, 6th edn. 2003, with permission from
Oxford University Press. Image supplied by Peggy Frith.

- Hypercoagulable states
  - Antithrombin III deficiency
  - Antiphospholipid syndrome
  - Protein S deficiency
  - Protein C deficiency
  - Factor V leiden mutation
- Orbital tumours
- Vasculitis

What is the association between retinal vein occlusion and glaucoma?

Patients with glaucoma are five times more likely to develop retinal vein occlusion than those
without glaucoma.

What are the complications of retinal vein occlusion?

- Permanent loss of vision
- Neovascularization*
- Rubeosis iridis**
- Rubeotic glaucoma***
- Vitreous haemorrhage
- Traction retinal detachment

---

* Neovascularization usually occurs after 1 month and is seen in up to 20% of cases of central retinal vein
occlusion and 1% of branch retinal vein occlusion.
** This is neovascularization over the root of the iris, and usually visualized using a slit-lamp.
*** This is acute glaucoma secondary to rubeotic iridis, which interferes with absorption of the vitreous.

Case 151 ◆ **Retinal Artery Occlusion**

CASE PRESENTATION 1

*The **retina is pale and oedematous**.[1] The **retinal arterioles are attenuated and scanty**.[2] There is **boxcar segmentation of the retinal veins**.[3] There is a **cherry-red spot at the macula**.[4] The patient is blind in the affected eye.[5]*

*The diagnosis is **central retinal artery occlusion**.[6]*

Clinical notes

1. The typical fundoscopic changes of central retinal artery occlusion usually develop after an hour following the acute occlusion and often resolve in 5–10 days. The retina becomes pale (milky white or yellow-white in appearance) and oedematous. This results from ischaemic necrosis of the inner two-thirds of the retina, and this appearance is most marked in the posterior pole, due to increased thickness of the nerve fibre layer and ganglion cells in this area. As the fundoscopic appearances resolve, the pale disc of optic atrophy may be present.

2. This results from the reflex vasoconstriction of the retinal arterial tree.

3. Boxcar segmentation of sausage-linked segmentation can affect retinal veins, or sometimes the retinal arteries. This implies sluggish flow, and indicates severe obstruction. This is most commonly observed in branch retinal artery occlusion. Other causes of boxcar segmentation are hyperviscosity syndromes.

4. The retina is pale due to obstruction of the retinal artery, whilst the choroidal circulation remains intact (ciliary arteries). This results in a bright red spot that appears at the thinnest part of the retina, the macula. Again, the cherry-red spot usually develops after an hour following the acute occlusion. The cilioretinal arteries are anatomical variants, which supply the macula, are present in 14% of the population and 25% of patients with central retinal artery occlusion. These cilioretinal arteries supply most or all of the macula in 10% of the population. In these individuals, the cherry-red spot will not be seen.

5. It is important to determine the severity of loss of vision, i.e. able to count fingers, detect hand movements, light perception or complete loss of vision). This is important as prognosis for complete recovery is directly related to initial loss of vision.

6. Emboli can be seen in approximately 20% of cases in central retinal artery occlusion. The causes of central retinal artery occlusion are list below. Having made the diagnosis, tell the examiner that you would like to look for:

    (a) **Hypertension**: measure blood pressure; features of hypertensive retinopathy in unaffected eye

    (b) **Diabetes**: finger tip skin pricks (glucose testing); features of diabetic retinopathy in unaffected eye

    (c) **Carotid atherosclerosis**: carotid bruits

    (d) **Atrial fibrillation**: irregular pulse; features of mitral valve disease

    (e) **Endocarditis**: heart murmurs; stigmata of endocarditis

    (f) **Giant cell arteritis**: loss of temporal pulse; temporal tenderness (look for this in patients >60 years)

CASE PRESENTATION 2

*The **retina is pale in the superior temporal pole of the retina**.[1] The **retinal arterioles are attenuated and scanty** in this area. There is **boxcar segmentation of the retinal veins**.[2] There is an **inferior nasal field defect**.[3]*

The diagnosis is **branch retinal artery occlusion** (involving the **superior temporal artery**).

Clinical notes

1. Branch retinal artery occlusion occurs when there is occlusion in a more distal branch of the retinal artery. This often involves the temporal retinal branches. The retinal pallor and arteriolar attenuation is confined to the affected area.
2. Boxcar segmentation is more commonly observed in branch retinal artery occlusion.
3. Branch retinal artery occlusion is often associated with a visual field defect, and will correspond to a region of retinal infarction.

Questions commonly asked by examiners

What are the causes of retinal artery occlusion?

- Hypertension
- Diabetes
- Atherosclerosis
- Carotid stenosis
- Cardiogenic embolism
    - Atrial fibrillation
    - Endocarditis
    - Myxoma
    - Paradoxical embolism
    - Left ventricular thrombus
- Giant cell arteritis
- Hypercoagulable states
- Cholesterol embolism
- Polyarteritis nodosa
- Thromboangitis obliterans
- Sickle cell disease
- Glaucoma
- Syphilis
- Behcet disease
- Migraine
- Vasospasm
- Trauma

What are the presenting symptoms of retinal artery occlusion?

Patients with central retinal artery occlusion often present with acute, persistent, and painless loss of vision. In branch retinal artery occlusions, visual loss often goes unnoticed (especially if a small areas of the visual fields are affected).

What is 'amaurosis fugax'?

This is a transient occlusion of the retinal artery or its branches that manifests as transient, painless, unilateral loss of vision.

What is the most common cause in younger patients?

Cardiogenic embolism is the most common cause in patients less than 40 years of age.

What do you know about the pathophysiology of central retinal artery occlusion?

This occurs due to infarction of the inner two-thirds of the retina. The ophthalmic artery is the first branch of the internal carotid artery and enters the orbit through the optic canal. The central retinal artery is the first intraorbital branch of the ophthalmic artery. The posterior ciliary arteries are short branches that branch distally from the ophthalmic artery and supply the choroid. In 14% of the population, there are cilioretinal arteries that branch from the posterior ciliary arteries and provide an additional blood supply to the macula. In 10% of the population, these cilioretinal arteries supply most of the macula. When the central retinal artery is occluded, there is oedema of the inner layers of the retina with ischaemic necrosis. The retina becomes opacified and pale. Pigmentary changes are not seen, as the retinal pigment epithelium is unaffected. In most patients, the choroidal circulation remains intact, and this manifests as a cherry-red spot at the thinnest part of the retina, the macula. However, in 10% of the population, where the choroidal circulation is derived primarily from the cilioretinal arteries, the cherry-red macula will not be seen.

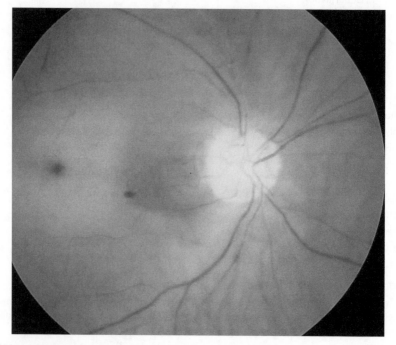

Figure 151.1 Central retinal artery occlusion (see colour plate section).
Reproduced from Sundaram et al. Training in Ophthalmology. 2009, with permission from Oxford University Press.

What is the treatment for central retinal artery occlusion?

- Ocular massage (helps dislodge the embolus)
- Lowering intraocular pressure (oral or intravenous acetazolamide)*
- Carbogen therapy (inhalation of 95% O_2 and 5% CO_2)**
- Anterior chamber paracentesis*

---

* A reduction in intraocular pressure improves perfusion
** CO_2 dilates retinal arterioles, whilst O_2 improves oxygenation of ischaemic tissues

Case 152 ◆ **Retinitis Pigmentosa**

CASE PRESENTATION

There is retinal pigmentation in the peripheries,[1] with **black-brown pigmentation** *in a characteristic pattern resembling* **bone spicules**.[2] *The optic disc are normal.[3] There are no cataracts.[4] The* **visual fields are constricted**.[5]

The diagnosis is **retinitis pigmentosa**.[6]

Clinical notes

1. Although retinal pigmentation can be widespread, it is often in the peripheral retina. This can be missed, if not looked for carefully. Retinitis punctate albescens is a variant, which is associated with yellow deposits (as opposed to black-brown) deep in the retina.
2. This is the characteristic pattern seen in retinitis pigmentosa.
3. Retinitis pigmentosa can lead to consecutive optic atrophy. It is important to look for this.
4. Up to 50% of patients have cataracts (posterior subcapsular). It is important to look for this.
5. As the condition progresses, the visual fields can become markedly constricted.
6. Although retinitis pigmentosa can occur in isolation, it can be associated with systemic disease. Look for:
   (a) **Hearing aids**: hearing loss is the most common systemic association; seen in 30% of patients (see below)
   (b) **Polydactyly**: a feature of Bardet-Biedl syndrome (see below)

Questions commonly asked by examiners

How common is retinitis pigmentosa?

The prevalence is 1 in 4000, with over a 1 million people affected worldwide.

What visual symptoms are associated with this condition?

- Nyctalopia (night blindness)
- Peripheral vision loss (tunnel vision)
- Photopsia (flashes of light)

What is the pathophysiology of retinitis pigmentosa?

Retinitis pigmentosa is associated with degeneration and apoptosis of rods and cones in the retina. The rod photoreceptors mediate achromatic vision in starlight or moonlight, whereas cone photoreceptors are important for colour vision and fine acuity in daylight. In most forms of retinitis pigmentosa, the rod photoreceptors are predominantly affected, which are most densely located in the mid periphery of the retina, thus night blindness and loss of peripheral vision are the earliest symptoms. In some forms, both rod and cone photoreceptors are equally affected. Rarely, the cone photoreceptors are predominantly affected, thus loss of visual acuity and colour vision are the earliest symptoms. There are many mechanisms and pathways that lead to photoreceptor apoptosis, and over a 100 different genetic mutations have been identified.

What is the cause of retinal pigmentation?

Pigment deposits are created when the retinal pigment epithelium (a pigmented layer next to the photoreceptors) migrates to the neural layer in response to photoreceptor apoptosis.

What do you know about the conditions associated with retinitis pigmentosa?

Usher syndrome

- Autosomal recessive condition (11 different genetic mutations have been identified)
- Most common syndrome associated with retinitis pigmentosa
- Hearing loss can be profound (sometimes complete) at birth, often associated with vestibular ataxia (type 1)
- Hearing loss can be mild–moderate at birth, and progress during life (type 2)
- Hearing can be normal at birth and gradual loss occurs in youth or adulthood (type 3)
- No specific treatments exist, other than early detection and patient education

Refsum's disease

- Autosomal recessive condition (chromosome 10)
- Phytanic acid oxidase deficiency leads to accumulation of phytanic acid in plasma and tissues
- Phytanic acid exogenous in origin, derived primarily from chlorophyll (green vegetables) but is also derived to a lesser extent from phytol (animal fats)
- Phytanic acid replaces essential fatty acids in lipid moieties of different tissues
- Main complications include peripheral sensorimotor neuropathy, cataracts, nystagmus, cerebellar ataxia, sensorineural deafness, retinitis pigmentosa, cardiomyopathy, and ichthyosis
- Treatment is to eliminate dietary phytanic acid, i.e. green vegetables (chlorophyll) and animal fat (phytol)
- Plasmapharesis can be used for those with severe clinical status

Abetalipoproteinaemia

- Also known as Bassen-Korzweig syndrome
- Deficiency of apolipoprotein B that leads to fat malabsorption and deficiencies of fat-soluble vitamins
- Features include steatorrhoea, mental retardation, spinocerebellar degeneration, and retinitis pigmentosa
- There are low levels of plasma chylomicrons and acanthocytes are seen on the blood film
- High dose therapy with vitamins A and E can limit retinal degeneration and can be vision-saving if commenced early

Kearns-Sayre syndrome

- Mitochondrial genetic defect (deletions in mitochondrial DNA)
- Characterized by a triad of (a) age less than 20 years, (b) chronic progressive external ophthalmoplegia, and (c) retinitis pigmentosa
- Other features include ptosis, cataracts, heart block, cerebellar ataxia, myopathy, diabetes, hypoparathyroidism, bilateral sensorineural deafness, growth retardation, dementia, encephalopathy, and renal tubular acidosis (type 2)

Bardet-Biedl syndrome

- Autosomal recessive (10 genes have been identified, account for 70% of cases)
- Accounts for 5–6% of cases of retinitis pigmentosa
- Polydactyly, short stature, truncal obesity, hypogonadism, cognitive impairment, and renal disease
- Renal disease manifests as calyceal cysts, interstitial nephritis, and can progress to end-stage renal failure requiring renal transplantation

Alport's syndrome

- Different modes of inheritance: X-linked dominant (80%), autosomal recessive (15%) and autosomal recessive (5%)
- Mutations in the gene that encodes collagen IV, lead to abnormalities in (a) glomerular basement membrane—haematuria and glomerulosclerosis; (b) eyes—anterior lenticonus, subcapsular cataracts, and peri-macular flecks; and (c) cochlea—bilateral sensorineural deafness (initially for high frequencies)

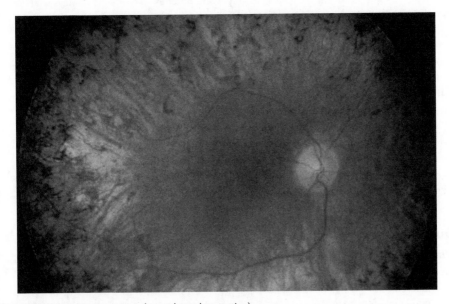

Figure 152.1 Retinitis pigmentosa (see colour plate section).
Reproduced from Sundaram et al. Training in Ophthalmology. 2009, with permission from Oxford University Press.

Waardenburg syndrome

- Autosomal dominant condition
- Features include convergent strabismus, prominent broad nasal root, hypertrichosis of medial eyebrows, heterochromia of the irides, white forelock, sensorineural deafness, and retinitis pigmentosa

Neuronal ceroid lipofuscinosis

- Also known as Batten disease
- Encompass a group of neurodegenerative lysosomal storage disorders
- Features include seizures, dementia, and progressive vision loss

What is the best diagnostic test for retinitis pigmentosa?

The electroretinogram (ERG) provides an objective measure of rod and cone function, and can detect even mild impairment of photoreceptor function. ERG amplitudes are useful for accurate diagnosis, assessment of severity, following the course of disease and measuring response to treatment.

Case 153 ◆ Old Choroiditis

CASE PRESENTATION

There are areas of focal atrophy manifesting as **grey-white patches**,[1] *around which there is scattered* **retinal pigmentation**.[2]

The diagnosis is **old choroiditis**[3]

Clinical notes

1. The atrophy of the choroidoretina exposes the underlying sclera, which can manifest as white, grey-white, or yellow patches.
2. This occurs secondary to proliferation of the retinal pigment epithelium.
3. There are many causes of choroiditis. The following may be easily looked for:
   - (a) **Tuberculosis**: apical lung signs
   - (b) **Syphilis**: Argyll-Robertson pupil; tabes dorsalis; aortic regurgitation
   - (c) **Sarcoidosis**: erythema nodosum; lupus pernio; lympahdenopathy; interstitial lung disease

Questions commonly asked by examiners

What are the causes of choroiditis?

Infectious causes

- Tuberculosis
- Toxoplasmosis
- Toxocariasis
- Baylisascaris

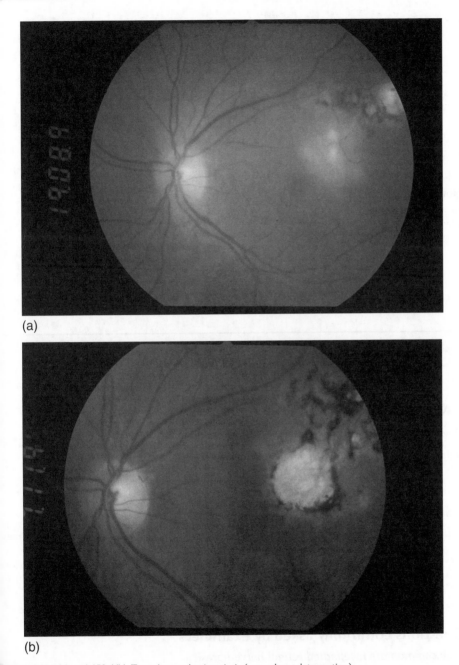

(a)

(b)

Figure 153.1(a) and 153.1(b) Toxoplasma chorioretintis (see colour plate section).
Reproduced from Sundaram et al. Training in Ophthalmology. 2009, with permission from
Oxford University Press.

- Syphilis
- Lyme disease
- Congenital rubella
- Candidiasis
- Histoplasmosis
- Cryptococcus
- CMV
- EBV
- VZV
- HIV

Non-infectious causes

- Sarcoidosis
- Behcet disease
- Juvenile rheumatoid arthritis
- Trauma
- Laser photocoagulation therapy*

Case 154 ◆ **Myelinated Nerve Fibres**

CASE PRESENTATION

There are **bright white**, **streaky patches** with **feathery edges**,[1] adjacent to the margins of the optic disc.[2]

The appearances are inkeeping with **myelinated nerve fibres**.[3]

Clinical notes

1. Myelinated retinal nerve fibres appear as bright white patches corresponding to the distribution of the ganglion fibres

2. They are usually continuous with the optic disc, and if extensive, the disc margin and emerging vessels may become obscured. This appearance may be mistaken for papilloedema (pseudopapilloedema). Myelinated nerve fibres may develop in the periphery, away from the optic disc.

3. Myelinated nerve fibres are usually unilateral, but cases where they are bilateral have been reported.

Questions commonly asked by examiners

How common are myelinated retinal nerve fibres?

These affect 1% of the population.

---

* Often the appearance of laser photocoagulation scars for diabetic retinopathy are confused with those of old choroiditis. In fact, laser photocoagulation results in atrophy of the choroidoretina, and therefore is a form of old choroiditis. Laser photocoagulation scars may be distinguished due to their regular and uniform appearance and the presence of other features of diabetic retinopathy.

What is the cause of myelinated retinal nerve fibres?

The normal retina is not myelinated, because it lacks oligodendroglia, the cells responsible for myelination in the central nervous system. During normal prenatal development, retinal ganglion axon myelination starts centrally in the lateral geniculate body and proceeds anteriorly to the optic tracts, chiasm, and nerves. This process of myelination normally stops shortly after birth at the lamina cribrosa. The anomalous distribution of oligodendroglia in the retina is thought to be responsible for myelinated retinal nerve fibres. Initially it was thought that the lamina cribrosa acted as a barrier to myelination, but myelinated nerve fibres have been reported in patients with intact lamina cribrosa, and furthermore, myelinated nerve fibres have been observed in the periphery away from the optic disc, thus refuting this speculation.

What is the clinical significance of myelinated retinal nerve fibres?

They are usually considered to be a benign fundoscopic finding. However, myelinated nerve fibres have been associated with:

- Visual field defects
- Severe myopia
- Amblyopia
- Strabismus
- Nystagmus
- Macular aplasia
- Keratoconus
- Epiretinal membranes
- Vitreous haemorrhage

What conditions are more commonly associated with myelinated nerve fibres?

- Neurofibromatosis
- Down's syndrome
- Gorlin's syndrome

Case 155 ◆ **Cataract**

CASE PRESENTATION

There is a **lens opacity** visible in the right eye.[1] On examination of the red reflex, there is **diminution of the red reflex**.[2] A **black opacity** is seen in the lens **against a reddish hue of the reflex**. This **moves upwards on upward gaze**.[3] The **visual acuity is reduced** in the right eye.

The diagnosis is a right-sided **cataract** (located in the **anterior half of the lens**).[4]

Clinical notes

1. Cataracts may be seen easily with the unaided eye. This should make the diagnosis straightforward. Large dense cataracts will cause a white pupil.

2. Examining the red reflex is important. With small cataracts, the red reflex will be reduced. In larger dense cataracts, the red reflex will be absent.

3. This examination technique can be applied to small cataracts, in which there is some degree of red reflex (as opposed to a total loss). When examining the red reflex with +4 dioptres at approximately 20cm from the eye, the cataract will manifest as a black opacity surrounded by the red tinge of the reflex. Ask the patient to look up. If it moves up on upward gaze, then it is located in the anterior half of the lens (anterior capsular cataracts). If it moves down on upward gaze, then it is located in the posterior half of the lens (posterior capsular cataracts). The position of cataracts located in the centre (nuclear cataracts) will not be affected. This simple manoeuvre helps localize cataracts, and will impress examiners. See below for typical locations of cataracts.

4. There are many causes of cataracts (listed below). Establishing a diagnosis of cataracts is relatively straightforward. Try to find the possible cause:

(a) **Senile cataracts**: patient age; arcus senilis

(b) **Diabetes**: diabetic finger tip skin pricks (glucose testing); features of diabetic retinopathy in unaffected eye

(c) **Cushing's syndrome**: moon face; centripetal obesity; buffalo hump; striae; purpura; proximal myopathy

(d) **Myotonic dystrophy**: frontal balding; temporalis wasting; partial ptosis

(e) **Hypoparathyroidism**: Chvostek's and Trousseau's signs

(f) **Bardet-Biedl syndrome**: retinal pigmentation; polydactyly; short stature; truncal obesity

(g) **Refsum's disease**: peripheral neuropathy; nystagmus; cerebellar signs, hearing aid (deafness); ichthyosis

(h) **Homocystinuria**: marfanoid habitus; downward lens dislocation; livedo reticularis

(i) **Turner's syndrome**: short stature; webbed neck; cubitus valgus; widely spaced nipples; high arch palate

(j) **Down's syndrome**: round face; epicanthic folds; flat occiput; protruding tongue; single palmar crease; 5th finger clinodactyly; wide sandal gap

(k) **Fabry's disease**: arthropathy; angiokeratoma; restrictive cardiomyopathy

(l) **Wilson's disease**: tremor; chorea; dysarthria (akinetic rigid syndrome); arthropathy; features of chronic liver disease

(m) **Drugs**: tell the examiner you would like to take a drug history (see below)

Questions commonly asked by examiners

What are the causes of cataracts?
Congenital

- Toxoplasmosis
- Rubella
- CMV
- HSV
- Syphilis
- Myotonic dystrophy
- Homocystinuria
- Down's syndrome
- Patau's syndrome
- Edward's syndrome
- Turner's syndrome

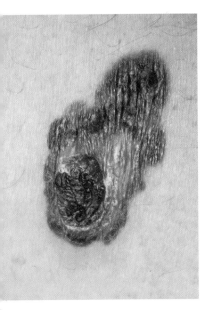

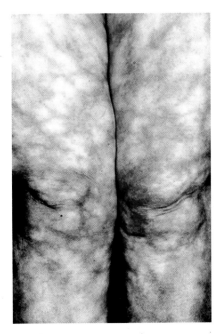

Plate 1 Chronic plaque psoriasis.
Reproduced from Collier et al, Oxford
Handbook of Clinical Specialties 7th edition,
2006, with permission from Oxford University
Press.

Plate 3 A "net-like" pattern of
discoloration gives the classical appearance of
livedo reticularis.
Reproduced from Longmore et al, Oxford
Hanbook of Clinical Medicine 7th edition, 2007,
with permission from Oxford University Press.

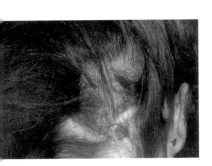

Plate 2 Multiple peripheral neurofibromata.
Reproduced from Sybert, V.P., Genetic Skin Disorders,
1997, with permission from Oxford University Press.

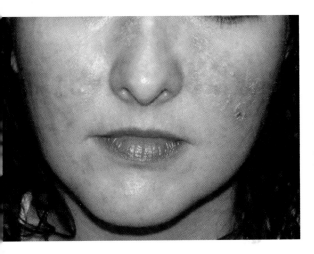

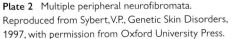

Plate 4 The characteristic malar
"butterfly" rash in systemic lupus
erythematosus. Note sparing of
the nasolabial folds.
Reproduced from Longmore
et al, Oxford Handbook of Clinical
Medicine 7th edition, 2007, with
permission from Oxford University
Press.

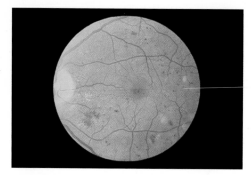

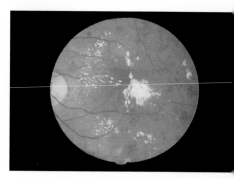

Plate 5 Background diabetic retinopathy.
Reproduced from Warrell et al, Oxford Textbook of
Medicine, Volume 3, 4th edition, 2003, with permission
from Oxford University Press.

Plate 6 Diabetic maculopathy with hard exudates visible at the macula.
Reproduced from Warrell et al, Oxford Textbook of
Medicine, Volume 3, 4th edition, 2003, with permission
from Oxford University Press.

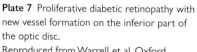

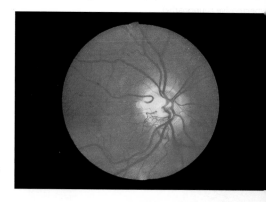

Plate 7 Proliferative diabetic retinopathy with
new vessel formation on the inferior part of
the optic disc.
Reproduced from Warrell et al, Oxford
Textbook of Medicine, Volume 3, 4th edition,
2003, with permission from Oxford University
Press.

Plate 8 Pan-retinal photocoagulation
laser treatment for proliferative diabetic
retinopathy.
Reproduced from Sundaram et al,
Training in Ophthalmology, 2009, with
permission from Oxford University
Press.

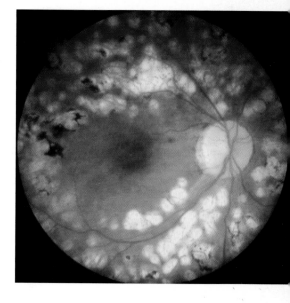

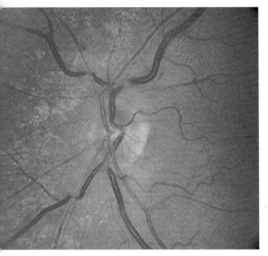

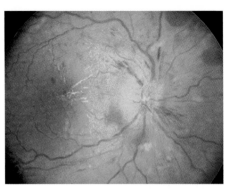

Plate 10 Arteriolar narrowing, cotton wool spots, blot haemmorhages, macular star and papilloedema (Grade 4 hypertensive retinopathy).
Reproduced from Sundaram et al, Training in Ophthalmology, 2009, with permission from Oxford University Press.

e 9 Arteriolar narrowing and arteriovenous nipping (Grade pertensive retinopathy).
roduced from Sundaram et al, Training in Ophthalmology, 9, with permission from Oxford University Press.

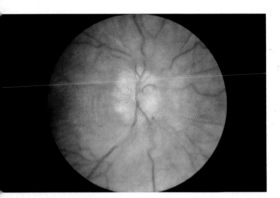

Plate 11 Chronic papilloedema.
Reproduced from Sundaram et al, Training in Ophthalmology, 2009, with permission from Oxford University Press.

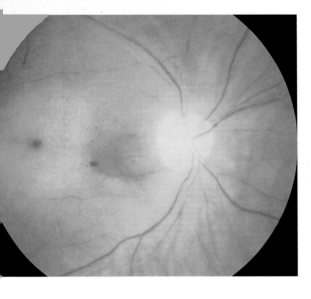

Plate 12 Central retinal artery occlusion.
Reproduced from Sundaram et al, Training in Ophthalmology, 2009, with permission from Oxford University Press.

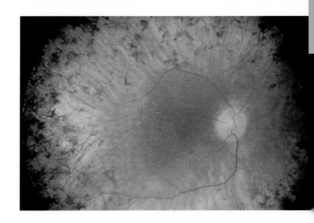

Plate 13 Retinitis pigmentosa. Reproduced from Sundaram et al, Training in Ophthalmology, 2009, with permission from Oxford University Press.

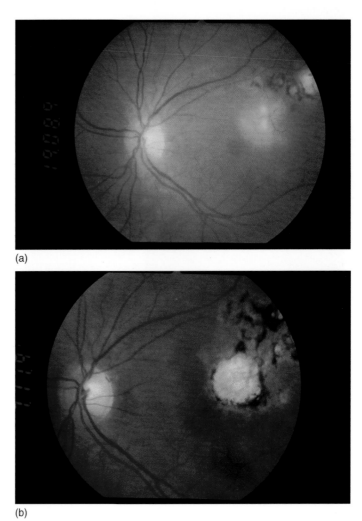

(a)

(b)

Plate 14 (a) and (b) Toxoplasma chorioretintis. Reproduced from Sundaram et al. Training in Ophthalmology. 2009, with permission from Oxford University Press.

Alport's syndrome

Fabry's disease

Wilson's disease

Refsum's disease

Bardet-Biedl syndrome

Autosomal dominant trait

Acquired

Age

Trauma

Uveitis

Diabetes

Cushing's syndrome

Hypoparathyroidism

Radiation

Cysticercosis

Onchocerciasis

Toxoplasmosis

Leprosy

Atopic dermatitis

Drugs (see below)

What drugs can cause cataracts?

Drugs most commonly implicated:

- Corticosteroids (oral, intravenous, topical, and inhaled)
- Chlorpromazine
- Chloroquine
- Busulphan
- Chlorambucil

Others drugs (weak association):

- Tamoxifen
- Tricyclic antidepressants
- Potassium-sparing diuretics
- Amiodarone
- Tetracyclines
- Allopurinol
- Psoralens

What do you know about the structure of the lens?

The lens is a crystalline structure made up of a central core (lens nucleus) surrounded by an outer cortex (lens cortex). A layer of metabolically active epithelial cells covers the anterior surface of the lens. This synthesizes protein for lens fibres, transports amino acids and maintains a cation pump to keep the lens clear. The entire lens is enclosed within a lens capsule.

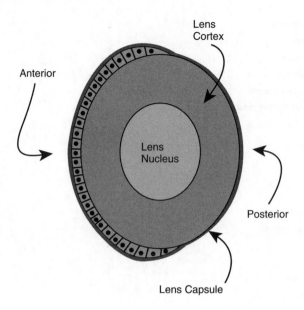

Figure 155.1

Where are cataracts located within the lens, and can you give specific examples?

Type of cataract	Location	Example
Anterior cortical cataract	Anterior portion of the lens cortex	Congenital
Anterior capsular cataract	Anterior part of the capsule	Senile cataract, chlorpromazine, uveitis
Anterior subcapsular cataract	Below the anterior capsule	Wilson's disease, amiodarone
Nuclear cataract	Lens nucleus	Senile cataract, congenital rubella, galactosaemia, steroids
Posterior cortical cataract	Posterior portion of the lens cortex	Congenital
Posterior capsular cataract	Posterior part of the capsule	Congenital
Posterior subcapsular cataract	Below the posterior capsule	Myotonic dystrophy, diabetes, steroids, radiation

What is the treatment for cataracts?
Intracapsular cataract extraction (ICCE)
This involves extraction of the whole lens including the posterior capsule, and placing the artificial lens in the anterior chamber or suturing it to the posterior chamber.

- **Advantages**: abolishes the risk of subsequent capsular opacity and less sophisticated equipment is necessary
- **Disadvantages**: larger incisions, increased post-operative complications

xtracapsular cataract extraction (ECCE)

his involves extraction of the lens through an opening in the anterior capsule whilst leaving the osterior capsule. The intact posterior capsule anchors the artificial lens.

Advantages: better anatomical placement of the artificial lens, smaller incisions, decreased post-operative complications

Disadvantages: a requirement is that the zonule ligaments must be intact and provide adequate support

he lens can be removed:

manually (standard ECCE)

by ultrasound driven needle to fragment and then aspirate the lens (phaecoemulsification)

Case 156 ◆ **Glaucoma**

CASE PRESENTATION

*here is **cupping of the optic disc**.[1] The **visual fields are constricted**.[2]*

*he diagnosis is **chronic (open-angle) glaucoma**.*

Clinical notes

1. Cupping of the optic disc (a hollowed-out appearance of the optic disc) is an important feature of chronic glaucoma. Cupping itself is not indicative of glaucoma, and it is more *an increase in cupping as the patient ages* that is an indicator of glaucoma. Stable cupping can occur due to hereditary factors without glaucoma. Generally, a cup: disc ratio >0.5 is a useful threshold for suspicion of glaucoma. As the disc cups posteriorly, the margins of the disc are steep and overhang the cupped portion of the disc. The retinal vessels as they climb up the sides of the cup appear hidden and this gives the appearance of vessels being broken off at the disc margin.

2. Classically an arcuate scotoma develops which progresses to generalized constriction of the visual fields and patients complain of tunnel vision. Sometimes, there may be a unilateral or bilateral nasal field defect.

Questions commonly asked by examiners

What are the causes of constricted visual fields (tunnel vision)?

Common causes

Retinitis pigmentosa

Photocoagulation scars (in the peripheries)

Old choroiditis

Chronic glaucoma

Papilloedema

Alcohol intoxication

Hallucinogenic drugs

Migraine

Rare causes

- Altitude sickness
- Snake venom (Black Mamba snakebite)
- Sustained high accelerations (common in aerobatic or fighter pilots)

What is the definition of glaucoma?

Glaucoma is defined as a disturbance of the structure or function of the optic nerve, where progressive loss of retinal ganglion cell axons results in characteristic atrophic changes in the optic nerve, which may also lead to specific visual field defects over time, and irreversible blindness if left untreated.*

What is the normal range for intraocular pressure?

The normal intraocular pressure is 10–20mmHg.

What do you know about chronic glaucoma (primary open-angle)?

This is the most common form of glaucoma. It is a chronic and progressive form of optic neuropathy that leads to characteristic visual field abnormalities in the presence of open anterior chamber angles. An elevated intraocular pressure is often associated with this condition, but is not a requirement for diagnosis. An elevated intraocular pressure is now considered as a risk factor for this condition. Other risk factors include myopia, female sex, age >40 years, black race, and family history. The exact mechanism of elevation of intraocular pressure is not known.

What do you know about acute glaucoma (primary angle-closure)?

Aqueous humor is produced by the ciliary body in the posterior chamber of the eye, which diffuses through the pupil, and into the anterior chamber. From here, the fluid is drained via the trabecular meshwork and Schlemm canal within the angle. In acute glaucoma, there is closure of the drainage angle and the obstruction to drainage of the aqueous humor results in an acute marked elevation in intraocular pressure. Risk factors include hyperopia, age >40 years, black race, and family history.

Patients present with an acutely painful red eye and this must be treated within 24 hours to prevent permanent blindness. It is an ophthalmological emergency. The onset of acute glaucoma is often in the evening, when lower light levels cause mydriasis, and folds of the peripheral iris block the angle. The signs that suggest a rapid rise in intraocular pressure include conjunctival redness, corneal oedema, a shallow anterior chamber, and a mid-dilated pupil (4–6mm) that reacts poorly to light.

What are the causes of secondary glaucoma?

Pretabecular

- Neovascularization (rubeotic glaucoma)
- Pseudoexfoliation (the deposition of white fluffy material within the anterior segment of the eye)
- Pigment dispersion syndrome (pigmentary glaucoma)

Trabecular

- Uveitis
- Scleritis

Post-trabecular

- Raised episcleral venous pressure, e.g. carotico-cavernous fistula and cavernous sinus thrombosis

---

* Glaucoma is more accurately described as an optic neuropathy than a disease of raised intraocular pressure. Controversy exists as to whether intraocular pressure should be included in the definition, as some patients can exhibit the characteristic optic nerve damage and visual field defects while having a normal intraocular pressure within the normal range.

What is the treatment for chronic glaucoma (primary open-angle)?

Medical treatment

α-agonists (topical)

β-blockers (topical)

Miotic agents (topical)

Prostaglandins (topical)

Carbonic anhydrase inhibitors (topical and systemic)

- Increase aqueous outflow: α-agonists, miotic agents, and prostaglandins
- Decrease aqueous production: α-agonists, β-blockers, and carbonic anhydrase inhibitors

Surgical treatment

Argon laser trabeculoplasty

Selective laser trabeculoplasty

Trabeculectomy

Drainage implant surgery

Ciliary body ablation

What is the management of acute glaucoma (primary angle-closure)?

Immediate management

Place patient in supine position*

Intravenous acetazolamide

Topical β-blocker

Topical steroids

Analgesia

Anti-emetics

Subsequent management

Pilocarpine (miotic agent)**

Hyperosmotic agents (glycerol PO or mannitol IV)***

Definitive management

Laser peripheral iridotomy****

---

* In the supine position, the lens falls away from the iris decreasing pupillary block.

** One hour after the initial management, miotic agents help open the angle. In the initial stages (<1 hour), the elevated pressure in the anterior chamber causes a pressure-induced ischaemic paralysis of the iris, during which time the pilocarpine would be ineffective.

*** If the intraocular pressure is not reduced 30 minutes after pilocarpine, an osmotic agent must be considered.

**** Laser peripheral iridotomy is the definitive treatment for acute angle-closure glaucoma. It should be performed 24–48 hours after the intraocular pressure is controlled. A laser is used to create a tiny hole in the peripheral iris through which aqueous humor can flow and reach the angle.

Case 157 ◆ **Drusen**

CASE PRESENTATION

*There are discrete, **pale yellow spots**[1] scattered around the **macula and posterior pole of the eye**.[2] These are not associated with **pigmentary changes**.[3] The visual acuity is normal.[4] There is no visual field defect.[4]*

*The diagnosis is **drusen**, which is associated with age-related macular degeneration.[5]*

Clinical notes

1. Drusen are yellow, yellow-white, or yellow-grey spots that represent accumulation of extracellular material between the retinal pigment epithelium and Bruch's membrane.

2. Drusen is usually scattered around the macula and posterior pole of the eye. It is important to note the number of drusen present and the presence of large drusen. When there are greater than 5 drusen and at least 63μm in diameter, this suggests age-related macular degeneration.

3. Look for retinal pigmentation, particularly in the posterior pole. As drusen enlarge and merge together there is shallow elevation of the retinal pigment epithelium, which overlies Bruch's membrane. This results in degeneration of the retinal pigment epithelium that manifests as retinal hyperpigmentation. Pigmentary changes are associated with age-related macular degeneration.

4. It is important to check both visual acuity and visual fields. Reduced visual acuity and visual field defect are seen in age-related macular degeneration. This occurs when the retinal pigment epithelium degenerates with secondary loss of overlying photoreceptor cells.

5. Having recognized drusen, it is important to decide if this is age-related macular degeneration. Features suggesting the later are:
   (a) Number of drusen >5
   (b) Large drusen (>63μm in diameter)
   (c) Retinal pigmentation
   (d) Reduced visual acuity

Questions commonly asked by examiners

How common is drusen?

The presence of drusen is normal with increasing age. Most individuals aged over 50 years have at least one small drusen (<63μm) in one or both eyes.

What are the constituents of the deposits seen in drusen?

Drusen are composed of vitronectin, lipids, amyloid associated proteins, complement factors, and trace elements (predominantly zinc).

What are the mechanisms that lead to formation of drusen?

Recent evidence suggests that drusen results from inflammation in the subretinal space.

- Complement factor H gene polymorphism has a strong association with age-related macular degeneration. The complement factor H is an anti-inflammatory agent that binds to activated complement C3b, thus protecting host cells from complement-mediated damage.

Among the trace elements present in drusen, the zinc concentrations are high. Zinc may play a role in drusen formation by inhibiting complement factor H.

How common is age-related macular degeneration?

This is the most common cause of blindness in people aged over 60 years. It accounts for 50% of the blind registrations in the UK.

What do you know about the different types of age-related macular degeneration?

There are two main types of age-related macular degeneration:

'Dry' age-related macular degeneration

This is the most common form of age-related macular degeneration. Increasing numbers (>5) of large (>63μm) drusen are present in the region of the macula and in the posterior pole of the eye. As they enlarge, there is detachment and degeneration of the retinal pigment epithelium with secondary loss of overlying photoreceptor cells. This results in pigmentary changes in the retina and is associated with loss of visual acuity and visual field defects. As drusen are located between the retinal pigment epithelium and its blood supply, the choriocapillaris, it is thought that drusen deprive the retinal pigment epithelium and photoreceptors of oxygen and nutrients.

'Wet' age-related macular degeneration

This form of age-related macular degeneration is associated with a more rapid loss of vision. It may present on a background of the 'dry' form. Choroidal neovascularization occurs across Bruch's membrane over the retinal pigment epithelium and extend into the subretinal space. This can result in exudates, retinal detachment, and haemorrhages with subsequent formation of fibrovascular scars.

What do you know about the genetics of age-related macular degeneration?

There is an increased incidence of age-related macular degeneration in patients with a family history. The inheritance is unclear. In some cases an autosomal dominant pattern has been demonstrated. The following genes have been implicated:

Complement factor H (chromosome 1)
Complement factor B (chromosome 6)
Complement factor 2 (chromosome 6)
LOC387715 (chromosome 10)

What are the risk factors for age-related macular degeneration?

Risk factor	Notes
Age	Increased prevalence after 60 years of age
Smoking	2–4-fold greater risk; may persist up to 20 years after stopping smoking
Hypertension	In patients with only one eye involvement, the risk of second eye involvement appears to be higher with uncontrolled hypertension. The Beaver Dam study showed that controlled and uncontrolled hypertension was associated with a 2-fold and 3-fold increased risk of developing age-related macular degeneration, respectively.
Genetics	A positive family history (see above)
Sunlight	Prolonged sunlight exposure is associated with increased risk of earlier development
Cataract surgery	The natural crystalline lens absorbs UV light (300–400nm) throughout life. As the lens yellows with age, it absorbs blue light (400–500nm). Both UV and blue light are phototoxic to the retina. Cataract surgery removes the aged yellow lens, thus increasing the amount of harmful light reaching the retina.

What treatment options are available for age-related macular degeneration?

'Dry' age-related macular degeneration

- Patient education
- Stop smoking
- Control blood pressure
- Diets rich in carotenoids (fresh fruit and vegetable)
- Anti-oxidant supplements (β-carotene, vitamin B and C, zinc, and lutein)
- Avoid sunlight exposure to eyes (use sunglasses or hat)
- Visual aids
- Blind registration

'Wet' age-related macular degeneration

As above for 'dry' age-related macular degeneration, but more specific therapies include:

- Laser photocoagulation therapy. An argon laser is used to ablate the neovascular membrane. Recurrence after treatment is common (50% recurrence at 5 years), and is often associated with more severe visual loss. Laser photocoagulation destroys the overlying retina resulting in an immediate central scotoma. Therefore, it is not recommended for subfoveal regions. It remains a treatment option for juxtafoveal and extrafoveal neovascularization.

- Photodynamic therapy. A photosensitizing drug (verteporfin)* is given intravenously and passes to the choroid and is preferentially absorbed by the rapidly dividing vessels in the neovascular membrane. This is followed by diode laser therapy that activates the dye and induces a photochemical reaction that releases free radicals. This causes endothelial damage and occlusion of the abnormal vessels. The neovascular membrane is selectively destroyed, thus sparing the retina. Most patients need 3–5 treatments over a 2-year period.

- Anti-angiogenic therapy (VEGF inhibitors). Vascular endothelial growth factor (VEGF) is a mediator of angiogenesis and promotes neovascularization. VEGF inhibitor therapy has shown promising results in patients with age-related macular degeneration. Available agents include pegaptanib, ranibizumab, and bevacizumab.

What are the new emerging non-pharmacological therapies for age-related macular degeneration?

- **Transpupillary thermotherapy.** This involves near-infrared long-pulse diode laser therapy to the neovascular membrane. The beam has lower intensity than conventional argon laser therapy. There is minimal uptake by the overlying retina, thus the damage is relatively specific, affecting mainly the abnormal vessels.

- **Diode feeder vessel photocoagulation.** This involves an indocyanogreen dye infusion with laser therapy directed at the stalk of the abnormal vessels.

- **Surgery.** Surgical treatment has high complication rates, and is not performed routinely. It is difficult to demonstrate the efficacy of these procedures due to a limited number of trained surgeons. There are two main surgical techniques:
  - **Submacular surgery.** This involves removal of the neovascular membrane blow the retina.

---

* Verteporfin is a benzoporphyrin derivative with a high affinity for plasma lipoproteins, and is preferentially taken up by cells with low-density lipoprotein receptors. The high levels of LDL receptors on proliferating endothelial cells trap the Verteporfin within the neovascular membrane.

Macular translocation surgery. This is a novel strategy for neovascularization. The macula is detached from the underlying neovascular membrane and diseased retinal pigment epithelium. It is then reattached to a healthier part of the retina. To avoid diplopia, this is often done with extensive extra-ocular muscle surgery.

Case 158 ◆ **Ocular prosthesis**

CASE PRESENTATION

The right **eyeball has a glazed appearance.**[1] The **light reflex is absent** on the right. The right **pupillary reflexes (both direct and consensual) are absent.** The patient is **blind** in the right eye.[2]

This patient has an **ocular prosthesis** on the right.[3]

Clinical notes

A glass eye is commonly encountered in the short cases of the MRCP (PACES) examination. They may be obvious, especially with older eye implants. In the current era, it is common for surgeons to attach the extra-ocular muscles to the implant. This creates proper volume of the orbit and allows natural eye movements. In such cases it may become difficult to distinguish a natural eye from an artificial one. If the candidate is not prepared to encounter such a case, it can cause considerable confusion in the examination.

1. The first clue to an ocular prosthesis may be the glazed appearance of the prosthesis. Although they are commonly referred to as 'glass eyes', they are made of medical grade acrylic, hydroxyapatite, polyethylene, and in some cases, cryolite glass.
2. The triad of absent light reflex, absent pupillary reflexes, and complete blindness should make the diagnosis of an ocular prosthesis straightforward.
3. Although, the term 'glass eye' is commonly used, it is best avoided—as not all implants are made of glass!

Questions commonly asked by examiners

What the indications for eye removal?
- Malignancy
  - Melanoma
  - Retinoblastoma
- Trauma
- End stage glaucoma
- Painful blind eye
  - Glaucoma
  - Endopthalmitis
  - Uveitis
  - Band keratopathy
- Congenital cystic eye

Case 159 ◆ Vitreous Opacities

CASE PRESENTATION 1

There are **tiny, white, oval-shaped vitreous opacities**.[1] They **move predictably with ocular movements**, *indicating that they are* **adherent to the vitreous framework**.[2]

The diagnosis is **asteroid hyalosis (Benson's disease)**.

CASE PRESENTATION 2

There are **tiny, yellow vitreous opacities**.[1] *They have an* **angular, crystalline appearance**. *They* **float freely in the vitreous**, *moving* **unpredictably with ocular movements** *and* **settle at the bottom of the vitreous when the eye is not moving**, *indicating that they are* **not adherent to the vitreous framework**.[2]

The diagnosis is **synchysis scintillans**.

Clinical notes

The most common vitreous opacity encountered in the MRCP (PACES) examination is blood seen in association with diabetic retinopathy and retinal vein occlusion. The above cases are rare, but have been encountered in the examination, and are therefore worth a brief mention.

1. To examine the vitreous, the ophthalmoscope must be focused in front of the retina. Look carefully at the distribution, shape, and colour of the opacities.
2. To determine if they are adherent to the vitreous framework or moving freely within the vitreous, ask the patient to look up and down, and observe carefully for the movement of the opacities. This requires practice.

Questions commonly asked by examiners

What are the differences between asteroid hyalosis and synchysis scintillans?

	Asteroid hyalosis	Synchysis scintillans
Sides affected	Often unilateral	Often bilateral
Colour of opacities	White opacities	Yellow-golden opacities
Shape of opacities	Oval or round appearance	Angulated and crystalline appearance
Composition of opacities	Calcium soaps (palmitate and stearate)	Cholesterol
Relationship to vitreous	Adherent to vitreous framework	Float freely in vitreous
Associations	Diabetes	Previous trauma or eye surgery

NDEX